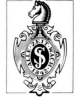

K. Maurer (Ed.)

Topographic Brain Mapping of EEG and Evoked Potentials

Foreword by F. H. Duffy

With 290 Figures, Partly in Colour

Springer-Verlag
Berlin Heidelberg New York
London Paris Tokyo

Prof. Dr. Konrad Maurer
Department of Psychiatry
University of Würzburg
Füchsleinstraße 15
8700 Würzburg, FRG

ISBN 3-540-17802-3 Springer-Verlag Berlin Heidelberg New York
ISBN 0-387-17802-3 Springer-Verlag New York Berlin Heidelberg

Library of Congress Cataloging-in-Publication Data. Topographic brain mapping of EEG and evoked potentials / K. Maurer (editor); foreword by F.H. Duffy. p. cm. Includes bibliographies and index. ISBN 0-387-17802-3 (U.S.)
1. Brain mapping. 2. Electroencephalography. 3. Evoked potentials (Electrophysiology) I. Maurer, Konrad, 1943– . [DNLM: 1. Brain Mapping. 2. Electroencephalography. 3. Evoked Potentials. WL150 T6748] RC386.6.B7T67 1988 612'.813 – dc19 DNLM/DLC

This work is subject to copyright. All rights are reserved, whether the whole or part of the material is concerned, specifically those of translation, reprinting, re-use of illustrations, broadcasting, reproduction by photocopying machine or similar means, and storage in data banks. Duplication of this publication or parts thereof is only permitted under the provisions of the German Copyright Law of September 9, 1965, in its version of June 24, 1985, and a copyright fee must always be paid. Violations fall under the prosecution act of the German Copyright Law.

© Springer-Verlag Berlin Heidelberg 1989
Printed in Germany

The use of registered names, trademarks, etc. in this publication does not imply, even in the absence of a specifc statement, that such names are exempt from the relevant protective laws and regulations and therefore free for general use.

Product Liability: The publisher can give no guarantee for information about drug dosage and application thereof contained in this book. In every individual case the respective user must check its accuracy by consulting other pharmaceutical literature.

Reproduction of figures: Chemigraphia, Gebr. Czech GmbH & Co., München

Typesetting, printing and bookbinding: Universitätsdruckerei Stürtz AG, Würzburg
2125/3130-543210. Printed on acid-free paper

Topographic Mapping:
Thoughts on the Past and the Future

Comments overheard at the Würzburg conference on topographic mapping reflected great enthusiasm and the feeling that neurophysiology had been dealt a fresh lease of life. One elder statesman of electrophysiology was noted as saying, "It is now clear that our field will survive into the 21st century." The merging of quantified EEG with topographic mapping and their application to clinical and research aspects of brain function is indeed an exciting development. One has only to inspect the contents of this volume to gain a flavor of the current directions in the field.

On the other hand there are disturbing signs. One might expect this new and highly technological field to be populated by young persons fresh from university programs in biomedical engineering. Although such individuals are represented, the primary moving forces, including those present at the Würzburg meeting, remain those who opened up the field many years ago – those who early on „knew" what mapping and quantification had to offer. As a result there is an overrepresentation of seasoned investigators and a worrisome lack of younger workers in our field.

It could be argued that this is too harsh a criticism and that our field has just reached the point where computing power has permitted major new developments. But this is not completely true. As early as 1969 complex topographic mapping systems were already being described by Estrin and Uzgalis and by Harris et al. It could be argued that such systems were based on mainframe computers which were located in remote computer centers and thereby difficult to access and that computing power was not as readily available in that era as it is now. Although this is true to some degree, we do not concur with the view that lack of convenient access to computing power was the only factor restraining development. Inquisitive minds always seem to find a way to obtain what they require.

Instead, we subscribe to the view that education of physicians has lagged substantially behind modern technology and that most classically educated neurologists and psychiatrists were then, and remain now, unequipped to appreciate what computers can do for them. Many practicing neurophysiologists still appear to lack a working comprehension of electric field theory and multivariate statistics – essential elements for understanding and appraisal of developments in the field. On one hand this leads to computer phobia, which often manifests itself by inappropriate criticism. On the other hand it may also lead to the inappropriately optimistic and uncritical use of some of the commercially available quantified EEG systems. Fortunately, today's ubiquitous personal computer is changing this. The power of yesterday's mainframe computer can now be made available on anyone's desk for a few thousand dollars. But it is sad to see technology driving intellectual curiosity when it should be the other way around.

Extrapolating from advances in electrophysiology as reported at the Würzburg conference, in this volume, and elsewhere in the modern literature, it is possible to make some predictions:

1. From scalp recordings of brain electrical activity it will become possible to reliably locate regions of brain activated by specific cognitive paradigms or functional activities.
2. From scalp recordings of focal epileptic spikes it will be possible to accurately locate the dipole source in three dimensions.
3. Topographic analysis of epileptic discharges will advance our understanding of epileptic pathophysiology as well as assist in diagnostic categorization.
4. Serial studies will allow us to predict changing neurological status with better definition than is now possible.
5. Multivariate statistics will provide objective means for automatic classification of patients with increasing reliability into a larger number of more complex diagnostic categories.
6. As the cost/performance ratio continues to drop, routine EEG studies will include the availability of complex topographic and other multivariate analyses.
7. Given the recent advances in superconductivity at more readily achievable temperatures, magnetoencephalography (MEG) will become a more practical tool, taking its place alongside EEG.

For these and other advances to proceed optimally, however, we must be assured of a new generation of clinicians and researchers whose education is such that it allows them to appreciate and participate in these developments. It is not enough to forge ahead ourselves. It is our responsibility and privilege to attract and train "new blood."

The Würzburg conference was a major step in bringing these modern advances in electrophysiology to the psychiatrists and neurologists who will profit from them. Credit goes to its organizer, Konrad Maurer, who recognized the need and generated the personal energy to actualize such a productive symposium.

F. H. DUFFY

Preface

Imaging procedures have been used for many years and are becoming increasingly important in a number of medical disciplines. This is due to recent technological advances, primarily computerization. The methods employed in CNS diagnostics are collectively referred to as "neuroimaging" and include procedures for investigating both cerebral morphology and cerebral function, such as computed tomography (CT), magnetic resonance imaging (MRI), positron emission tomography (PET), and single-photon emission computed tomography (SPECT). Topographic mapping of electroencephalograms (EEG) and evoked potentials represents one of the functional procedures and permits topographic imaging of EEG, evoked potentials, and magnetic fields. The latter application includes not only magnetic fields evoked by stimuli relating to different sensory modalities, but also endogenous and motor fields resulting from spontaneous brain magnetic activity, as recorded by magnetoencephalograms (MEG), the magnetic complement of the EEG. The advantage of recording electric and magnetic fields over other neuroimaging procedures is that these techniques are completely noninvasive and have extremely short analysis times (in the millisecond range).

The aim of this book is to clarify the current state of this emerging technology, to assess its potential for substantive contributions to brain research, to delineate areas for further research and, over all, to envisage clinical applications in disciplines such as psychiatry, neurology, and neuropsychology.

The impetus for this book was an international symposium entitled "Topographic Brain Mapping of EEG and Evoked Potentials" held in Würzburg, Federal Republic of Germany, under the auspices of the Department of Psychiatry, University of Würzburg. Participants presenting their data were asked to prepare a contribution to this book delineating their recent research activities and clinical results. Altogether, 59 chapters written by a total of 141 authors are presented here. These authors, representing research laboratories and clinics in many parts of Europe, Japan, and the United States, include many of the original pioneers as well as current experts in the field of electric and magnetic brain mapping.

The book is clearly organized, with a view toward educating the reader, beginning with a historical introduction on the past and future of brain mapping and a section dealing with the state of the art. The following sections cover methodological, clinical, psychophysiologic, psychiatric, and magnetoencephalographic aspects, as well as mapping of evoked potentials. To facilitate entry into this exciting field and to guide newcomers, F.H. Duffy and I have prepared guidelines on the implementation of topographic mapping. It is our hope that this volume will provide the impetus for the formulation of further guidelines in this field. In light of the difficulties involved in establishing universally applicable, concrete principles for the use of brain mapping methods, the main intention of our guidelines is to raise key issues that should be considered by those attempting to formulate future standards.

The reader will also find that the various chapters present a stimulating range of viewpoints. Special care has been taken to elucidate both clinical applications and exciting research on the location and components of the equivalent dipole. In conjunction with magnetoencephalography, this opens the possibility of studying not only surface electrical activity but also of determining the intracerebral location of brain activity and the direction of polarity. As already mentioned by Duffy in his foreword, magnetoencephalography will become a more practical tool owing to recent advances in superconductivity. It was therefore a special wish on my part to include a section on magnetoencephalographic aspects in order to introduce readers to this field.

Through the high quality of their scientific and clinical data, all the authors have made valuable contributions both to the symposium and to this volume. I wish to express my sincere thanks to all of them. I would also like to thank Prof. Dr. H. Beckmann, Director of the Department of Psychiatry, for making it possible to hold the symposium at the Psychiatric Clinic in Würzburg. I am also grateful to Dr. T. Dierks and Dr. R. Ihl and to my secretary Mrs. M. Möslein for their efforts in organizing the symposium and editing this volume.

My sincere thanks go to Dr. T. Thiekötter, Dr. S. Kentner, and Mr. W. Bischoff-Samide of Springer-Verlag, who made it possible to produce this book with an abundance of lavish color illustrations.

As editor of this volume, it is my hope that the book will help to promote mapping of EEG, MEG, and evoked potentials as a technique of neuroimaging and to enable it to take a prominent place in diagnostics and therapy monitoring for all disciplines concerned with the treatment of CNS diseases and conditions.

K. MAURER

Contents

Section I State of the Art

Establishment of Guidelines for the Use of Topographic Mapping
in Clinical Neurophysiology: A Philosophical Approach
F.H. DUFFY and K. MAURER 3

From Graphein to Topos: Past and Future of Brain Mapping
H. PETSCHE. With 1 Figure 11

Topographic Mapping of Brain Electrical Activity:
Clinical Applications and Issues
F.H. DUFFY. With 13 Figures 19

From Mapping to the Analysis and Interpretation
of EEG/EP Maps
D. LEHMANN. With 13 Figures 53

Topographic Mapping of Generators of Somatosensory Evoked
Potentials
J.E. DESMEDT. With 8 Figures 76

Neurometric Topographic Mapping of EEG and Evoked Potential
Features: Application to Clinical Diagnosis
and Cognitive Evaluation
E.R. JOHN, L.S. PRICHEP, J. FRIEDMAN, and P. EASTON
With 18 Figures 90

Advances in Brain Theory Give New Directions to the Use of
the Technologies of Brain Mapping in Behavioral Studies
W.J. FREEMAN and K. MAURER. With 1 Figure 118

Section II Methodological Aspects

Advanced Programming Techniques for Dynamic Brain Activity
Mapping on Personal Computers
U. BRANDL and D. WENZEL. With 5 Figures 129

The Use of Derived Map Parameters in Alpha Blocking
W. DE RIJKE and S.L. VISSER. With 3 Figures 136

The Effect of Source Extension on the Location and Components
of the Equivalent Dipole
J.C. DE MUNCK and H. SPEKREIJSE. With 4 Figures 141

A Simple Model to Aid the Examination of Brain Mapping Systems
and the Teaching of Topography
A.L. WINTER. With 3 Figures 147

The Use of Cross-Correlation in the Display of Paroxysmal Events
in the EEG: A Preliminary Report
G. SPIEL, F. BENNINGER, M. FEUCHT, and U. ZYCH. With 3 Figures 152

Joint Studies of Event-Related Brain Potentials and
^{99m}Tc-Hexamethyl-propyleneamineoxime SPECT on
Sensory-Guided Hand Tracking
W. LANG, M. LANG, I. PODREKA, E. SUESS, C. MÜLLER, M. STEINER,
and L. DEECKE. With 4 Figures 159

Section III Clinical Aspects

A Battery Approach to Clinical Utilisation of Topographic
Brain Mapping
H.L. HAMBURGER. With 32 Figures 167

Topography of Background EEG Rhythms in Normal Subjects
and in Patients with Cerebrovascular Disorders
D. SAMSON-DOLLFUS, C. DELMER, Y. VASCHALDE, E. DREANO,
and D. FODIL. With 2 Figures 185

P300 and Coma
B.M. REUTER and D.B. LINKE. With 2 Figures 192

Structure Differences of Topographical EEG Mappings
R.H. JINDRA and R. VOLLMER. With 2 Figures 197

Topographic Brain Mapping and Conventional Evoked Potential
to Checkerboard Reversal and Semantic Visual Stimulation in a
Dyslexic Boy with Amblyopia
D. WENZEL, U. BRANDL, and E. KRAUS-MACKIW. With 5 Figures . 201

EEG Mapping in Patients with Transient Ischemic Attacks:
A Follow-Up Study
E. KOERNER, E. OTT, P. KAISERFELD, G. PFURTSCHELLER, R. WOLF,
G. LINDINGER, and H. LECHNER. With 7 Figures 209

EEG Mapping in Pathological Aging and Dementia: Utility for
Diagnosis and Therapeutic Evaluation
B. GUEGUEN, P. ETEVENON, D. PLANCON, J. GACHES,
J. DE RECONDO, and P. RONDOT. With 2 Figures 219

Topographic Characteristics of EEG During a Saturation Dive to
a 31 ATA Helium-Oxygen Environment with Specific Reference
to Fmθ or FIRDA
S. MATSUOKA, C. KADOYA, S. OKUDA, S. WADA, and M. MORI
With 6 Figures 226

Spectral and Frequency Analysis of the Central EEG Activity
in Parkinson's Disease Patients with Alzheimer's Disease:
The Development During Nootropic Therapy
E.W. FÜNFGELD. With 6 Figures 233

EEG and EP Mapping in Patients with Senile Dementia
of Alzheimer Type Before and After Treatment with Pyritinol
R. IHL, K. MAURER, T. DIERKS, and W. WANNENMACHER
With 8 Figures 241

EEG Mapping in Epilepsy
J. GACHES and B. GUEGUEN. With 4 Figures 249

Topographic Representation of Brainstem Lesions: Brainstem
Auditory Evoked Potentials Compared with Nuclear Magnetic
Resonance Imaging in Multiple Sclerosis
K. BAUM, W. SCHEULER, U. HEGERL, W. GIRKE, and W. SCHÖRNER
With 1 Figure. 256

Topographic EEG Features During Deep Isoflurane Anesthesia in
Patients with Major Depressive Disorders
G. CARL, T. DIERKS, W. ENGELHARDT, and K. MAURER
With 2 Figures 259

Flash Visual Evoked Potential Topographic Mapping:
Normative and Clinical Data
E.J. HAMMOND, C.P. BARBER, and B.J. WILDER. With 5 Figures . . 265

Event-Related Potentials in Patients with Brain Tumors
and Traumatic Head Injuries
H.M. OLBRICH, H.E. NAU, J. FRITZE, and E. LODEMANN
With 2 Figures 273

Mapping of EEG in Patients with Intracranial Structural Lesions
H. POIMANN, K. MAURER, and T. DIERKS. With 5 Figures 278

Topographic Brain Mapping and Neuroendocrine Parameters in
a Patient with Addison's Disease and a Depressive Syndrome
Before and After Treatment with Hydrocortisone
R. RUPPRECHT, T. DIERKS, G. REIFSCHNEIDER, F. v. BAUMGARTEN,
K. MAURER, and J. PICHL. With 2 Figures 285

Dexfenfluramine Profile in Quantitative EEG
and Its Topographical Aspects
C. SEBBAN, K. LE ROCH, G. BENKEMOUN, C. DEBOUZY,
and P. BAUD. With 5 Figures 288

Synchrony (Measured by Cross-Correlation) in Children
with Cognitive Impairments
G. SPIEL, F. BENNINGER, and M. FEUCHT. With 1 Figure. 296

Section IV Psychophysiological Aspects

Cortical Activation Pattern During Reading and Recognition of Words Studied with Dynamic Event-Releated Desynchronization Mapping
G. PFURTSCHELLER and W. KLIMESCH. With 1 Figure 303

Topography of Preparation- and Performance-Related Slow Negative Potential Shifts in Verbal and Spatial Tasks
F. UHL, W. LANG, M. LANG, A. KORNHUBER, and L. DEECKE
With 3 Figures 314

Topographic Brain Mapping of Transient Visual Attention
A. TAGHAVY, C.F.A. KÜGLER, and H. LÖSSLEIN. With 3 Figures . 318

Patterns of Event-Related Brain Potentials in Paired Associative Learning Tasks: Learning and Directed Attention
M. LANG, W. LANG, F. UHL, and A. KORNHUBER. With 2 Figures . 323

Brain Lateralization in Stress Reactions
D.B. LINKE, B.M. REUTER, and M. KURTHEN. With 1 Figure . . . 326

EEG Dynamic Cartography of Wakefulness, Sleep and Dreams: A Movie
P. ETEVENON. With 1 Figure 329

Section V Evoked Potential Mapping

Visual Evoked Potential Topography: Physiological and Cognitive Components
W. SKRANDIES. With 11 Figures 337

Localization of the Visually Evoked Response: The Pattern Appearance Response
B.W. VAN DIJK and H. SPEKREIJSE. With 4 Figures 360

N100 Frontal Component and Influence of Reference Location in Pattern Visual Evoked Potential Studied with the Area Display Technique
M. GUIDI, O. SCARPINO, F. ANGELERI, and R.G. BICKFORD
With 6 Figures 366

Scalp Topography of Red LED Flash-Evoked Potentials: Normal and Clinical Data
E.J. HAMMOND, C.P. BARBER, and B.J. WILDER. With 6 Figures . . 373

Topographic Mapping of Somatosensory Representation Areas
H. EMMERT and K.A. FLÜGEL. With 4 Figures 383

Early Cortical Somatosensory and N1 Auditory Evoked Responses: Analysis with Potential Maps, Scalp Current Density Maps and Three-Concentric-Shell Head Models
F. PERRIN, O. BERTRAND, and J. PERNIER. With 3 Figures 390

The Topography of the N70 Component of the Visual Evoked
Potential in Humans
I. BÓDIS-WOLLNER, L. MYLIN, and S. FRKOVIĆ. With 4 Figures . . 396

Surface Maps and Generators of Brainstem Auditory Evoked
Potential Waves I, III, and V
F. GRANDORI. With 2 Figures 407

Topographic Brain Mapping and Long Latency Somatosensory
Evoked Potentials of Posterior Tibial Nerve
and Dorsal Nerve of Penis
W.H. SCHERB, G. GALLWITZ, J. KNEIP-SCHERB, W. BÄHREN,
and J. KRIEBEL. With 4 Figures 412

Section VI Psychiatric Aspects

The Neuropsychology of Schizophrenia in the Context
of Topographical Mapping of Electrocortical Activity
J. GRUZELIER and D. LIDDIARD. With 3 Figures 421

EEG Mapping in Psychiatry: Studies on Type I/II Schizophrenia
Using Motor Activation
W. GÜNTHER, R. STEINBERG, R. PETSCH, P. STRECK, and J. KUGLER
With 2 Figures 438

Coherence Mapping Reveals Differences in the EEG Between
Psychiatric Patients and Healthy Persons
H. POCKBERGER, K. THAU, A. LOVREK, H. PETSCHE,
and P. PAPPELSBERGER. With 2 Figures 451

Mapping of Evoked Potentials in Normals and Patients with
Psychiatric Diseases
K. MAURER, T. DIERKS, R. IHL, and G. LAUX. With 11 Figures . . 458

Event-Related Potential (N100) Studies in Depressed Patients
Treated with Electroconvulsive Therapy
J.A. COFFMAN and M.W. TORELLO. With 1 Figure 474

EEG Imaging of Brain Activity in Clinical Psychopharmacology
B. SALETU. With 9 Figures 482

Evaluation and Interpretation of Topographic EEG Data
in Schizophrenic Patients
T. DIERKS, K. MAURER, R. IHL, and A. SCHMIDTKE. With 5 Figures 507

EEG Mapping During Cholinergic Drug Challenge with RS-86
J. FRITZE, T. DIERKS, and K. MAURER. With 2 Figures 518

Topographic Mapping of Event-Related Potentials as a Diagnostic
Tool for Identification of Dyslexic Persons
J. LYCKLAMA À NIJEHOLT, W. VAN DRONGELEN,
and B.E.J. HILHORST. With 2 Figures 522

Topographic EEG Brain Maps and Mental Performance Under
Hypoxia After Placebo and Pyritinol
B. SALETU, P. ANDERER, K. KINSPERGER, and J. GRÜNBERGER
With 5 Figures 527

Section VII Magnetoencephalographic Aspects

Cortical Auditory Evoked Magnetic Fields: Mapping of Time and
Frequency Domain Aspects
M. HOKE, K. LEHNERTZ, B. LÜTKENHÖNER, and C. PANTEV
With 16 Figures 537

Mapping of MEG Amplitude Spectra: Its Significance for
the Diagnosis of Focal Epilepsy
C.E. ELGER, M. HOKE, K. LEHNERTZ, C. PANTEV, B. LÜTKENHÖNER,
P.A. ANNINOS, and G. ANOGIANAKIS. With 2 Figures 565

Subject Index 571

List of Contributors

The addresses are given at the beginning of each contribution

Anderer, P. 527
Angeleri, F. 366
Anninos, P.A. 565
Anogianakis, G. 565
Bähren, W. 412
Barber, C.P. 265, 373
Baud, P. 288
Baum, K. 256
Baumgarten, F.v. 285
Benkemoun, G. 288
Benninger, F. 152, 296
Bertrand, O. 390
Bickford, R.G. 366
Bódis-Wollner, I. 396
Brandl, U. 129, 201
Carl, G. 259
Coffman, J.A. 474
de Munck, J.C. 141
de Recondo, J. 219
de Rijke, W. 136
Debouzy, C. 288
Deecke, L. 159, 314
Delmer, C. 185
Desmedt, J.E. 76
Dierks, T. 241, 259, 278, 285, 458, 507, 518
Dreano, E. 185
Duffy, F.H. 3, 19
Easton, P. 90
Elger, C.E. 565
Emmert, H. 383
Engelhardt, W. 259
Etevenon, P. 219, 329

Feucht, M. 152, 296
Flügel, K.A. 383
Fodil, D. 185
Freeman, W.J. 118
Friedman, J. 90
Fritze, J. 273, 518
Frković, S. 396
Fünfgeld, E.W. 233
Gaches, J. 219, 249
Gallwitz, G. 412
Girke, W. 256
Grandori, F. 407
Grünberger, J. 527
Gruzelier, J. 421
Gueguen, B. 219, 249
Günther, W. 438
Guidi, M. 366
Hamburger, H.L. 167
Hammond, E.J. 265, 373
Hegerl, U. 256
Hilhorst, B.E.J. 522
Hoke, M. 537, 565
Ihl, R. 241, 458, 507
Jindra, R.H. 197
John, E.R. 90
Kadoya, C. 226
Kaiserfeld, P. 209
Kinsperger, K. 527
Klimesch, W. 303
Kneip-Scherb, J. 412
Koerner, E. 209
Kornhuber, A. 314, 323

Kraus-Mackiw, E. 201
Kriebel, J. 412
Kügler, C.F.A. 318
Kugler, J. 438
Kurthen, M. 326
Lang, M. 159, 314, 323
Lang, W. 159, 314, 323
Laux, G. 458
Le Roch, K. 288
Lechner, H. 209
Lehmann, D. 53
Lehnertz, K. 537, 565
Liddiard, D. 421
Lindinger, G. 209
Linke, D.B. 192, 326
Lodemann, E. 273
Lösslein, H. 318
Lovrek, A. 451
Lütkenhöner, B. 537, 565
Lycklama à Nijeholt, J. 522
Matsuoka, S. 226
Maurer, K. 3, 118, 241, 259, 278, 285, 458, 507, 518
Mori, M. 226
Müller, C. 159
Mylin, L. 396
Nau, H.E. 273
Okuda, S. 226
Olbrich, H.M. 273
Ott, E. 209
Pantev, C. 537, 565

Pappelsberger, P. 451
Pernier, J. 390
Perrin, F. 390
Petsch, R. 438
Petsche, H. 11, 451
Pfurtscheller, G. 209, 303
Pichl, J. 285
Plancon, D. 219
Pockberger, H. 451
Podreka, I. 159
Poimann, H. 278
Prichep, L.S. 90
Reifschneider, G. 285
Reuter, B.M. 192, 326
Rondot, P. 219
Rupprecht, R. 285
Saletu, B. 482, 527
Samson-Dollfus, D. 185
Scarpino, O. 366
Scherb, W.H. 412
Scheuler, W. 256
Schmidtke, A. 507
Schörner, W. 256
Sebban, C. 288
Skrandies, W. 337
Spekreijse, H. 141, 360
Spiel, G. 152, 296
Steinberg, R. 438
Steiner, M. 159
Streck, P. 438
Suess, E. 159
Taghavy, A. 318
Thau, K. 451
Torello, M.W. 474
Uhl, F. 314, 323
van Dijk, B.W. 360
van Drongelen, W. 522
Vaschalde, Y. 185
Visser, S.L. 136
Vollmer, R. 197
Wada, S. 226
Wannenmacher, W. 241
Wenzel, D. 129, 201
Wilder, B.J. 265, 373
Winter, A.L. 147
Wolf, R. 209
Zych, U. 152

Section I State of the Art

Establishment of Guidelines for the Use of Topographic Mapping in Clinical Neurophysiology: A Philosophical Approach

F.H. Duffy[1] and K. Maurer[2]

Introduction

The past several years have seen the increasing use of topographic mapping in clinical neurophysiology, especially in conjunction with techniques from quantified EEG to detect "abnormalities."

To generalize, there appear to be three differing ways in which mapping is used clinically. (1) Maps of spectrally analyzed EEG, sometimes along with evoked potentials (EP), are visually inspected and clinical impressions are written on the basis of these data alone. (2) Maps of EP and EEG are similarly inspected but are interpreted together with the underlying standard EEG polygraphic data. Maps are often referenced to a normative data base to assist in the detection of abnormality. The final clinical impression incorporates the standard EEG, the spectral EEG and EP maps, and the maps reflecting deviation from a normative data base. (3) Raw data and maps are used primarily for illustrative purposes. Subjects are studied under prescribed paradigms. Data from EEG and EP are automatically analyzed in reference to a data base and patients are classified into one or more clinical groupings on the basis of previously prepared discriminant functions.

Given such a diverse approach to clinical mapping it would be difficult to establish universal concrete guidelines. The intention here is therefore to raise key issues that should be considered by those attempting to set out such guidelines. The views expressed are those of the authors named above and do not necessarily represent a consensus of the many contributors to this book. On the other hand, care has been taken to incorporate suggestions made by many respected mapping practitioners, to whom gratitude is owed for many hours of productive dialogue.

Personnel

Technician

The technician is critical in the good clinical practice of topographic mapping. To begin with, s/he must already possess sufficient skill to perform classic EEG

[1] BEAM Laboratory, Department of Neurology, The Children's Hospital and Harvard Medical School, 300 Longwood Avenue, Boston, MA 02115, USA
[2] Department of Psychiatry, University of Würzburg, Füchsleinstraße 15, 8700 Würzburg, Federal Republic of Germany

studies, including accurate, measured low-impedance electrode placement. S/he must be knowledgeable about EEG and capable of detecting state change (e.g., drowsiness) and artifacts (e.g., electrode pop, eye contamination, muscle), as well as classic EEG abnormalities (e.g., discharges, focal slowing). Given these basic skills s/he must also receive specialized training in:
- Operation and maintenance of the requisite computer-based equipment
- Application of artifact-detecting electrodes
- Reduction of eye blink, eye movement, electrode artifact, and muscle artifact
- Control of state, i.e., maintenance of wakefulness when called for
- Management of specific behavioral paradigms while collecting data
- Removal of artifact-contaminated segments from EEG prior to spectral analysis

Reader

The reader must be a physician (usually a neurologist, a psychiatrist, or a Ph.D.) with special training in neurophysiology. S/he must have experience in reading clinical EEG. Given this basic skill s/he must receive specialized training in:
- Operation of the requisite computer-based equipment
- The basics of signal analysis (e.g., sampling rates, DC zero finding, spectral analysis)
- Recognition of state change effects upon mapped data
- Statistics as applied to mapping, including the t and Z statistic, data normality, effects of multiple measurements, and discriminant analysis
- Discrimination of "real" from "artifactual" data

Equipment and Data Manipulation

General Operating Environment

An ideal computer system for processing mapping data would contain adequate memory space and disk storage so as to allow data gathering and analyses to proceed without need for frequent interruptions to "onload" or "offload" data. The operating environment should not require the technicians or physician to have an intimate knowledge of operating system syntax. Ideally, interaction should occur through keyboard, touch-screen, or "mouse" response to menus and/or prompts. There should be provision for ready archiving of the final processed data and/or the raw input data on removable disk or tape, and for monitoring ongoing EEG activity during data gathering. There should be hard copy output capability for the basic EEG and EP data as well as the maps. An ordinary EEG record should be produced during data gathering for topographic mapping. The EEG provides critical information concerning data quality (e.g., artifact, state control) as well as information best appreciated by visual inspection (e.g., discharges). Alternatively, EEG may be stored on disk and displayed on a graphics terminal with resolution equalling that of a paper record.

Data Collection

Mapping systems should provide a normative data base gathered under standardized conditions. Accordingly, each system must provide for the collection of data from patients in the same manner. EEG machines produced by different manufacturers currently have differing bandpass filtering characteristics. Accordingly, mapping systems should either provide or require an appropriate EEG machine, or provide selectable filtering characteristics to convert output from differing EEG amplifiers to the required standard. Use of an EEG machine with different filtering characteristics than the apparatus used to gather control data can result in false impressions of increased or decreased EEG slowing and increased or decreased EP latency shift. Similarly, the appropriate visual and acoustic stimulators should be provided or required. Users should be provided with detailed stimulus and data-gathering parameters to ensure compatibility. Systems should facilitate the creation of standard EEG during data gathering for initial artifact control and later clinical analyses.

Color Graphics: Display Perspective

It is widely recognized that the use of color can both enhance and distort the clinical information contained in the data. Ideally, color scales should be chosen so as to give an inherent sense of maximum value (e.g., bright white), electrical zero (e.g., black), polarity (e.g., red positive, blue negative), and gradient (e.g., rainbow colors). Gradation of color change should appear more or less uniform so as not to create the impression that any particular color step is more meaningful than any other. Colors should not be repeated; this distorts the sense of gradient (i.e., which color change indicates "more" and which "less").

The simplest display perspective is an equal-area projection as seen from the vertex. This basic view should be provided by all systems. Side, front, and rear views are optional; when available they should be clearly specified as equal-area or perspective views. All views should provide the option of showing electrode location. Demonstration of underlying anatomical landmarks is optional. Finally, it would be highly desirable to provide a user interface to facilitate creation of new, specialized perspectives with placement of electrodes at desired positions.

Electrode Number and Location: Reference Location

It is currently common in mapping to employ a reduced number of channels by eliminating artifact-prone electrodes (e.g., FP1, FP2, T3, T4) and/or the midline electrodes (e.g., FZ, CZ, PZ, OZ). This practice is to be discouraged, since artifact may extend past these electrodes but be hard to recognize when FP1–T4 are not utilized. Moreover, most maps of normal subject data show maximal values along the midline, so the use of the midline electrodes is critical to accuracy. Furthermore, placements of extra electrodes positioned so as to permit discrimination of artifact is encouraged. Optimally, these electrodes should delineate vertical eye movement, horizontal eye movement, temporal muscle activity, and occipital muscle activity. Thus the minimum number of electrodes for basic screening should be the 19 of the 10–20 system plus at least four additional ones to monitor artifact, for a total of 23. Systems with 24 to 32 or more channels are preferred.

There can be no answer to the question, "What is the optimal number of electrodes?" without consideration of the purpose. For example, it may well be possible to follow diffuse encephalopathy with one or two electrodes. On the other hand, the precise localization of an epileptic focus may require a very dense array.

Reference location is a controversial issue with no perfect solution. For example, single reference points (e.g., ipsilateral ear or mastoid, linked ears, nasion) suffer from the fact that they may be electrically active, with artifact or real brain signals. "Reference-free" techniques such as the "average reference" and "Laplacian transformation" should be available as alternatives. For example, the average reference technique works well for small regions of the scalp in normal subjects. However, it proves less useful when the whole head is studied in the clinical situation, where a pathological signal may appear under one or two electrodes but appear to be spread across the head by the averaging process. Laplacian transformation produces a truly reference-free display, but also has disadvantages. By the process of differentiation, low spatial frequency information may be lost. Moreover, under certain circumstances spatial differentiation may produce complexities which are hard to decipher.

As there are no published studies demonstrating superiority of any one particular reference location over all others, it is desirable for a topographic mapping system to permit the use of several reference conventions, i.e., more than one single-locus reference, the average reference, and Laplacian transformation.

Interpolation Techniques

Satisfactory visualization of mapped data requires a process of interpolation so that regions between electrodes can be assigned appropriate colors and hues for display. There exists no unanimity among investigators as to which interpolation technique is best (e.g., three- or four-point linear, inverse distance to the power n, polynomial approximation). In general, those techniques that weight distant electrodes produce smoother topographic distributions but less accurate data, while those that weight the nearest electrodes produce coarser images but more accurate data. Decisions concerning the efficacy of one particular algorithm should be based not upon underyling theory but upon actual comparison with real data. Until one algorithm is shown to be superior to all others, clinical mapping systems should provide a choice of algorithms. Ultimately, the need for interpolation will be reduced as means for employing larger numbers of real electrodes are developed.

Normative Data Base

A normative data base is necessary in any clinical mapping system. However, the normative data must have been collected properly. The data base must provide different controls for different age groups, reflecting the sensitivity of EEG and EP data to age. Subjects in the data base must have been collected by some reproducible procedure, i.e., random selection from a large population, with >70% acceptance, and must satisfy, medical criteria of health. Two practices to be avoided are: (1) selection of subjects solely on the basis of response to advertisement and (2) acceptance of referred patients who appear "normal." The first tends to attract subjects who are out of work for reasons such as drug abuse or personality disorder, and the second also skews the population toward pathology. Also to be avoided is the selection or rejection of subjects on the basis of the appearance of their data, as this may skew the population toward a preconceived notion of "normality."

Precise details of the nature of the normative data base (e.g., subject selection and rejection criteria, number) must be made known by the supplier. Moreover, all systems must provide the user with the option of forming his/her own control group.

Data Manipulation

Calibration. Every system should provide means for a complete system calibration at the start of each study. A minimal requirement would be the ability to inject a known single-frequency sine wave of calibrated amplitude (e.g., 10 Hz and 100 µV peak to peak) at the front end of each polygraph amplifier so as to individually calculate each channel's gain. Better would be to calculate gain at many or all frequencies by means of multiple sine waves, white noise, etc. Additionally, measurements of distortion, phase differential, cross-talk, and bandpass limits are desirable. Bandpass 3-db points, roll-off, noise figure, and filter type should be specified for all amplifiers.

Normalization. For optimal use with parametric statistical procedures such as the Z or t statistic, data should have normal or Gaussian distribution. However, several factors may affect data so as to render them non-Gaussian. The first factor is the data itself. Alpha amplitude may never go below zero but may at times be much larger than a normative mean value. In this situation, the distribution about the mean value may be skewed. Unfortunately, careful studies of the actual distributions are not complete, so no agreed corrections can be made. Another factor influencing normality of distribution is the expression of spectral value as a function of squared microvolts. Because the distribution of squared values is inherently non-Guassian, an appropriate correction should be applied (e.g., square root spectra, logarithmic transformation, arcsine correction). A third factor is the use of percentage spectral data. Alpha, for example, is expressed as a percentage of total spectral power. Percentage data has the advantage of being independent of system calibration, but suffers from producing operationally dependent figures, i.e., percentage alpha is a function of all other frequencies as well as alpha. Percentage data is also inherently non-Gaussian, and corrections should be applied. Corrections may be quite complex when data is expressed as percent squared microvolts.

It is recognized that there is much controversy concerning data normalization. Mapping systems should be required to make available all standard data normalization procedures. Moreover, systems should provide for incorporating new transformations as they become available.

Further Data Computations. Although their clinical utility has not been unequivocally established, there exist a number of EEG-derived numerical parameters that may be of value. These include coefficient of variation, symmetry functions, mobility, Hjorth parameters, and coherence. Complete systems should include the ability to calculate these parameters and provide means to readily add more as they are developed.

Artifact Removal. Prior to submission for spectral analysis, EEG should be screened for artifact (e.g., blinks, eye movements, electrode pop, mains interference, myogenic signals, movements, etc) and affected segments removed. There is no on-line automated technique that performs this complex task as well as the human eye. Accordingly, although automated artifact rejection is desirable either as an on-line or off-line system, provision for visual analysis must also provided; every system should enable storage of collected data and redisplay for artifact removal purposes. This is usually accomplished by means of hard disk. Careful consideration need be given to length of epoch for submission to spectral analysis. Longer epochs, on the order of 8–10 s, increase the probability of artifact inclusion. Shorter epochs, on the order of 2 s, maximize the likelihood of finding artifact-free segments; however, they decrease the accuracy of low-frequency spectral estimation. Optimally, systems should provide options for recording differing segment lengths.

Evoked potential data are more difficult to screen for artifact. It is usual for a system to provide single-trial elimination on the basis of a user-supplied overvoltage criterion. Such a system will detect and eliminate gross eye blinks and muscle and movement artifacts. Recently, techniques have been developed for single-trial EP estimation. Inclusion of such methods is desirable.

Conduct and Evaluation of Studies

Electrode Application

Accuracy begins with proper electrode positioning; careful measurement is mandatory. Electrode type and number may vary, but the means of attachment must be secure. And, as previously discussed, the use of electrode to monitor eye movement and muscle artifact is strongly recommended.

Calibration

As previously discussed, a full system calibration should be performed at the commencement of each study.

State and Artifact Control

Great care must be taken to ensure proper maintenance and identification of the patient's state and level of attentiveness. If a normative data base is to be used, the homeostatic state of the subject must match that of the individuals used in the collection of control group data. It is well known that drowsiness and inattention can effect EEG spectral content and long-latency EP morphology. This is largely the responsibility of the technician but requires verification by the reader. The polygraphic EEG record can be most useful here.

It is also the technician's responsibility to recognize the occurrence of artifact and take steps to reduce or eliminate it. Various strategies such as visual fixation targets, "blink holidays," proper positioning, and frequent interrogation must be part of a good technician's repertoire.

Data Evaluation

Inspection of the EEG tracing by the reader is important to ensure the appropriate subject state, absence of artifact, and technical adequacy of data. Moreover, it is recognized that much more may be visible in EEG than can be adequately reflected by spectral analysis alone. Accordingly, the EEG must be clinically interpreted. Spectral data and long-latency EP data, if used, should be evaluated with the assistance of age-matched normative control data. Prior to topographic analysis, the underlying spectral and EP recordings should be visually inspected to ensure freedom from artifact and unusual features. A final evaluation should combine the findings of EEG, spectral and EP data.

It is widely recognized that the statistical inspection of multiple maps involves the risk of "capitalization upon chance." Thus the finding of a statistically significant abnormality in a single map may be due to chance alone, or to artifact rather than pathology. For an abnormality to be considered clinically significant, it must appear repeatedly across the differing study states. It is also very useful to repeat each study section two or more times and check whether findings remain constant.

Although automatic subject classification, if properly designed, may obviate the need to inspect data from a topographic perspective, it does not relieve the reader of two key responsibilities: (1) The discriminant function must be appropriate for the given patient. The reader must be assured that the criteria used to select the subjects/patients in establishing the discriminant function pertain to the patient presently being studied. (2) The reader must ensure that the behavioral paradigms used were properly executed and that the patient's state was correct. For example, drowsiness may produce change mimicking pathology.

Summary

We make the following key recommendations regarding the design of guidelines for the clinical use of topographic mapping:
1. Personnel already trained in neurophysiological procedures must receive additional specialized training.
2. Standard EEGs should be peformed at the time of data gathering for artifact and state control. These should be clinically interpreted as well.
3. A normative data base is mandatory. Normative data should be collected by reproducible means on the basis of specific criteria. Differing data bases are required for differing age groups.
4. Equipment used to evaluate patients should be technically or equivalent to that used to gather normative data.
5. At least 19 scalp and four artifact electrodes should be used.
6. As a minimal requirement for topographic maps a vertex-view, equal-area display format should be provided.
7. More than one technique for electrode referencing, interpolation, and data normalization should be available.
8. All systems should facilitate the detection and elimination of artifact prior to map formation.
9. Every system must provide means for complete calibration.
10. Clinical studies should include repetitions so as to avoid false conclusions based on chance findings.
11. Systems providing means for automatic classification must detail inclusion and exclusion criteria to ensure appropriate use.

From Graphein to Topos:
Past and Future of Brain Mapping

H. Petsche[1]

History is able to teach us scientists, among others, that the results obtained in every epoch are determined primarily by the technological means available at the time in question – another reason to be cautious of every scientific "truth." Any claim that a given finding is true or untrue should be abandoned. Only statements whether findings are sound or unsound with respect to the methods available at their times should be admitted.

As a lifelong companion of EEG topography I would like to show up the complex and sometimes quirky ways the human mind has taken to find compromises between its conceptions of those brain processes that enable us to behave as human beings and the prevailing technological constraints on the construction of equipment appropriate to test our hypotheses. When considering the course of scientific ideas in our field, I also hope to be able to make clear that not only have hypotheses about the brain influenced the way technological aids for their study have been developed, but also the reverse is true: the technological facilities available have largely guided our investigation of the functioning of the brain in certain directions. All our findings depend largely, if not exclusively, on the setup of our experiments and the equipment used to perform them. This, most impressively, teaches us the history of the sciences.

At the beginning of all attempts at utilization of the EEG is the concept of an analogy between the cortex and a geographic map. This notion lends itself at least as much to the production of nonsense as to the initiation of valuable hypotheses. To my knowledge, this concept was first promoted by Franz Joseph Gall, a German anatomist (1758–1828) reputed to be a founder of "phrenology" or "cranioscopy." An eminent anatomist, Gall was first in claiming that the white matter principally differs in function from the grey matter by serving to transmit information to lower levels of the central nervous system. However, it was not this that made him famous, but rather his erroneous conviction that different regions of the cortex have different restricted functions and therefore that their size must be correlated with different traits of character, which can thus be determined from examination of models of the skull. Physicians in the early nineteenth century generally had such skulls on display in their practices. They served, so to speak, as a forerunner of the EEG that came but a century thereafter.

Gall's hypothesis, as funny as it may seem to us today, probably originated in efforts, much pursued in the period of enlightenment, to recognize human traits of character, emotionality and mental condition from careful observation of facial expression. One of the most prominent advocates of this doctrine

---

[1] Institut für Neurophysiologie, Universität Wien, Währingerstr. 17, 1090 Wien, Austria

was Johann Caspar Lavater (1741–1801). It is no wonder that such ideas were also applied to the cortex, which was known by this time to house essential human properties. Thus Gall's ideas found ready acceptance and were able to flourish throughout the world.

Today's brain mapping seems to be appropriate for putting these early and nebulous ideas on a sound scientific base and for starting voyages of exploration to the brain.

It is perhaps not well enough known that in fact Pavlov may be considered as another father of brain mapping. In 1926, he wrote:

If one could observe the activity of the brain through the skull, one would see a continuously changing light-spot whisking over the hemispheres and surrounded by darker shadows arrested sometimes here, sometimes there and then again jumping to other regions. In this way the ceaselessly changing function of the consciousness seems to be activated from a central place.

At that time, Pavlov's statement sounded like the dream of a scientist who could afford such flights of fancy, as he was not personally involved in the hard, arid and still unprofitable attempts at recording brain activities. Although it had been known since Caton (1875) that the brain always produces weak electrical oscillations, the path from the early and cumbersome recordings from the exposed brains of animals to recordings from the intact human skull was long, stony and full of disillusionment.

Hans Berger trod this path, taking his first steps along it in 1900. Berger's main intention was to look for correlations between the EEG and mental events. It took no less than 29 years before he felt safe enough to publish his conclusions that the manifestations he was recording with his primitive instruments reflected, in reality, the voltage oscillations of the brain (Berger 1929). Throughout his life, Berger was convinced that the EEG has something to do with mental processes. This belief set him clearly apart from the general conviction of his colleagues and successors, who believed the EEG to represent but the noise of the mental apparatus.

In Berger's days, dreaming of looking through the skull to see "the potential fields interwoven like the warp and woof of a shimmering fabric," as Grey Walter expressed it (1953), was left to non-electroencephalographers such as Pavlov. An insider such as Berger was happy if he succeeded in writing or recording (Greek: *graphein*) from just two points of the skull. Fairly soon after Berger, however, it became clear that the next step to take would be simultaneous recordings from several points of the skull.

Almost at the same time, the first steps into topography were made (Greek *topos*, location). Among the forerunners of brain mapping, three scientists have to be mentioned who emphasized the spatial dimension in electroencephalography.

One of the first to do so was Adrian, who not only confirmed Berger's discovery of the alpha rhythm but also claimed that the alpha focus, occipitoparietally and close to the midline, has a frontal antifocus, behaving with respect to the occipitoparietal focus like the sun to the full moon: the more the former sinks, the more the latter rises (Adrian and Yamagiwa 1935). The same authors also observed, along a line of electrodes, that the alpha waves undergo phase shifts and seem to move along the skull.

From Graphein to Topos: Past and Future of Brain Mapping

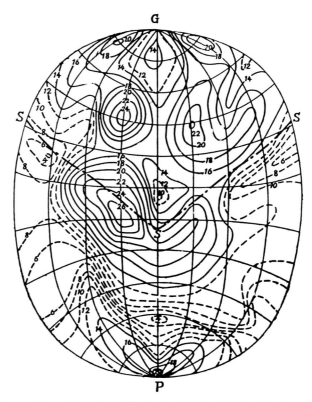

Fig. 1. Bioelectric brain map of man. Lines of equal amplitudes in μV. *G*, glabella; *S*, sulcus centralis, *P*, protuberantia occipitalis externa. (From Motokawa 1942)

Particular emphasis was laid on this phenomenon by Motokawa, an almost forgotten EEG pioneer, who built the first EEG amplifier in Japan in the 1940s and, in the following years, published a series of most remarkable papers. Motokawa was also the first to develop and use statistical analysis for the quantification of EEG data (Motokawa 1942). Most important in this context are his papers on the alpha phase recorded from 12 equidistant electrodes placed on the meridian of the skull, which he usually presented in the form of amplitude-phase vectors. The striking discontinuity of the phase diagrams between frontal and parietal areas is due to the marked differences in the structure and thickness of these two cortical areas (Motokawa and Tuziguti 1944).

Motokawa (1944) also succeeded in measuring the average alpha amplitude from not less than 90 equally distributed points on the skull, from which he recorded successively in 27 persons, and found a characteristic distribution of the alpha fields. To my knowledge, this was the very first EEG map: it dates from 1940 (Fig. 1).

Kornmüller's contribution to the understanding of the importance of the spatial parameter of the EEG was his findings in rabbits. The rabbit cortex is not gyrated and thus offers optimal conditions for examining questions concerning the dependence of the EEG on cortical structure. From 1932 to 1936, Kornmüller published data about characteristic differences of the EEG he had recorded from different areas, which he called *Feldeigenströme,* area-specific currents. Such differences actually exist, even if they are not in fact so clear-cut as in those early publications (Kornmüller 1937).

After these early voices, six independent groups of researchers started, in the early 1950s, to design displays for visualizing spatiotemporal details that are not detectable with the routine EEG. After the most sophisticated of these devices, designed by Grey Walter and Shipton in 1951, they can be called "toposcopes," from greek *topos*, place, and *skopein*, to view. The principal aim of these investigators was to learn more about the interdependence of the EEG in different regions of the skull.

The earliest and simplest model was designed by Goldman's group (Goldman et al. 1948). In this method, a square array of 16 electrodes was mounted on the skull (or even on the chest, to record from the heart); the signals were displayed on cathode ray tubes as brightness oscillations. No further papers were published by this group, but their ideas were taken up by Lilly (1950), who developed what he called the Bavatron (brain activity visualization in areas), which consisted of an array of 25 light spots on a screen. His main purpose was to find out how closely electrodes have to be placed to yield the essential information of how a cortical zone functions. With this device, Lilly was able to gain some insights into the electrical structure of evoked potentials in animals. However, the application of his method was limited, mainly because of the large quantities of recording film needed and the time-consuming evaluation of the data.

Livanov's "encephaloscope" was based on the same principle. He used an array of 5×10 electrodes and worked on humans and on rabbits (Livanov and Ananiev 1955).

Quite different in design was Grey Walter and Shipton's equipment built in 1951, which was used exclusively in man. Basically, it consisted of an arrangement of 22 small cathode ray tubes, each one displaying information from a bipolar recording from the head; the arrangement of the tubes corresponded to the placement of the electrode pairs on the head. In their first model, each tube displayed a rotating vector, like the hand of a clock. The brilliance of these signals was modulated by the amplitude of the EEG, so that when the speed of rotation of these vectors was equalled – by hand – to the frequency of the dominant rhythm of the EEG, one segment of the tube was consistently bright. Thus, phase differences of the alpha could be detected by the different positions of the bright segments displayed by the different tubes. In 1957 Shipton improved this system, replacing the rotating vector with a helical scan. This had the advantage that longer exposure times could be chosen, but the shortcoming that evaluation by the naked eye became even more difficult.

The two remaining groups of toposcopists, namely Rémond's and ours, restricted themselves intentionally to only one instead of two dimensions and recorded only from ranges of equidistant electrodes, in order to make their systems more suited for limited questions. Rémond's original idea, the basis of his "chrono-topogrammes," was to measure simultaneously the potential gradients between successive electrodes along a range of nine electrodes at equal time intervals (Rémond 1955). Rémond, too, used his system exclusively in man.

Finally, our own method (Petsche and Marko 1955), which we applied to both man and animals, was based on the same principle: 16 electrodes were placed along the cortex of a rabbit at 2-mm intervals and the potential oscillations with respect to a common reference electrode were conducted to glow modulators, their outputs being arranged in the same way, projecting onto a film. The zero crossings of the potential fluctuations were recorded on the film, running at 10 cm/s. With this device, mainly epileptic phenomena in the rabbit were studied.

Detailed descriptions of these methods may be found in Petsche and Shaw (1972). All these methods were more or less seriously restricted by the still fairly primitive technology of those days, not to mention the great expense more sophisticated systems would have required. In subsequent years a few more studies in this direction were undertaken, including those by Estrin and Uzgalis (1969), Yasuda (1961), and particularly DeMott, with his 400 channels (1966); however, with the exception of Lehmann's work on the human alpha and evoked potentials (1969) none of these methods seems to have decisively influenced EEG research. I think one reason for this was that none of them was simple enough (and also cheap and versatile enough) to become incorporated into clinical research and into EEG routine work, as for instance the recording of evoked potentials has become incorporated today.

This symposium is one proof more that such methods have now found their way to the EEG laboratories in hospitals. Certainly, more time will elapse before standard methods will be used in the clinic; but not nearly as long as it took for electroencephalography to become standard at every larger hospital.

The overwhelming invasion of the EEG by mapping methods demonstrates that scientists dealing with the EEG have become aware of the fact that traditional electroencephalography has neglected one essential aspect, namely location.

However, do we still need the EEG for locating brain processes at all? Much more efficient methods are available today to locate a tumor or an insult, for instance computer tomography or nuclear magnetic resonance. Neurosurgeons rely more and more on these modern brain-imaging techniques than on the EEG. However, this is only one side of the coin. The EEG has lost nothing of its significance in unraveling functional conditions of the brain. This holds not only for epilepsy, where the EEG is still the most important guide for the physician, but also for direct or indirect metabolic, vascular and other changes in the brain. In these respects, the EEG will most likely remain the leading method in the years to come, causing the least discomfort to the patient.

I am convinced that brain mapping – also in this respect – will contribute to improvement of diagnostic efficacy and remain a guide for therapy. Concerning this latter point, I am thinking not only of the epilepsies: pilot studies in my institute showed fairly specific topographic changes of power and coherence in a group of schizophrenic patients under drug therapy (Pockberger et al. 1984). It also turned out that drug-dependent changes of these parameters may take several weeks to develop and display clear topographic differences. Unfortunately, the pharmaco-EEG does not yet play a consistent role in clinical work. Most likely this will change as soon as brain mapping becomes feasible on a broad basis to study the action of drugs on the brain.

The increasing power of modern mapping methods is mainly due to the fact that computers have become so much more sophisticated and, simultaneously, smaller and cheaper. This has not only promoted and increased the number of data to be processed simultaneously but also opened the way to even greater sophistication of statistical analysis. Computerization of both the gathering and the statistical analysis of data from the brain was necessary to pick up the thread of Berger's original ideas.

As already mentioned, the vigor of the EEG lies in detecting functional changes. Therefore, one main stream of mapping techniques will most likely develop into the research of higher achievements of the brain, such as reading, performing mental arithmetic, listening etc. By means of probability mapping and the study of power and coherence changes in five frequency bands, characteristic changes were found for reading, performing mental arithmetic, listening to a text, listening to music and the like (Petsche et al. 1987). These findings support the view that mapping may contribute greatly to the diagnosis and localization of deficient higher brain achievements, such as aphasias. It may also contribute to a better understanding of the brain processes in psychoses. I would mention here the work of Duffy et al. (1979), Etevenon et al. (1985) and Buchsbaum et al. (1986).

I think that future techniques of brain mapping will aim at somewhat different targets than the early toposcopists had in mind: whereas these pioneers strove for a representation of the instantaneous behavior of the potential fields, today it seems probably more promising to average parameters and perform statistical evaluations. The inclusion of coherence estimates has also proved useful.

All this leads to the need for probability maps, which, to my knowledge, were first constructed by Roy John and his group (Roy John et al. 1977). One of Roy John's aims seems to be an atlas of average brain maps for different kinds of mental activities, to be used as a standard for better estimating the nature of patients' deficits. This seems to me one feasible way toward automatic analysis of the EEG, at least as far as the structure of its background activity is concerned.

For the detection of localized particularities, and especially for the recognition of artifacts, however, the evaluation of the row EEG by the naked eye will probably never become dispensable.

Let us now turn away from clinical neurological and psychiatric problems and consider psychology. In my opinion, brain mapping will soon become one of the most powerful tools for the neuropsychologist who wants to do brain research. It already supports cognition research and will do so even more strongly in the future. Quite a number of papers have already been published in this field.

But apart from this, mapping techniques together with statistics seem to have become most useful tools for studying how traits of intelligence and personality are embodied in the EEG. The lifelong work by Giannitrapani (1985), even if performed for the most part using less sophisticated technology than now available, provides evidence that certain personality traits, as defined by psychological tests, may actually be reflected by certain traits of the EEG. It may be hoped that a better definition of the complex and hardly manageable concept of "intelligence" will one day be feasible. The same holds true for the kindred concept of "musicality," which can also be conceived of as a special domain of intelligence and which has particularly occupied my attention of late (Petsche et al. 1985).

However, I wish to end with a warning.

Eleven years ago (Petsche 1976), I wrote: Computers, paradoxical as it may sound, frequently decrease the efficiency of the work, for nothing is more difficult than to sift the chaff from the wheat considering the huge number of data put out by the computer. The search for significant results has been becoming increasingly difficult. I even dare to claim that, since the computer has come to dominate electroencephalography, it has become much more difficult to distinguish efficient from foolish problems. I see only one way of escaping this danger: namely to keep in mind the physiologically and clinically relevant problems and not be become entangled in problems created by the computer. For the very anticipation the clinical neurologist has been putting in electroencephalography, is to have a diagnostic aim supplying optimal information about the functioning of the patient's brain.

This warning has not lost its significance. A second admonition in this era of proliferating topographic brain mapping systems is called for: never neglect the raw EEG data, as the entire wealth of experience rests on them.

With these two warnings in mind, a hopeful future for the EEG can be foreseen. With the step from *graphein*, to write, to *topos*, location, conceding equal rights to the two parameters of time and space, electroencephalography has crossed the threshold from adolescence to adulthood.

References

Adrian ED, Yamagiwa BHC (1935) The origin of the Berger rhythm. Brain 58:323–351

Berger H (1929) Über das Elektrenkephalogramm des Menschen. Arch Psychiatr Nervenkr 87:527–570

Buchsbaum MS, Hazlett E, Sicotte N, Ball R, Johnson S (1986) Geometric and scaling issues in topographic electroencephalography. In: Duffy FH (ed) Topographic mapping of brain electrical activity. Butterworth, Boston, pp 325–337

Caton R (1875) The electric currents of the brain. Br Med J 2:278

DeMott DW (1966) Cortical micro-toposcopy. Med Res Eng 5:23–29

Duffy FH, Bartels PH, Burchfield JL (1981) Significance probability mapping. Electroencephalogr Clin Neurophysiol 51:455–462

Duffy FH, Burchfield JL, Lombroso CT (1979) Brain electrical activity mapping (BEAM). Ann Neurol 5:309–321

Estrin T, Uzgalis R (1969) Computerised display of spatio-temporal EEG patterns. IEEE Trans Biomed Eng 16:192–196

Etevenon P, Gaches J, Debouzy C, Gueguen B, Peron Magnan P (1985) EEG cartography. I. By means of mini- or micro-computers. Neuropsychobiology 13:141–146

Giannitrapani D (1985) The electrophysiology of intellectual functions. Karger, Basel

Goldmann S, Vivian WE, Chien CK, Bowes HN (1948) Electronic mapping of the activity of the heart and brain. Science 24:720–723

Kornmüller AE (1937) Die bioelektrischen Erscheinungen der Hirnrindenfelder. Thieme, Leipzig

Lehmann D (1971) Multichannel topography of human alpha EEG fields. Electroencephalogr Clin Neurophysiol 31:439–449

Lilly CA (1950) A method of recording the moving electrical potential gradients in the brain: the 25 channel bavatron and electroiconograms. Conference on Electronics in Nucleonics and Medicine. Am Inst Electron Eng New York, pp 37–43

Livanov MN, Ananiev WM (1955) Electrophysiological study of the spread of activity in the rabbit cerebral cortex. Fiziol ZH SSSR 41:461–469

Motokawa K (1942) Die Analyse der Perioden im normalen Elektroencephalogramm des Menschen. Tohoku J Exp Med 42:9–20

Motokawa K (1944) Die Verteilung der elektrischen Aktivität auf der Kopfschwarte und ihre Beziehung zur Cytoarchitektonik der Großhirnrinde des Menschen. Jpn J Med Sci Biol 3 (10):99–111

Motokawa K, Tuziguti K (1944) Über Vektordiagramme für die gehirnelektrischen Erscheinungen des Menschen. Tohoku J Exp Med 48:73–86

Pavlov JP (1926) Die höchste Nerventätigkeit (das Verhalten) von Tieren. Bergmann, München

Petsche H (1976) Topography of the EEG: survey and prospects. Clin Neurol Neurosurg 79:15–28

Petsche H, Marko A (1955) Toposkopische Untersuchungen zur Ausbreitung des Alpharhythmus. Z Nervenheilk, Wien 12:87–100

Petsche H, Shaw JC (1972) EEG topography. In: Brazier MAB, Walter DO (eds) Evaluation of bioelectrical data from brain, nerve and muscle, II B. Elsevier, Amsterdam, pp 1–84 (Handbook of electroencephalography and clinical neurophysiology, vol 5)

Petsche H, Pockberger H, Rappelsberger P (1985) Musikrezeption, EEG und musikalische Vorbildung. Z EEG-EMG 16:183–190

Petsche H, Rappelsberger P, Pockberger H (1987) EEG-Veränderungen beim Lesen. In: Weinmann HM (ed) Zugang zum Verständnis höherer Hirnfunktionen durch das EEG. Zuckschwerdt, München, pp 59–74

Pockberger H, Rappelsberger P, Petsche H, Thau K, Küfferle B (1984) Computer-assisted EEG topography as a tool in the evaluation of actions of psychoactive drugs in patients. Neuropsychobiology 12:183–187

Rémond A (1955) Orientations et tendances des méthodes topographiques dans l'étude de l'activité électrique du cerveau. Rev Neurol (Paris) 93:399–432

Roy John E, Karmel BZ, Corning WC, Easton P, Brown D, Ahn H, John M, Harmony T, Prichep L, Toro A, Gerson I, Bartlett F, Thatcher R, Kaye H, Valdes P, Schwartz E (1977) Neurometrics. Science 196:1393–1410

Shipton HW (1957) An improved electrotoposcope. Electroencephalogr Clin Neurophysiol 9:182

Walter WG (1953) Third International EEG Congress. Symposium I on recent developments in electroencephalographic techniques. Elsevier, Amsterdam, pp 7–16

Walter WG, Shipton HW (1951) A new toposcopic display system. Electroencephalogr Clin Neurophysiol 3:281–292

Yasuda T (1961) EEG analysis with decatron toposcope. Tohoku J Exp Med 74:258–264

Topographic Mapping of Brain Electrical Activity: Clinical Applications and Issues

F.H. DUFFY[1]

Why Mapping?

Among those employing cartography there is universal enthusiasm, and the comment is often heard that computerized quantification and mapping will carry neurophysiology into the 21st century. The number of manufacturers offering mapping devices has moved from zero in 1984 to 14 as of early 1987. The reasons behind the general optimism are worthy of review.

Electroencephalographic Data

Similar enthusiasm was felt for EEG in the late 1930s or early 1940s. The discovery of a scalp-recorded rhythm responsive to eye closure (alpha) (Berger 1929) and the demonstration of electrographic concomitants of epilepsy (spike and wave) (Gibbs et al. 1935) led to the belief that EEG would prove to be a major clinical and scientific tool for the study of normal and pathologic brain function. Although EEG fulfilled its promise vis-à-vis epilepsy and certain other clinical conditions, it failed to become a major universal neuroscientific tool. Most normal and many abnormal brain states failed to produce an EEG signature as characteristic as the discharge of epilepsy.

For some years, we and other electroencephalographers have clung to the belief that the problem was not an inherent lack of EEG sensitivity. Rather, we postulated the limiting factor to be analytic, i.e., reliance upon unaided visual inspection. In short, we felt there was more useful information in EEG than could be detected and quantified by visual inspection.

Our approach to the development of a method to extract more information from brain electrical activity was, first, to summarize the processes by which an electrocephalographer went about reading an EEG and, second, to implement these processes in modern hardware/software configuration. Visual analysis appears to proceed of a five-part process involving:

1. Search for discontinuities
2. Spectral analyses of frequency content
3. Temporal summation over time
4. Spatial topographic analyses
5. Statistical analyses

---

[1] BEAM Laboratory, Department of Neurology, The Children's Hospital and Harvard Medical School, 300 Longwood Avenue, Boston, MA 02115, USA

Visual screening of data for discontinuities such as spikes, sharp waves, and artifact is the traditional first step, and its success no doubt accounts for the major role EEG plays in the diagnosis and management of epilepsy. Even computerized spike detection algorithms rely upon visual inspection as the "gold standard" (Gotman 1982; Gotman and Gloor 1976). Accordingly, we have not attempted to improve upon this area of relative strength. Once the presence or absence of spikes has been determined, the next traditional step is to analyze EEG background activity. This process involves an estimation of frequency content (e.g., delta, theta, alpha, and beta), its consistency or lack of consistency over time, and its spatial extent. Success in the extraction of information from EEG background by visual inspection has been more limited, and it is in this area where a computerized approach appeared to us to be of greatest potential value.

Spectral analysis has been available by computer for some time (Cooley and Tukey 1965) and has been extensively used for EEG analyses. This technique not only summarizes frequency content, but may also be applied to EEG epochs of differing lengths, thereby summarizing spectral content over time (Bickford et al. 1973). Now, long EEG segments are usually broken down into shorter segments ranging from one to ten seconds. Results of spectral analyses on these subsegments are typically averaged to represent the mean EEG spectral content. At the same time, the standard deviation (SD) of each spectral band can be derived. The coefficient of variation (the SD divided by the mean) constitutes a useful parameter of spectral variability. It can be thought of as a measure of paroxysmal activity within a spectral band (Duffy 1986). The obvious next step is to map these data so as to condense both spectral and spatial information into single images.

Evoked Potential Data

Analysis of long-latency evoked potential (EP) data raises similar issues. The demonstration of signal averaging in the 1950s (Dawson 1950; Halliday 1987) spawned the expectation that these long-latency waves of apparent cortical origin would rival or at least complement clinical EEG. Unfortunately, long-latency EP data proved to be exceptionally difficult to analyze by simple unaided visual inspection (Callaway 1969; Chiappa 1983). Clinical attention turned to the subsequently discovered short-latency auditory evoked response (AER) (Jewett and Williston 1971) where individual components have distinct anatomical relationships to underlying brainstem gray matter nuclei. Not only are long-latency components not clearly associated with identifiable anatomical structures, there is evidence from the animal data that single surface components represent the superimposition of waves from multiple spatially dispersed neural generators (Arezzo et al. 1975). Indeed, it is sometimes difficult to define long-latency EP components reliably across subjects. Jeffreys and Axford (1972) were the first to suggest that in defining a component one must take into account not only amplitude and latency, but spatial extent as well. With this in mind, it seems the obvious next step is to create a series of maps from sets of multichannel

EP data so as to define spatiotemporal relationships more carefully by viewing the resulting cartooned images (Duffy 1982; Duffy et al. 1979).

But mapping of EEG and EP data is not the final step, for maps alone do not address the issue of detecting abnormalities. The final step is to compare unknown data to control or reference data. This important step obviates the need to maintain an image of normality in one's mind. We have referred to the process by which unknown topographic data are transformed into images of deviation from normal as significance probability mapping, or SPM (Duffy et al. 1981).

Map Making

Interpolation, Color, Electrode Number, Reference

Topographic mapping of EEG data is not new, with pioneering systems having been demonstrated in the 1950s and 1960s (Estrin and Uzgalis 1969; Harris et al. 1969; Walter and Shipton 1951). The lag of clinical implementation to the 1980s probably reflected historically the relative inaccessability of computing power, especially that devoted to image processing. Dramatic reductions in cost and size have placed powerful and sophisticated systems within the reach of individual laboratories, if not individual desk tops. These ongoing evolutionary developments have greatly facilitated the complex computational tasks that have to be performed in quantified EEG and EP analysis involving topographic mapping.

Our approach to mapping, first described in 1979, involved "nearest three point linear interpolation" of data from 20 standard electrode placements onto a 64 by 64 matrix, as illustrated in Fig. 1 (Duffy et al. 1979). The resulting matrix values are displayed on a video monitor in color-coded "gray scale."

There have been almost as many approaches to interpolation as there have been authors. Methods have differed as to the number of electrodes used and the weighting factor for each electrode. To understand differences, it is best to examine two extreme cases. In the first, only nearby electrodes are employed to interpolate an unknown point, and they are not heavily weighted. This gives rise to a punctate display with regions of similar value surrounding each electrode location. In the second extreme, many electrodes are used, and distant electrodes are given significant weighting. This results in a pleasing display, but by its inherent smoothing, local details may be blurred. The optimal interpolation is yet to be agreed upon, and until such time as consensus is achieved we have adopted one making minimal assumptions, i.e., an unknown point is best estimated by the three nearest real data values on a linear basis. The key is to recall that *all* interpolation techniques are approximations. Justification for one particular interpolation technique should not stop with a theoretical discussion. Values created by the interpolation algorithm should be put to a test, i.e., compared to real values from extra electrodes placed over the spot to be interpolated.

Some years ago, as part of our early experiments with differing interpolation techniques, we investigated the magnitude of error introduced by our interpola-

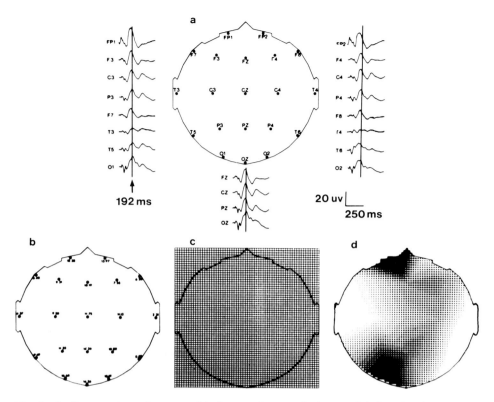

Fig. 1a–d. Construction of topographic images from evoked potential data by the BEAM (brain electrical activity mapping) methodology. Example of the construction of a topographic map for EP data. Mean EPs are formed from each of 20 recording sites. Each EP is divided into 128 4-ms intervals, and the mean voltage value for each interval is calculated. **a** The individual EPs for the electrode locations indicated on the head diagram. **b** The mean voltage values at these locations for the interval beginning 192 ms after the stimulus (the *vertical line* in **a** indicates this time on the EPs). **c** Next the head region is treated as a 64 × 64 matrix, yielding 4096 spatial domains. Each domain is assigned a voltage value by linear interpolation from the three nearest known points. **d** Finally, for display, the raw voltage values are fitted to a discrete-level equal-interval intensity scale. Although a VER is used to illustrate the mapping process, the same procedure is used for mapping other data, including the AER

tion method. We placed a single electrode at the center of the triangle formed by CZ, C3, and P3. We compared the actual value found at this point with the interpolated value over 50 trials for fast Fourier transform (FFT) data and 50 trials for EP data. There was no significant difference between the interpolated and actual values for either modality. By no means does this establish interpolation as equivalent to actual measurement, nor does it establish three-point linear interpolation as the best method. It merely suggests that this method is adequate for routine clinical measurement. Much theoretical and practical work has yet to be done here.

The use of color, the standard for modern image processing when available, has become surprisingly controversial in topographic mapping, although widely employed. It is our observation that there are two classes of abuse leading to a "mistrust" of colored images that is often discussed at seminars and occasionally in print (Bickford and Allen 1986). In the first place, color juxtaposition is useful in emphasizing distinctions. The emphasis of a contour threshold by color, when justified on the basis of the underlying data structure, is most valuable. However, the incautious or improper juxtaposition of contrasting colors may lead to the visual impression of an important threshold when, in fact, none exists! In the second place, the proper use of color sequences can provide a sense of the gradient of the field. Random and/or repetitive color sequences, however, may be confusing and even misleading. This often happens when a PC-based color display device runs out of color so previous colors must be repeated, often slightly modified, as by cross-matching, etc.

To say that color should not be employed because it can be abused would be much like saying that one ought not to have children because they can be abused. In our opinion, color can add to a topographic image much as it does to ordinary vision. The point is to use color properly!

Closely linked with the issue of interpolation is that of the correct number of real electrodes to employ. What is often forgotten in such discussions is the question "For what purpose?" It is possible that one could follow the course of a patient with a metabolic encephalopathy with from one to four electrodes. This derives from the observation that metabolic derangements ordinarily produce diffuse change observable at most locations, hence, few spatial samplings are necessary to detect its presence. In contrast, if one undertakes the more refined task of discriminating topographically by means of EPs between stimulation of adjacent digits on the same hand, then a much denser electrode array of 81 electrodes overlying one somatomotor area is required (Duff 1980). Once again, much more theoretical and practical work is needed in this area. Until such time as this work is completed, we have based our mapping on the standard 10–20 electrode placement (Jasper 1958) augmented by additional artifact-monitoring placements. In our experience, the transition from 16 to 20 electrodes provided more definition for our clinical studies. We have tried going from 20 to 28 or more electrodes, but are not yet convinced that this is useful. Surprisingly, there has been little emphasis on the number and placement of artifact electrodes. In our opinion, this is a crucial issue in the detection and elimination or reduction of eye and muscle activity contamination.

As is true for EEG and EP data, there is no ideal and certainly no universally agreed upon electrode reference location for topographic mapping studies. Every known anatomical location (i.e., ears, mastoid, face, chin, chest) has known advantages and disadvantages. Two techniques have recently gained attention and have been used in mapping. The first is the common average reference (Lehmann 1986; Offner 1950). The biggest disadvantage of this technique is seen in the clinical situation where focal pathology exists and values from the abnormal region will influence values from uninvolved regions. The second is the "source derivation" or Laplacian method, where data are replaced by

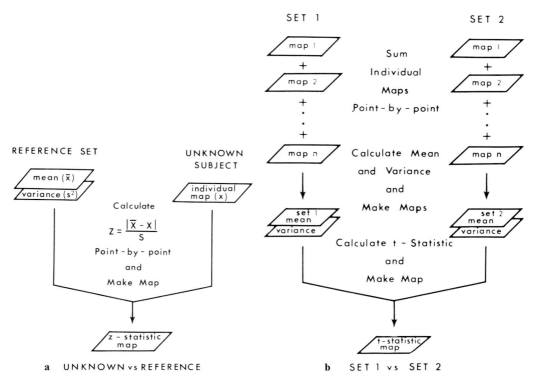

Fig. 2a, b. Topographic imaging of abnormality: significance probability mapping (SPM). **a** The formation of a Z-statistic SPM. The Z transform represents the number of SD by which an individual observation differs from the mean of a reference set. For BEAM, the Z statistic is calculated individually for each of the 20–32 scalp electrodes between the data of a subject and that of a normative control population. The resulting 20–32 Z values are then interpolated according to the procedure shown in Fig. 1 to produce the Z-SPM. The product is a display of a subject's deviation from normal in units of SD in such a way that the spatial relations of the original BEAM image are retained. Z-SPMs are ordinarily used in clinical practice to define abnormality in individual subjects. **b** The formation of a *t*-statistic SPM. Student's *t* statistic quantifies the separation between two sets of measures, taking into account not only the difference between the mean value of each group but also the variability within each group. Thus the *t* value is lower for the same difference in group mean when the variance in either or both groups increases. For BEAM, the *t* statistic is calculated individually for each of the 20–32 scalp electrodes between the data from one group of subjects and the data from another group. The resulting 20–32 *t* values are then mapped as per Fig. 1 to produce the *t*-SPM. The product is a topographic display of where the brain electrical activity of one group differs from that of another. Ordinarily *t*-SPMs are used in research to delineate where a pathological population differs from a control population

their second spatial derivative (Hjorth 1975, 1986). This truly reference-free approach has the advantage of visualizing current sources and sinks. In certain circumstances, this may provide important new information on source localization, especially in the auditory system of the newborn infant (Vaughan, work in progress). However, the process of mathematical differentiation inherently increases noise as well as signal. In our limited experience with the Laplacian method, we have found it produces images more complex, more confusing, and less intuitive than those yielded by mapping of unprocessed data. Nonetheless, both the average reference technique and the Laplacian method are valid and important additions to mapping and should be available on all systems. Only experience will clarify their value relative to more conventional reference electrode placements. Until this is established, most mapping systems used for clinical work should allow many or all of these reference options.

Significance Probability Mapping

The essence of the clinical application of topographic mapping is the detection and localization of abnormalities. Whereas there is certainly much to gain from the visual inspection of EP and spectral EEG images, one is often struck by their complexity. Although symmetry is expected, minor asymmetries are not uncommon. It can be difficult to determine when a perceived asymmetry is within the normal range of variation and when it is out of bounds. To assist the clinician in this often difficult task, we developed SPM. Figure 2 graphically depicts this statistical imaging technique. Essentially, a patient's data are replaced by the number of standard deviations separating them from the data of an age-matched normative control population. This relieves the clinician of the burden of having to mentally reference what a normal topographic map should look like for a given spectral band, age group, etc.

The key to this process is the availability of a normative population. The time and effort involved in gathering such data are repaid many times in the value they add to clinical investigation. In establishing a data base, however, there are many important issues, some of which are addressed in the following two sections.

Statistical Issues

Normative Data Base

In the formation of a normative data base, three issues stand out: (1) need for age-appropriate samples, (2) population sampling technique, and (3) exclusionary criteria. It is widely recognized that development is an important factor in establishing "normative" data. The EEG of the child differs markedly from that of the adult (John et al. 1980). Moreover, the rate of change of EEG and EP characteristics is quite non-linear (Duffy et al. 1984b; Dustman and Snyder 1981). For example, it may not be unreasonable to compare a 45-year-old man to the mean of a group ranging 5 years either side of this age. However, the analogous age range for a 10-year-old might span, maximally, plus or minus 2 years. For a newborn infant, it may span plus or minus 1 week. The use of an inappropriately large age span causes two problems: first, the resulting large SD will tend to reduce sensitivity; second, subjects at one or the other extreme end of the age range will have a biased difference from the group mean value. This may artificially increase or decrease the likelihood of detection of an apparent abnormality.

Population sampling is a crucial issue. Ideally, one would follow rules standardly utilized for the determination of characteristics of large populations. For example, it is usual to predict election results in the USA by a controlled sampling of voters such that accuracy within a few percent error can be obtained from samples as low as several thousand. This requires a specific preplanned sampling schedule and acquiescence on the part of all polled. Unfortunately, this approach would be unlikely to work for the collection of electrophysiologic data. First, the collection of such large amounts of data might take years. Second, and more important, by no means would everyone respond positively to a request to spend a half a day away from work in a neurophysiology lab to have paste smeared in their hair and endure a series of benign but boring tasks such as having a strobe light flashed in the eyes or listening to several hundred tone pips for a minimal remuneration – usually $ 20 or $ 50. It would be hard to imagine many successful businessmen in their 40s agreeing to time away from work for such a study. On the other hand, it is not hard to imagine someone out of work due to drug, emotional, alcohol, or intellectual problems readily agreeing to be studied. Many such individuals have concerns about the state of their brain, find the study a welcome change in their otherwise boring lives, and value the small payment. By such unintentional mechanisms the recruited population could become skewed away from a truly representative sample.

We have turned away from the "large random sample" approach toward a more practical one. Rather than attempt to establish a "representative" subsample of the entire population (for the reasons given above), we have instead turned to a "benchmark" approach. The benchmark is based upon medical health. One recruits subjects from as wide a population base as practical and then carefully screens each subject for "health". Our experience has been that the tighter one's exclusionary criteria, the more stable the population. The goal is to choose subjects who are as "healthy as we ourselves would like to be". All our adult subjects are seen by an internist, a neurologist, and a psychologist. Subjects are excluded if their histories or examinations show evidence of any of the following:

Diabetes	Genetic abnormality	Abnormal vision
Drug abuse	Clinical depression	Recognized learning
Encephalitis	Hypertension	disability
Myocardial infarction	Severe head injury	Psychiatric hospitalization
Severe headaches	Coma	
Cancer	Stroke	Schizophrenia
Abnormal audition	Abnormal pulmonary	(thought disorder)
Mental retardation	function	Alcoholism
	Abnormal hepatic	Meningitis
	function	Epilepsy

Moreover, all subjects must be drug-free (recreational and therapeutic) at time of study for at least 24 h. They must not have used alcohol, sleep inducers, or antihistamines and must not be taking chronic medications, e.g., tranquilizers. All subjects must have classically normal medical, neurological, and psychological screening examinations. Should the medical or neurological review of systems be positive, subjects are excluded if the demarcated items suggest central nervous system involvement.

We commonly approach organizations (e.g., unions, veterans' organizations, fraternal orders, companies) for permission to approach their members and perform initial screening via telephone. Placing advertisements in a local newspaper is usually less productive, since experience has shown that the proportion of non-acceptable subjects rises. Subjects who pass this initial screening come for a half a day of further screening examination. For those who pass these hurdles, the final decision is taken by the EEG technician at the time of study, often several days later. Several subjects have confided to the technician how they "fooled the doctors" and concealed crucial historical details!

As expected, the ratio of subjects accepted to those recruited drops among older individuals, reflecting the higher ambient disease level in those groups. Thus, far fewer subjects in their 70s and 80s fulfill our criteria than in their 20s and 30s. Such a population of "optimally healthy" subjects has been termed "super controls." It is certainly true that optimally healthy 70-year-old subjects are not representative of the "norm." However, such a healthy population establishes a reliable benchmark against which comparisons can be made.

It has been suggested that our criteria are too strict and should be "loosened." The problem with this is the decision of what to loosen. What may happen is that what gets loosened could be a function of the characteristics of the local population source. One center may wish to include patients with asymptomatic hypertension, another those with a history of alcoholism, another depression, etc. Not only would such loosening increase the group SD (or covariance) and thereby reduce sensitivity, but these groups would not be comparable among centers and might be difficult to reproduce.

Until such time as large, truly representative populations can be gathered and studied, we argue for optimal health as the best benchmark population criterion. As a corollary to this, there is no substitute for the careful examination of every subject that enters a normative data base. It should not be necessary to say that subjects should *not* be excluded for apparent abnormalities in their neurophysiologic data – unless caused by technical flaws or artifact. To do so would be to form a group based upon one's *a priori* concept of neurophysiologic normality. Screening neurophysiologic data is no substitute for screening subjects *prior* to gathering data. In our experience, there are a surprising number of truly normal subjects with technically perfect data who demonstrate unusual asymmetries. It is important to include such subjects to ensure a proper estimate of normal variability. Failure to do so results in an excessively small range of variation and the potential detection of abnormality in normal subjects.

Detection of Abnormality: General Approaches

There appear to be three approaches to the detection of abnormality from electrotopographic data.

The first involves the unaided visual inspection of maps derived from EP or spectral analyzed EEG data. This approach is a natural extension of classic electroencephalography where the analytic power of the human visual system has proven itself of value. Its major disadvantage derives from the limitations of human vision. Some asymmetry or other topographic irregularity is often seen in normals. In our experience, it may be very difficult to tell by inspection alone when an individual topographic aberration falls out of normal bounds, i.e., becomes "abnormal." It is not uncommon for clinicians to be falsely lured to regions highlighted by a dramatic color transition. Bad experience with this is no doubt a reason behind the widespread chromophobia often expressed at meetings on mapping.

The second approach involves the use of SPM, which produces a map of "abnormality" in units of SD from normal. In our experience, this otherwise helpful tool may be subject to misuse and misinterpretation if slavishly used in an uncritical manner. The basic problem is that the clinician must remain responsible for deciding when a statistical abnormality becomes a clinical abnormality. There are four basic causes of statistical abnormality that should be ignored:

1. Artifact (blink, muscle)
2. State change (drowsiness)
3. Random chance
4. Inadequate data base

The ability to recognize such confounding effects requires training and often the ability of a good detective. Reaching false conclusions by the uncritical use of SPM appears, in our experience, a primary cause of mistrust of topographic mapping in clinical neurology and psychiatry, of calls for better control of data base formations, of calls for more conservative statistical measures, and of pleas for caution. We shall address these issues below.

The third approach, although primarily quantitative, relies much less on the topographic map per se than it does upon the extraction of numerical measures from EEG and EP data. Its intent is to obviate the need for expert clinical interpretation. On the basis of prior studies, diagnostic rules are set up to place a patient into one of two differing diagnostic categories. The process is based upon measures extracted from neurophysiologic data and employs a previously defined discriminant function to perform the automated classification. This is clearly the ultimate use of neurophysiologic data for clinical diagnoses. Inherently this approach relies upon the excellence of the original two-group comparison. Success is very much a function of the expertise frozen in the final discriminant function.

Resistance to this automated approach comes from those who feel uncomfortable relying totally upon the expertise of others. To some degree, the resistance may be emotional, as it is for chromophobia. On the other hand, real issues remain. For example, a discriminant function will classify any subject into one of the only two outcomes it has available. A patient with a stroke will be classified as "depressed" or "demented" if presented to the "depression vs dementia" discriminant function whether or not the patient is actually depressed or demented. Thus, although the clinician is removed from the actual details of the classification process, he or she must be very much involved in selection of an appropriate discriminant function, i.e., in the appropriateness of a given discriminant function to a given patient. To make this decision, not only must the clinician know the patient, he or she must be confident in the knowledge of the detailed makeup of the original groups used to form the discriminant function.

The major drawback to this approach is that there are virtually an infinite number of clinical dichotomies, but a limited number of proven discriminant functions. Time and effort will ultimately reveal the practical value of this promising approach.

Detection of Abnormality: Our Philosophy and Approach

A cornerstone of our approach is the belief that neurophysiologic data are not "diagnostic", but may provide important information to aid in the formation of a diagnosis. It is the clinician who makes the diagnosis, not the machine. This is a generalization of the well-known statement that the EEG does not diagnose epilepsy, but may confirm or extend the clinician's presumptive diagnosis.

As the clinician reads an EEG, he or she searches for important features, e.g., spikes, focal slowing, generalized slowing, hemispheric asymmetry. The presence or absence of such findings are folded into the patient's history, to make a diagnosis. Our approach is to make such abnormal features more visually obvious by topographic mapping and to facilitate their detection in the face of normal variation by SPM. This process is extended to long-latency EP as well as EEG data. Once again, it is the clinician who must make "diagnostic" use of such data. The value of this quantified topographic approach is in its augmented sensitivity to abnormality. But as previously indicated, the heightened sensitivity applies to artifact as well, and the multiple statistical assessments raise the issue of capitalization on chance findings.

Real VS Chance Findings. The typical clinical study in our laboratory generates data from EEG separately in the "eyes open" and "eyes closed" awake states and from EP separately to flash and click. This results in a large amount of data. The spectrally analyzed EEG data from 20 channels, in two states, and over six spectral bands produce 240 variables ($20 \times 2 \times 6$). The EP data from 20 channels, for two modalities, and over 11 40-ms latency ranges produce 440 variables ($20 \times 2 \times 11$). Thus, each clinical study produces 680 variables ($240 + 440$). For an n of 680, it is virtually certain that at least one variable will appear significant by chance alone (Maus and Endresen 1979). Indeed, at the 0.05 probability level, 19–35 variables, and at the 0.01 level 2–10 variables are to be expected to reach significance by chance alone! How is one to discriminate "real" from "chance?" That this problem is not unique to topographic mapping is illustrated by applying the same scenario to classic EEG reading. Given a 20-min 16-channel recording, if we assume that the EEG reader can estimate spectral content in four spectral bands every 4s, then 19 200 variables are produced [(20 × 60)/4 × 16 × 4]. Clearly, EEG is of established clinical value, so this statistical quandary must be in some way manageable.

It is also clear that there is no way, on the basis of a single set of comparisons, of determining with certainty which variables achieve significance by chance and which reflect "real" difference. Maus and Endreson (1979) suggest the use of a limited number of variables and adjustment of significance levels upward as a function of the number of variables. Based upon the binomial theorem for a 10% level of significance for all tests combined and 680 variables, one would have to demand a significance level of 0.00016: $p = 1. - (0.9)**(11/680)$. However, reduction of variables would presuppose knowledge of those which could be omitted. Setting the detection level at the $p < 0.00016$ level would be equally undesirable, as few variables would be likely to reach that level. Should one wish to retain a criterion level at $p < 0.05$, then one would have to limit oneself to at most two variables; for $p < 0.01$, 10 variables. On the surface, it would seem to be an unsolvable problem.

However, a moment's reflection reveals a solution. The hallmark of chance results is randomness and of real results, reproducibility. Accordingly, a repetitive study should show the same results if they are real and differing results if they are due to random chance. Clearly this is what an electroencephalographer does when reading an EEG. Every few pages, he or she forms an "opinion" and matches it against the next few pages. Eventually, changes that are random chance stand out against patterns that remain constant and are presumed to be real. This same technique applies to the use of SPM. One searches for spatial patterns that are constant across state, involve more than one electrode, and reach high levels of significance. Conversely, scattered spatial patterns of low significance involving only a single electrode are ignored. If the reader is in doubt, testing of a given state or all states can be repeated.

These overall statistical issues are part of a branch of statistics known as exploratory data analyses, or EDA. In his excellent text, Tukey (1977) advises on the use of separate exploratory (first-step) analyses to develop hypotheses and confirmatory (second-step) analyses to test these hypotheses. It is a demanding task to repeat analyses, but the only way to be sure.

Non-Normal Distributions. A second statistical issue concerns the observation that many neurophysiologic variables are non-normal (not Gaussian) in their distribution. Parametric statistics, such as the Student's *t* test or the Z transformation, assume a normal distribution. Thus, the finding of non-normal distributions raises questions concerning the appropriateness of such parametric tests. The most common solution for spectral analyzed EEG data is to recast spectral energy as relative or percentage energy. These recast values are then mathematically transformed to improve Gaussianity. Although this approach has proven successful in certain laboratories, it has failed in others (Coben et al. 1985; John et al. 1977). John et al. (1977) report restoration of Gaussianity by the ln x(l-x) transformation. Coben et al. (1985) failed to make EEG spectral distributions more Gaussian by the ln x(l-x), square root, or arc sine corrections.

The use of relative (percent) rather than absolute spectral values raises an additional complication, namely, the lack of operational independence between resulting values. For example, absolute theta is an independent variable; percent theta however, is a function of, hence dependent upon, not only theta but all other frequencies as well. Thus, a real increase in alpha produces not only an increase in percent alpha, but also a decrease in the percentage of all other frequencies. It is clear that the final word regarding correction for non-normal distributions remains to be spoken. Until then, one can take heart from the statement in Steger's well-known text (1971, p. 42) that the t test "... has the advantage of having been demonstrated empirically to be relatively robust in the face of violations of the assumptions of normality and equality of variances."

Issues of Artifact

In our experience, the most common errors in the clinical interpretation of topographic mapping studies stem from misreading of artifact. Just as mapping makes the underlying spatial structure of neurophysiologic data more visible, so it enhances the visibility of artifact. Just as SPM highlights brain-generated deviations from normal, so it delineates artifact. Indeed, artifact may produce some of the largest Z values, as will be shown.

The subject of artifact is so important that it warrants a review of techniques used in its management. The first step is to eliminate it at the source. In our experience, electrode artifact is prevented by secure attachment of the electrodes with collodion, impedance reduction to below 5 kΩ by skin abrasion, and frequent impedance checks to pick up early signs of failure. To reduce muscle artifact, subjects should be seated in a reclining chair designed so as to support the head, neck, and trunk comfortably, thereby reducing the need to maintain postural tonus. Eye blink and eye movement are especially troublesome. During collection of "eyes open" EEG, subjects are asked to fixate on a target and suppress blinks. Every so often, as requested by either the subject or the technician, the subject blinks frequently on command (a "blink holiday") and then continues blink suppression. Eye movement and blink can thereby be managed in all but the most difficult patient. During eye closure, however, many subjects continue to blink and others develop a low-amplitude vertical nystagmus, especially when fully alert; characteristically subjects are totally unaware of such movements. Through closed lids, of course, fixation targets are of no value. We have found that the placement of thin gauze pads lightly over the closed lids may reduce or eliminate these phenomena. Presumably flicking of the eyelashes against the gauze provides sufficient feedback for subjects to become aware of and partially suppress such movements. Ironically, it is often harder to control eye movements in the eyes closed than in the eyes open state.

The appropriate control of a subject's state is crucial. A considerable effort is made by the technologist to ensure the fully alert state throughout all study conditions, EEG and EP alike. To do this, the technologist relies upon frequent breaks, subject interrogation, and EEG monitoring. At the first sign of drowsiness, the subject is alerted, if necessary walked up and down the hall, and, as a last resort, given coffee or tea. Patients who seem exceptionally fatigued

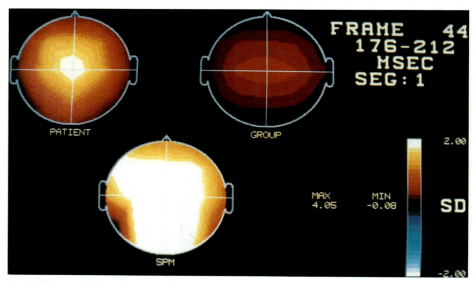

Fig. 3. Effects of drowsiness on the AER. Three BEAM images are shown. For each image, the head is seen as a schematic outline in vertex view. The nose is above, left ear to the left, right ear to the right, and occiput below. The three head outlines represent: *upper left*, data from the subject; *upper right*, data from an age-appropriate control group; *below*, the significance probability map (SPM). Data in this figure are from a 31-year-old male referred with the clinical diagnosis "atypical depression, rule out temporal lobe epilepsy." Data shown span the time epoch 176–216 ms, a full 40 ms. Note that the patient shows a prominent central positive vertex wave which is not as well developed in the group. Inspections of underlying waveforms (not shown) or visualization of cartoon images of the basic AER maps both demonstrate that the patient's EP has delayed positive vertex waves. This is statistically manifest in the lower SPM, where the deviation from normal reaches 4.05 SD by the Z transformation. All the regions shown in *white* are above 2 SD from normal. The *color key* for the SPM is shown to the right. The patient's EEG data demonstrated drowsiness during the period that the stimuli were delivered to form the AER. Excessive delayed symmetrical vertex wave abnormalities are characteristic of state change, such as drowsiness. Vertex wave abnormalities in general are seen in drowsiness, as a result of medications, or as a sign of diffuse encephalopathy. This example illustrates a major statistical abnormality. It is not, however, of clinical significance

are allowed to sleep for up to 30 min. This, plus ambulation and coffee, perk up all but the most somnolent patient. State control is crucial during EP as well as EEG states. It is usual for the repetitive stimulation involved in EP generation to induce drowsiness, so great care must be taken and stimulation stopped when signs of sleepiness are seen.

The appropriate placement of additional electrodes so that they are maximally sensitive to artifact is important for several reasons. First, they allow for on-line, real-time monitoring by the technician at time of recording. Second, when the raw EEG is visually inspected off-line, these electrodes allow more accurate identification of artifact to aid in its elimination prior to subsequent spectral analyses – a process we have termed "deglitching." Third, it is often useful to include the artifact electrodes as part of the topographic display. Activity of artifactual origin will most often be of highest amplitude and thereby

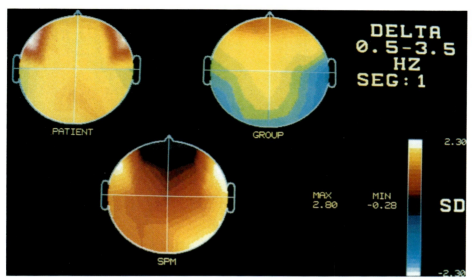

Fig. 4. Effects of horizontal eye-movement. Three BEAM images in the same format as for Fig. 3. In this case, spectrally analyzed EEG delta activity from 0.5 to 3.5 Hz is shown. Data are derived from a 33-year-old female with the diagnosis of uncomplicated depression. Note the prominent bilateral anterior temporal augmentation of delta activity which reaches significance (see SPM below) by a maximum of 2.80 SD. Visual inspection of the eye movement channels of the standard polygraph demonstrates that this apparent anterior temporal slow activity results from uncontrollable horizontal eye movement. This figure illustrates the classic topographic distribution of horizontal eye movement, which could be recognized in the background EEG by its characteristic pattern

most visible in these electrodes. Fourth, the statistical comparisons may also be carried forward on these electrodes. Intergroup or subject vs group difference reaching greater significance in these electrodes than in adjacent scalp electrodes signifies the presence of extracerebral artifact and renders invalid otherwise apparently significant differences seen over the adjacent scalp regions.

Even without extra electrodes, topographic displays make artifact more readily apparent than inspection of polygraphic tracings. For example, Fig. 3 shows a large centrally placed positive vertex wave abnormality during an AER reaching a maximum of over 5 SD from the age-matched normative control group in a patient with "atypical depression." The majority of electrodes are more than 2 SD from normal, and the SPM summarizes a full 40-ms epoch. Thus, this is statistically a very significant finding. Clinically, however it is within normal limits, for this subject was exceptionally drowsy during the AER and could not be maintained in the alert state. Delayed EP vertex activity is commonly associated with drowsiness, medications, and diffuse encephalopathy. Because each clinical study includes the initial standard interpretation of the extensive EEG tracing produced during all states, the neurophysiologist responsible for interpreting the data was aware of the drowsiness and correctly interpreted this statistically significant but clinically trivial finding.

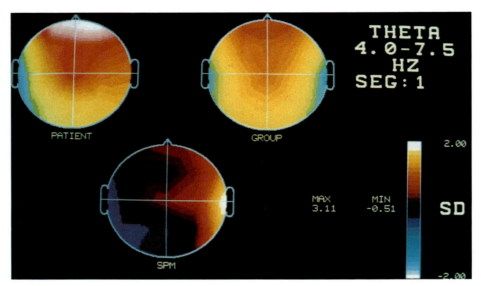

Fig. 5. Topographic artifact of lateralized EKG. Three BEAM images in the same format as Fig. 3. Spectrally analyzed EEG theta is displayed in a 32-year-old male with a history of panic attacks. Note the large augmentation of theta in the right temporal region, reaching a maxima in the right midtemporal focus of 3.11 SD. Ordinarily, this would be interpreted as an indication of organic pathology in the right temporal lobe. However, the EEG taken during this study demonstrated high-voltage EKG artifact, most marked over the right hemisphere in the temporal region. Accordingly, the temporal lobe abnormality seen in the SPM was interpreted as an artifact of uncontrolled EKG contamination. It is unusual to see EKG greater over the right hemisphere, but this is occasionally observed

Figure 4 shows large bilateral anterior temporal deviations from normal for the EEG delta range (2.80 SD) in a patient referred with the diagnosis of "depression, rule out temporal lobe epilepsy." Once again, the neurophysiologist correctly identified these findings as characteristic of horizontal eye movement artifact on the basis of the specific topographic characteristics of the "abnormality" and on the basis of the accompanying EEG tracing, where the artifact channels showed evidence of uncontrolled horizontal eye movement.

Figure 5 shows an extensive right midtemporal abnormality (3.11 SD of EEG theta, in a patient referred for elucidation of recurrent panic attacks. Once again, the EEG tracing demonstrated the presence of unreducible EKG artifact, unusually greatest over the right hemicranium, maximal in the right midtemporal region. On this basis, the neurophysiologist correctly interpreted this otherwise potentially interesting finding as probable artifact.

Figure 6 shows an unusually prominent left central positivity at 36 ms of the AER in a patient with clinical depression. Although it involves only one electrode, the Z score was extremely high (9.96 SD), warranting an explanation. During AER recording, the EEG record demonstrated high-voltage muscle activity in the left temporal area, which the technologist had been unable to reduce despite much effort. The left central EP waveform showed a "spike"

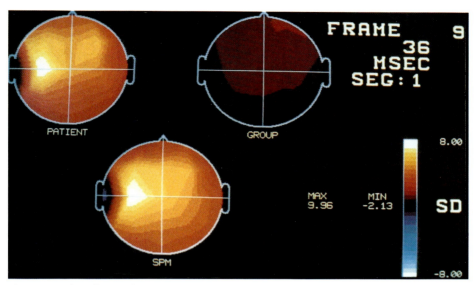

Fig. 6. Muscle spike artifact in the AER. Three BEAM images in the same format as for Fig. 3. The AER activity at 36 ms is illustrated for a 51-year-old woman with a history of bipolar depression. Notice the prominent left central positivity. Notice the dramatic abnormality in SPM consisting of augmented left central positive activity, by 9.96 SD, and the concurrent negative abnormality in the left midtemporal region of just 2.13 SD. Examination of the underlying EEG demonstrated dramatically asymmetrical background muscle artifact which could not be removed despite many attempts. Inspection of the left central AER tracing (not shown) demonstrated a spike of activity at approximately 35–40 ms. The topographic display shown above is characteristic for the muscle microreflex, reported by Bickford, seen following auditory or other stimulation in the face of augmented muscle tension

at 36 ms. This finding, therefore, represents a time-locked myogenic artifact of the sort originally reported in the 1960s (Bickford 1968; Bickford et al. 1964a, b; Cody et al. 1964).

Figure 7 demonstrates an asymmetrically increased negativity primarily in the right occipital region for a 40-ms epoch of the late AER that reaches 3.83 SD and involves at least four electrodes. The referring diagnosis was bipolar depression. Although statistically significant, the EEG record revealed markedly asymmetrical alpha, greater on the right. The right occipital AER waveform revealed a striking time-locked alpha component that was not seen on the left. On the basis of these data, the neurophysiologist correctly presumed this statistically prominent finding to be an artifact of asymmetrical time-locked alpha seen in this patient and of no more clinical significance than the alpha asymmetry. Time-locked alpha often contaminates the late portions of long-latency EPs when subjects are drowsy or fatigued.

Other forms of artifact often have characteristic spatial signatures. For example, vertical eye movement or eye blink produces a crescent-shaped abnormality primarily in the prefrontal regions for EEG delta and for the late flash visual evoked response (VER) if time-locked. A bad electrode stands out as a dramatic isolated geometric shape in both spectral and EP maps. This is analogous to

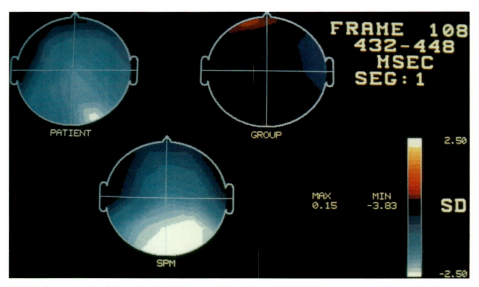

Fig. 7. Asymmetrical time-locked alpha artifact. Three BEAM images according to the format of Fig. 3. Data are illustrated for 40 ms of the AER beginning at 432 ms for a 56-year-old woman with bipolar depression. Notice the asymmetrical augmented negativity in the right occipital region and the slightly broader regional abnormality by SPM, reaching 3.83 SD from normal. Inspection of the background EEG revealed high-voltage asymmetrical alpha, much greater on the right, during auditory stimulation. Inspection of the posterior AER tracings revealed alpha time-locking, also much more prominent on the right. The statistical abnormality demonstrated above is interpreted as representing asymmetrical time-locked alpha, a normal phenomenon seen in drowsiness, but usually more symmetrical. The significance of this abnormality in the AER is no more than the significance of the underlying alpha asymmetry in the waking background record. Ordinarily, time-locked alpha is most common during visual stimulation, but more rarely is seen in response to auditory stimulation. In its usual form, positive and negative deviations from normal are seen occipitally, with a period of approximately 100 ms

the statement that electrode artifacts in EEG have "no field." Temporal muscle artifact often produces apparent augmentation of beta activity. The distribution is characteristically maximal and often limited to the midtemporal electrode. The degree of abnormality produced by muscle in the SPM generally increases with increasing frequency, consistent with the very high frequency content of the electromyograph (EMG).

To assist in evaluation of EP data, we always analyze a time epoch in advance of stimulation of at least 512 ms. This crucial prestimulus epoch serves three purposes: First, it allows for an estimation of the adequacy of signal averaging. It should appear as a horizontal straight line. If it shows a signal, then the amplitude of this signal is an error signal affecting the post-stimulus EP. Any apparent change of post-stimulus EP that is within the level of the prestimulus noise base must be considered artifact. It is also not uncommon to find more prestimulus noise in EPs from electrodes overlying regions of pathology. Only by reviewing this epoch can one be sure that post-stimulus EP changes are not due to background noise. Second, the prestimulus epoch forms a basis for calculating the baseline or DC zero voltage reference point. In our experience, the typical 50-ms epoch used for this purpose by many laboratories is inadequate if the prestimulus epoch contains any residual noise at all. Third, inspection of the prestimulus epoch allows one to detect the presence of time-locked artifact. Most often this is of two types – time-locked anticipatory eye blink and unintentional anticipatory event-related potentials (ERPs) such as the contingent negative variable (CNV). With AC-coupled amplifiers, the return from the negative CNV to baseline may produce an apparent positive deflection just before or at time of stimulation. This can seriously distort one's DC baseline estimate if not recognized.

Role of Group Comparison Studies

It is, unfortunately, no rare experience to learn of a study showing "significant group difference" between normals and a particular disease entity (disease X), only to find the results of no practical value in the "diagnosis of individual subjects" with disease X. There are two major reasons for this all too common disappointment. The first explanation stems from the fact that group difference concentrates on the separation between the multivariate mean (centroids) of the two groups. "Diagnosis", however, depends upon the actual distribution of subjects in the two groups, especially the presence or absence of population overlap. Although centroid separation and population overlap are clearly related, it is certainly possible with real data to have a significant group centroid difference, but with non-trivial population overlap. The second explanation stems from the fact that although a discriminant function may indeed separate patients with disease X from normals it may also classify patients with hypothetical diseases Y and Z as having disease X. These are issues of sensitivity (ability to discriminate disease X from normality) and specificity (ability to separate disease X from Y from Z) (Ransohoff and Feinstein 1978).

Among our research publications are papers showing topographic difference between normals and patients with dyslexia (Duffy et al. 1980; Duffy and McAnulty 1985), schizophrenia (Morihisa et al. 1983; Morstyn et al. 1983a, b), Alzheimer's disease (Duffy et al. 1984a), and poorer functioning newborn infants (Duffy and Als 1983). These studies were intended to advance our understanding of the basic neurophysiology of these important clinical problems. These studies were not intended to establish "diagnostic" criteria and not intended to demonstrate that one can "diagnose" these disease conditions with brain electrical activity mapping (BEAM) data. Although our findings may speak for the sensitivity of neurophysiologic data in recognizing these disease entities, they were not designed to say anything about diagnostic specificity. To develop useful discriminant functions to diagnose dyslexia, for example, one would need separate classifiers of children with all other forms of learning disability alone and in combination. It would take many, many person-years of work and major financial outlay to carry this out. Moreover, even if successful, it would not be obvious that neurophysiologic classifiers were any better than more common neuropsychologially based classifiers. Accordingly, our research efforts have been organized more to provide basic information about disease processes than to provide information of immediate value to the process of automated classification.

Clinical Usefulness of BEAM

Introduction

So if BEAM studies are not intended to be "diagnostic," of what clinical value are they? As per our previous discussion, the goal is not to diagnose, but to provide important pieces of information useful in establishing a diagnosis. As a simple example, take the case of a patient referred for BEAM study with the diagnosis of headache who already has a normal anatomical study (CT scan, magnetic resonance imaging). The referring clinician expects and certainly hopes for a normal result. However, should there prove to be, for example, evidence of diffuse slowing – a sign of possible encephalopathy – then the clinician would have new and important information requiring a fuller diagnostic evaluation. In our experience, the advantage of our quantified topographic approach to neurophysiologic evaluation over standard EEG lies in increased sensitivity and increased objectivity (SPM). These points are best illustrated by the following brief case studies.

Examples

School Problems, Age 11. An 11-year-old boy was referred from a local school system for evaluation of poor academic performance. The school's educational psychologist felt the boy had poor organization skills and speculated that his problem resided in poor function of the right hemisphere, especially the right frontal lobe. In our laboratory at The Children's Hospital, the neuropsychologist's evaluation resulted in a different conclusion. She felt that his right hemispheric performance was normal (good block design and figure copy), but he had language difficulties (6 year level on the Boston Naming Test and poor syntactic comprehension) and an attentional problem (poor arithmetic ability, digit span, and coding). She postulated a left temporal – left frontal deficit. Unfortunately, the resulting disagreement brought the boy's educational program to a halt pending resolution. A BEAM study was performed, the results of which are shown in Fig. 8. In Fig. 8A, the asymmetry of theta greater on the left (or reduced on the right) in the frontal regions. In Fig. 8B, the SPM shows clear augmentation of left frontal and left temporal theta by a maximum of 4.39 SD. This finding established the credibility of the hospital neuropsychologist's report, and the appropriate support for the boy's attentional and language problems were provided. Although BEAM studies are not often necessary in the management of learning disabilities, for selected cases they may be most helpful.

Topographic Mapping of Brain Electrical Activity: Clinical Applications and Issues

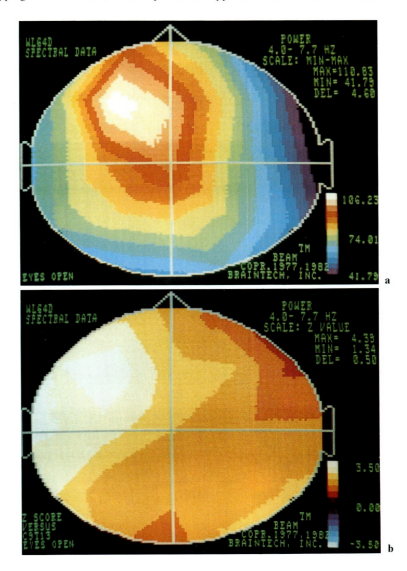

Fig. 8a, b. Two topographic maps of brain electrical activity constructed on a different machine than illustrated in Fig. 3. The display convention is nonetheless similar. The data illustrated are derived from an 11-year-old male with a history of school problems. A conflict arose in the course of his evaluation, with one psychologist feeling that the boy's difficulty derived from abnormalities in the right hemisphere, especially in the frontal area. Another psychologist believed the boy's difficulties arose from language and attentional problems involving the left frontal and temporal region. **a** The BEAM study demonstrated an asymmetry of theta activity, greatest in the left frontal region. **b** The corresponding SPM demonstrated augmented theta activity, more over the left hemisphere, by a maximum of 4.39 SD greatest in the left frontal and midtemporal regions. These data were taken as evidence to support the contention of left frontal and temporal lobe abnormalities

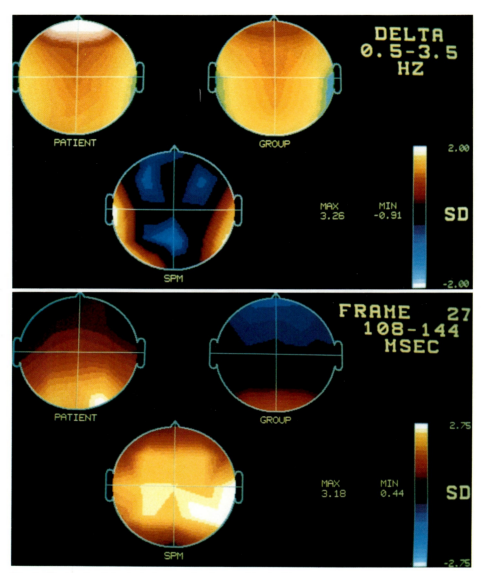

Fig. 9. Electrophysiological abnormality in psychiatric illness. Data are in the format of Figure 3. The patient is a 42-year-old female health professional with a history of severe depression nonreactive to standard pharmacotherapy. BEAM data demonstrated surprising augmentation of bilateral temporal theta activity, by a maximum of 3.26 SD. Furthermore, the VER demonstrated augmented right posterior temporal and right parietal positive activity over 40 ms, beginning at 108 ms, that reached 3.18 SD from normal. Subsequent neurological examination revealed a mild left hemisparesis and extracted a history that had not previously been disclosed of a suicide attempt resulting in head injury and prolonged coma. The patient responded well to medications more appropriate for organic depression than for uncomplicated, endogenous depression

Unexpected Pathology in a Depressed Patient, Age 42. A 42-year-old female health professional was referred for a BEAM study for evaluation of chronic depression. Results of her study are shown in Fig. 9. Note the markedly increased bitemporal theta, reaching 3.26 SD from normal. Note, also that the VER showed an abnormal augmentation of right posterior temporal and right parietal positive activity by 3.18 SD. Although right posterior abnormalities are occasionally noted in uncomplicated depression, such prominent abnormalities as shown here are out of the ordinary. As a result of the study, a neurological consultation was obtained. Examination revealed mild but definite increases in left-sided reflexes, with a left Babinski response. Historical questioning revealed a past history of alcoholism and suicide attempts, none of which had been previously disclosed. One suicide attempt had resulted in a severe head injury with coma for over 24 h. The neurologist presumed that the mild left hemiparesis and electrophysiological abnormalities stemmed from the head injury. Mild ventricular enlargement was noted by CT scan, slightly more prominent in the right temporal lobe. The psychiatrist switched his therapeutic approach from common mood-elevating drugs to those believed to be more effective in organically based depression, with considerable improvement in patient response.

This study illustrates how BEAM may find unexpected evidence of neurologic disease in psychiatric patients.

Personality of Temporal Lobe Epilepsy Syndrome, Age 29. A 29-year-old female was referred for BEAM evaluation of "chronic ruminative syndrome" unresponsive to medication. Her classic EEG was read as "borderline normal due to possible slowing in excess for normal." No seizure discharges were seen. Results of her first BEAM study are shown in Fig. 10A, B. Note the globally increased theta, with the entire head more than 2.97 SD above normal but with an accentuation in the right posterior quadrant (8.23 SD) involving the mid- and right parietal regions and the right posterior temporal region (Fig. 10A). The findings were similar for eyes open and eyes closed. Note the same region highlighted as abnormal (3.41 SD) for the 40-ms VER epoch starting at 172 ms (Fig. 10B). There were eight additional abnormal EP epochs. The classic neurological examination was normal, as was a CT scan. However, the patient presented with an unusual personality profile. She kept a diary, actually bringing it in to report to her neurologist on her thoughts about her obsessional concerns. She reported extreme moral concerns, a history of alternating hypo- and hypersexuality, and periods of religious pre-occupation. She was very verbal and would persist in one topic once she started talking ("stickiness"). In short, she presented with the classic picture of the personality of temporal lobe epilepsy (Bear 1979; Bear and Fedio 1977). However, she denied a history of seizures. Upon detailed questioning, however, she admitted "fainting" three times as a teenager. Each time, she felt a strange feeling in her back and stomach that moved up to her mouth. She recalled being very much afraid, being unable to communicate, and then "fainting." On the basis of the prominent BEAM findings and probable past history of partial complex seizures, it was decided to start her on carbamazepine.

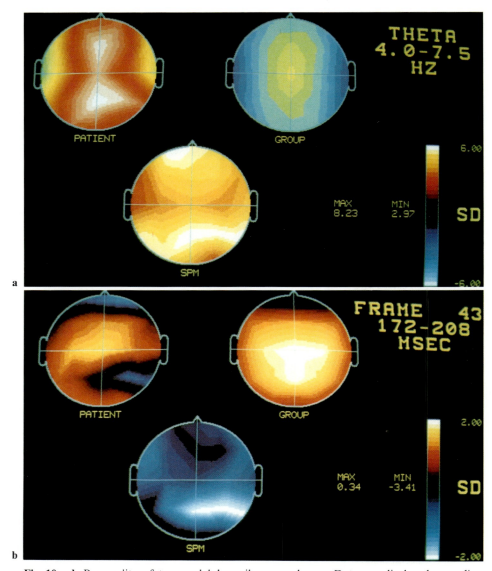

Fig. 10a–d. Personality of temporal lobe epilepsy syndrome. Data are displayed according to the convention of Figure 3. The patient is a 29-year-old female referred for BEAM with a complaint of chronic ruminative condition. **a** Theta activity was augmented globally by a minimum of 2.97 SD. **b** This augmentation reached a maximum of 8.23 SD in the right parietal and posterior temporal regions. This region is also implicated by the VER study, where differences were seen during the 172–208 ms epoch of −3.41 SD. Eight additional regions of abnormality were demonstrated in the evoked responses (not shown). On the basis of these unexpected abnormalities, this patient was referred for neurological evaluation, which revealed a behavioral disorder characteristic of personality of temporal lobe epilepsy syndrome. However, the patient denied epilepsy. Only by detailed and persistent questioning was a history

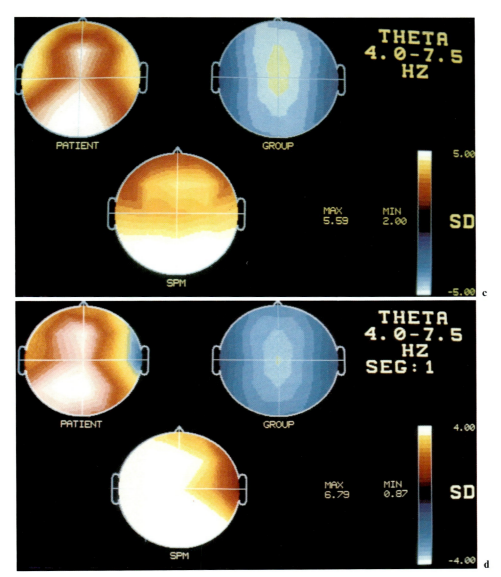

suggestive of seizures in the teenage years finally elicited. Were it not for the BEAM study, these historical details would not have been obtained. The patient was placed on carbamazepine, with improvement clinically and in the 6-month follow-up BEAM data (c). Here, theta is still abnormal, but by a lesser amount (5.59 SD). Six months later, due to continuing improvement, the patient discontinued medications. An additional 6 months later, she returned for a follow-up BEAM, which showed for the first time discharges in the left temporal lobe on classic EEG (not shown) and a differing pattern of theta augmentation now involving left temporal lobe, by 6.79 SD (d). The patient reported the clinical return of probable partial complex seizures. Restarting of carbamazepine rapidly improved the patient's clinical status

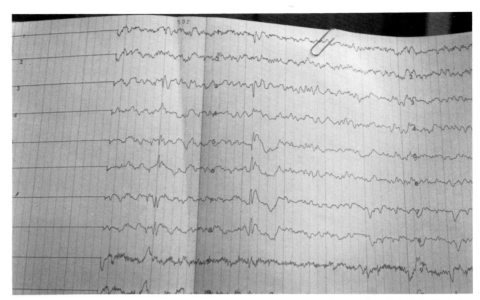

Fig. 11. The EEG of a 7-year-old boy with clinical history of attentional deficit disorder and generalized seizures beginning with left body phenomena. The EEG shown is the parasagittal monopolar montage referenced to a face electrode. From top to bottom, the illustrated channels are F4, F3, C4, C3, P4, P3, O2, O1, FP2, FP1. Note the obvious bilateral occipital spike wave discharge. Note, also, the accompanying positive discharge from the right central electrode. Topographic distributions of this discharge are seen in Fig. 12

Six months later, she was reevaluated. The classic EEG report was unchanged. By spectral analysis (Fig. 10C), theta was still increased by SPM, but somewhat less than before, now by 5.39 SD. Only one EP abnormality was noted. She was clinically much improved. Heretofore, she had been supported by her family, only being able to work as a part-time secretary despite the fact that she had graduated at the top of her class at a quality local university. Now she had started her own acting workshop, had pupils working for her, had decided to discontinue family support and no longer had time for her

Fig. 12a–p. Spike topography. Sixteen BEAM images in the format of Fig. 3. In each case, however, the maps displayed are the topographic distribution of unanalyzed EEG activity from the 7-year-old patient described in the text and in the legend of Fig. 11. Furthermore, the location of the underlying electrodes is illustrated in each image by small circles. **a** The topographic distribution of resting background activity 8 ms prior to the start of the discharge shown in Fig. 11. **b–p.** The changing topographic distribution of positive (*red*) and negative (*blue*) activities every 4 ms for a total of 56 ms. Note the obvious onset, as described in the text, of a horizontal dipole, with the occipital region negative and the right central region positive. There is apparent dipole "rotation," with the negative end becoming vertical and appearing prominently at the surface. Continued rotation essentially reverses the dipole polarity, with the occipital region eventually becoming positive and the right central region negative. This figure represents the power of BEAM in the microdissection of the topographic distribution of left epileptic spikes. The clinical utility of such displays has yet to be fully determined

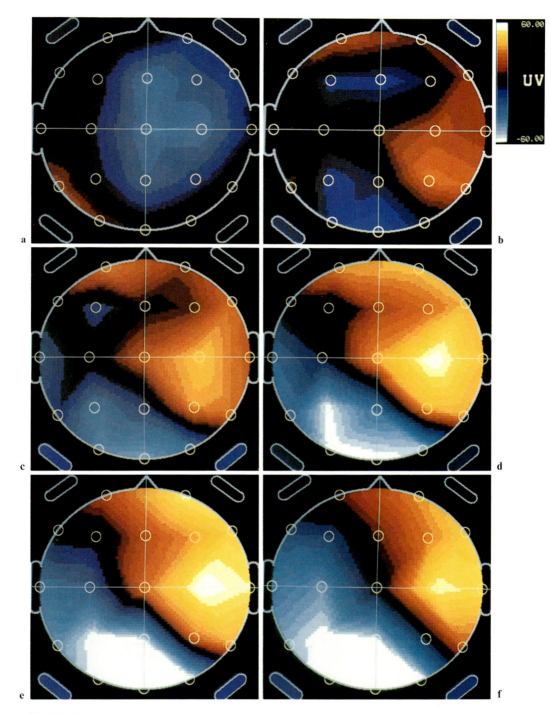

Fig. 12a–f

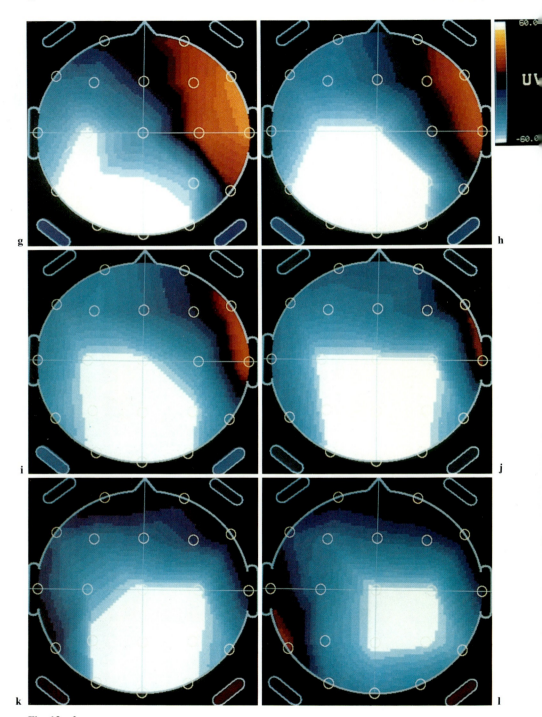

Fig. 12g–l

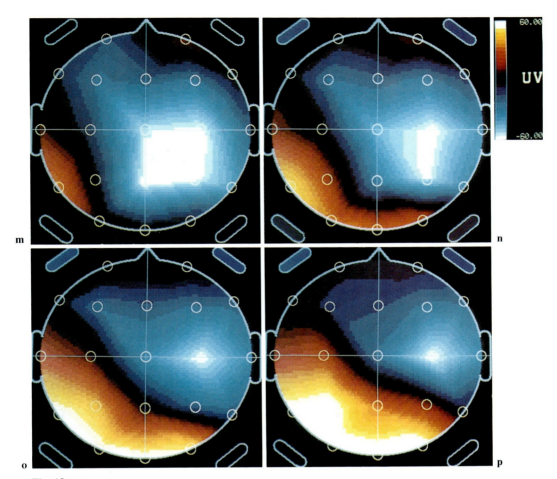

Fig. 12 m–p

diary. She did very well. In fact, she felt so well she cancelled her follow-up appointment scheduled for six months later.

After an additional 6 months, she called for a return appointment and evaluation. This time, her EEG was distinctly abnormal, showing, for the first time, clear left temporal discharges. Her BEAM data revealed increased theta slowing by 6.79 SD, involving the left hemisphere – especially the left temporal lobe – more extensively than before (Fig. 10 D). She had begun her diary again. She reported that 3 months before, she had discontinued her carbamazepine. She felt so well, she felt the medications were no longer necessary. Subsequently, things "didn't go well." In fact, 2 months later she had two "fainting spells" of the sort she had not had since her teenage years. She was restarted on carbamazepine, with restoration of her well-being.

This study demonstrates, once again, the ability of BEAM data to suggest alternative diagnoses and therapies in patients with behavioral dysfunction.

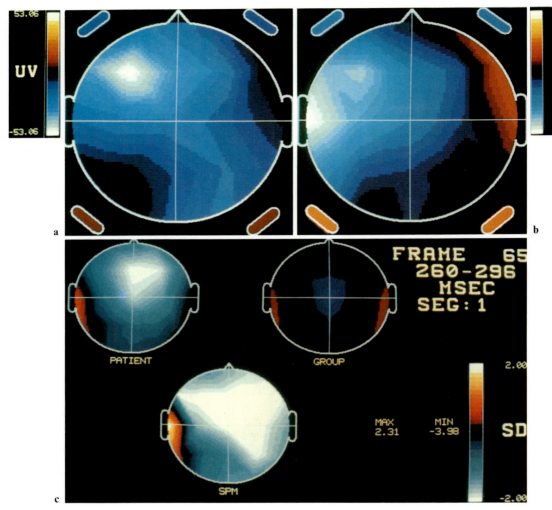

Fig. 13a–c. Data, displayed according to the convention of Fig. 3, derived from an 8-year-old boy who presented with clinical signs and symptoms consistent with the Sylvian Seizure Syndrome, generally believed to be a benign, self-limited disorder. In contrast to the usual findings, however, the distribution of activity at the onset of a typical spike was maximal in the left frontal region (**a**) and moved secondarily to the left midtemporal region (**b**). Ordinarily, discharges in this syndrome commence in the centroparietal, not frontal, regions. Although spectral and VER data were normal (not shown), the AER demonstrated a very large "dipole" abnormality, with augmented left temporal positivity, by 2.31 SD, and broadly increased frontal and hemispheric negativity, by 3.98 SD. This degree of abnormality is unusual in the Sylvian Seizure Syndrome. Owing to these unusual BEAM findings, radiographic studies were performed, revealing a left thalamic tumor. Had it not been for the topographic deviations from the normal pattern, prompt radiographic investigations would not have been performed

Spike-Wave Topography, Age 7. Figure 11 shows a page of the EEG of a 7-year-old child with attentional deficit disorder and generalized seizures of left-sided onset. Note the prominent bi-occipital spike-wave discharge. Also, note the apparent positive spike evident in the right central (C4) electrode. Figure 12 shows 16 topographic images taken at 8 ms before discharge onset (A) and every 4 ms thereafter out to 56 ms (B-P). Note the simultaneous onset of occipital negativity and right central positivity (B-F). The epileptic dipole of origin is clearly horizontal in position. Note from G through P, however, a complete polarity reversal, as if the dipole has rotated, pointing the negative end out halfway through (I-L). We do not suggest physical rotation of a static dipole source, which would, of course, be impossible. Rather, we suggest that as the epileptic dipole layer extends, the complex infoldings of cortex alter the net dipole position, simulating rotation.

This example shows how much detailed information can be made visible via serial topographic maps of EEG transient phenomena, such as spikes. The presence of dipole rotation was completely unexpected on the basis of the EEG tracing alone.

Abnormality in a Patient with Sylvian Seizure Syndrome, Age 8. An 8-year-old boy was referred for minor seizures involving peculiar facial sensations and difficulty in speaking. Nocturnal grand mal seizures were reported. The classic EEG demonstrated focal discharges emanating from the left frontotemporal-midtemporal region (not shown). The clinical diagnosis was Sylvian Seizure Syndrome, generally a mild, self-limited epileptic syndrome (Lombroso 1967). Spike topography revealed a discharge beginning in the left frontal region (Fig. 13A), but quickly reaching maximal value in the left midtemporal region 20 ms later (Fig. 13B). This was an unusual finding for this syndrome as, in our experience, virtually all patients demonstrate central parietal onset. The BEAM spectral and VER studies were normal (not shown). However, the AER demonstrated a large abnormality over 40 ms, starting at 260 ms. During this epoch, the left midtemporal region was excessively positive, by 2.31 SD, while both frontal regions and much of the right hemisphere were excessively negative, by 3.98 SD. We refer to the appearance of both negative and positive deviations from normal on SPM as a "dipole abnormality." It is almost always associated with pathology. Given these two atypical findings for Sylvian Seizure Syndrome, a CT scan was obtained. It revealed a subtle, but definite left thalamic tumor. This finding was confirmed by magnetic resonance imaging.

This study demonstrates the role BEAM can play in the refinement of a neurological diagnosis. Had it not been for the unusual BEAM findings, it is not likely this patient would have undergone CT scan so promptly.

Closing Remarks

The introduction of computer-generated and color-scaled topographic maps of brain electrical activity in the late 1970s and early 1980s was met with a bipolar response on the part of the neurological and psychiatric communities.

On the one hand, "advocates" believed it to be a whole new way of viewing brain function and predicted it would rapidly replace the antiquated specialty of EEG. On the other hand, many "skeptics" felt it to be nothing more than a sophisticated computer game, a gimmick destined to fail when put to real clinical tests by serious investigators. Time has mellowed both extremes of viewpoint, although a dichotomy still exists. The growing number of conferences, books, and articles dealing with topographic mapping – not to mention the many companies now manufacturing mapping equipment – attests to the fact that interest in mapping is growing, not declining. On the other hand, it appears clear that mapping will not replace classic EEG. In our opinion, mapping is an alternative way of viewing EEG and EP data which provides new and important perspectives. However, there remains much that can be better seen and quantified in classic polygraphic tracings. As time progresses, mapping will be seen to be less and less a separate diagnostic entity and more and more an important adjunct to clinical neurophysiology. As the costs of computers and computer graphics continue to fall, mapping will become more ubiquitous. Far from replacing EEG, mapping will enlarge the field, increasing its complexity and placing new demands upon clinician training. Electroencephalographers have spent years extracting information in the time domain. Now tools are available to examine data simultaneously in time and space.

But the story has just begun. There remain many important, unanswered questions. To name but a few: How many electrodes should be used and how should they be referenced? What constitutes an optimal control group? How can one best determine whether deviations from normal are due to real difference or chance? What is the role to be played by fully automatized diagnosis? Is there a clinical value to mapping the topographic distribution of epileptic spikes? Can dipole sources be reliably and rapidly estimated in depth from surface maps of electrical activity? It is an exciting time. The field is at its beginning, and it is not yet time to summarize.

Acknowledgement. I wish to thank the parents, patients and subjects for their participation; the members of the BEAM Laboratory for their quality performance at all times; David McAnulty for his expert editorial assistance; and, finally, all those who contributed their time and efforts to the Würzburg Symposium.

References

Arezzo JA, Pickoff A, Vaughan HGJ (1975) The sources and intracerebral distribution of auditory evoked potentials in the alert rhesus monkey. Brain Res 90:57–73
Bear DM (1979) Temporal lobe epilepsy – a syndrome of sensory-limbic hyperconnection. Cortex 15:357–384
Bear DM, Fedio P (1977) Quantitative analysis of interictal behavior in temporal lobe epilepsy. Arch Neurol 34:454–467
Berger H (1929) Über das Elektrenkephalogram des Menschen: I. Mitteilung. Arch Psychiatr Nervenkr 87:527–528
Bickford RG (1968) Properties of the microreflex system – human and animal studies. Proc Int Union Physiol Sci 7

Bickford RG, Allen B (1986) A simple add-on personal computer procedure for color displays of electrophysiological data: advantages and pitfalls. In: Duffy FH (ed) Topographic mapping of brain electrical activity. Butterworths, Boston

Bickford RG, Cody DT, Jacobsen JL, Lambert EH (1964a) Fast motor systems in man: physiopathology of the sonomotor response. Trans Am Neurol Assoc 89:56–58

Bickford RG, Jacobson JL, Cody DT (1964b) Nature of average evoked potentials to sound and other stimuli in man. Ann NY Acad Sci 112:204–223

Bickford RG, Brimmer J, Berger L (1973) Application of a compressed spectral array in clinical EEG. Raven, New York

Callaway E (1969) Diagnostic uses of the averaged evoked potential. In: Donchin E (ed) Average evoked potentials. NASA, Washington DC

Chiappa KH (1983) Evoked potentials in clinical medicine. Raven, New York

Coben L, Danziger W, Storandt M (1985) A longitudinal EEG study of mild senile dementia of Alzheimer type: changes at 1 year and at 2.5 years. Electroencephalogr Clin Neurophysiol 61:101–112

Cody DT, Jacobson JL, Walker JC, Bickford RG (1964) Averaged evoked myogenic and cortical potentials to sound in man. Ann Otol Rhinol Laryngol 73:763–777

Cooley JW, Tukey JW (1965) An algorithm for the machine calculation of Fourier series. Math Comp 19:297–301

Dawson GD (1950) Cerebral responses to nerve stimulation in man. Br Med Bull 6:326–329

Duff TA (1980) Topography of scalph recorded potentials by stimulation of the digits. Electroencephalogr Clin Neurophysiol 49:452–460

Duffy FH (1982) Topographic display of evoked potentials: clinical applications of brain electrical activity mapping (BEAM). Ann NY Acad Sci 388:193–196

Duffy FH (1986) Brain electrical activity mapping: issues and answers. In: Duffy FH (ed) Topographic mapping of brain electrical activity. Butterworths, Boston

Duffy FH, Als H (1983) Neurophysiological assessment of the neonate: an approach combining brain electrical activity mapping (BEAM) with behavioral assessment (APIB). In: Brazelton TB (ed) New approaches to developmental screening of infants. Elsevier, New York

Duffy FH, McAnulty G (1985) Brain electrical activity mapping (BEAM): search for a physiological signature of dyslexia. In: Duffy FH, Geschwind N (eds) Dyslexia: a neuroscientific approach to clinical evaluation. Little Brown, Boston

Duffy FH, Burchfiel JL, Lombroso CT (1979) Brain electrical activity mapping (BEAM): a method for extending the clinical utility of EEG and evoked potential data. Ann Neurol 5:309–321

Duffy FH, Denckla MB, Bartels P, Sandini G (1980) Dyslexia: regional differences in brain electrical activity by topographic mapping. Ann Neurol 7:412–420

Duffy FH, Bartels PH, Burchfiel JL (1981) Significance probability mapping: an aid in the topographic analysis of brain electrical activity. Electroencephalogr Clin Neurophysiol 51:455–462

Duffy FH, Albert MS, McAnulty G (1984a) Brain electrical activity in patients with presenile and senile dementia of the Alzheimer's type. Ann Neurol 16:439–448

Duffy FH, Albert MS, McAnulty G, Garvey AJ (1984b) Age-related differences in brain electrical activity mapping of healthy subjects. Ann Neurol 16:430–438

Dustman RE, Snyder EW (1981) Life-span changes in visually evoked potentials at central scalp. Neurobiol Aging 2:303–308

Estrin T, Uzgalis R (1969) Computer display of spatio-temporal EEG patterns. IEEE Trans Biomed Eng 16:192–196

Gibbs FA, Davis H, Lennox WG (1935) The electroencephalogram in epilepsy and in conditions of impaired consciousness. Arch Neurol Psychiatry 34:1133–1135

Gotman J (1982) Automatic recognition of epileptic seizures in the EEG. Electroencephalogr Clin Neurophysiol 54:530–540

Gotman J, Gloor P (1967) Automatic recognition and quantification of interictal epileptic activity in the human scalp. Electroencephalogr Clin Neurophysiol 41:513–529

Halliday AM (1987) Fourth Dawson memorial lecture. Clin Evoked Potentials 5:2–10

Harris JA, Melby GM, Bickford RG (1969) Computer-controlled multidimensional display device for investigation and modeling of physiologic systems. Comput Biomed Res 2:519–538

Hjorth B (1975) An on-line transformation of scalp potentials into orthogonal source derivations. Electroencephalogr Clin Neurophysiol 39:526–530

Hjorth B (1986) Physical aspects of EEG data as a basis for topographic mapping. In: Duffy FH (ed) Topographic mapping of brain electrical activity. Butterworths, Boston

Jasper HH (1958) The ten-twenty system of the International Federation. Electroencephalogr Clin Neurophysiol 10:371–375

Jeffreys DA, Axford JG (1972) Source locations of pattern-specific components of human visual evoked potentials. Exp Brain Res 16:1–40

Jewett DL, Williston JS (1971) Auditory-evoked far fields averaged from the scalp of humans. Brain 94:681–696

John ER, Karmel BZ, Corning WC et al. (1977) Neurometrics. Science 196:1393–1410

John ER, Ahn H, Prichep L (1980) Developmental equations for the electroencephalogram. Science 210:1255–1258

Lehmann D (1986) Spatial analysis of EEG and evoked potential data. In: Duffy FH (ed) Topographic mapping brain electrical activity. Butterworths, Boston

Lombroso C (1967) Sylvian seizures and mid temporal spike foci in children. Arch Neurol 17:52–57

Maus A, Endresen J (1979) Misuse of computer-generated results. Med Biol Eng Comput 17:126–129

Morihisa JM, Duffy FH, Wyatt RJ (1983) Brain electrical activity mapping (BEAM) in schizophrenia patients. Arch Gen Psychiatry 40:719–728

Morstyn R, Duffy FH, McCarley RW (1983a) Altered P300 topography in schizophrenia. Arch Gen Psychiatry 40:729–734

Morstyn R, Duffy FH, McCarley RW (1983b) Altered topography of EEG spectral content in schizophrenia. Electroencephalogr Clin Neurophysiol 65:263–271

Offner FF (1950) The EEG as potential mapping: the value of the average monopolar reference. Electroencephalogr Clin Neurophysiol 2:215–216

Ransohoff DF, Feinstein AR (1978) Problems of spectrum and bias in evaluating the efficacy of diagnostic tests. N Engl J Med 299:926–930

Steger JA (1971) Readings in statistics. Holt Rinehart and Winston, New York

Tukey JW (1977) Exploratory data analysis. Addison-Wesley, Reading

Walter WG, Shipton HW (1951) A new topographic display system. Electroencephalogr Clin Neurophysiol 3:281–292

From Mapping to the Analysis and Interpretation of EEG/EP Maps*

D. Lehmann[1]

Functional States of the Brain and Brain Electric Fields

The organization of the neuronal activity of the brain varies over time, depending on determinants such as maturational stage, circadian activity cycle, metabolic condition, motivational state, newly arriving information in conjunction with related, past context experiences, drugs, and disease (Koukkou et al. 1980). A every moment in time, there exists a particular global, brain functional state which is the consequence of the interaction between newly received information (Koukkou-Lehmann 1987) and spontaneous ("housekeeping") activity. In turn, the momentary functional state (Koukkou and Lehmann 1983) constrains and shapes the elaboration of, and the responses to newly arriving information, and constrains and shapes access within the brain to information-processing strategies and to context information which was stored earlier ("state-dependent learning and recall"). Classical examples are wakefulness and sleep, or childhood and adulthood, with their different modes of information processing. These gross functional states ough to be seen as composed of local and temporal microstates. A global brain state is thus made up from a large number of local, mementary states of the various cortical and subcortical functional analyzers and processors (Koella 1982). Concerning the temporal dimension, there is good evidence that as a consequence of newly arriving information, series of different, brief brain states are initiated which manifest different steps and aspects of the processing of the information, and which are referred to as "components" in evoked potential/event-related potential (EP) work. Likewise, "spontaneous" EEG activity is hypothesized to consist of a sequence of similarly brief epochs of stationary spatial electric patterns (maps) which manifest different functional states (Lehmann et al. 1987).

The spatial pattern of the neuronal activity at each moment in time is the representation of the momentary functional brain state, which is manifest as a particular spatial configuration of the brain electric field. Different configurations ("landscapes") of the brain electric field are accounted for by the activity of different neural populations, and therefore are expected to manifest different steps or modes of information processing, which by the same token implies constraints of the reactivity of the system to subsequently arriving information. The distribution of the brain field on the scalp can be measured as EEG or evoked/event-related potential (EP) data.

---

* This work was supported by grants from the Swiss National Science Foundation and the Sandoz Foundation, Basel
[1] Department of Neurology, University Hospital, 8091 Zürich, Switzerland

We consider only the landscape of the mapped field distribution near and around the brain; the configuration of this landscape is the important information about brain activity which manifests the brain's functional state. Points far away from the brain cannot be expected to contribute information about the brain, and information about the electric relation between these latter far-away points and the points near the brain does not alter the landscape which is constituted by the points near the brain.

Mapping

Mapping is the only way to convey three-dimensional information in an immediately understandable form (Fig. 1). The time series of momentary maps of the brain electric field constitute an unbiased way to display the brain electric field data if mapping has been done correctly and if the maps are read adequately.

If spatial sampling of the brain electric field has been adequate following the Nyquist constraints, polynomial interpolations between measured locations (e.g., Ashida et al. 1984) are preferable over linear interpolations for reconstruction of the true features of the landscape of the maps. In general it is said that if linear interpolation is used, i.e. if the data are shown as sampled, the sampling rate should be at least 5 times higher than the Nyquist rate in order to avoid gross deviations of the map from the original. As an example, presume that the peak of a landscape occurs nearly halfway between the midline electrode and a left lateral neighbor electrode but slightly closer to the lateral electrode. Linear interpolation will produce a field peak at the lateral electrode. The error in peak location in a linear interpolation, then, is nearly half the interelectrode distance. It is commonly assumed that interelectrode distances below about 2 cm do not contribute worthwhile detail to EEG findings. However, systematic reports about the spatial frequencies present in human scalp-recorded brain field maps are not yet available; the available reports refer to space-time interactions, i.e., presumed wave propagations. In our pilot computations of spatial fast fourier transforms (FFT) in momentary maps, power appeared to recede into the noise level at around one wave per 6 cm. Spatial frequency resolution is poor by nature, since the entire available scalp extension is only about 35 cm from nasion to inion. It is also to be considered that close electrode spacing for high spatial frequencies will require very many electrodes to cover the entire scalp area, and that there are practical limits to the closeness of spacing. If space is severely undersampled, only linear interpolation should be used. Interpolated locations should only be used for further analysis if it is certain that spatial sampling and interpolation procedures were adequate.

Maps of Momentary EEG and EP Data

At each point in time, a unique map of the momentary electric landscape of the brain's activity can be constructed from the recorded data. The landscape of this map is independent from the chosen reference electrode (similar to the

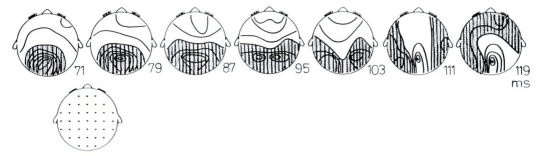

Fig. 1. Sequence of 3/s flash evoked average potential maps, 71–119 ms latency post-stimulus. Thirty-seven channels were recorded simultaneously with 750 samples/s/channel. For the array, see the schematic. Equipotential contour lines at steps of 2 µV; *hatched* negative, *white* positive to average reference. (From Lehmann 1972)

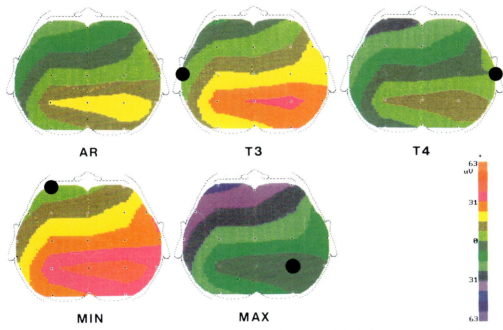

Fig. 2. A momentary map (one single time frame of a map series) during spontaneous alpha-EEG. Different electrodes were chosen as reference for the display of the same map (recomputations, using a BioLogic system). Color and microvolt level of the equipotential areas are changed by the references, but the landscapes remain identical: the voltage differences between the recorded points, and therefore the landscape, are not changed. Minor changes of the shape of the displayed contour lines result from cutting the landscapes at somewhat different amplitudes for the different references; if all contour lines were shown, identical shapes would be visible. – The different references (*black dots*) are: *AR*, average reference (spatial high-pass filter); *T3*, T3; *T4*, T4; *MIN*, Fp1, the location of lowest potential in the map; the map therefore appears "all positive"; *MAX*, P4, the location of highest potential in the map: hence, an "all negative" map results. The 21 electrode positions are indicated by dots; the voltage color scale is shown on the right

geographical landscape which is independent from the choice of the point which is called zero) – only the color of the equipotential areas or the values of the equipotential lines depend on the reference, not their shapes or their configurations or their equipotential-line distances (Fig. 2). The only information of relevance is the configuration and the strength (the landscape and the hilliness) of these momentary maps.

On the other hand, the landscape of the momentary maps depends completely on the chosen baselines (Lehmann, 1987). The baseline problem is not related to the reference problem. If other than zero potential difference (technical zero) between locations is used as baseline, the interpretation of the momentary maps must consider this. The popular prestimulus baselines in EP work accordingly lead to displays of the amount of landscape change which occurred between the map at prestimulus time and the map at the investigated latency; baselines other than technical zero cannot produce maps of the momentary landscape, but produce maps of differences between two landscapes.

Assessment of Maps: Extracted Landscape Descriptors for Reduction in Space

The spatial configuration or landscape of a map may be operationalized by the question where the peak(s) and the trough(s) are within the map, how large the potential difference between these highest and lowest points is, and how steep the slopes of the potential gradients are. These landscape descriptors are reference-independent.

The maximal potential difference within a map, or "potential range" (Lehmann and Skrandies 1980) assesses the magnitude or strength of the landscape relief (Fig. 3A, see also Fig. 10); this measure is directly related to the "map hilliness" (Lehmann 1971) or "global field power" (Lehmann and Skrandies 1980) which are discussed in the section on global field power below.

The description of the landscape configuration of a map by the locations of its two extreme potentials (Lehmann 1971, 1981; Lehmann and Julesz 1978; Lehmann and Skrandies 1984) can be used with ease for any number of recording electrodes (Fig. 4); it implies a reduction factor of 10 for 20 recording electrodes, a factor of more than 30 for 64 electrodes. The two-extreme-description is based on the observation that many – but certainly not all – momentary maps often appear to be grossly concentric around a maximum and a minimum. In order to conveniently survey an entire EP map series one might plot the time-space trajectories of the locations on the maps' maximum potential and the maps' minimum potential (Lehmann et al. 1977; Brandeis and Lehmann 1986): the locations are projected onto the anterior-posterior and right-left axes of the head, and plotted as function of time (example in Fig. 3b). Two-dimensional Fourier transforms of momentary maps are per se no data reduction, but emphasize certain properties of the mapped data.

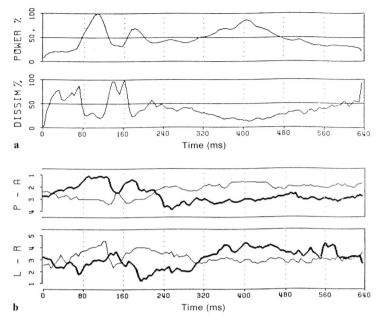

Fig. 3a, b. Survey of an EP map sequence. **a** Global field power of each map (*top*) and global dissimilarity between successive maps (*bottom*) as function of time. Magnitudes (*vertical*) were scaled so that the largest value equals 100%. **b** Space-time trajectories of the locations of the maps minimum (heavy) and maximum (thin) locations. The locations are projected onto an anterior-posterior axis (*top*) and onto a right-left axis (*bottom*) and plotted as function of time. Event-related map series, averaged over 16 average ($n=35$) map series of a normal subject in a "P3" paradigm. Electrode array as in Fig. 13; sampling rate 500/s/channel. (From D. Brandeis, A. Horst, R. Müller and D. Lehmann, in preparation)

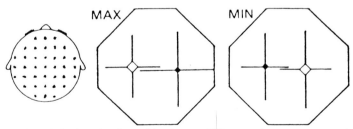

Fig. 4. Map description and statistical evaluation of landscape differences between averaged evoked maps, using extracted locations of maximum and minimum potential. The mean locations over 11 averages with stimuli to the right hemiretina (*open squares*) and 11 to the left hemiretina (*solid dots*) and the standard deviations of the locations of the maximum and minimum potential in the map at 225 ms latency are shown. Stimuli were the appearance of a binocularly disparate (visual depth) target shown to the right or left hemiretina as dynamic random-dot stereogram. The U-test significance of the topographical differences between right and left hemiretinal stimuli was $p<0.005$. Note that the original maps showed much steeper gradients around the minimum than the maximum location, indicative of a closer proximity of the negativity to the recording surface (i.e., the negativity was the spatially closest response component). Simultaneous recording from 37 electrodes; array in inset. (From Lehmann and Julesz 1978)

Equivalent Model Dipoles for Reduction in Space

Instead of describing the major features of the map landscape by the locations of the two extreme voltages, an equivalent best-fit dipole generator might be determined. This reduces the map to six parameters (three for location, two for angles and one for strength). Many maps are fairly well described by one or two dipoles, and the procedure is interesting as a systematic spatial data reduction. However, since in reality there are always very many generator sources and since there is no unique solution to the "inverse problem" of determining the sources from knowledge of the surface of the electric field, practically useful results require additional information or constraints on the question or acceptance of assumptions, even though some studies demonstrate good agreement with expected source locations (Lehmann et al. 1982; Grandori 1984).

Measuring Global Dissimilarity Between Maps

Global dissimilarity between two or more maps (Lehmann and Skrandies 1980) is the mean of the voltage differences at all electrodes. If landscape is to be assessed without any influence of magnitude (hilliness), the maps (momentary or power maps) must first be scaled to unity global field power. Of course, for momentary maps, global dissimilarity requires data recomputation into voltages against the average reference or into current source density values.

Global dissimilarity can be used to recognize times of changes of map landscape in a map series: global dissimilarity between two maps when computed as series over time between pairs of successive maps results in a curve which shows distinct peak values of dissimilarity separated by stretches of low dissimilarity (Lehmann 1986). It is important to note that, as Fig. 3 shows, times of relative similarity tend to coincide with times of high global field power, and conversely that times of high dissimilarity tend to coincide with times of low global field power (Lehmann and Skrandies 1980). This tendency also exists during spontaneous EEG activity (Lehmann et al. 1987). This finding agrees with the direct observation that spontaneous and evoked potential map series show relatively sudden changes of landscape, then stay stable for longer times (Lehmann 1981; Lehmann and Skrandies 1979, 1984; Brandeis and Lehmann 1986). This is accounted for by the fact that in general, there are no wavefronts in the maps, and no continuous propagations of major map landmarks over extensive distances on the scalp over time. Rather, the maps change over time in the manner of a volcanic landscape, with occasional or periodic eruptions within some preferred areas.

Maps of FFT Power

Fast Fourier transform power maps (Ueno et al. 1975) are concerned with EEG (or sometimes EP) data over time. These maps of FFT band power correspond to the maps of the standard deviation of the average of all momentary maps

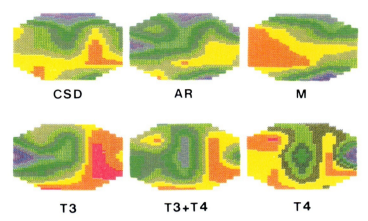

Fig. 5. Effect of the choice of the reference on the landscapes of the maps of the spatial distribution of power. Data comprise the 3–4 Hz temporal frequency band during a 2-s epoch of pathological EEG in an epileptic patient. Before FFT computation, the data epoch was recomputed (using a BioLogic system) into voltages vs the average reference (*AR*), into current source densities (*CSD*), into voltages vs combined mandibulae (*M*), vs T3 (*T3*), vs the mean of T3 and T4 (*T3 + T4*) and vs T4 (*T4*). Twenty-one-electrode array as in Fig. 2. Equipower areas in equal steps from high to low, from red to yellow, green, blue. Note that the resulting maps of power landscapes are very different, depending on the chosen reference. Note also that the average reference power map resembles the current source density power map. (Recording and display on a Bio-logic system)

over time (Fig. 3B in Lehmann 1975). Contrary to maps of the momentary electric landscape, the landscapes of maps of FFT band power depend on the chosen reference as shown in Fig. 5 (see also Lehmann 1984, Lehmann et al. 1986), quite as conventional waveshapes depend on the reference. This is so because the electric relationship between different locations changes over time, and the arbitrary assignment of zero variance might be given with equal right to any real electrode (Katznelson 1981). There are as many different (and correct) maps of band power as there are electrodes in the recorded area. The landscapes of these different maps of band power can be very different; at any case, the chosen reference location by definition always shows zero power. Since brain-remote references (right ear, left ear, chin, neck, chest, etc.) are not electrically identical, they also produce different maps of FFT band power.

On the other hand, the maps of the landscapes of FFT band power do not depend on the baselines. Only a map of the power at 0 Hz temporal frequency would be determined by the baseline; traditionally 0 Hz temporal frequency (DC) is disregarded in conventional EEG work.

Even though the Fourier transform of the data over time permits the reconstitution of the original data by the inverse procedure and, accordingly, contains the complete information about the momentary landscapes, mapping of FFT power is ambiguous because only one half of the available information is displayed after FFT. The crucial other half, the phase angle information, is missing (Lehmann et al. 1986). Therefore, only maps of FFT band power which were computed from data which were first treated over space (average reference or current source density computation) can be used for unique statements about functional-physiological aspects. Like any other maps, the maps of FFT power might be assessed using the reference-independent extraction parameters which were mentioned above.

For a comprehensive and unbiased display of the results of Fourier transformations, vector diagrams ("Nyquist diagrams") are recommended, where amplitude (power) and phase relationships between the electrode positions within the recorded field, and the problems with interpreting these relations become immediately obvious (discussed, e.g., in Lehmann et al. 1986).

Review of Reference and Baseline Effects

In summary, the baseline question is to be distinguished from the reference question. The landscape of momentary maps ("EP maps") depends on the chosen baselines, and does not depend on the chosen reference (the reference, however, determines the magnitude and polarity of local values – it supplies a constant offset for the entire map). The landscape of band power maps depends on the reference, and does not depend on the baselines (except for a map of 0 Hz power). If momentary maps are compared (over subjects, times, conditions), the magnitude and polarity of the differences at the electrode sites depend on the reference.

Accordingly, it is advisable to transform the data into reference-independent values before further treatment. The recommended technique is recomputation into average reference voltages (spatial DC rejection).

Treatments Over Space

In order to obtain reference-independent data for the individual electrode positions on the head, the potential differences which were obtained as original records against any reference must be spatially transformed (Lehmann 1987). These transforms are in principle spatial frequency high-pass procedures.

The computation of voltages against the *average reference* (i.e. the mean of all momentarily measured potentials within the area of interest) means a rejection of the time-varying offset or spatial DC component that was measured between the arbitrarily chosen reference and all other positions (Offner 1950; Rémond 1960; Lehmann 1971, 1975, 1987; Bertrand et al. 1985). The procedure is comparable to the traditional rejection of the DC component over time when time-oriented recording is performed. The average reference computation produces momentary voltage field maps which, when averaged over time, show a standard deviation whose landscape corresponds to the landscape of the locations of the maximal and the minimal potential values accumulated from all momentary maps during the analysis epoch. (The mean of all maps during an extended analysis epoch will always tend to a completely flat field.) An example is shown in Fig. 6.

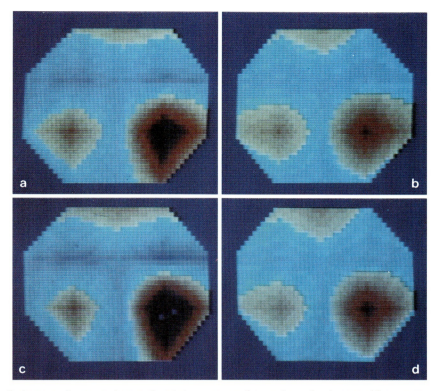

Fig. 6a–d. A map of extracted map descriptors averaged over time closely resembles a map based on the complete data. The figure shows the results from a digitally band-passed 24-s epoch of 8–12 Hz alpha-EEG collected from a normal subject during rest with eyes closed. Sixteen channels; 128 samples/channel/s; digitally filtered to 8–12 Hz. Color coding of local values from low to high amplitudes (µV) or extremes occurrence rate: dark blue, light blue, yellow, red, black. Head seen from above, left ear on left. **a** Complete data set (all time points, all space points) mapping the standard deviation of the mean of all 3072 maps, using the average reference; this corresponds to the map of the square root of band power. **b** Reduced set (all time points, one-eighth of space points) mapping only the locations of the maximum and minimum potential of each of the 3072 maps. **c** Reduced set (one-sixth of the time points, all space points) mapping the standard deviation of the mean of only the maps at the times of maximal global field power (see Fig. 10), but using all space points. **d** Reduced set (one-sixth of the time points, one-eight of the space points) mapping only the locations of the maxima and minima of only the maps at maximal global field power, combining the reductions of **b** and **c**. Note the similarities of the maps even after the 1:50 data reduction in **d**, and note that only the average reference power map (see Fig. 5) resembles the distribution maps of the reference-free extracted features (maxima and minima)

The computation of voltage *gradients* for each position likewise eliminates the recording reference, but results in a magnitude and an angle of the local voltage gradient for each position. This two-number result for each position makes further data analysis more complicated. In practice, therefore, the angle is often disregarded or preselected, and only the magnitude is used, or vice versa. The computation of the local gradient means the computation of the first spatial derivative of the field.

The computation of *current source density* (or "*source derivation*") likewise eliminates the recording reference, and gives a one-number statement for the current flow in or out of the brain (only perpendicular to the surface) at the electrode positions (Hjorth 1975; Thickbroom et al. 1984). The computation of the current density means the computation of the second spatial derivative (the local curvature) of the potential field. The resulting field map is comparable to the usual magnetoencephalographic (MEG) measurements (Cohen and Cuffin 1983) when rotated in space by 90°, and yields very localized and "sharpened" landscapes. Computation of current density results in a reduced area of the map, even though currently popular strategies extrapolate to the originally recorded area border.

It is of interest that, generally speaking, computations of the first and second spatial derivative are equivalent to spatial high-pass filter procedures: Spatial low-frequency features will be suppressed, and the narrowly localized spatial features become more prominent. The user must decide whether it is appropriate to disregard low spatial frequencies when, for example, he or she chooses current source density values instead of voltages us the average reference.

Waveshapes of EEG and EP Data

Traditionally, the brain's electric activity has been displayed as time series of voltages ("trace," "waveshape," "curve") recorded between two electrodes. If recordings are obtained from n electrodes, $n*(n-1)$ waveshapes of voltages are possible because the measured voltages cannot be ascribed only to one of the two electrodes of a channel (Lehmann 1981, 1984; Lehmann and Skrandies 1984). Nevertheless, the limited number of available channels has led to the general convention to record and analyze only $n-1$ preselected waveshapes, by preselecting one of the electrodes as a common zero reference or by preselecting certain combinations of the electrodes. Since there is no possible physical proof for electrical inactivity of any recording point (Katznelson 1981), or for a priori superior importance of any direction of gradient, these preselection procedures imply an arbitrary reduction of the result space before analysis, and therefore cannot lead to physiologically meaningful and comprehensive functional interpretations. If waveshapes are to be analyzed, treatment over space must precede treatment over time. Treatments over space which lead to locally unique values are spatial DC rejection ("average reference" computation) or the first derivative (gradient) or the second derivative (current density, "source derivation") of the momentary field data. Such treatments when plotted over time result in n unique waveshapes for n electrodes, i.e., produce values which are unique for given locations (for gradient values, only magnitude, not angle, can be conveniently treated in the form of waveshapes).

Diagnostics VS Functional Interpretation

For clinical or other diagnostics, i.e. for the experience-based heuristic classification of EEG/EP data into one of several groups of pathology, reference-independence and comprehensiveness is not necessary. In fact, selective information, if sufficient, is to be preferred for classification, in order to avoid unnecessary and costly additional data or analysis. Results obtained with preselected or weighted data are not wrong – they are merely not comprehensive, and might lead to very misleading interpretations, although they lead to correct classifications. A case in point is, for example, the EEG coherence between left and right parietal areas during REM and non-REM sleep: The value during REM sleep is higher than during non-REM sleep with Cz as reference, but lower with the ear as reference (Appendix B in Dumermuth et al. 1983). Although both statements are internally compatible (for reasons not to be discussed here, see Lehmann et al. 1986), a functional interpretation suggested by considering only one of the statements might be very misleading.

EEG/EP Result Space vs Brain Space

Scalp maps of the electric (and magnetic) brain field are very suggestive as to brain localization of the generating sources, and many reports study this question. We would like to advocate caution in this work. Firstly, since there is no unique solution to the so-called "inverse problem" of detecting the sources of a field if more than one generator is involved, and secondly, because most brain processes beyond the immediate input stage are assumed to involve extended cortical and subcortical areas.

In practical work, the location of a "hot area" in an EEG or EP map might be very misleading. Figure 7 illustrates the classical case of visual pattern-evoked potential fields:

The visual stimulation of a lateral hemiretina leads to activation of the ipsilateral visual processing areas, as is well known in anatomy and physiology. However, depending on the type and on the retinal extent of the stimulus which is given to the *same* lateral hemiretina, the scalp-recorded, averaged, EP field might show an ipsilateral or a contralateral "hot area." If a large (16 deg) pattern reversal stimulus is used, the hot area appears over the hemisphere contralateral to the stimulated hemiretina and hemisphere (i.e., ipsilateral to the stimulated visual hemifield), as shown in the upper row of Fig. 7. The opposite hemispheric lateralization is obtained when stimulating the *same* lateral hemiretina with a small, "on" or "on/off" checkerboard pattern followed by a long-lasting unpatterned visual field, as shown in the lower row of Fig. 7. A similar seemingly "correct" map lateralization is obtained by hemiretinal flash stimuli (Lehmann et al. 1969) and with small dynamic random-dot stereo stimuli (Fig. 4; see also Lehmann and Julesz 1978).

It might be observed that areas of steepest field gradients indicate more reliably the "correct" location of the generators (see also Skrandies, this volume,

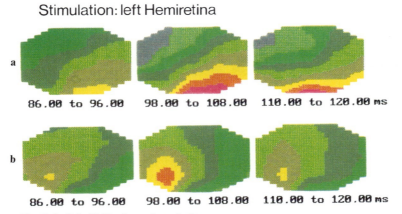

Fig. 7. Left half. For legend see facing page

Fig. 7a, b. Maps of the brain electric field do not directly reflect the generator location. The figure shows visual checkerboard reversal-evoked average ($n=93$) potential maps from a normal subject. Four stimulus conditions were used: **left** or **right** hemiretinal stimulation, and **a** a large target (16 deg field, 55 min checks) as pattern reversal at 2/s, or **b** a small target (7 deg field, 24 min checks) as 52 ms pattern "on" and 470 ms pattern "off" stimuli. For each stimulus condition, three mean maps (six successive data points each) are shown covering 86–120 ms latency; 21-electrode recording. Note that stimulation of a given hemisphere results in "hot spots" over opposite hemispheres depending on the size and type of the stimulus. (Recording and display on a BioLogic system)

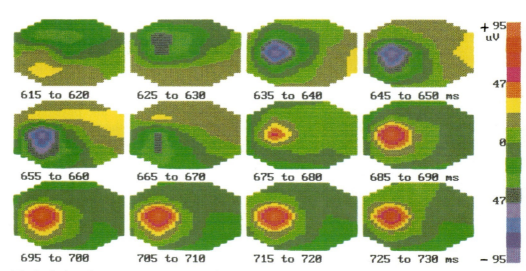

Fig. 8. Series of momentary maps covering 115 ms during an epileptic EEG "spike." For electrode array see Fig. 2; 200 samples/s/channel; display vs average reference; voltage color scale on the right. Note the spatial progression of the map's minimum from anterior left to central left areas, then a very quick polarity reversal around 665 to 670 ms, and the subsequent relatively stable landscapes of the maps. (Recording and display on a BioLogic system)

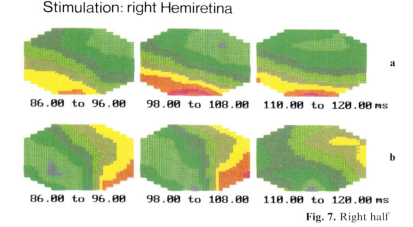

Fig. 7. Right half

p. 337), and that the reduction of the maps to equivalent model dipole generators tends to yield "correct" results (Lehmann et al. 1982). The physiological interpretation of these results is relatively simple and is based on the orientation, not the location, of the mean generating process (see Skrandies and Lehmann 1982), but in practice it is important that even an apparently straightforward situation such as hemiretinal stimuli produces maps whose landscapes cannot simply be read as images of brain anatomy.

Accordingly, the very suggestive map sequences obtained when epileptic spikes are displayed deserve cautious interpretation. The maps in Fig. 8 suggest a change of the location of extreme values over the lateral left hemisphere. The change of the minimum location over time might, however, be accounted for by a mere rotation of the generating process at a constant brain location, between the map maximum and minimum in frame 665–670 ms.

Reducing EEG and EP Map Series by Traditional Time-Oriented Strategies

Mapping of EEG and EP data is neither data reduction nor data analysis – rather, map display increases the total amount of data by a large factor (of over 100 to 1000), because locations between actually measured locations must be filled in on the screen by some method. For survey and analysis, the mapped data typically need to be reduced. Reduction is possible in time and in space.

Conventional Reductions in Time for Spontaneous EEG

Although FFTs do not in themselves constitute data reduction, in practical applications of FFT the procedures work as data reduction in time, because conventional strategies immediately average transforms over several successive data epochs in order to increase the reliability of the estimate. Typical are averages over five to ten epochs of 2–4 s duration (stationarity over time is assumed, often not tested), and since only the power and not the phase information is used for mapping, a reduction factor of 10 to 20 is achieved. Averaging over frequency bands (reducing frequency resolution), say from 0.25 Hz (4-s epochs) to conventional bands of about 4 Hz offers another reduction factor of 16 and brings total reduction in our example to the substantial factor of 320. In some applications (vigilance, sleep studies), much longer periods extending over many minutes are averaged. We are still left with maps of FFT band power of the many locations which have been measured. These locations must not be treated blindly as to their spatial relationships in further analyses, e.g., in analyses of variance (ANOVAs). There is obviously a difference in whether a decrease of the measurement between condition A and condition B occurs at two neighboring electrode locations, or whether the decrease occurs at locations far apart from each other. In the former case, the landscape of the difference between A and B will be very different from that in the latter case. Space-oriented reduction and analysis takes the configuration of the landscapes of the maps into account, whereas conventional multivariate analysis, multiple cross-correlations or coherence computations between channels do not consider spatial vicinity or remoteness of the electrodes involved.

Conventional Reductions in Time for EP Data

"Components" are recognized in the recorded waveshapes, and the maps at maximal amplitude of the waveshapes are examined. The conventional procedure implies selecting "classical" waveshapes – for example for visual EP data an occipital-to-ear recording – and determining the times of maximal or minimal amplitude. This approach is arbitrary because of the preselection of the examined waveshape(s). Since it is possible to record $n*(n-1)$ equally correct voltage waveshapes from n electrodes, all waveshapes would have to be searched for peak (trough) latencies if blind weighting is to be avoided; no unique latency can be found this way, even if narrow time windows are used, since latencies in waveshapes recorded from the same electrode against various others will differ (Lehmann and Skrandies 1980). Even with use of locally unique waveshapes, as obtained by spatial transformation of the data (average reference; current density), that result in only n waveshapes for the peak- or trough-searching procedures, the ambivalence of the component latency will persist for the different locations.

Global Field Power for Reduction of Map Series in the Time Dimension

The concept of the strength of a brain process as marker of the most important time point(s), which is the rationale for the traditional search strategy for component identification, might be applied in a generalized form to the data in the

From Mapping to the Analysis and Interpretation of EEG/EP Maps 67

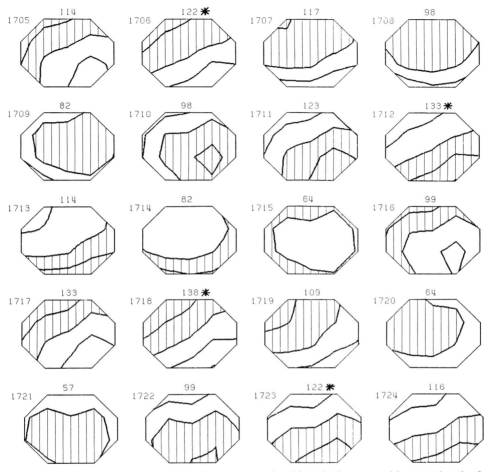

Fig. 9. Series of momentary maps from a normal subject during rest with eyes closed of a normal subject, covering about $1^1/_2$ conventional alpha cycles (152 ms). Recording in 16 channels between Cz and Oz (for array see Fig. 13) with 128 samples/s/channel, i.e., maps at 8-ms intervals (continuously numbered at upper left corner). Equipotential lines at 10-μV steps; *white* positive, *hatched* negative vs average reference. *Numbers above each map* give value of global field power; maps with maximal values are marked by *asterisks*. Note that the maps at successive times of maximal global field power show generally similar landscapes but inverted polarity. From a study with H. Ozaki and I. Pal (see Lehmann et al., in press)

entire maps. This is supported by the observation that sequences of momentary evoked maps (Lehmann 1972; Lehmann et al. 1977) and of momentary spontaneous maps (Lehmann 1971, 1972) show landscapes of unequal electric strength (see, e.g., Figs. 7, 8): some are hilly with steep gradients, others are more flat. The hilly maps, those with a more pronounced landscape, recommend themselves, since obviously the landscape in these maps is most clearly defined, or in other words, the signal-to-noise ratio is favorable.

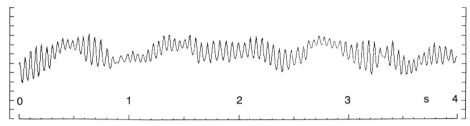

Fig. 10. Global field power during spontaneous alpha activity recorded from a normal subject with eyes closed. Recording from 16 electrodes; 256 samples/s/channel; digitally FIR filtered to the temporal 8–12 Hz band. Note the ca. 20-Hz periodicity of the electric strength of the maps. Total analysis time was 4 seconds (s)

The momentary electric strength of the mapped landscape can be measured (without resorting to a preselected reference) as the mean of all possibly measurable potential differences between the electrodes within the recorded area ($n*(n-1)$ potential differences), given about equal interelectrode distances. This measure of "global field power" (Lehmann and Skrandies 1980) is directly related to the mean of all absolute, local voltages measured vs the average reference ("map hilliness," Lehmann 1971). The curve of the behavior of global field power over time is closely similar to that of the maximal potential difference within the field or "potential range" (the voltage between map maximum and minimum values, wherever those might occur) which also does not require a preselected reference (Lehmann and Skrandies 1980, 1984). In conventional parlance, the "map hilliness" or "field power" is the standard deviation of all momentarily measured values (which implies the computation of their mean value over space, i.e., of the so-called average reference).

The maps selected at times of maximal hilliness (Figs. 3, 10) tend to be representative for entire epochs. Figure 9 shows an example of spontaneous EEG data where times of maximal field power are marked. The spatial distribution of band power computed from all data points in time and space (Fig. 6a) is very similar to the spatial distribution of the standard deviation of the mean of the selected maps at only the times of maximal global field power (Fig. 6c), and even similar to that of the locations of the maximal and minimal map potentials extracted from only the maps at maximal global field power (Fig. 6d).

Global field power has been used for meaningful reduction of map series in several of our studies (Lehmann and Skrandies 1979, 1980; Adachi and Lehmann 1983; Skrandies and Lehmann 1982), where one time point within a time window needed to be determined as a meaningful ERP latency for further statistics about the characteristics of the map landscapes. The time of maximal global field power within a time window of interest meaningfully determines the selection of one of the many maps for comparisons over conditions or subjects.

Figure 11 shows an example of the latency difference of the so-called P100 component evoked by checkerboard reversal stimuli to the upper and to the lower hemiretina in one subject, determined with global field power while analyz-

From Mapping to the Analysis and Interpretation of EEG/EP Maps 69

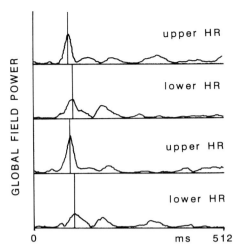

Fig. 11. Global field power of map series evoked by checkerboard pattern reversal stimuli (16 deg target field, 55 min checks) shown binocularly to the upper or lower hemiretina (HR) of a normal subject. Twenty-one-electrode array as in Fig. 2. Normal subject, sequential runs with 93 stimuli each. *Vertical lines* mark times of maximal value of global field power

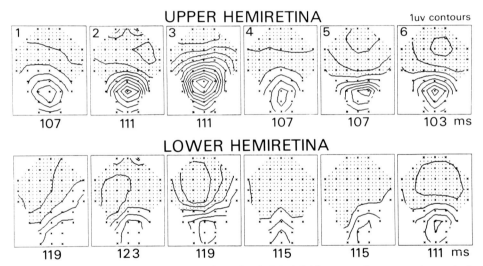

Fig. 12. Momentary maps at the times of maximal global field power of a map series evoked by checkerboard reversal stimuli (16 deg target field, 55 min checks) to the upper and to the lower hemiretina in six normal subjects. Recordings with 45 electrodes as indicated, between 30% nasion-inion and 3 cm below inion. Head seen from above, nose up, left ear left. Positive areas *white*, negative areas *dotted* relative to average reference; contour lines in steps of 1 µV. Note earlier latencies and spatially more anterior location of maximum potential for upper hemiretinal stimuli, but note also the variability over subjects. (Results from a study with W. Skrandies)

ing 20 simultaneously recorded channels. Figure 12 illustrates EP maps recorded from six different subjects with 45 channels at the times of maximal global field power during upper and lower hemiretinal stimulation.

The measure of global field power is applicable to any number of recordings channels and is therefore useful for objective data assessment in routine work, where latency differences between channels are often observed even when only four channels are considered (Lehmann and Skrandies 1979; Adachi and Lehmann 1983; Skrandies 1987).

Space-Oriented Segmentation for Reduction of Map Series in the Time Dimension

The rationale of maximal electric strength of the landscape for the definition of the occurrence of a step in information processing is not completely satisfying: One could well argue that a particular step in information processing might involve a major decision, even though it is executed by a small number of neural elements. If neural elements in a particular geometric constellation become active, an electric field of a particular configuration will be present. If this field configuration changes, then a geometrically different population of neural elements must be active. As discussed above, it is reasonable to assume that a different neural population will perform a different processing task or operate in a different mode.

Following this line of thought, a meaningful way to reduce a map series in time is to segment it into epochs of stable landscapes that (possibly) show unequal durations; as soon as the landscape changes, a new segment starts. Each segment might represent a mode or step of information processing, characterized by a particular state of global activity. The momentary strength of the landscape might be disregarded completely in this argument. The task then is to recognize changes of the momentary landscape (the spatial pattern).

We have used the two reference-independent locations of the extreme potential values (maximum and minimum) within each map as phenomenological descriptors of the major characteristics of the map's landscape, resulting in a spatial reduction of data. This approach is related to reducing map data to one equivalent current dipole, but without further assumptions and without thereby suggesting brain locations of real generators.

EP Map Series

For the segmentation of a series of EP maps, a spatial window is erected around the locations of the maximum and the minimum in the first map of the series. Then the orbits or trajectories of the locations of the maximum and the minimum within the mapped area are plotted over time. As soon as one extreme leaves its spatial window, the segment is terminated, and a new segment starts for which the windows are reset around the new extreme locations (Lehmann 1984; Lehmann and Skrandies 1984; Brandeis and Lehmann 1986).

This adaptive space-oriented segmentation for identification of microstates was applied to brain electric field data collected from humans in an experimental paradigm where visual figures (triangles) consisting of "subjective" or "illusory" contours ("Kanisza figures") were briefly and repeatedly presented to the

16 subjects, alternating every 512 ms with the brief presentation of a "control" figure which consisted of the same visual elements in a different arrangement so as not to create the illusory triangle figure. The subject "attended" (counted silently) either the illusory figure or the control figure; the alternating figure in a given run thereby became an "ignored" target. The stimuli were shown either to the right or to the left visual field. Adaptive segmentation of the grand mean EP map series during the interstimulus interval yielded five segments that were analyzed for landscape differences between stimulus conditions. All maps which belonged to segment (as identified in the grand data) were averaged for each condition and subject. The maximum and minimum (extreme) locations as descriptors of each of these mean maps were then extracted, averaged over subjects and used for further statistical testing for significance of landscape differences between conditions using conventional ANOVA statistics. It turned out that "subjective figure" stimuli evoked field maps which in analyzed segments 1, 2 and 4 showed larger anterior-posterior distances between extreme voltage locations than "control figure" stimuli, and "attended" stimuli showed larger anterior-posterior extreme distances in segments 1, 3 and 4 than "ignored" stimuli. These results support the hypothesis that voluntary attention activates a brain functional resource that is automatically implemented when viewing a target with illusory contours, at least during segments 1 (168–200 ms) and 4 (296–376 ms) after stimulus presentation (see preliminary report in Brandeis and Lehmann 1986).

Spontaneous EEG Map Series

In adaptive segmentation of series of spontaneous EEG maps into time epochs of stationary microstates, one needs to consider that a brain state in terms of spontaneous activity is characterized by iterative reversals of polarity of the stationary landscape: periodic polarity reversal is considered to be inherent to all spontaneous activity. The periodic polarity reversals are associated with periodic variations of the global field power, for instance for alpha-EEG-dominated activity around 20 peaks per second (Figs. 9, 10). The signal-to-noise ratio of the momentary landscapes is obviously highest at the moments of peak global field power. It can be shown (Lehmann et al. 1987) that the maps collected and averaged exclusively at the moments of maximal global field power are very similar to the maps of FFT-computed band power using all available time points (Fig. 6).

Accordingly, the recognition of a brain microstate during spontaneous activity uses a modification of the extremes location approach discussed above for EP map series; this modification considers only maps at the moments of maximal global field power, and disregards polarity. As long as the two extremes remain within their spatial windows, the segment continues; if at a new frame one or both are outside of the windows, the segment terminates and new windows are erected. We found that during 2 min relaxed wakefulness with closed eyes, these spontaneous microstates in the alpha frequency band had a mean duration of 210 ms over six normal subjects; 50% of the entire time was covered

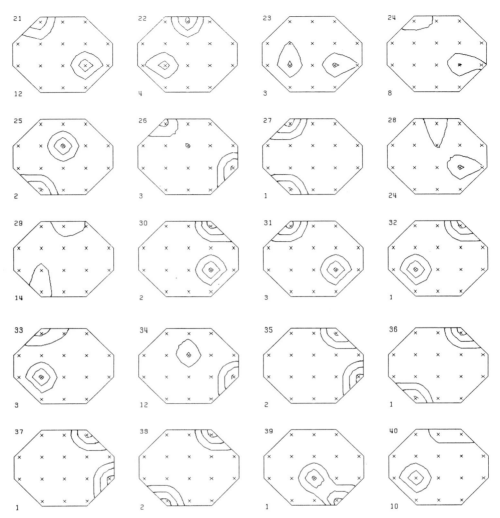

Fig. 13. Adaptive segmentation of spontaneous EEG map series using spatial criteria. The maps show the accumulated locations of the extreme potentials at the times of peak field power during successive segments. The figure illustrates the maps of 20 successive segments (microstates) of spontaneous EEG recorded with 16 electrodes during 5.5 s from a normal subject during rest with eyes closed. Digitally filtered 8–12 Hz band; head seen from above, left ear left, nose up. Electrode positions marked; most anterior electrode at Cz, most posterior 0.5 cm above inion. The number to the left *below* each map indicates the number of peak times of global field power (see Fig. 10) during which the segment lasted (this number multiplied by 50 is the approximate duration of the segment in milliseconds). The number to the left *above* each map is the serial segment number. Note that some types of maps (microstates) occurred several times, others once, some lasted for short times, others for long times. (Results from a study done with H. Ozaki and I. Pal; see also Lehmann et al. 1987)

by segments longer than 323 ms; the longest microstate segment lasted for 2656 ms (Lehmann et al. 1987). These typical segment durations are in the range of Libet's (1982) consciousness time and of minimum times in perception (e.g., Fig. 13 in Michaels and Turvey 1979). Our Fig. 13 shows a short sequence of maps of microstates as detected in the ongoing, spontaneous EEG during relaxation in a normal subject.

The functional significance of the adaptive segments of spontaneous activity was examined in a study of selective reaction time involving eight subjects, where rare and frequent tones of different pitch were presented and the subjects had to react to the rare tones. The segment type which existed at the moment of occurrence of each rare tone and the reaction time was determined. Each subject responded to 337 rare tones. Over subjects, there were similar differences in reaction time for the 26 different segment types which occurred in all subjects (Friedman ANOVA $\chi^2 = 40.6$, df $= 25$, $p < 0.025$). Thus, the behavior effect of information varies, depending on the different functional microstates as defined by the momentary EEG field map.

Brain electric microstates might serve as a common concept for EEG and EP analysis; certain types of spontaneously occurring segments might have map landscapes which are similar to those in event-related segments of known significance and this might be ascribed a putative significance in spontaneous EEG. Comprehensive analysis of spontaneous EEG over gross changes of vigilance could first use adaptive time segmentation (based on conventional temporal criteria) of the global field power curve to identify the borders of the gross states, then use the adaptive time segmentation (based on spatial criteria) to identify the microstates. Psychotic and other thought disorders might involve aberrant concatenation or aberrant occurrence frequencies of the different brain microstates.

Conclusion

The brain electric-magnetic field is a very sensitive indicator of brain functional states (information processing steps or modes) offering an extremely high temporal resolution. Mapping of EEG/EP data or analysis results leads to comprehensible display of the three- or more-dimensional information. Electric field result space is not directly related to brain space.

Landscapes of momentary (EP or EEG) brain maps depend on the baselines, not on the reference (only color or voltage offset depends on reference). Landscapes of FFT power maps depend on the reference, not on the baseline. Comparisons between momentary maps depend on the reference. Power maps vs the average reference display reference-independent and interpretable characteristics of the analysis epoch, i.e., the mean locations of the maximal and minimal voltages of all momentary maps.

In itself, mapping is neither data reduction nor data analysis. Analysis of EEG/EP data must extract reference-independent parameters from the field data if functional-physiological interpretation is the goal, for comprehensive assessment and statistical comparisons over subjects, conditions or times.

Data-reducing parameters for systematic survey and formal statistics in space are the locations of map maximal and minimal potential; in time, global field power (map hilliness). Global map dissimilarity compares two or more maps using one number. Map series can be adaptively segmented in time using map landscape descriptors that lead to the identification of functional brain microstates via stationary landscapes in evoked/event-related and in spontaneous brain activity. The functional significance of the microstates can be experimentally examined.

References

Adachi-Usami E, Lehmann D. (1983) Monocular and binocular evoked average potential field topography: upper and lower hemiretinal stimuli. Exp Brain Res 50:341–346

Ashida H, Tatsuno J, Okamoto J, Maru E (1984) Field mapping of EEG by unbiased polynomial interpolation. Comput Biomed Res 17:267–276

Bertrand O, Perrin F, Pernier J (1985) A theoretical justification of the average reference in topographic evoked potential studies. Electroencephalogr Clin Neurophysiol 62:462–464

Brandeis D, Lehmann D (1986) Event-related potentials of the brain and cognitive processes: approaches and applications. Neuropsychologia 24:151–168

Cohen D, Cuffin BN (1983) Demonstration of useful differences between magnetoencephalogram and electroencephalogram. Electroencephalogr Clin Neurophysiol 56:38–41

Dumermuth G, Lange B, Lehmann D, Meier CA, Dinkelmann R, Molinari L (1983) Spectral analysis of all-night sleep EEG in healthy adults. J Neurol 22:322–339

Grandori F (1984) Dipole localization methods (DLM) and auditory evoked brainstem potentials. Rev Laryngol Otol Rhinol (Bord) 105 (Suppl):171–178

Hjorth B (1975) On-line transformation of EEG scalp potentials into orthogonal source derivations. Electroencephalogr Clin Neurophysiol 39:526–530

Katznelson RD (1981) EEG recording, electrode placement and aspects of generator localization. In: Nunez P, Katznelson R (eds) Electric fields of the brain. Oxford University Press, London, pp 176–213

Koella WP (1982) A modern neurobiological concept of vigilance. Experientia 38:1426–1437

Koukkou-Lehmann M (1987) Hirnmechanismen normalen und schizophrenen Denkens. Springer, Berlin Heidelberg New York Tokyo

Koukkou M, Lehmann D (1983) Dreaming: the functional state-shift hypothesis. Br J Psychiatry 142:122–231

Koukkou M, Lehmann D, Angst J (1980) (eds) Functional states of the brain: their determinants. Elsevier, Amsterdam

Lehmann D (1971) Multichannel topography of human alpha EEG fields. Electroencephalogr Clin Neurophysiol 31:439–449

Lehmann D (1972) Human scalp EEG fields: evoked, alpha, sleep and spike-wave patterns. In: Petsche HH, Brazier MAB (eds) Synchronization of EEG activity in epilepsies. Springer, Berlin Heidelberg New York, pp 301–325

Lehmann D (1975) EEG phase differences and their physiological significance in scalp field studies. In: Dolce E, Künkel HH (eds) Computerized EEG analysis (CEAN). Fischer, Stuttgart, pp 102–110

Lehmann D (1981) Spatial analysis of evoked and spontaneous EEG potentials. In: Yamaguchi N, Fujisawa K (eds) Recent advances in EEG and EMG data processing. Elsevier, Amsterdam, pp 117–132

Lehmann D (1984) EEG assessment of brain activity: spatial aspects, segmentation and imaging. Int J Psychophysiol 1:267–276

Lehmann D (1986) Mapping, spatial analysis and adaptive time segmentation of EEG/EP data. In: Shagass C, Josiassen RC, Roemer RA (eds) Brain electrical potentials and psychopathology. Elsevier, Amsterdam, pp 27–46

Lehmann D, Julesz B (1978) Lateralized cortical potentials evoked in humans by dynamic random dot stereograms. Vision Res 1:1265–1271

Lehmann D, Skrandies W (1979) Multichannel mapping of spatial distributions of scalp potential fields evoked by checkerboard stimuli to different retinal areas. In: Lehmann D, Callaway E (eds) Human evoked potentials: applications and problems. Plenum, London, pp 201–214

Lehmann D, Skrandies W (1980) Reference-free identification of components of checkerboard-evoked multichannel potential fields. Electroencephalogr Clin Neurophysiol 48:609–621

Lehmann D, Skrandies W (1984) Spatial analysis of evoked potentials in man – an overview. Progr Neurobiol 23:227–250

Lehmann D, Kavanagh RN, Fender DH (1969) Field studies of averaged visually evoked EEG potentials in a patient with split chiasm. Electroencephalogr Clin Neurophysiol 26:193–199

Lehmann D, Meles H, Mir Z (1977) Average multichannel potential fields evoked from upper and lower hemi-retina: latency differences. Electroencephalogr Clin Neurophysiol 43:725–731

Lehmann D, Darcey TM, Skrandies W (1982) Intracerebral scalp fields evoked by hemiretinal checkerboard reversal, and modeling of their dipole generators. In: Courjon J, Maugiere F, Revol M (eds) Clinical application of evoked potentials in neurology. Raven, New York, pp 41–48

Lehmann D, Ozaki H, Pal I (1986) Averaging of spectral power and phase via vector diagram best fits without reference electrode or reference channel. Electroencephalogr Clin Neurophysiol 64:350–363

Lehmann D (1987) Principles of spatial analysis. In: Gevins A, Rémond A (eds) Handbook of electroencephalography and clinical neurophysiology, vol 1: Methods of analysis of brain electrical and magnetic signals. Elsevier, Amsterdam, pp 309–354

Lehmann D, Ozaki H, Pal I (1987) EEG alpha map series: brain micro-states by space-oriented adaptive segmentation. Electroencephalogr Clin Neurophysiol 67:271–288

Libet B (1982) Brain stimulation of the study of neuronal functions for conscious experience. Hum Neurobiol 1:235–242

Michaels CF, Turvey MT (1979) Central sources of visual masking: indexing structures supporting seeing at a single, brief glance. Psychol Res 41:1–61

Offner FF (1950) The EEG as potential mapping: the value of the average monopolar reference. Electroencephalogr Clin Neurophysiol 2:215–216

Rémond A (1960) Poursuit de la significance en EEG. I. Problème de la référence spatiale. Rev Neurol 102:412–415

Skrandies W (1987) The upper and lower visual field of man: electrophysiological and functional differences. Prog Sens Physiol 8:1–93

Skrandies W, Lehmann D (1982) Spatial principal components of multichannel maps evoked by lateral visual half-field stimuli. Electroencephalogr Clin Neurophysiol 54:662–667

Thickbroom GW, Mastaglia FL, Carroll WM, Davies HD (1984) Source derivation: application to topographic mapping of visual evoked potentials. Electroencephalogr Clin Neurophysiol 59:279–285

Ueno S, Matsuoka S, Mizoguchi T, Nagashima M, Cheng C (1975) Topographic computer display of abnormal EEG in patients with CNS diseases. Memoirs of the Faculty of Engineering Kyushu University 34:195–209

Topographic Mapping of Generators of Somatosensory Evoked Potentials*

J.E. Desmedt[1]

Introduction

The current interest in somatosensory evoked potentials (SEP) after electrical stimulation of peripheral nerves in humans results from the feasibility of noninvasive studies involving electronic averaging. Such spinal or brain averaged responses do not represent variations of membrane potentials at single neurons, but are compound profiles built up of a sequence of distinct components. Physiological analysis of the corresponding neural generators is important, since data obtained in other mammals cannot be safely extrapolated to man. A robust data base on human responses is essential for their changes in health or disease to be understood and used for clinical diagnosis or investigations of the electrophysiological correlates of psychological processes such as selective attention or memory (see Callaway et al. 1978; Desmedt 1979; Hillyard and Kutas 1983).

Background Data on Recording of Evoked Potentials

Volume Conduction of Potentials in the Brain

Evoked potentials recorded from the body surface are small (about 1 µV) and present complex spatial distributions. They must be interpreted in conjunction with the properties of potential fields in conductive media. Phasic changes of extracellular potential fields are produced by volume conduction either of a synchronized volley of action potentials in nerve trunk or corticipetal tract (Lorente de N 1947), or of postsynaptic potentials generated in the geometrically coherent assemblies of soma-dendrites (Eccles 1951).

Lorente de N (1947) distinguished several pertinent sets of geometric parameters. A spike volley in a tract of parallel nerve fibers can be viewed as equivalent to a propagated dipole and it represents a good example of an "open field" system that can generate recordable extracellular potential fields in the volume conductor. Beyond the termination of such a tract, volume conduction of the dipole is recorded as a positive-going approach wave without subsequent negativity ("killed end" recording).

---

* This research has been supported by the Fonds de la Recherche Scientifique Médicale, Belgium

[1] Brain Research Unit, University of Brussels, Boulevard de Waterloo 115, 1000 Brussels, Belgium

Coherent gemetrical orientation of the individual nerve fibers in the tract is required for observing sizeable volume conduction at a distance. Cancellation of individual potentials fields would occur if the individual fibers were oriented in different directions. Noncoherent geometry is actually prevailing in many central nuclei and it corresponds to the "closed field" system of Lorente de N (1947). For example, depolarization of neurons in a nuclear structure with dendrites radiating in different directions would produce inward flows of current toward the center of the nucleus, but virtually no recordable potential difference outside its anatomical boundaries (Klee and Rall 1977).

Early interpretations of brain waves in electroencephalography (EEG) considered summation of action potentials as a possibility. Eccles (1951) made an essential contribution when he proposed that cortical EEG potentials were rather related to the excitatory postsynaptic potentials generated in the geometrically coherent apical dendrites of cortical pyramidal neurons. These indeed represent an "open-field" system (see Towe 1966; Humphrey 1968; Creutzfeldt et al. 1969; Klee and Rall 1977; Mitzdorf 1985).

Nearfield and Farfield Potentials

Human SEP studies have only recently identified the true practical relevance of volume conduction of potentials generated at a distance from the recording electrodes. This important issue has been clarified by the use of noncephalic reference recording (Cracco and Cracco 1976; Desmedt and Cheron 1980).

As a rule, electrophysiological recordings use differential amplifiers to reject in-phase (common mode) interference. Therefore, all recordings are in fact bipolar and they measure the potential difference between the "active" electrode connected to grid 1 and the "reference" electrode connected to grid 2 of the amplifier. If the reference is placed on the head, it also picks up brain potentials and subtracts them from the brain potentials derived by the "active" electrode at another head site.

Moreover, both electrodes are influenced to a similar extent by the widespread potential fields that are volume-conducted from distant (subcortical) neural generators, so that these potentials cancel out in such montages. Such severe distortions are avoided when using a noncephalic reference placed on the hand or shoulder on the nonstimulated side.

Noncephalic reference recording ensures that any open field generator producing a potential difference at the scalp will indeed be manifested in the recorded trace. Then, one can conveniently distinguish between "nearfield" and "farfield" potentials (Jewett and Williston 1981).

Most cortical SEP generators are located near the brain convexity right under the skull (this is not the case for all auditory or visual areas in man) and they can be considered as relatively nearfield for scalp recording. The scalp electrodes are nevertheless 12–30 mm away from the active cortex which results in attentuation by a factor of about 10 to 80 for scalp as compared to direct cortical recordings (Domino et al. 1964). The SEP potential gradients are somewhat smoothed out because of the distance from cortex to scalp, but this does not prevent distinct cortical generators from being mapped out (Desmedt and Cheron 1981 b; Mauguière et al. 1983 a; Desmedt et al. 1987). Spinal potentials recorded through electrodes over the neck or back can also be considered nearfield.

By contrast, subcortical SEP generators are even more distant from the scalp. Hence, their volume-conducted field potentials are smaller and present much smaller potential gradients over the scalp. Electronic averaging which increases the signal-to-noise ratio is indeed a powerful technique for disclosing even these very small farfield potentials. The terms nearfield and farfield are convenient to use but they should not imply a strict dichotomy, since they relate in fact to a continuum of voltage distributions (for more or less distant neural generators of different strengths and orientations) in the volume conductor of the head.

Thus, scalp-recorded brain potentials relate to open field generators, and the extent to which any generator will be represented in the averaged response depends on several factors: geometry of the active neural units (Klee and Rall 1977); temporal synchronization, duration and spatial distribution of the transmembrane currents in these neural units ("size" of resulting dipole) (Humphrey 1968); and amount of summation or cancellation or field potentials volume-conducted from multiple concomitant sources.

Methods

The data were acquired from normal subjects of either sex and of 20–35 years who had given informed consent and were free from neurological disease. The subjects were selected from a larger group on the basis of good yields for SEP averaging and ability to relax fully so as to minimize muscle and blink interference. They lay comfortably on a couch in a soundproofed, electrically shielded and air-conditioned room at 24° C. The procedure was noninvasive and carried no risk. Electrical square pulses of 0.2 ms duration and 3–10 mA were delivered either to the left median nerve at the wrist (about thumb twitch threshold), or to fingers. The upper limb temperature was 35–37° C.

Scalp, earlobe and neck sites were recorded with sterile unvarnished stainless steel needles of 0.2 mm diameter inserted subcutaneously. The reference electrode was placed on the right hand or shoulder. Early SEP components include high-frequency transients that require the system bandpass to extend from about 1 Hz to 3 kHz (Desmedt et al. 1974). Later components involve fewer high-frequency transients and will not be distorted with low pass set at 100 or 200 Hz. Differential amplifiers were used in conjunction with a PDP 11–34 averaging computer, using bin width of 125 or 250 μs (details in Desmedt 1977; Desmedt and Cheron 1980, 1981 a, b; Desmedt et al. 1987 a). The last-named paper discusses in detail current issues and methods for bit-mapped imaging of potential fields. SEP components were labeled from their positive (P) or negative (N) polarity and modal peak latency in normal adults of average body size.

Results

Early SEP Components

Noncephalic reference recording of SEPs to upper limb stimulation discloses characteristic response profiles at the neck (Fig. 1 B, C) and at the scalp (Fig. 1 A). The initial positivity P9 seen at both sites is followed by the N11 and N13 negativities at the neck, but by two positive dips P11 and P14, followed in turn by the N18 negativity, at the scalp.

The P9 farfield precedes the arrival of the peripheral nerve volley at the cervical spinal cord and is generated by the volley as it travels in the brachial plexus (Desmedt and Cheron 1980; Desmedt and Nguyen 1984). P9 persists while all subsequent SEP components are lost in patients with dorsal spinal roots avulsed by traction injuries (Anziska and Cracco 1981).

The spinal entry time of the afferent volley fits with the onset of the negative N11 nearfield component recorded at the low posterior neck (Fig. 1 C) and

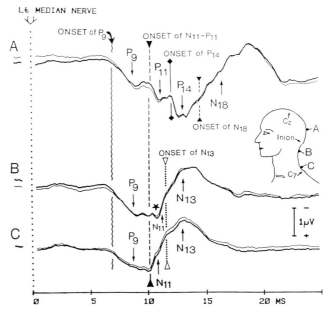

Fig. 1. SEPs after stimulation of left median nerve at the wrist. The two traces superimposed represent separate averages of different runs to show consistency of waveform for the same recording electrode. Noncephalic (NC) reference on the right hand dorsum. *A* Recording from posterior scalp above the inion (see schema). *B* Recording from upper posterior neck at the C2 vertebra. *C* recording from the lower posterior neck at the C6 vertebra. Negativity of the active electrode registers upward in this and subsequent figures. The vertical *wavy line* identifies onset of the P9 farfield. The vertical *interrupted line* identifies onset of neck N11 nearfield or scalp P11 farfield, which share the same generator. The shorter vertical *dotted line* identifies onset of the spinal N13. Notice that N13 onset (*B, C*) occurs about 1 ms before the P14 onset (*A*). N13 has a longer duration than P14. (From Desmedt and Nguyen 1984)

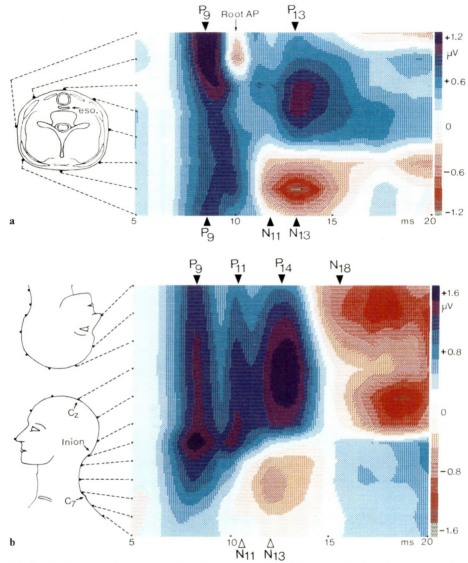

Fig. 2a, b. Bit-mapped color imaging of neck potential fields. Stimulation of the left median nerve at the wrist. Noncephalic reference on the dorsum of the right hand. Voltage increments are represented by different hues of blue-purple for positive or red for negative. **a** Spatiotemporal imaging of the changes in SEP fields over time. The mapping is based on eight electrodes placed in a horizontal plane at midneck (*ordinate*). The time (*abscissa*) is from 5 to 20 ms after the left median nerve stimulus. After the deep blue source around the neck at 9 ms (P9 farfield), a negativity develops at the back of the neck (N11 and N13) while a concomitant positivity appears at the anterior neck (P13). **b** Spatiotemporal imaging of SEP farfields. The mapping is based on 12 skin electrodes placed along the midline from the upper back to neck, scalp and tip of the nose (*ordinate*). The time (*abscissa*) is from 5 to 20 ms after the left median nerve stimulus. The three blue sources, corresponding respectively to the P9, P11 and P14 farfields have a vertical axis, indicating a stationary latency throughout the volume

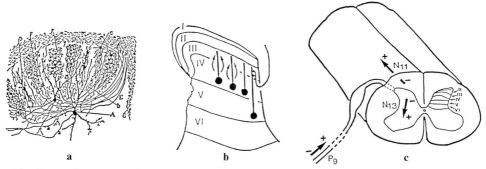

Fig. 3a–c. The N13 nearfield neural generator in the dorsal horn of the cervical spinal cord. **a** Drawing by Cajal (1909) of the bushy arborizations formed by the large diameter primary afferents which enter the dorsal horn from its mesial side. **b** Sketch of relay neurons of layers IV and V of the dorsal horn whose apical dendrites extend into layer III, where they receive excitatory synapses from the bushy aborizations of primary afferents from skin. Depolarization of these apical dendrites creates a coherent dipole sheet with negative at the back and positive in front. **c** Sketch of the equivalent dipoles reflected in the P9 farfield (oblique axis), in the N11 nearfield (longitudinal axis) and in the N13–P13 nearfields (horizontal axis)

also with the onset of the positive P11 farfield recorded over the scalp (Fig. 1A). Both N11 and P11 are thought to reflect the action potentials volley which ascends in the dorsal column. Actually, the onset latency of the N11 nearfield is somewhat later at the upper neck (where it is preceded by an approach positive dip) as compared to the lower neck. More distant scalp electrodes only register a P11 positive farfield, as they are situated beyond pathway termination in the cuneate nucleus (located about 1 cm *above* foramen magnum) (Desmedt and Cheron 1980; Desmedt and Nguyen 1984).

Noncephalic reference recording from posterior neck shows that a second negativity N13 is superimposed on N11 (see notch on ascending limb of the neck negativity). The significance of N13 was elucidated when it was shown to phase-reverse into a positive P13 in front of the spinal cord (noninvasive recordings with esophageal electrodes) (Desmedt and Cheron 1981a; Desmedt and Nguyen 1984).

Bit-mapped color imaging of SEP field topography around the neck volume conductor reveals (a) the circular positivity of the P9 brachial plexus farfield; (b) the negativities of N11 and N13 at the posterior neck; and (c) the concomitant P13 positivity at the anterior neck (Fig. 2a). These and other data substantiate the segmental nature of the N13–P13 generator whose equivalent dipole

---

conductor of neck and head. Whereas P9 extends down to lower neck, P11 encroaches only over the upper neck (see approach positive dip in Fig. 1B) while P14 does not extend further down than the inion. From about 10 ms after the stimulus, the neck negative field (*red*) is seen to extend progressively from lower to upper neck (propagation of N11 nearfield). After 15 ms, the whole scalp goes negative (widespread N18 brainstem response). (From Desmedt and Nguyen 1984).

has an axis at right angles to that of the neck (Fig. 3c). The N13 generator involves excitatory postsynaptic potentials evoked by large diameter afferents from the skin (type A-alpha) traveling along the medial side of the dorsal horn over a few spinal segments and emitting branches which penetrate the dorsal horn and bend backwards to form the bushy terminals of Cajal in layer III (Fig. 3a). These terminals synapse onto the apical dendrites of relay neurons whose somata are located in layers IV and V (Fig. 3b). Depolarization of these dendrites creates a sink at the level of layer III and a source in deeper layers of the cervical spinal cord. Due to their consistent geometry, these soma-dendrites form an open field generator producing extracellular fields with negativity at the neck and positivity anteriorly (Desmedt 1984; Desmedt and Nguyen 1984). Because of its horizontal axis, the spinal N13–P13 generator does not produce any farfield at the top of the head which is at right angle to its own axis.

The third positive farfield, P14, is recorded all over the scalp as far back as the inion, but it is not seen at the posterior neck (Fig. 1a). Its neural generator is located above foramen magnum and corresponds to the afferent volley in the medial lemniscus (Desmedt and Cheron 1980, 1981a; Emerson et al. 1984). P14 persists in patients with thalamic lesions that eliminate all subsequent SEP response (Nakanishi et al. 1978; Chiappa et al. 1980; Anziska and Cracco 1981; Maugière et al. 1983b). Depth recording is also in line with a brainstem P14 generator (Suzuki and Mayanagi 1984).

Bit-mapped imaging of SEP farfields documents their widespread distribution and distinct extension over the neck (Fig. 2b). The farfield topography over an array of midline electrodes arranged from the back along the neck and scalp up to the tip of the nose strikingly discloses characteristic features, as seen in Fig. 2b, where noncephalic reference recording is used and the abscissa represents time in the spatiotemporal display. The positive farfields P9, P11 and P14 are each imaged as an elongated blue area whose axis is sharply vertical, indicating a stationary latency. This implies that their onset and peak correspond to the arrival of the volume-conducted afferent volley at precise levels along the somatosensory pathway. Each farfield extends virtually throughout the 180° solid angle of the volume conductor ahead of the direction of propagation of the corresponding action potentials volley, with a maximum voltage in the scalp area targeted by the axis of propagation. At the back, P14 fails to extend below the inion, which is in line with its generator being located above the foramen magnum. The P9 field extends much further down to the lower neck, which obviously relates to its brachial plexus generator projecting volume-conducted potentials throughout the neck and head. The P11 field encroaches over the high neck during its initial part and this corresponds to the approach positive dip of the upper neck response seen in Fig. 1B.

At the 10–11 ms latency, the imaging over the neck shows a clearly oblique boundary between blue (positive) and red (negative) areas. This obliquity in the spatiotemporal display indicates that the N11 negativity first appears at the low neck and subsequently propagates upward to the high neck. It is a striking illustration of the N11 latency shift from lower to upper neck as the afferent volley propagates up the dorsal column pathway.

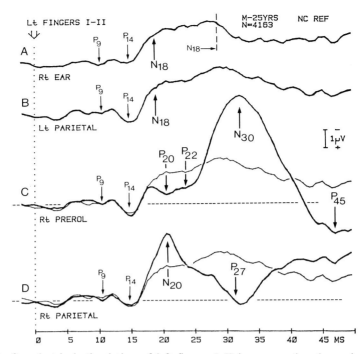

Fig. 4. Averaged SEP after electrical stimulation of left fingers I–II in a normal male aged 25 years. Noncephalic reference on right hand dorsum. *A* Right earlobe showing P9–P14 farfields and N18 (which lasts up to about 28 ms). *B* Left parietal scalp ipsilateral to fingers stimulated showing a large N18. *C* Right prerolandic scalp at 7 cm from midline (thick trace) superimposed on the left parietal trace which is used as "baseline" for identifying the N18 underlying the cortically generated components P20, P22 and N30. *D* Right parietal scalp superimposed on left parietal trace with cortical components N20 and P27. (From Desmedt et al. 1987)

The duration (horizontal extent) of the N13 field is longer than the duration of either the P11 or P14 fields at the scalp. This is in line with the fact that the spinal N13 nearfield reflects nonpropagated postsynaptic potentials in the apical dendrites of spinal interneurons (Fig. 3), whereas the positive farfields reflect spike volleys (Desmedt and Cheron 1981a, b; Desmedt and Nguyen 1984).

After about 15 ms, significant SEP fields occur, not at the neck, but over the head with a widespread N18 negativity (Fig. 2b). This is a major feature of the SEP response recorded with noncephalic reference (Desmedt and Cheron 1981b; Desmedt and Bourguet 1985). The N18 appears virtually in isolation at the parietal scalp ipsilateral to the upper limb stimulated (Fig. 4B) and also at the earlobes (Fig. 4A). At the contralateral parietal scalp, the N20 and P27 focal cortical responses are seen to diverge and superimpose on this N18 "baseline" (Fig. 4D). At the contralateral frontal scalp, the P20, P22 and N30 responses similarly superimpose on the N18 baseline (Fig. 4C). N18 actually reflects subcortical generators because, in patients with a unilateral thalamic

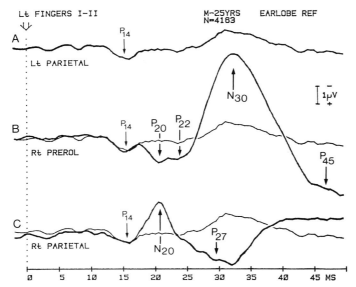

Fig. 5. Same experiment as Fig. 4, but with right earlobe reference recording. *A* Left parietal (ipsilateral) scalp showing no early response after the P14 farfield except for a small negativity diffusing from the front. *B* Right prerolandic scalp (*thick trace*) superimposed on the left parietal trace showing cortical components P20, P22 and P30. *C* Right parietal scalp (*thick trace*) superimposed on the left parietal trace showing N20 and P27. (From Desmedt et al. 1987)

lesion, stimulation on the affected side elicits a bilateral N18 (mean total duration 19 ms) while all subsequent SEP components are lost (Mauguière et al. 1983b). N18 is thought to be generated in brainstem nuclei with open field geometry, such as the superior colliculus, which receive short-latency lemniscal input. Depth recordings also suggest a brainstem generator for N18 (Hashimoto 1984).

Figure 5 presents the SEP data of Fig. 4, but with earlobe reference. This is roughly equivalent to subtracting the N18 response (also present at the earlobe) from the scalp traces. For bit-mapped imaging, it is indeed more convenient to display earlobe than noncephalic reference data in order to avoid the prolonged negative shift of the baseline. Earlobe reference recording is indeed compatible with the differentiation of focal cortical SEP responses.

Figure 6 presents a series of frozen maps at the stated latencies after stimulation of left fingers. With noncephalic reference (A–F), the scalp goes negative just after the P14 farfield (A), and the positive components P20 (C), P22 (D), P27 (E) and P45 (F) are seen as relative reductions from the (red) negative background.

Only P45 (F) reaches actual positive levels (blue). With earlobe reference (G–L), the baseline remains virtually at about zero and the positive components P20 (I), P22 (J), P27 (K) and P45 (L), depicted in blue, are clearly differentiated from the negative components N20 (I) and N30 (K) (Desmedt et al. 1987).

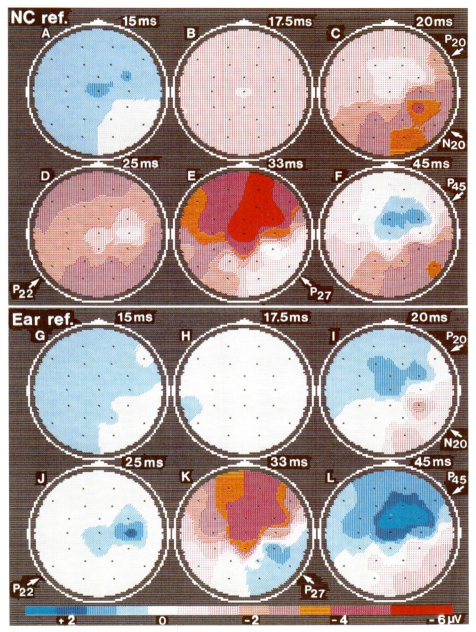

Fig. 6A–L. Bit-mapped color imaging of SEP after stimulation of left fingers I–II in the same experiment. Frozen maps based on 27 recording channels at latencies indicated. Each map includes 4000 pixels calculated by interpolation of averaged data at the four nearest electrodes using third power of distance for weighting. The voltage steps of the color scale (*red* negative, *blue* positive) are too large to provide enough detail for smaller components. **A–F,** Noncephalic reference recording in which the large N18 drives all maps into the red and the positive components P20, P22, P27 and P45 appear as reductions from ambient negativity. **G–L,** Right earlobe reference recording of same data in which the baseline remains close to zero. (From Desmedt et al. 1987)

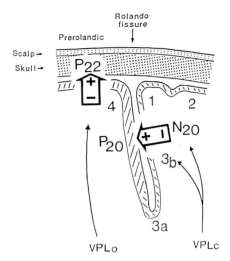

Fig. 7. Cartoon of perirolandic SEP generators about 20 ms after contralateral median nerve or fingers stimulation. Parasagittal section through fissure of Rolando (drawn roughly to scale) with cortical areas 2, 1, 3b, 3a, and 4. Thalamocortical inputs from the ventroposterolateral caudal nucleus (VPLc) to parietal cortex or from the ventroposterolateral oral nucleus (VPLo) to motor area 4 are sketched. A tangential dipole in area 3_b in the posterior bank of the fissure of Rolando (about 25 mm from the scalp surface) concomitantly generates the parietal N20 and the frontal P20 fields. A radial dipole in motor area 4 generates the prerolandic P22 field with distinct spatiotemporal features. (From Desmedt et al. 1987)

Though confusing at first sight, the maps obtained with noncephalic reference recording (Fig. 6A–F) are consistent with those recorded with earlobe reference.

The data are also pertinent to current issues about dipole generators of early cortical SEP (see Desmedt et al. 1987a). Briefly, the diffuse frontal positivity P20 concomitant with the parietal N20 (Fig. 6C, I) reflects an equivalent dipole which is tangential to the scalp surface and located in parietal area 3b, at about 25 mm from scalp in the posterior bank of the Rolando fissure (Fig. 7). The neurons columns have indeed an anteroposterior orientation in area 3b which is a major recipient of cutaneous inputs from the ventroposterolateral caudal nucleus (Jones 1983). The oblique line of polarity reversal between the N20 and P20 fields roughly corresponds to the orientation of the fissure of Rolando (Deiber et al. 1986). Magnetic recordings assessed the tangential dipole depth and disproved the possible subcortical origin of N20 (Okada et al. 1984). A separate generator is involved in the prerolandic P22 field (Fig. 6D, J), displayed as concentric positive isopotentials with no adjacent negativity (Desmedt and Bourguet 1985). This corresponds to a cortical dipole sheet with radial orientation with respect to the scalp (Fig. 7).

Cognitive SEP Components in Selective Attention Tasks

Components invoked during cognitive processing must be differentiated from obligatory, or exogenous, components which are evoked by identical sensory stimuli in the absence of any perceptual task. Cognitive SEP components, including very early ERP events, were analyzed in randomly intermixed runs of nontarget stimuli and target stimuli which were delivered to several fingers of the left hand.

In attended runs, the subject pressed a microswitch key with the right index finger for each target. Control no-task runs in counterbalanced sequences involved identical stimuli delivered alone ($p = 1.0$) with instructions to disregard

Rare Target

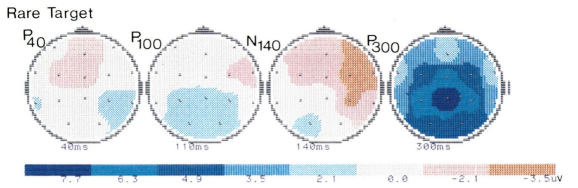

Fig. 8. Bit-mapped imaging of cognition-related components in the contralateral parietal SEP to left target finger stimulus. Subtraction mapping obtained by algebraic subtraction of control maps at the same latency (identical finger stimuli delivered in a homogeneous 100% series in no-task runs) from the selective attention maps evoked by target finger stimuli. The frozen maps display the cognitive P40, P100, N140 and P300 components. The latency of each frozen map is indicated

these stimuli altogether. The cognitive components were identified by subtraction mapping, namely by subtracting the control no-task maps from the maps recorded in selective attention runs (Desmedt et al. 1987b).

Figure 8 presents frozen "subtraction maps" at latencies chosen to display a number of cognitive SEP components. The first item is the P40 positivity that appears shortly after arrival of the target input at the parietal cortex. P40 shows a remarkably restricted distribution over the contralateral parietal scalp (Fig. 8) (Desmedt et al. 1983). The second component P100 (Desmedt and Robertson 1977) presents a more extensive scalp topography. Independent evidence shows that P100 has distinct features that makes it a separate cognitive event from P40. The third component N140 has a remarkable precentral topography. Thereafter, the P300 presents a rather symmetrical topography with the expected postcentral maximum.

On the basis of previous work, researchers had considered that cognition-related potential changes did not occur earlier than about 70 ms after the stimulus (Hillyard et al. 1973; Desmedt and Robertson 1977; Hillyard and Kutas 1983). This view must now be changed, since the somatosensory P40 represents a robust earlier signa associated with target analysis (Desmedt et al. 1983, 1987b). P40 cannot thought to be a result of some stimulus identification process because it is too early, only a few milliseconds after the afferent volley actually reaches the parietal cortex. Rather, P40 must reflect an anticipatory mechanism that primes the receiving cortex for the expected target.

The subsequent cognitive components, P100 and N140, are consistent features of cognitive SEP (Fig. 8) (Desmedt and Robertson 1977).

They presumably reflect steps in the perceptual processing which leads to target identification. The reason why a major component such as P100 has a positive polarity, whereas equivalent components are negative for auditory or visual targets, remains obscure. These components precede the P300 which other evcidence has shown to be a postdecisional event reflecting "closure" of the cognitive channel (Desmedt and Debecker 1979). The widespread topography of P300 (Fig. 8) as well as its surface-positive polarity seem to be compatible with this view insofar as part of the P300 neural generators are located in the cortex. An additional component generator of P300 has been demonstrated in the hippocampal formation (Halgren et al. 1980).

References

Anziska B, Cracco RQ (1981) Short latency SEPs to median nerve stimulation: comparison of recording methods and origin of components. Electroencephalogr Clin Neurophysiol 52:531–539

Callaway E, Tueting P, Koslow S (eds) (1978) Event-related potentials in man. Academic, New York

Chiappa KH, Choi SK, Young RR (1980) Short-latency somatosensory evoked potentials following median nerve stimulation in patients with neurological lesions. In: Desmedt JE (ed) Clinical uses of cerebral, brainstem and spinal somatosensory evoked potentials. Prog Clin Neurophysiol 7:264–281

Cracco RQ, Cracco JB (1976) Somatosensory evoked potentials in man: farfield potentials. Electroencephalogr Clin Neurophysiol 41:460–466

Creutzfeldt O, Watanabe S, Lux HD (1969) Relations between EEG phenomena and potentials in single cells. Electroencephalogr Clin Neurophysiol 20:1–18

Deiber MP, Giard MH, Mauguière F (1986) Separate generators with distinct orientations for N20 and P22 somatosensory evoked potentials to finger stimulation. Electroencephalogr Clin Neurophysiol 65:321–334

Desmedt JE (1977) Some observations on the methodology of cerebral evoked potentials in man. In: Desmedt JE (ed) Attention, voluntary contraction and event-related cerebral potentials. Prog Clin Neurophysiol 1:12–29

Desmedt JE (ed) (1979) Cognitive components in cerebral event-related potentials and selective attention. Progr Clin Neurophysiol, vol 6. Karger, Basel

Desmedt JE (1984) Non-invasive analysis of the spinal cord generators activated by somatosensory input in man: nearfield and farfield potentials. In: Creutzfeldt O, Schmidt RF, Willis WD (eds) Sensory motor integration in the nervous system. Springer, Berlin Heidelberg New York, pp 45–62 (Experimental brain research series, vol 9)

Desmedt JE, Robertson D (1977) Differential enhancement of early and late components of the cerebral somatosensory evoked potentials during fast sequential cognitive tasks in man. J Physiol (Lond) 271:761–782

Desmedt JE, Debecker J (1979) Waveform and neural mechanism of the decision P350 elicited without pre-stimulus CNV or readiness potential in random sequences of near-threshold auditory clicks and finger stimuli. Electroencephalogr Clin Neurophysiol 47:648–670

Desmedt JE, Cheron G (1980) Central somatosensory conduction in man: neural generators and interpeak latencies of the farfield components recorded from neck and right or left scalp and earlobes. Electroencephalogr Clin Neurophysiol 50:382–403

Desmedt JE, Cheron G (1981a) Prevertebral (oesophageal) recording of subcortical somatosensory evoked potentials in man: the spinal P13 component and the dual nature of the spinal generators. Electroencephalogr Clin Neurophysiol 52:257–275

Desmedt JE, Cheron G (1981b) Non-cephalic reference recording of early somatosensory potentials to finger stimulation in adult or aging man: differentiation of widespread N18 and contralateral N20 from the prerolandic P22 and N30 components. Electroencephalogr Clin Neurophysiol 52:553–570

Desmedt JE, Nguyen TH (1984) Bit-mapped color imaging of the potential fields of propagated and segmental subcortical components of somatosensory evoked potentials in man. Electroencephalogr Clin Neurophysiol 58:481–497

Desmedt JE, Bourguet M (1985) Color imaging of scalp topography of parietal and frontal components of somatosensory evoked potentials to stimulation of median or posterior tibial nerve in man. Electroencephalogr Clin Neurophysiol 62:1–17

Desmedt JE, Brunko E, Debecker J, Carmeliet J (1974) The system bandpass required to avoid distortion of early components when averaging somatosensory evoked potentials. Electroencephalogr Clin Neurophysiol 37:407–410

Desmedt JE, Nguyen TH, Bourguet M (1983) The cognitive P40, N60 and P100 components of somatosensory evoked potentials and the earliest electrical signs of sensory processing in man. Electroencephalogr Clin Neurophysiol 56:272–282

Desmedt JE, Hguyen TH, Bourguet M (1987) Bit-mapped color imaging of human evoked potentials with reference to the N20, P22, P27 and N30 somatosensory components. Electroencephalogr Clin Neurophysiol 68:1–19

Desmedt JE, Tomberg C, Zhu Y, Nguyen TH (1987b) Bit-mapped scalp field topographies of early and late cognitive components to somatosensory (finger) target stimuli. Electroenceph Clin Neurophysiol Suppl 40:170–177

Domino EF, Matsuoka S, Waltz J, Cooper I (1964) Simultaneous recordings from scalp and epidural somatosensory evoked response in man. Science 145:1199–1200

Eccles JC (1951) Interpretation of action potentials evoked in the cerebral cortex. Electroencephalogr Clin Neurophysiol 3:449–464

Emerson DG, Seyal M, Pedley TA (1984) Somatosensory evoked potentials following median nerve stimulation: the cervical components. Brain 107:169–182

Halgren E, Squires NK, Wilson CL, Rohrbaugh JW, Babb TL, Crandall PH (1980) Endogenous potentials generated in the human hippocampal formation and amygdala by infrequent events. Science 210:803–805

Hashimoto I (1984) Somatosensory evoked potentials from the human brainstem: origins of short-latency potentials. Electroencephalogr Clin Neurophysiol 57:221–227

Hillyard SA, Hink RF, Schwent VL, Picton TW (1973) Electrical signs of selective attention in the human brain. Science 182:177–179

Hillyard SA, Kutas M (1983) Electrophysiology of cognitive processing. Annu Rev Neurosci 34:33–61

Humphrey DR (1968) Re-analysis of the antidromic cortical response. On the contribution of cell discharge and PSPs to the evoked potentials. Electroencephalogr Clin Neurophysiol 25:421–442

Jewett DL, Williston JS (1971) Auditory evoked farfields averaged from the scalp in humans. Brain 94:681–696

Jones EG (1983) The nature of the afferent pathways conveying short-latency inputs to primate motor cortex. In: Desmedt JE (ed) Motor control mechanisms in health and disease. Raven, New York, pp 263–285

Klee M, Rall W (1977) Computed potentials of cortically arranged populations of neurons. J Neurophysiol 40:647–666

Lorente de NR (1947) Action potential of the motoneurons of the hypoglossus nucleus. J Cell Compar Physiol 29:207–287

Mauguière F, Desmedt JE, Courjon J (1983a) Astereognosis and dissociated loss of frontal or parietal components of somatosensory evoked potentials in hemispheric lesions. Brain 106:271–311

Mauguière F, Desmedt JE, Courjon J (1983b) Neural generators of N18 and P14 farfield somatosensory evoked potentials: patients with lesion of thalamus or thalamo-cortical radiations. Electroencephalogr Clin Neurophysiol 56:283–292

Mitzdorf U (1985) Current source density method and application in cat cerebral cortex: investigations of evoked potentials and EEG phenomena. Physiol Rev 65:37–100

Nakanishi T, Shimada Y, Sukata M, Toyokura Y (1978) The initial positive component of scalp-recorded somatosensory evoked potentials in normal subjects and in patients with neurological disorders. Electroencephalogr Clin Neurophysiol 45:26–34

Okada YC, Tanenbaum R, Williamson SJ, Kaufman L (1984) Somatotopic organization of the human somatosensory cortex revealed by neuromagnetic measurements. Exp Brain Res 56:197–205

Suzuki I, Mayanagi Y (1984) Intracranial recording of short-latency somatosensory evoked potentials in man: identification of origin of each component. Electroencephalogr Clin Neurophysiol 59:286–296

Towe AL (1966) On the nature of the primary evoked response. Exp Neurol 15:113–139

Neurometric Topographic Mapping of EEG and Evoked Potential Features: Application to Clinical Diagnosis and Cognitive Evaluation

E.R. JOHN[1,2], L.S. PRICHEP[1,2], J. FRIEDMAN[1], and P. EASTON[1]

Introduction

There is widespread agreement that topographic maps of EEG measures are difficult to evaluate unless referred to a normative data base. This raises the difficult question of how "normal" should be defined. Because the particular target of our method, which we call "neurometrics," was cognitive dysfunctions and psychiatric disorders, the instruments used to evaluate our "normal" subjects included an extensive psychiatric and neuropsychological test battery, a psychiatric as well as neurological examination, achievement tests, and determination of eye, hand, and foot dominance. Medical and psychosocial histories, pre- and perinatal data, and current and past school or work records were also evaluated. The subset of instruments used varied with age. Subjects with significant abnormal findings or events in their history which placed them at risk were excluded. Additional exclusion criteria included current use of prescription drugs, a history of head injury or loss of consciousness, any previous EEG or neurological examination, and febrile convulsions.

Obviously, normal results on medical or neurological examination alone would have been clearly inadequate for our purposes, since they have little predictive value for cognitive functions or psychiatric competence. Our concern was more to confirm the ability of the normal subject to function adequately within the demands of his life situation than to achieve some universally acceptable definition of normality. While we tried to avoid the tight variance of a "supranormal" reference group, we were not as concerned about false positives as we would have been if we had been developing a mass screening method. Most of the patients expected to be compared against these norms would have displayed symptoms bringing them to the attention of a physician; false negatives were of greater concern to us.

Our normative data base was derived from over 750 subjects between 6 and 90 years old, collected from six sites, using standardized methods and criteria.

Neurometric Analysis of the EEG

Statistical techniques must be used to compare an individual to a normative data base. For more than 10 years, we have used the Z-transform (see Fig. 1)

---

[1] Brain Research Laboratories, Department of Psychiatry, New York University Medical Center, 550 First Avenue, New York, NY 10016, USA
[2] Nathan S. Kline Research Institute Orangeburg, NY, USA

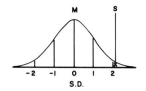

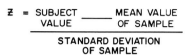

Fig. 1. Gaussian or bell-shaped distribution curve. *M*, mean; *S*, subject value; S.D., standard deviation. The Z-transform scales the deviation of a feature in an individual patient from the mean value of that feature in the population into S.D. intervals. The fraction of the area under the curve which lies less than that distance from the mean equals the probability that the patient belongs to the normal population. This assessment provides the basic statistical foundation for computerized evaluation of electrophysiological data to quantify the probability that a given EEG feature is abnormal, a method since adopted by many workers to advance beyond the ambiguous phenomenology of topographic maps of actual feature values (John et al. 1977).

Normalized or "Gaussian" Distributions

The precision of this statistic depends upon satisfying the assumption of a normal or gaussian distribution. In order to guarantee this, we examined the distributions of all of the 1 200 features we now extract from the EEG, found most to be non-gaussian, and constructed various transforms to achieve gaussianity for all of them, many of which have since been confirmed by other workers (John et al. 1983, 1987).

Figure 2 illustrates the extreme deviation from gaussianity displayed by some features extracted from normal subjects, as seen in the upper row of histograms. The lower row of histograms show the gaussian distributions achieved by appropriate transforms of each of these features.

Many of these features show significant correlation with age. Reliance upon a single value for the mean and standard deviation of such a variable will yield false positives which increase with deviation from the center of the age range, as well as false negatives because of the inflated estimate of variance. For this reason, the means and standard deviations of all of our 1 200 normative neurometric features have been described by polynomial age regression equations from age 6 to 90 years (John et al. 1983; John et al. 1987).

Some workers in this field have deprecated these bias-correcting procedures as "slavish adherence to formal statistical requirements," not actually needed because the Z-transform is so robust. Therefore, for this meeting we prepared an objective evaluation of whether these corrections have a practical clinical consequence.

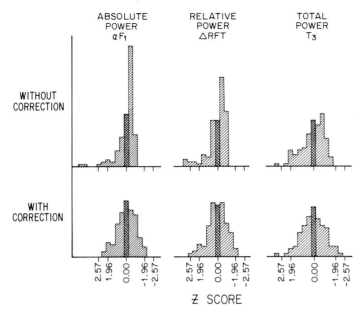

Fig. 2. Histograms of Z-values for three different EEG features without and with transformations to achieve gaussianity. Note marked skewedness of distributions before correction

The data shown in Fig. 3 demonstrate that respect for recognized statistical rules yields significantly improved sensitivity of quantitative EEG features. False-positive findings in normal subjects are less frequent when corrections are made for skewed distributions and age effects, while true-positive findings increase. The incidence of false negatives in the absence of these corrections is different for different clinical groups. Topographic mapping of statistically invalid data necessarily has less clinical utility than when legitimate statistical procedures are followed.

Multivariate Features

The functional organization of the brain is based upon complex relationships *among* its regions. Quantitative analyses restricted to the topographic mapping of *local* features yield little insight into subtle changes in organization. For this reason, we augmented our set of local or "univariate" features with a set of regional and systemic composite variables. We have normed the covariance structure of relationships between regions across features or among features within a region, using the Mahalanobis distance to quantify changes from normal relationships (John et al. 1983; John et al. 1987).

For example, consider the univariate features left parieto-occipital alpha and left parieto-occipital beta, shown in Fig. 4. If one considers these features

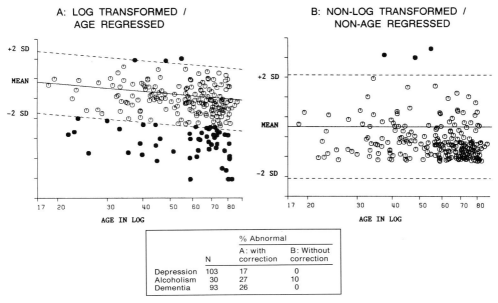

Fig. 3. Scatterplots for temporal coherence in the beta band between T3T5 and T4T6, shown with both age regression and log transform for gaussianity (*left*) and without either (*right*). *Dotted lines* represent ±2 S.D. from mean (*solid line*). *Solid circles* indicate cases displaying significantly abnormal values. *Bottom panel* tallies the percentage of patients found abnormal in each of three categories, with and without correction. Note the far greater sensitivity achieved when features are corrected for biases

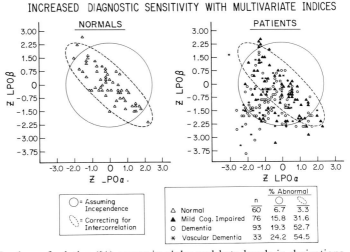

Fig. 4. Scatterplot for Z-values of relative (%) power in alpha and beta bands in derivations P301 for 60 normal subjects (*left graph*) and for 202 patients in three categories (*right graphs*). In each graph, the 95% confidence region is represented by the *circle* if the multivariate compression of the two features is computed as the square root of the sum of the squared Z-values, and by the *ellipse* if it is computed as the Mahalanobis distance. Note the far superior sensitivity achieved by taking the intercorrelations between features into account

to be independent, the 95% confidence interval of the two-dimensional composite feature defined by the square root of the sum of their squares is represented by the circle. The confidence interval shown by the ellipse reflects the high covariance normally found between these two features. Note how few false positives among an independent sample of normal subjects lie outside the ellipse, seen on the left side of Fig. 4. The data shown on the right side of Fig. 4 demonstrate the great increase in sensitivity to brain dysfunction achieved by taking normal covariation between features into account. Only the patients outside the *circle* would be identified as abnormal if independence were assumed between these two measures. When their normal covariance is utilized to define the composite feature, the patients outside the *ellipse* are classified as abnormal.

Cerebrovascular Disease

Properly constructed multivariate composite features, which we have normed to permit valid Z-transformation, are indispensable for the detection of subtle neurological or cognitive dysfunctions and for differential diagnosis of psychiatric disorders. For example, in collaboration with Drs. Jonkman, Poortvliet and DeWeerd in the Netherlands, we studied a population of patients with known cerebrovascular disease, all with compromised middle cerebral arteries (Jonkman et al. 1985). They were divided into four groups: two with persisting symptoms [completed stroke (CS) and persisting neurological symptoms (PNS)] and two which were asymptomatic at the time of study [reversed ischemic neurological deficit (RIND) and transient ischemic attack (TIA)].

In the CS patients, a high incidence of abnormality was found on most univariate as well as multivariate features. The same was true of the PNS patients. In the asymptomatic RIND patients, a much lower incidence of abnormality was found on univariate features. Many TIA patients showed no univariate abnormalities at all. In such cases, topographic maps would be normal. However, multivariate features consistently detected a high incidence of abnormality in asymptomatic as well as symptomatic patients.

Figure 5 compares the results obtained in these four groups of patients with quantitative EEG (black bars) and with radioactive Xenon measures of regional cerebral blood flow (rCBF; white bars). In the symptomatic CS and PNS patients, ^{133}Xe blood flow measures detected a high proportion of abnormalities, but in the asymptomatic RIND and TIA groups, the radio-xenon method was very insensitive. The composite neurometric measure "overall all frequencies" was consistently superior, detecting a high proportion of abnormal patients in all four groups, with only 3% false positives in a control group of normal subjects. Visual evaluation of the EEG tracings from these patients by two skilled electroencephalographers revealed abnormalities in only 57% of the total group, far below the neurometric accuracy.

Intraoperative topographic maps, which we obtained while monitoring neuroembolization of 92 arteriovenous malformations and clipping of 97 cerebral aneurysms, provide many examples of dramatic and essentially immediate cere-

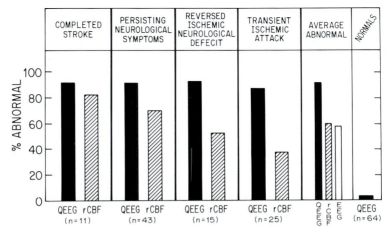

Fig. 5. Incidence of abnormal findings in four different categories of cerebrovascular patients using the neurometric multivariate feature "overall abnormality" [quantitative EEG (*QEEG*); *black bars*] and ^{133}Xe measurement of regional cerebral blood flow (*rCBF; shaded bars*). Note the consistently higher sensitivity of the neurometric measure and the low incidence of false positives. The *white bar* (EEG) in the Average Abnormal panel shows the percentage of patients in the total sample judged abnormal by two conventional electroencephalographers

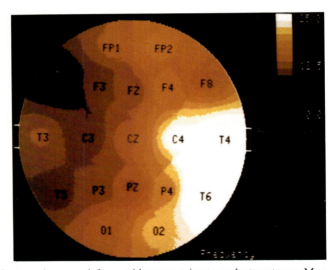

Fig. 6. Paradoxical effect of a test clamp on left carotid artery prior to endarterectomy. Map of relative (%) power in delta band showed an almost immediate increase of delta over extensive regions of the *right* hemisphere in this conscious, locally anesthetized patient. This reflects cerebral steal due to the fact that the right carotid artery was almost compromised. Scale (%)

bral steal reflecting widespread hemodynamic changes. Signs of cerebral ischemia, caused by localized occlusion, appear in multiple regions and are not restricted either to the site or even the side of the surgical maneuver. For example, consider the paradoxical effect of a test clamp on the left carotid prior

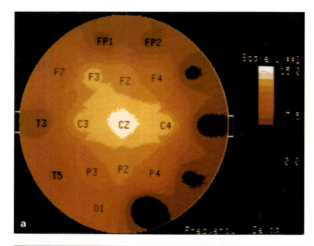
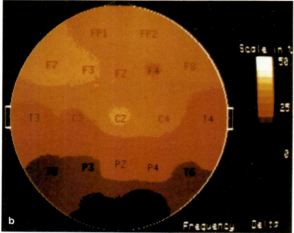
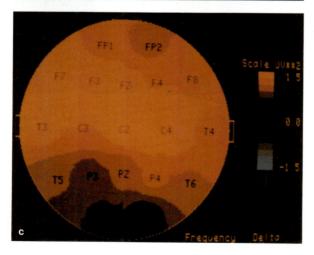

Table 1. Percentage accuracy of discriminant classification of right anterior vs right posterior subarachnoid hemorrhage (SAH) patients using two quantitative EEG composite variables. Results of jack-knife replication are shown in parentheses

Actual group	Predicted group membership	
	I	II
I. Right anterior SAH	100.00 (100.0)	0.0 (0.0)
II. Right posterior SAH	0.0 (0.0)	100.0 (100.0)

to endarterectomy, shown in Fig. 6, where signs of cerebral ischemia are seen over extensive regions on the right side. Multivariate features are well suited to detect even minimal effects of this sort.

Other examples of the utility of composite neurometric features in cerebrovascular disease come from patients with subarachnoid hemorrhages (SAH). Topographic maps of univariate features in SAH patients are of little value in localization of the hemorrhage.

The patient shown in Fig. 7, after SAH of the *right anterior* cerebral artery (ACA), does *not* display abnormal ipsilateral features in the topographic map of absolute power in the delta band (Fig. 7a), percent or relative delta power (Fig. 7b), or Z-transformed relative delta power (Fig. 7c). Compare these paradoxical results with those from the patient shown in Fig. 8 after SAH of the right *posterior* cerebral artery (PCA), who displayed very similar topographic maps for absolute delta power (Fig. 8A), relative delta power (Fig. 8B), and Z-transformed relative delta power (Fig. 8C). Clearly, the consequences of rupture of a major artery produce widespread EEG abnormalities. Localization of a cerebrovascular accident by topographic mapping of univariate features is unreliable.

Using the Mahalanobis distance features "anterior coherence of theta across all frequency bands between the anterior regions" and "total coherence between the posterior regions of the two hemispheres," we obtained 100% accurate discrimination between ACA and PCA patients (jack-knife replication in parentheses), as seen in Table 1. Thus, in spite of the ambiguous localization available from univariate features in cerebrovascular disease, multivariate features may permit meaningful localization.

Fig. 7 a–c. Widespread changes in topographic maps due to changes in cerebral hemodynamic regulation after subarachnoid hemorrhage (*SAH*) make localization based upon one univariate, feature extremely ambiguous. Compare absolute delta power (**a**), relative delta power (**b**), and Z-transformed relative delta power (**c**) in this patient after CT scan-confirmed SAH of *right anterior* cerebral artery with the data shown in Fig. 8 from a patient after SAH of the *right posterior* cerebral artery

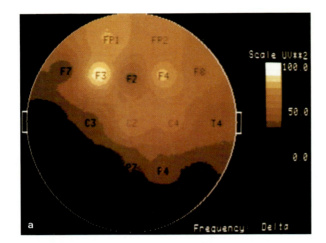

a

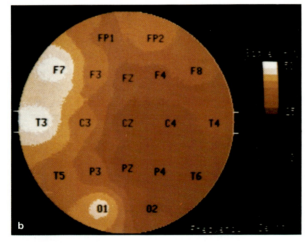

b

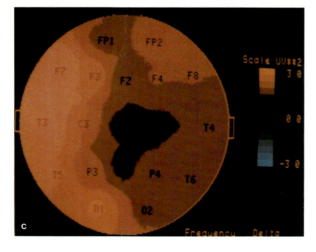

c

Psychiatric Disorders

It should be noted that the patients in the various groups discussed below, as well as our normal subjects, came from several different clinics. Recordings at different sites were made using equipment with identical recording parameters and standardized conditions. In all discriminant functions reported here, two split samples of every group were constructed which were counterbalanced for site of diagnosis and/or recording. One of these samples was used for the initial discriminant and one for the independent replication.

Differential Discriminant Analysis

The neurometric feature set, especially the multivariate features, permits accurate differential diagnosis of psychiatric disorders. Rates of false positives among normal individuals are acceptably low. A high incidence of abnormal findings occurs in patient populations, and values correlate well with clinical severity.

Figure 9 shows histograms of the value of the composite neurometric feature "overall theta excess" in normal subjects and elderly patients with mild (global dysfunction score = 2), moderate (GDS score = 3), and severe (GDS score = 4-7) cognitive dysfunction. The correlation between the level of cognitive impairment and increasing values of the multivariate feature is obvious, with analysis of variance (ANOVA) yielding $p < 0.0001$.

Groups of patients with different psychiatric disorders display distinctive neurometric profiles which can contribute to more accurate differential diagnosis (Prichep and John 1986; John et al. 1988). Figure 10 shows the accuracy achieved by a multiple discriminant function in differential classification of normal subjects and patients with primary depression, alcoholism, or dementia. The mean accuracy of this four-way discriminant was 78% for the initial samples (black bars) and 79% for the *independent* replication (white bars).

Table 2 shows the accuracy of classification of normal subjects versus patients with primary affective disorders, all examined in a depressed state. Mean accuracy was 92% for the initial samples (upper half) and 90.5% for the independent replication (lower half).

In another discriminant function using only the single multivariate feature "anterior coherence across all frequency bands," patients with primary affective disorders were identified with 73.5% accuracy.

Fig. 8a–c. Topographic maps from a patient after CT scan-confirmed SAH of *right posterior* cerebral artery. Compare absolute delta power (**a**), relative delta power (**b**), and Z-transformed relative delta power (**c**) with corresponding data in Fig. 7 from a patient after SAH of *right anterior* cerebral artery. No obvious differences can be readily discerned between the abnormal distributions of univariate features resulting from these vascular accidents located in different quadrants of the cerebral arterial system

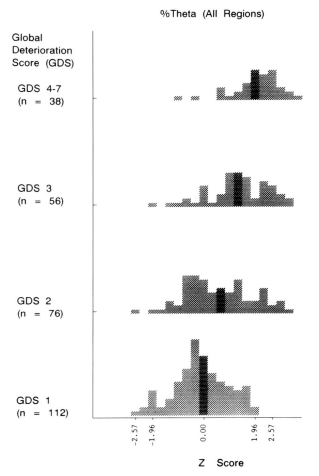

Fig. 9. Distributions of Z-scores for multivariate feature "relative (%) power in theta across all regions" for groups of elderly individuals showing a Global Dysfunction Score of 1 (normal), 2 (mild impairment), 3 (moderate impairment), and 4 or above (severe impairment). Note that the mean Z-score increases with greater impairment

The black bars in the left half of Fig. 11 show the accuracy of separation of unmedicated, unipolar versus bipolar depressed patients, all examined during a period of depression. The white bars represent independent replications. Overall accuracy was 85%, with the *independent* replication 86% accurate.

The right half of Fig. 11 shows the loss of discriminant accuracy between the same unipolar and bipolar depressed patients when non-log-transformed, non-age-regressed features were used. The initial discriminant results are shown as black bars, and the independent replication as white bars, with a mean accuracy of 70%.

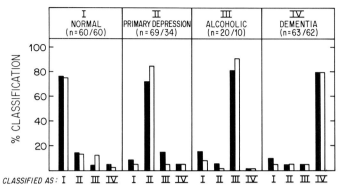

Fig. 10. Percentage of normal subjects (*I*) and patients with primary depression (*II*), alcoholism (*III*), or dementia (*IV*) classified as I, II, III, or IV by a four-way discriminant function. The first and second *numbers in parentheses* above each panel indicate the sample size of each group used as the training set in the initial discriminant (*black bars*) and as the test set in the independent replication (*open bars*). Average accuracy of this discriminant was 78%

Table 2. Discriminant classification of depression using neurometric quantitative EEG variables

Initial discriminant		Classification (%)	
Actual group	*n*	I	II
I Primary depression	69	*91*	9
II Normal adults	60	7	*93*
Independent replication			
Actual group	*n*	I	II
I Primary depression	34	*94*	6
II Normal adults	60	13	*87*

In preliminary studies, it was possible to discriminate between primary depression and unmedicated chronic schizophrenic patients with about 80% accuracy, with jack-knife replication at the same level.

Thus, accurate differential discrimination between subtle psychiatric disorders can be achieved if multivariate statistical techniques are carefully exploited. Once multiple discriminants have identified the diagnostically significant variables, topographic mapping of the major univariate features contributing to discrimination (selected from the much larger set of mappable variables) reveals patterns which are commonly encountered within patients with the same

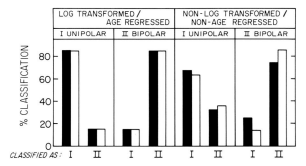

Fig. 11. Percentage of unipolar (*I*), and bipolar (*II*) classified as I or II by a two-way discriminant function. The *left* half shows results when features are corrected for non-gaussianity and age effects, while the *right* half shows results with failure to correct these biases. The first and second numbers indicate the sample size of each group used as the training set in the initial discriminant (*black bars*) and the test set in the independent replication (*open bars*). Note the higher specificity of the discriminant using corrected features. Mean accuracy was 85% with corrected but only 70% with uncorrected features. Unipolar $n=34/34$, bipolar $n=18/17$

disorder. However, such maps are not unique and may also be encountered in other disorders, as can be seen in Fig. 12.

The topographic maps in Fig. 12 depict the Z-transformed relative power in the beta band for different groups of patients. The normals ($n=60$), not illustrated, show average Z-values of relative beta power around zero. The average of the unipolar depressed ($n=68$), shown in Fig. 12a, displays a diffuse deficit of beta. This is one of the features which distinguishes them from the average of the bipolar depressed ($n=35$), shown in Fig. 12b, who display a diffuse excess of beta. However, this abnormal beta topography is not unique to these diseases. The average in Fig. 12c, with a significant diffuse beta deficit, comes from a group of 93 patients with dementia, not unipolar depression. The average in Fig. 12d, with a significant diffuse beta excess, comes from a group of 30 patients suffering from alcoholism, not from bipolar depression.

Thus, although the features yielded by quantitative analysis of the EEG permit highly accurate classification of patients by multivariate statistical methods (Prichep and John 1986; John et al. 1988), topographic maps of selected univariate features *do not* possess sufficient uniqueness to permit accurate differential diagnosis.

Neurometric Analysis of Evoked Potentials

Topographic maps of evoked potential (EP) features yield a phenomenology even more bewildering than those of the EEG, compounded by the multiplicity of time points in a "map movie." Apparently "abnormal" asymmetry can often be observed in one frame of the movie, while "normal" symmetry can

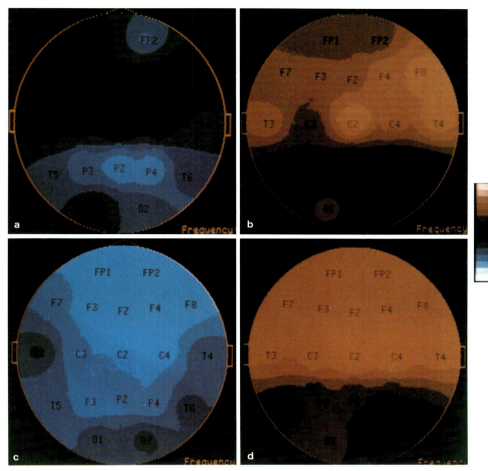

Fig. 12a–d. Topographic maps of Z-transformed relative beta power, averaged across different groups of patients: **a** Unipolar depressed ($n=68$); **b** bipolar depressed ($n=35$); **c** senile dementia ($n=93$); **d** alcoholism ($n=30$). Note that beta deficit characterizes both the unipolar depressed and the demented, while beta excess characterizes both the bipolar depressed and the alcoholics. Topographic maps of selected univariate features do not possess sufficient uniqueness to permit accurate differential diagnosis. Scale: **a, b** ±0.7; **c, d** ±1.5

be observed only a few milliseconds later. Visually impressive apparent pathology may be spurious, while reassuringly symmetrical maps may obscure pathology reflected primarily by latency shifts or amplitudes.

Quantitative descriptors of the EP, capable of decomposing the EP into standardized constituents analogous to the broad frequency bands which summarize so much clinically valuable information about the EEG, would greatly simplify the objective interpretation of this phenomenology. Some workers have attempted to make EP maps more interpretable by performing serial t tests

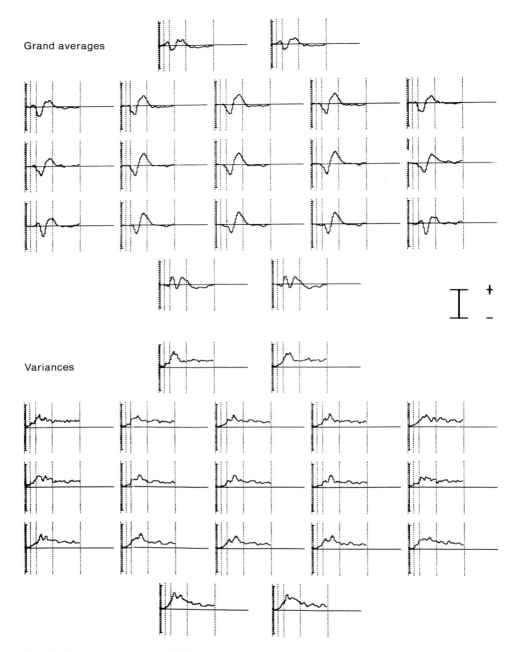

Fig. 13. Group grand average VEPs (*top*) and variance of grand average VEP (*bottom*) computed for each electrode of the international 10/20 system and displayed as a topographic array viewed from the top, face upward. Averages from 100 normal individuals, each derived from 100 stimuli, were combined in this computation. In this and all subsequent EP or factor displays, the *vertical lines* correspond to 50, 100, 250, and 500 ms. All waves were truncated at 500 ms, although the average interstimulus intervals and analysis epochs were 1 000 ms

against a "norm" consisting of a grand average EP across a sample of normal individuals.

In our opinion, two aspects of that procedure are inadequate. Aside from the statistical dubiousness of serial t tests across highly correlated sequential samples, the resulting map movies still resemble a kaleidoscope. The group grand average EP itself suffers from inherent shortcomings as a reference waveshape, as can be seen from Fig. 13.

The upper portion of Fig. 13 shows a group grand average visual EP (VEP) constructed from a sample of 60 normal individuals. The waveshapes are displayed in correspondence with the positions of the 10/20 electrode placement system from which they were recorded. The lower portion of Fig. 13 shows the variance of the group grand average VEPs across the set of averaged VEPs obtained from these 60 different persons, for the same electrode positions. Inspection of these variance curves reveals marked peaks reflecting inhomogeneity of variance at the corresponding latencies in the analysis epoch. Further, this inhomogeneity of variance differs widely across different leads. These data indicate that *VEPs across a large sample of normal individuals display a wide range of "normal" waveshapes,* that this diversity is particularly found in certain latency intervals, and that it varies from lead to lead. The same holds true for group grand average auditory EPs (AEPs), not illustrated here.

In view of these findings, it is not tenable to propose that *unique* "normal" VEP or AEP waveshapes exist and that group grand averages reveal the true morphology of those waveshapes and provide a valid reference. For these reasons, we studied the utility of factor analysis as a method to achieve decomposition of any EP into a set of standardized descriptors, each of which could be represented by a neurometric topographic map.

Signal-to-Noise Ratio of the EP

In the typical adult patient, the peak-to-peak amplitude of the ongoing EEG during computation of an average EP is about 50 µV, while the peak-to-peak amplitude of the averaged EP is about 15 µV. If 100 individual EPs were averaged, as is usually the case, the residual "noise" would be expected to be 5 µV, reflecting a reduction proportional to the square root of the sample size. Thus, after averaging 100 samples, the signal-to-noise ratio of the extracted average response waveshape is about 3:1. Only about 75% of the variance of an average EP is related to the true signal morphology, while the remaining 25% reflects unresolved noise.

Factor Analysis Procedure

For each of 130 normal individuals, averaged evoked responses were recorded from each of the 19 placements of the full 10/20 electrode system, relative to linked earlobes, in each of four different stimulus conditions. Four stimuli were used: blank flash, grid flash (7 lines/in), regular click and random click. The subjects were divided into two split-half groups, each of about 60–70 persons. Each stimulus was presented under two different conditions: while the subject was in the dark ("no video") and while watching a defocused television screen ("unfocused video plus"). One split-half group was assigned to each of these conditions: "no video" and "unfocused video plus". One hundred artifact-free responses were obtained from each subject to each of the four stimuli, yielding four different averaged EP waveshapes for each of the 19 electrodes.

Specific Factors

The sets of 1 140 averaged evoked responses (60 subjects times 19 electrodes) obtained from the two split halves were analyzed separately for each of the eight stimulus conditions. On each set of such data, a principal component analysis of the waveshapes was performed, followed by a Varimax rotation. In each analysis, the set of factors was selected which most parsimoniously accounted for approximately 75% of the total variance, in view of the estimated signal-to-noise ratio in the elements of the original EP set.

In each analysis, it was possible to account for or "span" very nearly 75% of the total variance with either six or seven factors. The number of factors required, the proportion of the variance accounted for by each separate factor, and the actual waveshapes of the individual factors were essentially identical for the two different split-half samples in each of the eight analyses.

These factors were called *specific factors*. Table 3 presents the number of specific factors required to span each of the eight sets of 1 140 averages and the variance of the total sample of 1 140 EPs which could be accounted for in each condition. These results indicated that the signal information $S_i(t)$ in the EPs from the average individual in the normal sample could be essentially completely described as:

Table 3. Evoked potential variance (%) accounted for by specific and general factors

	n	No. of factors	Specific factors %	Seven general factors %	Decreased accuracy %
No video:					
Regular click	67	7	77.4	76.0	1.4
Random click	68	7	74.2	72.7	1.5
Blank flash	69	6	74.0	75.3	−1.3
Seven lines/in grid	65	7	78.0	76.2	2.6
Unfocused video plus:					
Regular click	64	7	75.4	73.4	2.0
Random click	59	7	79.3	76.7	2.6
Blank flash	61	7	72.4	70.6	2.2
Seven lines/in grid	64	6	79.0	79.8	−0.8
Mean variance accounted for:			76.3	75.1	1.3

$$S_i(t) = \sum_{i=1}^{19} \sum_{j=1}^{7} A_{ij} F_j(t) \qquad (1)$$

where $S_i(t)$ = signal information S in EP waveshape of electrode i across analysis epoch t; $i = 1, \ldots 19$ = subscript of electrode; $j = 1, \ldots 7$ = subscript of factor; A_{ij} = factor score for contribution of jth factor to EP waveshape $S(t)$ in ith electrode; $F_j(t)$ = waveshape of jth factor across analysis epoch t.

In other words, the signal information, $S_i(t)$, in the waveshape of the average EP recorded from any electrode in any member of our normal sample could be reconstructed with an acceptable (and theoretically near-perfect) accuracy as a linear combination of six or seven specific factor waveshapes, $F_j(t)$, each multiplied by an optimal weighting coefficient or factor score, A_{ij}.

General Factors

It seems reasonable to suggest that the basic steps in processing of information about events in different sensory modalities, once afferent input has occurred, should be mediated by the same functional neuroanatomical systems, independent of the modality. Further, since aspects of complex stimuli in different modalities are perceived subjectively as simultaneous, the functional processing should proceed at the same rate for any modality. If we assume that the wave-

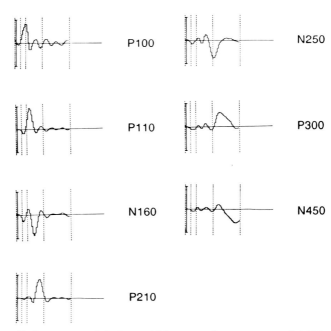

Fig. 14. Waveshapes of seven Varimax general factors which spanned an average of 1.3% less variance than each of eight sets of specific factors extracted from EPs elicited by four visual and four auditory stimulus conditions

shape of each factor represents the contribution of a particular functional neuroanatomical system, it should be possible to subsume the set of 54 *specific factors* describing the waveshapes obtained in the eight different conditions by a smaller set of *general factors* capable of describing the EPs elicited by *any* stimulus.

Accordingly, the 54 specific factor waveshapes were subjected to principal component analysis followed by a Varimax rotation. This procedure yielded seven general factors which spanned 92.4% of the variance of the specific factor set. The waveshapes of the 19 averaged evoked potentials from every one of the normal subjects in each of the eight different stimulus conditions were then reconstructed as linear combinations of these seven general factors. The general factors accounted for an average of only 1.3% less variance in each data set than the corresponding set of specific factors. These data are also presented in Table 3. The waveshapes of the seven general factors are shown in Fig. 14.

Functional Interpretation of General Factors: An Hypothesis

These results are compatible with the hypothesis stated above; that is, the set of neurophysiological processes which are activated and time-locked by presentation of stimuli in different sensory modalities appears to be independent of the modality of the stimulus. The clear temporal sequence of the general factors suggests that they may represent sequential stages of central information processing. These stages may correspond to brain mechanisms mediating identifiable functions such as sensory registration, attention, perception, cognition and semantic encoding. This notion is compatible with numerous EP studies indicating that experimental manipulation of these functions produces EP changes primarily manifested in sequential, relatively restricted latency intervals that correspond to the intervals of peak power of the general factors which we have identified.

It is noteworthy that although the general factors are capable of describing well any EP recorded in any electrode position, the factor scores which represent the relative contribution of each factor to an EP vary greatly *from lead to lead* within a given stimulus condition. Further, they are markedly different *between* sensory modalities within any electrode position. In other words, each factor score seems to have a characteristic value for *each brain region* and for *each stimulus modality* or condition.

Fig. 15a, b. Original (*top array*) and reconstructed (*bottom array*) averaged VEP waveshapes in two normal subjects whose data were collected at two different sites. Responses to 100 flash stimuli were averaged. Note the marked difference in actual waveshape among different electrode positions and between subjects, and the good approximation of the reconstruction to the original waves. **a** Subject RE434; **b** subject KN140

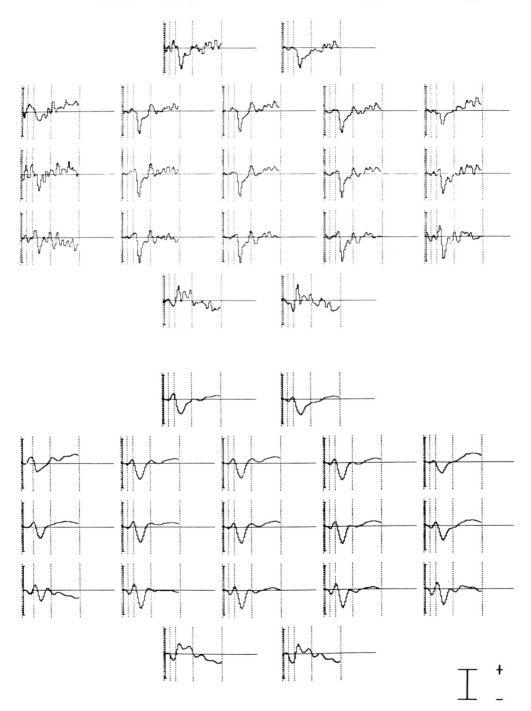

Fig. 15a

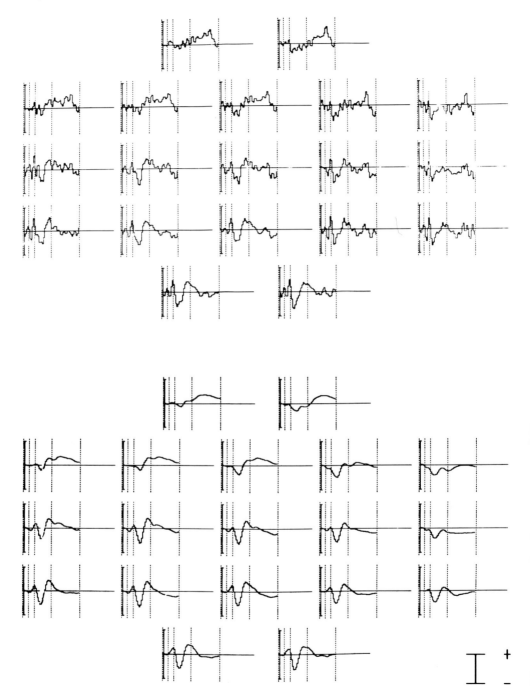

Fig. 15b. Legend see p. 108

Reconstruction of EPs from Individual Subjects

Figure 15 shows the averaged VEPs elicited by a 1/s blank flash in the 19 electrodes of the 10/20 system in two different normal subjects (Fig. 15a, b) as actually recorded (top) and as reconstructed using the seven general factors (bottom).

Figure 16 shows the averaged AEPs elicited by a 70-dB regular 1/s click in the 19 electrodes of the 10/20 system in the same two normal subjects (Fig. 16a, b) as actually recorded (top) and as reconstructed using the seven general factors (bottom).

Inspection of Figs. 15 and 16 reveals several important facts: (1) the EPs elicited in different leads by a particular stimulus are different within a given subject; (2) the EPs elicited in the same lead by visual and auditory stimuli are different within a given subject; (3) the EPs elicited by the same stimulus at the same electrode location in two normal subjects are different; (4) all of these apparently idiosyncratic waveshapes could be well described by the same seven general factors; (5) factor reconstruction yields a waveshape reminiscent of low pass filtering.

Figure 17 shows the waveshapes representing the residual variance of each EP reconstructed in Figs. 15 and 16. Residuals after VEP (top) and AEP (bottom) reconstruction in the two different subjects (left and right sides of the figure) are distributed across the whole latency domain and reflect residual ongoing EEG not time-locked to the stimuli and not removed by the averaging process.

Z-Transformation and Topographic Maps of Factor Scores

These findings indicated that topographic mapping of normalized factor scores, separately for each general factor, could provide a standardized set of EP descriptors. Each such descriptor would reflect a process which extends through some portion of the latency epoch and may correspond to a specific step in information processing. Such maps would constitute a quantitative and interpretable description of the EP in each brain region and might replace the qualitative phenomenology of EP map movies.

In order to normalize the factor scores, the distribution of raw factor scores for each factor for each lead in each stimulus condition was examined and adjusted to achieve gaussianity. The mean value and standard deviation were computed for each of these distributions. It now became possible to Z-transform the factor scores for each general factor in every electrode location which were required to reconstruct the average EP, $S_i(t)$, obtained by visual or auditory stimuli, such that:

$$S_i(t) = \sum_{i=1}^{19} \sum_{j=1}^{7} Z_{Aij} F_j(t) \qquad (2)$$

where Z_{Aij} = Z-transformed factor score Aij for contribution of jth factor to EP waveshape in ith electrode, and all other symbols are as in Eq. 1.

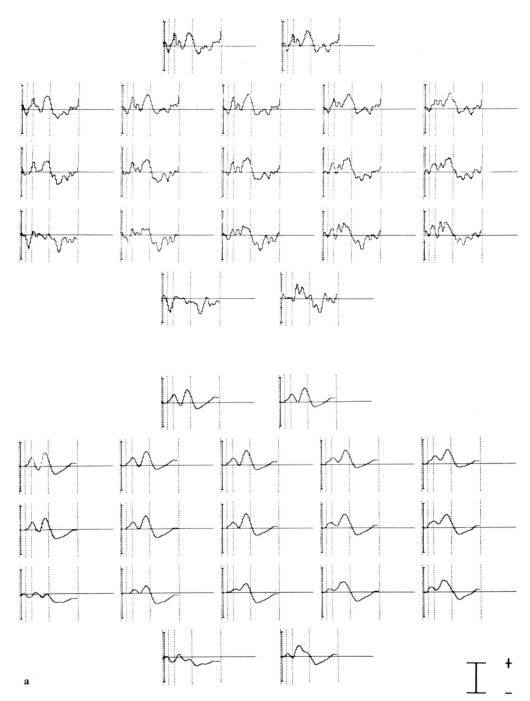

Fig. 16a, b. Original (*top array*) and reconstructed (*bottom array*) waveshapes in same two subjects as in Fig. 15, but for averaged AEPs rather than VEPs

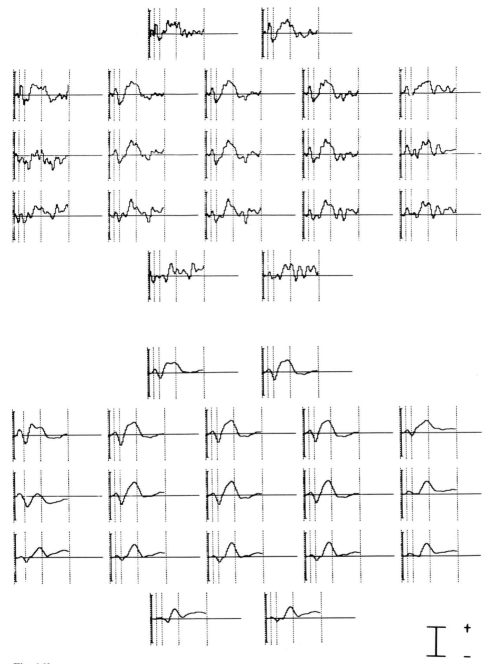

Fig. 16b

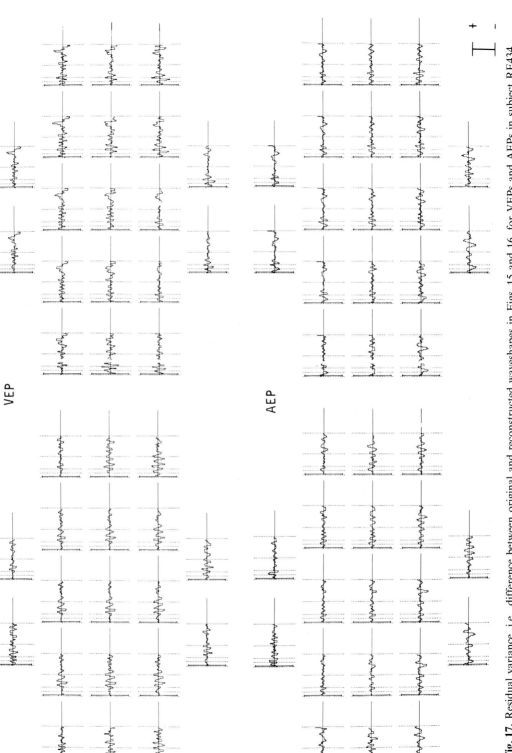

Fig. 17. Residual variance, i.e., difference between original and reconstructed waveshapes in Figs. 15 and 16, for VEPs and AEPs in subject RE434 (*left*) and subject KN140 (*right*)

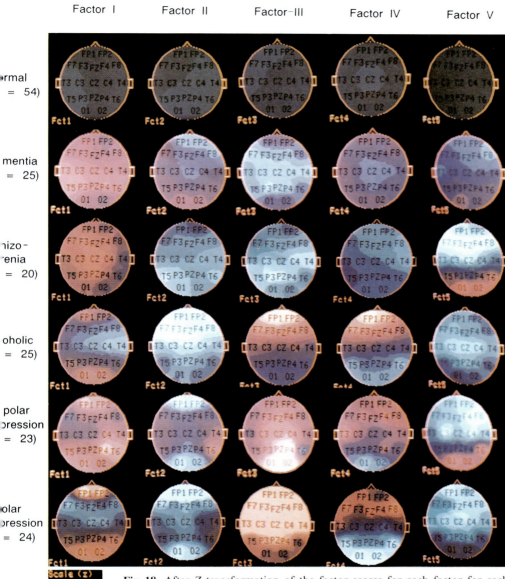

Fig. 18. After Z-transformation of the factor scores for each factor for each electrode, group average Z-score topographic maps were constructed by averaging the factor Z-scores within each of six groups separately for each factor and each electrode and interpolating the resulting values. Note the dramatic differences among groups with different disorders. In this figure, factor I was positive with a peak latency of 100 ms, factor II negative with peak at 160 ms, factor III positive with peak at 210 ms, factor IV positive with peak at 300 ms, and factor V negative with peak at 450 ms. All maps are color-coded with a Z-scale from ±0.7

Group Mean Factor Z-Score Topographic Maps for Different Groups of Patients

The utility of this method for detection of EP abnormalities is currently under evaluation. As a first step, we constructed the group mean factor Z-score topographic maps for the general factors with peak latencies and polarity corresponding to P100, N160, P210, P300, and N450, for a group of 54 normal subjects *not* used to construct the factor score norms, 25 patients with senile dementia, 20 non-medicated schizophrenic patients, 25 alcoholic patients, 23 patients with unipolar depression, and 24 patients with bipolar depression.

The resulting group average factor Z-score topographic maps, for blank flash VEPs, are seen in Fig. 18. No significant abnormalities are seen in the normal group average. Each of the patient groups shows clear abnormalities in their average map. The abnormalities for each factor are different among different brain regions and among pathologies. Similar results (not shown) were obtained for other stimulus conditions.

Conclusion

In the first part of this paper, we showed that multivariate statistical analyses of neurometric EEG data could be used for quite accurate classification of patients suffering from different psychiatric disorders. Statistically coded topographic maps revealed distinctive patterns of EEG abnormality among patients with the same disorder. However, such univariate feature maps were not *uniquely* characteristic of a particular disorder and, therefore, could not be used alone to achieve a reliable diagnosis. Multiple discriminant functions were constructed which could achieve high classification accuracy on independent replications.

In the second part of this paper, we presented a new method to obtain a standardized quantitative analysis of averaged evoked potentials. The resulting topographic maps of general factor Z-scores provide a description of the EPs elicited by visual or auditory stimuli which may correspond to distinct stages in information processing. These normalized factor score maps provide a concise statistical neurometric description of EPs, analogous to the description of the EEG frequency spectrum provided by normalized maps of activity in the delta, theta, alpha, and beta frequency bands.

Work is currently in progress to evaluate the sensitivity and specificity of these new EEG and EP descriptors for the detection and differential diagnosis of psychiatric disorders and to construct functional images of the differential involvement of brain regions in the mediation of different kinds of mental activity in normal subjects and in psychiatric patients.

References

John ER, Karmel BZ, Corning WC, Easton P, Brown D, Ahn H, John M, Harmony T, Prichep L, Toro A, Gerson I, Bartlett F, Thatcher R, Kaye H, Valdes P, Schwartz E (1977) Neurometrics: numerical taxonomy identifies different profiles of the brain functions within groups of behaviorally similar propel. Science 196:1393–1410

John ER, Prichep LS, Ahn H, Easton P, Fridman J, Kaye H (1983) Neurometric evaluation of cognitive dysfunctions and neurological disorders in children. Prog Neurobiol 21:239–290

John ER, Prichep LS, Easton P (1987) Normative data banks and neurometrics: basic concepts, current status and clinical applications. In: Remond A, Lopes da Silva F (eds) Computer analysis of EEG and other neurophysiological variables: clinical applications. Elsevier, Amsterdam (EEG handbook, vol 3)

John ER, Prichep LS, Friedman J, Easton P (in preparation) Neurometrics: Science

Jonkman EJ, Poortvliet DCJ, Veering MM, Weerd AW, John ER (1985) The use of neurometrics in the study of patients with cerebral ischemia. Electroencephalogr Clin Neurophysiol 61:333–341

Prichep LS, John ER (1986) Neurometrics: clinical applications. In: Lopes da Silva FH, Leeuwen van Storm W, Remond A (eds) Clinical applications of computer analysis of EEG and other neurophysiological signals. Elsevier, Amsterdam (EEG handbook, vol 2)

Advances in Brain Theory Give New Directions to the Use of the Technologies of Brain Mapping in Behavioral Studies*

W.J. Freeman[1] and K. Maurer[2]

Brain as a Dynamic System

The human brain, for all its complexity and power, is a physical and chemical system that performs its miracles in a physical and chemical world operating by the same dynamic laws. The entire profession of electroencephalography is based on the premise that observations and measurements of the electromagnetic fields of potential at the surface of the scalp and brain, when taken in close conjunction with measurements of behavior, will tell us something about how the brain works and in what ways it can malfunction in disordered states of behavior.

What we mean by "how the brain works" is an explanation in physicochemical terms of how the brain accepts external information from the outside world by way of its sensory receptors and transforms that input first to its own internal information content about the world and then to orderly sequences of muscular contraction. By way of an analogy with a machine, or more generally a homology with a naturally occurring "self-organizing" physicochemical system, we can say that the brain is a dynamic system that accepts input, operates on it to transform it in different ways, and then gives an output. The definition and description of each operation requires that we know enough about the space-time patterns of the input and of the output of each transforming step, so that we can say what must be done to change the former into the latter. For example, one may shine a spot of light onto the retina, measure the discharge patterns of the receptors and of the ganglion cells, and infer that the retina operates on its input (light patterns) to give spatially filtered patterns of action potentials on the optic tract that represent the "sharpened" (contrast-enhanced) stimulus images to the brain.

It is implicit in this description that two kinds of information are to be found in electroencephalograhic and magnetoencephalographic measurements of brain activity. One kind consists of the information content that is being operated on by the brain. Brain theory, including the experimental studies on which it is based, tells us that, except for the activity of sensory receptors,

---

* This work was supported by grant MH06686 from the National Institute of Mental Health. United States Public Health Service. The work with human subjects was done following the guidelines of the University of Würzburg.

[1] Department of Physiology-Anatomy, University of California, Berkeley, CA 94720, USA
[2] Department of Psychiatry, University of Würzburg, Füchsleinstraße 15, 8700 Würzburg, Federal Republic of Germany

this brain activity does not serve to represent sensory stimuli as they actually impinge on receptors. It serves to embody and convey concepts that the sensory stimuli release, trigger, or enter into. On the motor side the brain activity does not lay action patterns or "commands" onto motor neurons, but instead initiates conceptual trends or trajectories, which are shaped at the level of the spinal cord by proprioceptive feedback into specific movements that instantiate the concepts. Hence the correlates of brain activity are not specific stimuli and responses but are percepts and concepts that have been established by prior learning (Freeman 1975, 1979, 1981, 1983, 1987; Freeman and Skarda 1985; Skarda and Freeman 1987).

The other kind of information concerns not the content but the operations done on the content. It consists of the unfolding or manifestation of the operations being done on the conceptual information. When a stimulus is delivered to an area of cortex, it is amplified, normalized, integrated over time and space, sharpened, and then forced into a decision tree for the selection of an appropriate concept. These several operations are manifested by a collection of electrical events having specific signatures by which they can be identified and measured. Within the brain, one concept cascades into and through the next, meaning that one vortex of neural activity feeds into and triggers the next, each transition giving rise to its own characteristic signature or electrical "noise" as in the operation of a machine, until the output is brought to completion.

It is the business of brain mapping, among other tasks, to find, read and measure these signatures of brain operations. But in order that we interpret these signs correctly, we must know what the operations are, and for this we must know the "before" and "after" patterns of the conceptual neural information for each operation. In this task we are assisted by the findings of brain theory, which tell us where and how to look for this conceptual information; it is to be found not in the temporal patterns of brain waves, but in their spatial configurations. Brain theory tells us that concepts occur as brief (ca. 100 ms) wave packets, for which a common oscillatory waveform exists among hundreds of millions of neurons in domains of cortex that may extend over tens of square centimeters of cortical tissue. The content of the concept is expressed in the amplitude modulation of the common waveform in its entire spatial extent. The operations of formation, transmission and termination of the concept are expressed in the temporal amplitude modulation and temporal spectrum of the common waveform.

This distinguishing set of characteristics exists by virtue of the nature of the dynamics that gives rise to the neural activity of concepts. In essence the processes of generation are self-organizing. When a large collection of semiautonomous elements such as cortical neurons is allowed or encouraged to interact extensively, each with very many others in its surround, then a cooperative entity emerges that exists as a macroscopic or large-scale system having much larger spatial and temporal scales than its component have. The cooperative interaction gives rise to the common waveform that is found over the entire extent of the interactive mass of neurons, and that serves as the "carrier wave" of the conceptual information. This information does not appear in the unaveraged activity of single neurons, but only in large averages or sums;

but it is visible in the spatial patterns of the electroencephalogram (EEG), whose potentials are the sum of contributions from large numbers of the cooperating neurons within the reach of each recording electrode.

Behavioral Information in the EEG

Animal studies in the olfactory (Freeman and Viana di Prisco 1986) and visual (Freeman and van Dijk 1987) cortices have indicated that the carrier waves bearing the desired information tend to have irregular wave shapes, that are often aperiodic and may have wildly chaotic textures. While an occasion they show concentration of their energy into a narrow spectral peak (a "burst"), often, and especially in neocortex, the spectrum is broad and tapering at higher temporal frequencies. The minimal carrier frequency, which is determined in the main by the passive membrane time constants of the component neurons, appears to be about 15–20 Hz; the optimal is 40–50 Hz, well above the range commonly dealt with in scalp recording of the human EEG, and it seems likely that significant information exists at frequencies up to 80 Hz and beyond. These high frequencies are fully compatible with the short duration of the time segments in which the concepts exist: a time span of 100 ms allows only four cycles of a carrier wave at 40 Hz, which is insufficient to establish a phase pattern but is quite adequate to specify an amplitude pattern.

These properties of conceptual information (brief duration, broad spectrum with emphasis on high frequencies, wide spatial distribution, and spatial patterning of the amplitude of a common waveform) place such activity well beyond the reach of the conventional EEG. It is rendered even more inaccessible by contamination with muscle and movement artifacts, which also have broad spectra and strong energy content in the higher frequencies. However, the redeeming feature is the commonality of waveform over an extended area. This is not shared by electromyographic potentials, which have the phase lags and high spatial spectral frequencies characteristic of propagated action potentials. The EEG and the electromyogram (EMG) can be separated by the use of large electrode arrays and appropriately designed two-dimensional spatial filters for high-pass and low-pass filtering. The common waveform can be extracted by any of several forms of spatial ensemble averaging, which is related to but distinct from temporal ensemble averaging. The latter is used to derive averaged evoked potentials, but it cannot be used on the EEG owing to the chaotic nature of the EEG.

The technology of mapping of brain potentials provides the means for gaining access to the conceptual information that is present in the scalp potentials generated by the cerebral cortex. What is needed is the use of a large number of electrodes (for example, 64 in an 8×8 array, or 256 in a 16×16 array) at spacings on the order of 0.5 cm, yielding "windows" onto the brain of 4×4 cm or 8×8 cm. A high-speed multiplexer with an ADC is needed to digitize at rates of 500 samples/second/channel in order to gain the temporal resolution needed to examine high frequencies. Strong computer power is needed on line to extract the common carrier wave shape by adaptive filtering (Freeman and Viana di Prisco 1986) or by principle components analysis (PCA; Freeman and van Dijk 1987), to determine the amplitude coefficients by regression, and to process the amplitude patterns in the variety of ways needed to extract the conceptual information (Freeman 1987), and to validate it by behavioral assay. The proper temporal digitizing intervals and interelectrode spacings are determined by use of the Fourier transform of EEG data in order to identify spectral ranges and avoid aliassing. These capabilities are not fully within the reach of existing machines, but it is to be expected that they will become so within a very few years.

An Example from Brain Mapping

Some idea of what can be hoped for is provided by an example of scalp recording from a normal volunteer who was examined in the Psychiatric Clinic at the University of Würzburg. A set of 16 scalp electrodes was attached in the overall pattern of the 10–20 system, but with a spacing of 2 cm between electrodes, giving a window of 6×8 cm (Fig. 1). The array was placed over the left parietofrontal area so that the Rolandic fissure ran medially where normally the midsagittal line would run anteriorly, placing the left half of each pattern seen in Fig. 1 over the motor cortex and the right half over the primary somatosensory cortex in the areas devoted to the right hand and arm.

The subject was instructed to lie quietly with eyes shut and mouth open and to hold a buzzer and switch in the right hand waiting for a buzz at an unexpected time. The buzz at 150 Hz (faint but clearly audible) lasted 2 s, and at its end the subject was instructed to press the button on the switch lightly for 2 s and then relax. Records were taken continuously for several trials over a 10-s period for each trial. Four segments each 2 s in length were taken for off-line analysis from the times of waiting for the buzz to begin, waiting for it to end, pressing the switch, and relaxing immediately after releasing the switch but waiting to the told that the trial was over.

The example in Fig. 1 shows the spatial distributions of the spectral bands 4 Hz in width from 0 to 47 Hz in the four states. In both the beginning and end control periods the high concentration of spectral energy is seen to hold for 12 Hz and below. The fall-off in energy with increasing frequency is characteristic of what is called "1/f noise." The high energy content, mainly but not exclusively in the alpha band, is seen to persist in the two test periods, but there is the emergence of augmented activity in the 39–43 Hz band during the buzz (B), concentrated in the part of the array over the sensory cortex, and of activity in the 15–23 Hz region during pressing the switch (C), most markedly in the part of the array over the motor cortex. On repeated trials the spectral range in which the augmentation took place varied erratically, indicating that the Fourier decomposition offered by spectral analysis was not appropriate for capturing the invariants of this EEG activity.

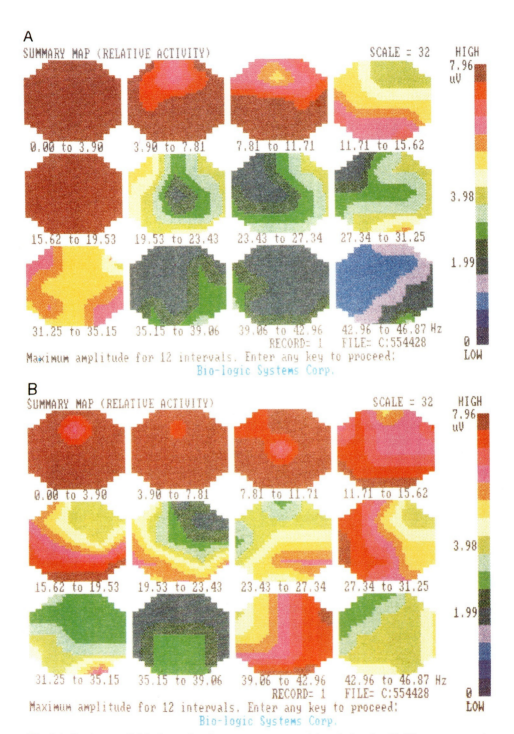

Fig. 1A–D. A set of 16 electrodes 2 cm apart was positioned (in the 10–20 arrangement) to form a 6 × 8 cm window over the left front parietal cortex of a normal volunteer subject. Upward was medial and left was anterior. Power spectra were computed for four 2-s segments of unaveraged EEG in a single behavioral task having four stages (see text). The spatial

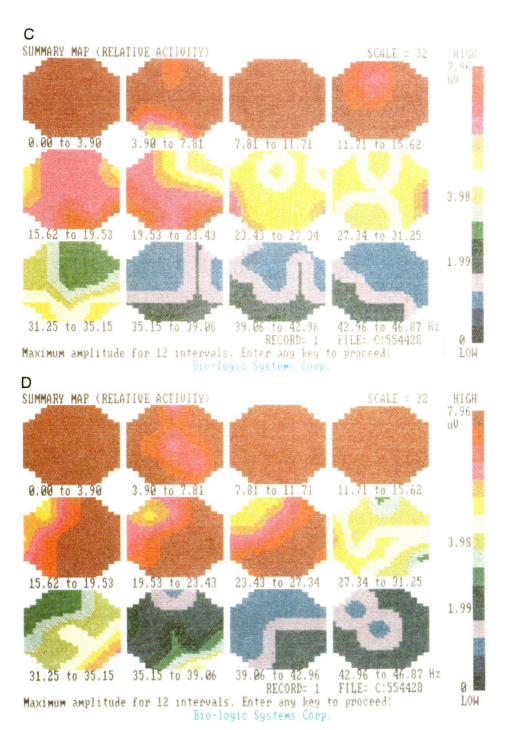

amplitude plots are shown for the 12 4-Hz intervals in each of four steps in a single behavioral task: **A** waiting for a sensory stimulus to begin; **B** sensing a vibration in the hand and waiting for it to end; **C** pressing a switch with the thumb for 2 s at the end of the buzz; **D** waiting to be told that the trial was ended

These anecdotal results show that activity of some degree of coherence (restriction to one or another 4- to 8-Hz spectral band) exists over an extended region of the scalp in temporal relation to a conceptual event and in spatial relation to a relevant part of the brain; that its amplitude is spatially inhomogeneous; and that it occupies a relatively high part of the temporal spectrum. They also reflect the serious limitations of the methods currently available. The present digitizing interval and computational capability restricts examination of the spectrum to 50 Hz or less. The forced reliance on spectral decomposition is not compatible with fine-grain temporal segmentation but forces use of a segment 2 s in length, which is 20-fold longer than is desired. The number of electrodes and channels is too small by a factor of 4–16, so that the spatial resolution is deficient and the window of observation is too small. Fourier decomposition is not appropriate for examining the fine structure of events that appear to have chaotic carrier waveforms. The carrier waveform is not retrieved; yet it must be retrieved without averaging across time, if the desired information content is to be detected in the amplitude of the carrier modulation. At best we can say only that we believe that interesting spatial patterns of activity may exist in the high-frequency "gamma" range of the scalp EEG of humans which have promise of revealing conceptual information content, if properly measured and analyzed (Sheer 1984). The requisite tools are available, but they must be adapted and extended in order to become adequate for the task.

Conclusions

The mapping of brain potentials has found its greatest use thus far in gross localization of activity, mainly in the search for focal epilepsy and space-occupying lesions, and to a lesser extent in confirming that brain activity in the occipital lobe accompanies a visual task, parietal activity a somesthetic task, and so forth. These uses involve low temporal and spatial resolution, so that small numbers of electrodes (16–32) suffice, and extensive time ensemble averaging is permissible, as in Fourier analysis and averaging of event-related potentials. One may question whether these uses are as effective for their purpose as are alternative methods involving computed axial tomography, nuclear magnetic resonance, positron emission tomography, and the use of radioisotopes to reveal metabolic activity and cerebral blood flow.

Theoretical analysis of brain functions and a wealth of experimental data show that conceptual information is generated and maintained in the cerebral cortex in the form of spatial patterns of cortical neural activity. It would seem obvious that the techniques developed for spatial mapping of brain activity would be immediately applicable to the task of reading and measuring these spatial patterns as revealed by the EEG and the magnetoencephalogram (MEG). In fact, only the EEG and the MEG have the spatial and temporal resolution that are essential to deriving estimates of these patterns; none of the other techniques can now or foreseeably be expected to serve this purpose, because they are much too slow and coarse.

However, theoretical analysis tells us that the desired conceptual information is to be found at high ranges of both the spatial and temporal spectra of brain activity, which are not normally examined by conventional techniques. Therefore, it is desirable that steps be taken to adapt existing devices and computer algorithms for analysis and graphic display to the requirements spelled out by brain theory. These include increased numbers of electrodes, closer spacing, faster digitizing, decreased reliance on Fourier analysis, and increased reliance on PCA and related procedures for extracting common waveforms from multiple simultaneously recorded traces (Freeman 1975, 1987; Gevins 1987).

The expected benefits will include better understanding of how information is generated, conveyed, expressed, transformed, and stored in the human brain. This knowledge will give better insight into the deep-lying mechanisms of human and animal intelligence, starting with concept formation (Skarda and Freeman 1987; Baird 1986). We may hope that when we can better understand how the normal brain functions, we can then use these same techniques to learn how abnormalities and instabilities develop that cause pathological behavior. First steps in this direction have led to a neurochemical hypothesis on the development of petit mal epilepsy in the limbic system of the brain, as an emergent instability leading to a degenerate state of hypersynchrony of brain activity (Freeman 1986). A rich field of study has been opened up for us by these new tools for brain mapping.

Summary

The development of new experimental techniques in mathematics has led to a renaissance in brain theory in which the brain is seen as a dynamic system subject to the laws of physics and chemistry that hold for other complex self-organizing systems of the natural world. These analytic approaches place heavy requirements on the observation and measurement of the behaviorally related information content of the brain as the basis for assessing its dynamic operations. The electroencephalogram (EEG) and the magnetoencephalogram (MEG) are well suited to provide the requisite information and have served this purpose in animal studies. The available results show that the behavioral information is present in the high-frequency "gamma" range of the EEG spectrum in the form of amplitude modulation of widespread broad-spectrum "carrier waves." The domains of common cooperative activity appear to be sufficiently broad spatially to be accessible in scalp recordings of the human EEG. The technology that is required to observe and measure these waves consists of electrode arrays, banks of amplifiers, machines for high-speed data processing, and computer graphics for display. This technology is now widely available, but it must be modified and extended to take full advantage of the wealth of information in the scalp EEG that brain theory predicts must be available for our clinical use.

References

Baird B (1986) Nonlinear dynamics of pattern formation and pattern recognition in the rabbit olfactory bulb. Physica 22D:150–175

Freeman WJ (1975) Mass action in the nervous system. Academic, New York

Freeman WJ (1979) EEG analysis gives model of neuronal template-matching mechanism for sensory search with olfactory bulb. Biol Cybern 35:221–234

Freeman WJ (1981) A physiological hypothesis on perception. Perspect Biol Med 24:561–592

Freeman WJ (1983) The physiology of mental images. Academic address. Biol Psychiatry 18:1107–1125

Freeman WJ (1986) Petit mal seizure spikes in olfactory bulb and cortex caused by runaway inhibition after exhaustion of excitation. Brain Res Rev 4:259–284

Freeman WJ (1987) Techniques used in the search for the physiological basis of the EEG. In: Gevins A, Remond A (eds) Handbook of EEG and Clin Neurophysiol, vol 3A, part 2. Elsevier, Amsterdam, pp 583–664

Freeman WJ, Skarda CA (1985) Nonlinear dynamics, perception, and the EEG; the neo-Sherringtonian view: Brain Res 10:147–175

Freeman WJ, Viana Di Prisco G (1986) EEG spatial pattern differences with discriminated odors manifest chaotic and limit cycle attractors in olfactory bulb of rabbits. In: Palm G, Aertson A (eds) Brain theory. Springer, Berlin Heidelberg New York Tokyo, pp 97–119

Freeman WJ, Van Dijk B (1987) Spatial patterns of visual cortical fast EEG during conditioned reflex in a rhesus working. Brain Res 422:267–276

Gevins AS (1987) Statistical pattern recognition. In: Gevins AS, Remond A (eds) Handbook of EEG and Clin Neurophysiol, vol 1. Elsevier, Amsterdam

Sheer DE (1984) Focussed arousal, 40 Hz EEG, and disfunction. In: Elbert T, Rochstroh B, Lutzenberger W, Birbaumer N (eds) Self-regulation of the brain and behavior. Springer, Berlin Heidelberg New York Tokyo, pp 64–84

Skarda CA, Freeman WJ (1987) How brains make chaos in order to make sense of the world. Brain Behav Sci 10:161–195

Section II Methodological Aspects

Advanced Programming Techniques for Dynamic Brain Activity Mapping on Personal Computers

U. BRANDL and D. WENZEL[1]

Introduction

Dynamic brain activity mapping means displaying a sequence of topographic brain maps as a movie. This is a simple and impressive way of studying the time course of EEG and evoked potential topography. Although dynamic brain activity mapping is only a qualitative method, we believe that it will be helpful in developing more sophisticated methods to derive clinically evident parameters from brain maps. As a counterpart to industrial solutions using extremely fast and expensive multiprocessor designs we introduce a software technique to speed up map display on a normal personal computer. This also offers the possibility of mapping and programming of innovative methods on the same machine.

Hardware Requirements

Displaying a single brain map means performing a lot of computation. Even greatly optimized mapping programs require a fast processor to produce sufficient display following rates. Some currently available personal computers offering sufficient speed are listed in Table 1. The most widespread system is the 80286-based IBM machine known as AT Standard. Its advantage is a huge market of hardware like analog-to-digital (A/D) converters, graphics devices, add-on memories and other equipment allowing tailoring of the computer to the users special requirements. Most of these devices are also usable with the new 32-bit 80386 machines. The 68000-based machines are also fast enough, but currently it is difficult to equip those systems with analog data-acquisition devices, so one needs a second computer to sample the EEG (this might be a way to upgrade an existing laboratory computer).

If the personal computer is used as a stand-along mapping system an A/D converter is required to sample EEG data. As you need high sampling rates in multichannel EEG recording, a DMA (direct memory access) sampling system such as the DT 2821 (Data Translation Corp.) is highly recommended. This converter allows sampling of 16 EEG channels, either triggered for evoked potentials or continuously for raw EEG or spectral mapping. If you need more than 16 channels you can use two of these converters simultaneously. Note the data throughput rates: a resolution of 0.5 ms in evoked potential mapping

---

[1] Universitäts-Kinderklinik, Loschgestraße 15, 8520 Erlangen, Federal Republic of Germany

Table 1. Currently available microprocessors implemented in personal computers offering sufficient processing speed

Processor	Computer	Bits	ADC available
80286	IBM AT	16	DT2821 (16 channels)
80386	Compaq	32	DT2821 (16 channels)
68000	McIntosh	32	No[a]
68000	Atari ST	32	No[a]

ADC, analog-to-digital conversion
[a] Usable as "mapping terminal" for existing PDP-11 or other laboratory computers

Table 2. Display systems for AT Standard personal computers

Graphics card	Type	Levels	Resolution
Hercules (recommended as standard)	Black/white	11	720 × 350 pixels (40 × 40 map)
IBM-EGA	Color*		640 × 350 pixels (80 × 80 map × 6)
DT-Video	Black/white[b] or color	64 256	512 × 512 pixels 512 × 512 pixels

Note that the monochrome Hercules card allows only one dot intensity. Map pixels must thus be built up from many points to achieve sufficient gray scale levels. So only two maps with a 40 × 40 pixel resolution can be displayed at a time while the other cards allow display of six maps at 80 × 80 pixels
[a] Palette selection of colors. Allows also 16 different gray values on color screen
[b] True analog gray values, no pixel density

requires a data throughput of 32000 Hz at 16 channels. As A/D converters are normally not designed for microvolt applications you need a preamplifier for each channel. This could be normal EEG equipment with analog outputs. Data also must be low-pass filtered before A/D conversion to avoid "aliasing," i.e., interference phenomena between signal and sampling frequencies. Next, your computer should be equipped with enough storage space. A hard disk of at least 20 megabytes and a memory of at least 1 megabyte should be present in your system. The graphics hardware should offer enough resolution to display the raw curves and easy addressing of any point on the screen to provide fast mapping. The (monochrome) (Hercules Graphics Card (or a compatible card) offers a resolution of 720 × 350 points, allowing a good presentation of four curves at a time and 11 well-distinguishable dot patterns to build a map gray scale. An increased amplitude resolution (more scale levels) can be provided by using a color graphics card (16 levels) or a video image processing system (256 levels, Table 2). But note that the transfer of color information greatly increases the computation time needed to display one brain map.

We thus recommend use of the monochrome graphics card for dynamic mapping and a high-resolution color graphics system as secondary screen for the display of static high-quality maps.

Analysis of the Mapping Process

The mapping process can be divided into four different procedures (see Fig. 1):
– Data acquisition and signal processing
– Calculation and display of maps

Data Acquisition and Preparation

Data acquisition means collecting EEG information and converting it into digital data. This is done by the A/D converter. The sampled data can either be processed immediately or be stored on a mass storage device for later off-line processing. For evoked potential mapping we recommend performance of data collection and averaging in one program. This requires storage space only for the averaged potential and offers good on-line monitoring of the experiment, as you can see the potential "grow" on the display.

If you want to map power spectra it is a good practice to store the raw, unprocessed EEG on disk and perform frequency analysis off line. This allows a visual check for artifacts or the selection of artifact-free segments before mapping. Note that every step of data processing can mask artifacts and often the most "interesting" maps are only the result of an electrode artifact. In addition, off-line frequency analysis allows overlapping time segments (see Bendat and Piersol 1971): For a power spectrum of 0.25 cps resolution you need segments of 4 s for Fourier transform. As EEG activity can change greatly within such a period, information can be improved by computing the power spectrum every second using overlapping 4-s intervals (0–4 s, 1–5 s, 2–6 s etc.).

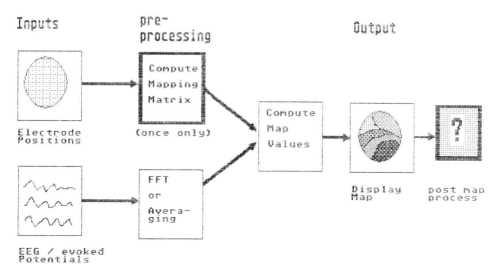

Fig. 1. Flow chart of the complete mapping process. If electrode positioning is variable electrode coordinates have to be considered as an input to the process. *FFT*, fast Fourier transform

As this method requires 16 Fourier transforms per second at 16 channels it greatly exceeds the speed limits of a personal computer and thus can be performed only off line on such systems.

Calculation of the Map

Calculation of a brain map is always an interpolation of values between electrodes. This process has two inputs:
- The preprocessed EEG (evoked potential, power spectrum)
- The head surface model and electrode positioning.

Normally the head surface model (a spheric surface) is projected onto a plane that is divided into a number of squares, called "pixels." The Hercules monochrome graphics card allows construction of maps of 40×40 pixels; in color graphics systems you can use twice that resolution in each direction. Computing the map means computing an interpolated value (voltage or power) for each pixel that it can be displayed. The most widespread interpolation method is the "four nearest neighbors" method: every pixel value is calculated from the values at the four surrounding electrodes weighted by the four pixel-to-electrode distances. A more recent method involves the use of a surface spline interpolation that allows estimation of maxima between electrodes at the price of greatly increased computation time. Note that the following general considerations for process optimization are largely independent of the interpolation method used. For a discussion of these methods see Buchsbaum et al. (1981) and Perrin et al. (1987).

Process Optimization

The whole mapping process described in the previous section requires over 3 s on an 8-MHz AT (see Fig. 2). Most of the time is spent on computing electrode-to-pixel distances. As these are constant during one experiment, they can be computed once only and held stored in memory while computing a sequence of maps. This reduces computation time to about 300 ms per map. But this is still too slow to get the effect of a moving picture. This section will discuss some techniques which allow us to overcome the speed limits of the personal computer.

Intermediate Storage of Maps

As memory chips have become so cheap that personal computers can be equipped with megabytes of memory it has become possible to calculate a large number of maps and store them in memory. At display time they need only to be recalled (Fig. 3): This reduces display time to 134 ms per map. One 40×40 pixel map having 16 levels can be stored in 800 bytes of memory. A 1-megabyte

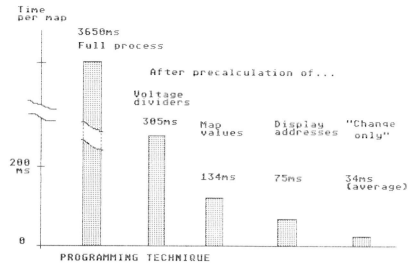

Fig. 2. Computation time for displaying a single brain map from a set of readily calculated electrode values. The time decreases with the optimizations discussed in the text

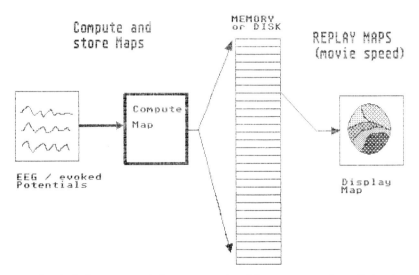

Fig. 3. Memory replay technique: computed maps are stored in memory and recalled only at display time to achieve movie speed. Fast hard disks can also be used to store long map sequences exceeding the machine's memory limits

AT can thus store a sequence of 750 maps beside the program that calculates and replays the maps. This is enough to store the whole time pass of an evoked potential.

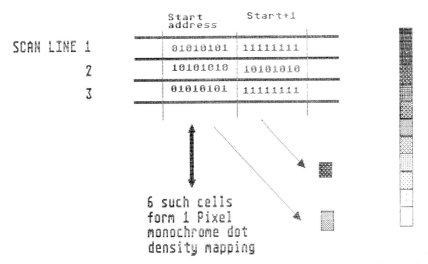

Fig. 4. Display organization for monochrome dot density gray scales and example reference bar for an 8 × 6 dot matrix

Precalculation of Display Addresses

In displaying maps on the Hercules card every pixel is represented by six memory cells arranged in successive horizontal scan lines (Fig. 4). Unfortunately, these lines do not have a continuous order in memory. The start address of a horizontal line for a given Y value is calculated by:

Start address $= (Y \bmod 4) * 8192 + int(Y/4) * 90$

where *mod* is the remainder, *int* the whole number part of a division. This calculation needs a lot of computation time as it is to be performed 9600 times per map. Precalculating the addresses and recalling them from a linear array again almost halves display time. Furthermore, it speeds up display, so that no vertical motion can be noticed during display refresh.

Avoidance of Redundant Operations

If you use a sufficient time resolution in dynamic brain mapping it is rare that brain activity has changed completely from one maps to the next. So only a part of the pixels have to be altered when displaying the next sequential map (Fig. 5). This replaces writing of 6 bytes using complex storage modes by a 1-byte comparsion if the map value has not changed. This reduces display time to an average of 34 ms (in VEP mapping) per map. As refresh time varies depending on the amount of changes, a delay should be used to get a constant picture frequency of 16–20 pictures per second, comparable to an amateur 8-mm movie.

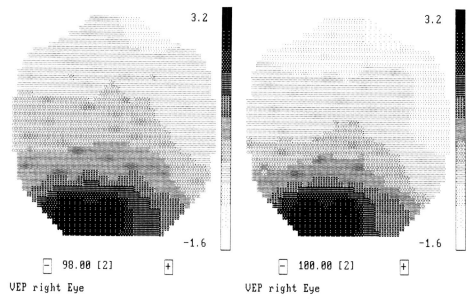

Fig. 5. Example of two VEP maps at latencies of 98 and 100 ms (P100). This illustrates the small amount of changes within 2 ms, allowing speed optimization by skipping unnecessary picture refreshes (see section "Avoidance of Redundant Operations")

Final Considerations

This paper has shown a method for displaying the time course of brain potential topography as a movie on personal computers. The discussed optimization techniques for the display of data are independent of the mapped data (evoked potentials, current densities, power spectra) and the interpolation method used.

References

Bendat JS, Piersol A (1971) Random data. Wiley, New York
Buchsbaum MS, Rigal F, Coppola R, Capelletti J, King C, Johnson J (1981) A new system for grey-level surface distribution maps of electrical activity. Electroencephalogr Clin Neurophysiol 53:237–242
IBM AT Personal Computers Technical Reference Manual (1984) IBM Part Number 6322509
Perrin F, Pernier J, Bertrand O, Girard MH, Echallier JF (1987) Mapping of scalp potentials by surface spline interpolation. Electroencephalogr Clin Neurophysiol 66:75–81

The Use of Derived Map Parameters in Alpha Blocking

W. DE RIJKE and S.L. VISSER[1]

To enhance the usefulness of topographic analysis of the EEG, given the great variability, it is mandatory to use statistical methods and not to be satisfied by similarities between beautiful colored brain maps and the grey tones of the brain scans, or by appearance or disappearance of the blue or red areas at physiologically expected locations.

Sophisticated methods of statistical analysis of the EEG topographic analysis have been applied by Skrandies and Lehmann (1982) and Duffy et al. (1984). Our method of coordinates is a simple first step to data reduction and statistical analysis.

To aid the quantification of localized phenomena in brain maps of the EEG, we want to introduce a number of simple parameters and report results of their use in alpha blocking in normal subjects.

Material and Methods

The alpha blocking reaction was studied in 19 young healthy normal adults. The 9 female and 10 male volunteers, aged 23–47 years, had no neurological diseases and were not on medication. The only selection criterion was their agreement to participate. The awake subjects lay on an examination bench in a quiet, dimly lit room. Nineteen surface electrodes, placed according to the 10–20 system except A1 and A2, were used in an average reference montage. The -3 dB points of the 6 dB/octave high- and low-pass filters were 0.3 and 30 Hz. Before each registration all channels were calibrated with a computer-generated 10000 times attenuated 10-Hz sinus. The amplification remained stable within 0.33% over months, and the differences between channels were less than 1%. Corrections were applied for those changes and differences.

The subjects were asked to relax and suppress eye movements as much as possible. For each subject, five 20.48-s epochs were digitized with a sampling rate of 100 Hz; epochs 1, 3 and 5 with eyes closed, epochs 2 and 4 with eyes open. The sampling of each epoch was started at the command to open or close the eyes. By a provisional eye movement artifact rejection method, only segments of 2.56 s in which the amplitudes in all derivations were between -100 and $+100$ µV were accepted; as soon as an amplitude in any channel was out of this range, a new segment of 2.56 s was started. The remaining

---

[1] Department of Clinical Neurophysiology, 01.13B1, Academic Hospital Free University, De Boelelaan 1117, 1081 HV Amsterdam, The Netherlands

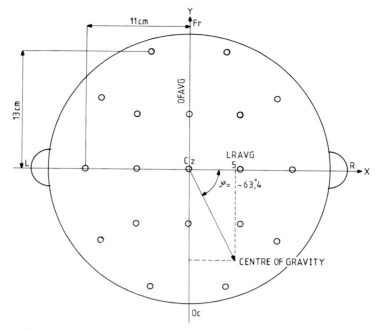

Fig. 1. Coordinate axes through Cz. X-axis from left to right, Y-axis from occipital to frontal

low-frequency artifacts had no appreciable effect on the alpha power in the occipital leads.

To calculate the frequency content of the signals, fast Fourier transform (FFT) was applied to the segments of 2.56 s of each derivation and the power of the 13 frequency bands between 8 Hz and 13 Hz was summed. The behavior of the topographic distribution of this quantity (alpha power) and its square root (alpha amplitude) is the subject of this investigation. For each segment of 2.56 s colored brain maps were plotted, so for each subject 40 maps could be admired. Besides the 19 power values P_i from which the maps were constructed, eight derived parameters D1 ... D8 were calculated; $\sum$ means $\sum_{i=1}^{19}$ (see Fig. 1 for the coordinate axes).

$D1 = \text{total power} = \sum P_i$
$D2 = \text{LRAVG} = \sum P_i X_i / D1$
$D3 = \text{LRSD} = \sqrt{\sum P_i X_i^2 / D1 - D2^2}$
$D4 = \text{OFAVG} = \sum P_i Y_i / D1$
$D5 = \text{OFSD} = \sqrt{\sum P_i Y_i^2 / D1 - D4^2}$
$D6 = R = \sqrt{D2^2 + D4^2}$
$D7 = \text{PHI} = \text{TAN}^{-1} D4/D2$
$D8 = \text{N50} = $ minimal number of electrodes summing to $D1/2$

Parameters D2 and D4 or D6 and D7 describe, in cartesian or polar coordinates respectively, the position of the center of gravity of a disk as in Fig. 1 to which weights are attached, proportional to the power, at the positions of the electrodes. D3 and D5 are comparable to standard deviations in describing the width of the power distribution in the left-right and occipital-frontal directions respectively. D7 is extended from its normal range of $\pm 90°$ to $\pm 180°$ by taking into account the signs of D2 and D4. In the case of the alpha blocking reaction, the power value in the O1 and O2 leads are the best discriminating parameters between eyes open and eyes closed. Certainly they will not be the optimal choice in other cases. Some of the proposed parameters should have about the same discriminating power as O1 and O2 in this investigation in order to be candidates for more general applicability.

Results and Discussion

For each subject a time plot was made for the power in each of the 19 derivations and the eight derived parameters (see Figs. 2 and 3 for a subject with clear alpha blocking).

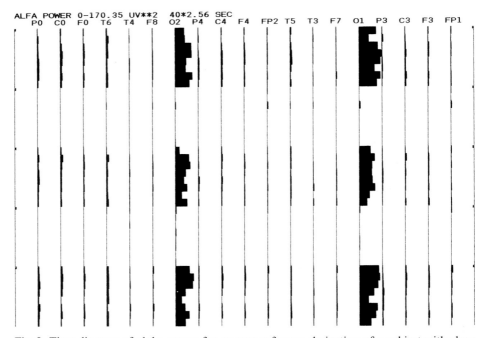

Fig. 2. Time diagram of alpha power for average reference derivation of a subject with clear alpha blocking. Each *bar* represents a segment of 2.56 s. *Epochs* of 20.48 s represent alternating eyes closed and open. Calibration: 170 µV* × 2 between the lines

The Use of Derived Map Parameters in Alpha Blocking 139

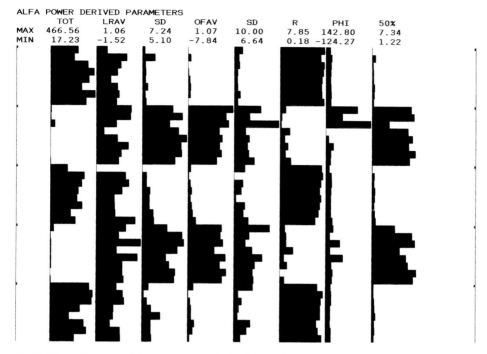

Fig. 3. Time diagram of the parameters derived from data plotted in Fig. 2. Calibration: the minimal (*left*) and maximal (*right*) are given above the curves

Table 1. a The *t* values averaged over 19 subjects for the comparison eyes closed – eyes open. **b** The *t* values of averaged maps and the parameters derived from these maps for the comparison eyes closed – eyes open

a	PR	AR	PS	AS	b	PR	AR	PS	AS
TOT	8	10	9	10		22	23	24	24
LRAVG	1	1	1	1		4	4	5	5
LRSD	−4	−4	−4	−2		−10	−12	−8	−6
OFAVG	−9	−8	−10	−10		−15	−14	−18	−17
OFSD	1	3	−2	0		4	7	−4	1
R	6	5	8	8		22	14	27	19
PHI	−4	−5	−4	−5		−2	−3	−2	−3
N50	−4	−4	−5	−7		−21	−17	−19	−18
O1	9	11	9	11		22	26	23	29
O2	9	12	9	13		26	31	28	33
Fz	7	8	3	3		19	23	5	9
Cz	7	8	5	6		21	27	8	11
Pz	5	6	6	7		10	13	11	14

P, power of the alpha band; A, amplitude alpha band; R, average reference; S, source reference

The differences between eyes open (24 segments of 2.56 s) and eyes closed (16 segments of 2.56 s) were expressed as t values (Student's test). The left column of Table 1a gives the t values averaged over 19 subjects. The other columns concern the same operations on the amplitude and for the source derivation, recalculated from the original average reference data. Table 1b gives the t values for averaged maps: for each of the 40 segments of 2.56 s and each electrode position the power (or amplitude) of the alpha band was averaged over the 19 subjects. For each of the 40 maps that could be constructed, the eight derived parameters were calculated. In general, the t values are higher for amplitude than for power, indicating that normalization of their probability distribution could benifit the discriminating power. Comparison of source and average reference results shows higher or the same t values at the back of the head and lower t values at other locations. This can be explained at least in part by the spread of alpha activity caused by the average reference montage. From Table 1a, b it can also been seen that the derived parameters TOT, OFAVG and R have only slightly less discriminating power than the occipital leads O1 and O2. Their usefulness in other experiments will be investigated.

References

Duffy FH, Albert MS, McAnnulty G, Garvey AJ (1984) Age related differences in brain electrical activity in healthy subjects. Ann Neurol 16:430–438

Skrandies W, Lehmann D (1982) Spatial principal components of multichannel maps evoked by lateral visual half-field stimuli. Electroencephalogr Clin Neurophysiol 54:662–667

The Effect of Source Extension on the Location and Components of the Equivalent Dipole

J.C. DE MUNCK and H. SPEKREIJSE[1]

Introduction

Evoked potentials and Electroencephalograms can be used to determine the location of brain activity and the direction of the polarity. For this purpose mathematical models are used in which the various regions in the head with different conductivity are represented by generalized forms like spheres and spheroids. In most models the source is described by a mathematical point dipole. Since there exists a one-to-one correspondence between visual field and area 17 of the visual cortex, in many evoked potential experiments with visual stimuli the size of the stimulus field is chosen as small as possible in order to activate only a small part of the cortex. In this way a point dipole is imitated at the cost of a lower signal-to-noise ratio.

To investigate whether these precautions are necessary, both the effect of source extension on the potential distribution measured at the scalp (the forward problem) and on the difference in the locations of the extended source and the equivalent dipole (the inverse problem) will be calculated. Studies have been reported in which the forward problem has been solved (Yeh and Martinek 1959; Rudy and Plonsey 1979) for a dipole layer, and in which the inverse problem was solved for several source configurations (Cuffin 1985). Among the dipole distributions studied by Cuffin are line sources and a non-radial dipole distribution of a disk. These examples are not very interesting from a physiological point of view because an extended area of the cortex can better be described by a radial dipole distribution on a sheet. Further, Cuffin's results are obtained by simulating electrode positions, which may seriously influence the results.

In the present study we have chosen an analytical approach which allows for a number of generalizations as described in De Munck et al. 1988.

The Mathematical Formulation of the Problem

The potential distributions due to the extended source ($\psi_L(\vec{x})$) and to the point dipole ($\psi_P(\vec{x})$) are calculated for the case that both sources are situated in a three-sphere volume conductor (Fig. 1). In this model the brain is described

---

[1] The Netherlands Ophthalmic Research Institute P.O. Box 12141, 1100 AC Amsterdam, The Netherlands

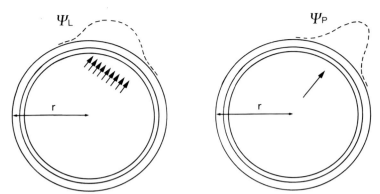

Fig. 1. View of the models. Both sources are assumed to be in a spherical symmetric volume conductor, *left*: the extended source, *right*: the point dipole. The *inner spheres* represent the brain, the *inner spherical shells* represent the skull and the *outer spherical shells* represent the skin. The outer sphere, with radius r, is the surface on which the potentials are measured. The *broken lines* give an impression of the potential distributions

by a sphere and the skull and the skin are described by concentric spherical layers. The point dipole parameters were adjusted such that the difference in power measured on a sphere is minimal. This statement can be expressed by the following equations

$$H = \oiint (\psi_L - \psi_P)^2 \, dS \tag{1}$$

$$\frac{\partial H}{\partial \vec{p}} = 0. \tag{2}$$

The position and orientation of the point dipole are represented by the vector $\vec{p}$. In Eqs. 1 and 2 the surface integral is over the outer sphere, i.e., the scalp. Ary et al. (1981) used the same approach to investigate the effect of layers with different conductivity on the equivalent dipole.

To determine the integrals, the potential distributions are expanded in spherical harmonics $Y_{nm\alpha}$:

$$\psi_L = \sum_{n=0}^{\infty} \sum_{m=0}^{n} \sum_{\alpha=0}^{1} A_{nm\alpha} Y_{nm\alpha} \tag{3}$$

$$\psi_P = \sum_{n=0}^{\infty} \sum_{m=0}^{n} \sum_{\alpha=0}^{1} B_{nm\alpha} Y_{nm\alpha} \tag{4}$$

The odd spherical harmonics are denoted by $\alpha = 0$ and the even ones by $\alpha = 1$. The coefficients of the layer potential, $A_{nm\alpha}$, depend on the position, the orientation and the extension of the dipole layer, and the coefficients of the point dipole $B_{nm\alpha}$ depend on the parameter $\vec{p}$. Since spherical harmonics

Effect of Source Extension on the Location and Components of the Equivalent Dipole 143

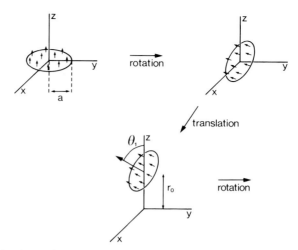

Fig. 2. Outline of the solution of the forward problem. First the potential distribution and the coefficients of the expansion of the spherical harmonics are calculated in a frame in which the calculations are easy. Next the effect of rotating and translating this disk on the coefficients is calculated

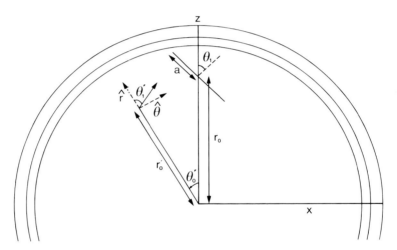

Fig. 3. Definition of the symbols. The dipole disk is located on the z-axis at a distance r_0 from the origin. It has a radius a and an orientation θ_1 with respect to the z-axis. The $x-z$ plane is a plane of mirror symmetry. The equivalent dipole is located at a distance r'_0 from the origin and at an angle θ'_0 from the z-axis, in the $x-z$ plane. The orientation of the point dipole θ'_0 is defined with respect to the local spherical coordinate frame

are orthogonal on a sphere, a summation over the coefficients replaces the integral when the expansion Eqs. 3 and 4 are substituted in the integral.

In a separate paper (De Munck et al. 1987) a method is presented to calculate the coefficients $A_{nm\alpha}$ for a circular symmetric disk with an arbitrary orientation and position with respect to a fixed coordinate frame. First, the coefficients are calculated with the disk in the $x-y$ plane and the point of symmetry in the origin (see Fig. 2). Next the disk is rotated and its effect on the coefficients is considered. Then the effect of translating the disk along the z-axis is calculated and finally the disk is rotated to its destination position.

The coefficients of the dipole $B_{nm\alpha}$ can be found in a straightforward way. Although in general a point dipole is described with six parameters, in our case the problem of finding the equivalent dipole is mathematically equivalent to solving a set of four equations with four parameters. This is so because a circular symmetric disk and a sphere always have a plane of mirror symmetry and the equivalent dipole must also lie in that plane. Therefore one position parameter and one component parameter are trivial.

It is numerically advantageous to put the point dipole on the z-axis when solving the inverse problem and to rotate the disk instead. After the parameters which minimize H have been found the disk is put on the z-axis and the point dipole is rotated over the corresponding angle off the z-axis (Fig. 3).

Results

This paper presents the results of the calculations for a normalized homogeneous dipole distribution on a disk with radius a (Table 1). In the table distance parameters are expressed in terms of the head radius and angle parameters are given in degrees. In the first and second columns the orientation and the radius of the disk are varied respectively. The depth of the disk was adjusted such that the upper edge of the disk was just under the skull. The fourth and fifth columns show the amplitude and the deviation in orientation of the equivalent dipole respectively. In the last two columns the depth deviation and separation angle are shown. For a definition of the symbols see Fig. 3.

The results show that the effect of source extension on the parameters of the equivalent dipole is very small. The table shows that the deviation in source strength and orientation is negligible. The most important parameters are the position patameters. It appears that for a disk with a radius of 0.2 times the head radius the depth error is smaller than 0.03. For a disk radius of 0.3 (i.e. a disk with a diameter larger than half the head radius) the error is smaller than 0.05. Also the deviation from the z-axis is very small. It is expected that for a deeper disk these deviations are even smaller. Similar results are obtained when the dipole disk and the point dipole are situated in a homogeneous sphere.

The choice of a homogeneous disk allows for a generalization because for a homogeneous radial dipole layer the potential is a function of the contour only (see, e.g., Van Oosterom 1978). So, our results are valid for any homogeneous dipole layer with a circular contour. This implies that we can expect to find deep sources when the activated area is highly curved (Fig. 4a). But if, on the other hand, the cortex activated is flat, we may conclude that the location of the equivalent dipole is not influenced by the source extension (Fig. 4b).

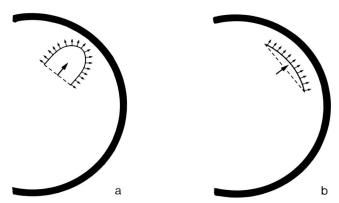

Fig. 4a, b. The locations of the equivalent dipoles with the cortex locally curved (**a**) or locally flat (**b**)

Table 1. Numerical results

θ_1	a	r_0	Amplitude	$\Delta\theta_1$	$r_0-r'_0$	θ'_0
0	0.1	0.838	1.006	0.0	0.0092	0.0
15	0.1	0.814	1.005	−0.54	0.0065	−0.244
30	0.1	0.791	1.005	−0.81	0.0027	−0.413
45	0.1	0.773	1.005	−0.81	−0.0011	−0.499
60	0.1	0.759	1.003	−0.59	−0.0035	−0.458
75	0.1	0.750	1.000	−0.30	−0.0040	−0.293
90	0.1	0.747	0.999	0.0	−0.0037	0.0
0	0.2	0.821	1.015	0.0	0.0284	0.0
15	0.2	0.773	1.013	−1.61	0.0190	−0.756
30	0.2	0.730	1.015	−2.33	−0.0077	−1.24
45	0.2	0.696	1.014	−2.29	−0.0028	−1.45
60	0.2	0.670	1.007	−1.39	−0.0082	−1.11
75	0.2	0.655	0.999	−0.22	−0.0087	−0.245
90	0.2	0.650	0.998	0.0	−0.0099	0.0
0	0.3	0.792	1.021	0.0	0.0485	0.0
15	0.3	0.720	1.019	−2.86	0.0316	−1.38
30	0.3	0.660	1.024	−4.10	0.0128	−2.24
45	0.3	0.613	1.025	−4.02	−0.0046	−2.61
60	0.3	0.579	1.016	−2.94	−0.0151	−2.34
75	0.3	0.559	1.003	−1.43	−0.0169	−0.137
90	0.3	0.553	0.997	0.0	−0.0159	0.0

The first three columns give several combinations of disk parameters and the other columns give the resulting equivalent dipole parameters. The distance from the center of the disk to the origin (third column) is so chosen that the upper tip of the disk is located just under the skull. The fourth column gives the amplitude of the equivalent dipole, under the assumption that the total disk strength equals 1. The fifth column shows the difference in orientation between the equivalent dipole and the disk, where $\Delta\theta_1 = \theta_1 - (\theta'_1 - \theta_0)$. The sixth column shows the difference in depth between the two sources, and the last column gives the separation angle between the equivalent dipole position and the symmetry point of the disk

We can conclude from these calculations that it appears to be unnecessary to choose small stimulus fields in visual evoked potential experiments to imitate a point dipole. The drawback, however, is that it is impossible to estimate the extent of the cortical area activated by measuring and analyzing surface potentials.

References

Ary JP, Klein SA, Fender DH (1981) Location of sources of evoked potentials: correction for skull and scalp thicknesses. IEEE Trans Biomed Eng 28:447–452

Cuffin BN (1985) A comparison of moving dipole inverse solutions using EEG's and MEG's. IEEE Trans Biomed Eng 32:905–910

De Munck JC, Van Dijk BW, Spekreijse H (1988) An analytic method to determine the effect of source modelling errors on the apparent location and direction of biological sources. J Appl Phys 63(3):944–956

Rudy Y, Plonsey R (1979) The eccentric spheres model as the basis for a study of the role of geometry and inhomogeneities in electrocardiography. IEEE Trans Biomed Eng 26:392–399

Van Oosterom A (1978) Cardiac potential distributions. Thesis, University of Amsterdam

Yeh GCK, Martinek J (1959) Multipole representation of an eccentric dipole and an eccentric double layer. Bull Math Biophys 21:33–60

A Simple Model to Aid the Examination of Brain Mapping Systems and the Teaching of Topography

A.L. WINTER[1]

The complexity of computer systems used for topographic mapping of brain electrical activity in experimental and clinical laboratories is a challenge to the philosophy that has been the backbone of scientific, technical and clinical work in the neurophysiological field for many decades. This requires that the user understands and is competent to test the fundamental functions of the machine and that the interpreter is equally competent to challenge the authenticity of the data.

The history of encephalography has shown that each new phase of technological development has necessitated the acquisition of new skills by the operator and reader, often just to identify artefacts in the data, for example in the development of ambulatory monitoring of EEG. Automated topographic mapping of brain electrical activity is certainly no exception and requires greater operative skills than any previous development. Basic problems of EEG procedures which lead to artefacts are just as relevant if not more so than before the introduction of automated mapping techniques. Unfortunately, an additional hazard presents itself. Seduction by clever technology that can produce pretty, coloured maps can lead colleagues who are unskilled in neuroscientific techniques to accept the results without question. The importance of this cannot be overestimated.

Experience has shown that it is important to test a mapping system routinely, and this should begin with examination of its amplifier characteristics in much the same way as frequency response and gain are checked on conventional EEG machines. Figure 1 shows examples of distortion of waveforms that have been found in commercial mapping systems, due either to use of multiple-pole filters of types not employed in conventional EEG or mistakes in notch filter design. A mapping system that displays amplitude measurements to 0.01 of a microvolt tends to instil confidence in the system's accuracy and capability of measurement. Unfortunately errors of amplifier gain as great as 20% have been found in such systems. Perhaps more important is the fact that an error may occur in the internal calibration programme itself and neither it nor the consequent error of gain will be apparent when calibration of the machine is checked according to the instruction manual. This demonstrates the necessity of using an accurate external calibration signal when comprehensively checking one of these systems, about which the manufacturers may claim, "There is no need to worry about calibration – the machine looks after itself".

It can be informative to apply a calibration signal to all channels simultaneously and map the voltage distribution at stepped intervals throughout the signal period. The maps should show a colour common to the whole head

---

[1] Burden Neurological Hospital and Institute, Bristol BS16 1QT, England

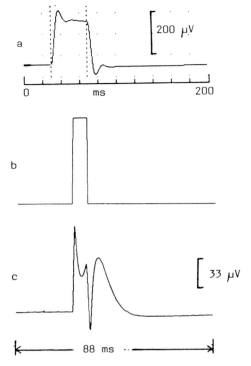

Fig. 1. a Response of the amplifiers of a commercial mapping system to a square wave input. **b** Square wave calibration signal applied to input of mapping system amplifiers referred to below. **c** Response of the amplifiers of another manufacturer's mapping system to the square wave shown above. (By permission of Ray Cooper, Burden Neurological Institute)

at any single point in time which should change according to the potential of the signal at each time step. Figure 2a shows maps of potential difference at successive 4 ms intervals during a single period of square wave signal applied synchronously to all channels. The erroneous contours on the maps display false evidence of localisation and temporal changes of voltage distribution, due to incorrect synchronisation of channel sampling.

Ideally, a mapping system should be tested by applying a known potential distribution to its input and checking that the map it produces agrees with the known topology. This requirement begs a model, and I have exhumed an idea of Grey Walter's from the steam age for the purpose and christened it "STEAM" (simple topographic electrical activity mapping). This model can be used for teaching basic principles of topography to students as well as being a useful model on which a brain mapping system can be tested.

The STEAM model is inexpensive to make, comprising a piece of synthetic sponge about 2 cm thick covered with fine linen and mounted on a wooden board. Elastic netting is stretched over the whole "head", which is basically circular and about 500 cm in diameter (Fig. 3). The sponge pad is made wet, initially with saline (2%–5%), to make it electrically conductive and thereafter kept moist (whilst in use) by finely spraying with water every few hours.

Sine wave electrical activity from an oscillator is applied to the model by means of a pair of pad-type EEG electrodes, simulating a dipole generator.

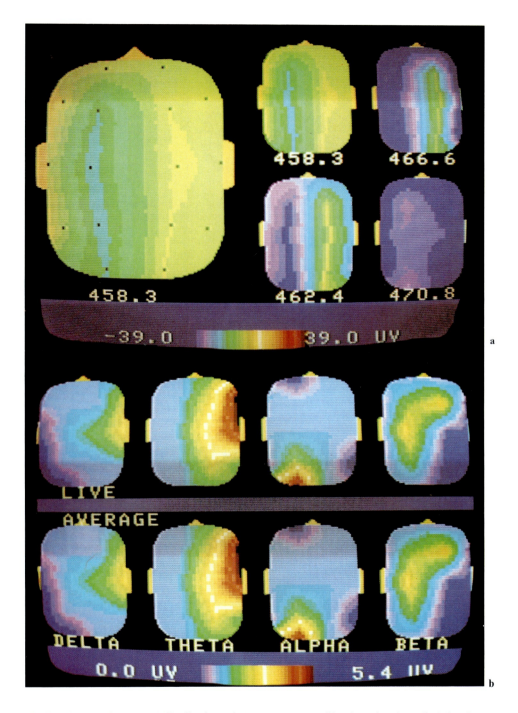

Fig. 2. a Maps of potential distribution of a square wave calibration signal applied simultaneously to the input of each channel (see text). **b** Topographic maps of spectrally analysed activity recorded from the STEAM model to which four electrical generators, each of different origin and frequency, were simultaneously applied

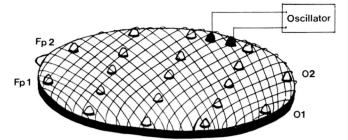

Fig. 3. Diagram of the STEAM model. Multiple electrical sources may be added where required in the same way as the one shown, and the complex topography mapped (see text)

The electrodes are held in place on the model, in the positions and orientation required, by the elastic netting.

Other pad electrodes, placed according to the 10–20 system, are used to record the activity conducted across the model. Multiple electrical dipoles, each from a separate oscillator of known frequency and voltage, may be applied simultaneously to specific regions of the model and the resulting potential fields mapped.

The STEAM model can be used to build a simulated profile of a patient's EEG activity, for demonstrating or teaching topography. The following steps represent an example of mapping quantified electrical activity of four spectral bands – delta (0.5–3.5 Hz), theta (3.5–8 Hz), alpha (8–13 Hz) and beta (13–25 Hz) – from the model. Each step made in building a simulated profile of a patient's EEG should be mapped. Unfortunately, restriction of colour plates does not permit publication in this chapter of the series of maps displaying each step of the following example, and only the final map is presented.

Step 1. Sine wave activity of delta frequency is applied from an oscillator to a pair of "input" electrodes placed near T4 on the model.

Step 2. Activity of theta frequency is applied from another oscillator, or the same oscillator if it has multiple outputs, to another pair of input electrodes more widely spaced near T4-F8.

Step 3. Activity of alpha frequency is applied to a pair of input electrodes placed near O1 such that the map of alpha activity shows greater amplitude of alpha activity in the left occipital region than the right. Orientation of the alpha dipole can be adjusted to achieve this if need be.

Step 4. Activity of beta frequency is applied to a pair of input electrodes placed near F4-C3.

The resulting stimulated profile of a patient with a right temporal delta focus, prominent theta activity in the right frontotemporal region and alpha and beta activity prominent in the "normal" hemisphere is shown in Fig. 2b. The simulated profile may be rebuilt using a different reference and the effects noted, orientation of the dipoles may be changed and numerous exercises developed. Transient signals may be applied to the model and maps may be made of voltage, power and symmetry from single and integrated data points.

Signal amplitude can be measured on the model, enabling the student to become familiar with the concept of spectral lines, their amplitude measurement and their relationship with colour scales displayed during compressed spectral array mapping. These simple exercises also check that the display software, and any subsequent modification to it, is functioning correctly.

In conclusion, I have little doubt that topographic mapping will in time further the understanding and assist and improve the diagnosis of cerebral disorders. However, I recommend colleagues who are on the verge of applying topographic mapping to experimental and clinical problems to be aware of the seductive powers of pretty maps, and to equip themselves with a square wave calibrator and a STEAM model as "tools of the trade".

The Use of Cross-Correlation in the Display of Paroxysmal Events in the EEG: A Preliminary Report

G. SPIEL[1,2], F. BENNINGER[2], M. FEUCHT[2], and U. ZYCH[2]

Introduction

EEG correlates of epileptic seizures show extremely varied morphological, temporal and topographical patterns, depending on the type of seizures as well as on a number of other parameters, especially age. Visual analysis of the EEG recordings is hampered by technical limitations of the writing systems, especially of paper speed. Moreover, the structural, temporal and topographical complexities of these paroxysmal EEG correlates are of such magnitude as to make adequate visual analysis virtually impossible. Such an analysis thus usually remains limited to the classification of the recorded patterns into one of a number of prototypical EEG seizure patterns (Dummermuth 1972) (localized-general, irregular-regular, asymmetric-symmetric, rhythmic-nonrhythmic) without sufficient consideration of the complexity of the paroxysmal changes, especially regarding their dynamic properties in the temporal and topographical domain.

For a more adequate analysis of these parameters a software package has been developed for computer-assisted examination and quantification of paroxysmal EEG changes, using cross-correlation techniques. The first results of mapping the temporal and topographical relationships of paroxysmal EEG events will be presented.

A quite similar technique was applied initially by Brazier (1972, 1973) and Gotman (1981, 1983) to study small time differences between EEG channels. The phenomena thus found were interpreted as originating from the propagation of neuronal activity between the recording sites.

There are, as well as the possibility of measuring small time differences between EEG channels with the cross-correlation function, other statistical methods:
- Computation of the phase and coherence spectra (e.g., Brazier 1972; Gotmann 1983), with the possibility of restricting the frequency range
- Computation of the average amount of mutual information (Mars 1982), with the advantage that linear as well as nonlinear relationships can be handled

We decided to use for the present the cross-correlation function because by this means also short paroxysmal events can be analyzed in detail and a segmentation of a complex paroxysmal discharge can be done, so that changes during

---

[1] Neurologische Universitätsklinik Wien, Lazarettgasse 14, A-1090 Wien, Austria
[2] Universitätsklinik für Neuropsychiatrie des Kindes- und Jugendalters, Währinger Gürtel 18–20, 1090 Wien, Austria

the evolving phenomenon of a paroxysm can be studied. The limitations of the application of the phase and coherence spectra concerning the shortest period which can be subjected to analysis can be deduced from the Nyquist paradigm and is clearly of great importance, especially if the low-frequency range should also be considered.

Methods

The covariance is a measure of the similarity of two signals; as it is also dependent on the respective amplitudes of the signals, two signals can have a large covariance, either because they are similar or because they are less similar but have large amplitudes. To make the covariance independent of the signal amplitudes it is divided by the square root of the product of the variance of each of the two signals. This normalized covariance is the correlation coefficient. If the two signals are of identical pattern the correlation coefficient is $+1$, even though they may be of different amplitudes. If they are identical but of opposite polarity, the correlation coefficient is -1. Any other degree of similarity will fall between $+1$ and -1. In the case of unsystematic linear relations between the two signals, a correlation coefficient near 0 can be expected.

By repeated shifting of one of the signals along the time axis stepwise using defined increments (lag), correlation analysis can be calculated between this displaced signal and the original one stepwise. The relation between the thus calculated correlation coefficients and the increasing time delay is the correlation function. Signals having similar patterns often occur at different parts of a system at different times. The correlation coefficient between two such signals will be a maximum if one signal can be displaced in time with respect to the other when they orignally fluctuate together. If the time difference is not known it may be derived by calculating the correlation coefficient for a number of values of time displacement between the two signals. The resulting relationship between the correlation coefficient and this time displacement is a correlation function. With this strategy can be distinguished not only the maximal possible similarity between two EEG epochs but also the time delay in the amount of lags thereby (Cooper et al. 1974; Bauer 1984).

EEG raw data (routine waking EEG examination, approximately 30 min duration, eyes closed, 10/20 system, bipolar and unipolar derivation, Beckmann ACCUTRACE 16, low-frequency filter, 0.3 s, high-frequency filter 70 Hz) are digitized at a sampling rate of 2 ms/point, recorded on to magnetic tape and analyzed off line (HP 1000 computer system, 2250 M&C processing system, 7912 disk, 7945 disk, 7970b digital tape unit, 2631 printer, 2645 terminal, 2623 terminal, 9278 plotter).

Only unipolar montage (referred to linked earlobes) was analyzed. In a first step a reference lead was chosen, usually that one with the most prominent (amplitude) and most distinct paroxysmal pattern or the one with the earliest onset according to visual examination. Starting from this reference on epoch of any suitable length was defined (window). Thus it becomes possible to examine a spike or a sharp wave discharge alone or in combination with the following graphic elements. In this way complex paroxysmal patterns can be split up into smaller segments. In a second step each lead was compared to all the others (120 comparisons possible) and correlation function was calculated for all of them. In a third step the maximal correlation coefficient of each correlation function was searched for, as well as the corresponding time delay (in lags). Both values were mapped in a matrix (the horizontal axis indicating time delay, the vertical axis correlation coefficient).

Subjects

The subjects chosen for this presentation were three children, aged 6–16 years, who were treated on an outpatient basis.

Patient 1. Female, age 9, suffered from partial complex and partial elementary seizures, age of seizure onset 8, kryptogenic. Visual examination of the EEG showed focal spike and wave discharges in the left centrotemporal area, sometimes also in the left frontal areas.

Patient 2. Male, age 6, had partial complex seizures, age of seizure onset 5, postencephalitic. EEG showed frequent irregular generalized spike and wave activity, maximal amplitude in the left hemisphere.

Patient 3. Female, age 16, generalized tonic-clonic seizures during the night, age of seizure onset 4, perinatal-residual. Interictal EEG showed visually bilateral synchronous spike and wave bursts, three per second, often limited to the frontotemporal areas, sometimes generalized.

Results

Patient 1. Three consecutive paroxysmal discharges that occurred within a period of 15 s during a routine EEG recording were analyzed. The first discharge seems to be located in a definitely circumscribed area (left central and temporal). Analysis of this pattern (C3 serving a reference point) demonstrates that no similar patterns occur within a period up to 40 ms before or after it.

The second more diffuse EEG pattern can be observed not only in the central and temporal regions, but also in other leads. Analysis of the first component (spike) of this complex pattern makes it evident that the event taking place in C3 and P3 at the same time is preceded by highly correlating patterns in contralateral areas (P4, T6). Here too, paroxysmal activity is not spreading to other areas within a period of 14 ms after.

Unlike the spike, the second component of this pattern is not preceded by these contralateral changes; on the contrary it is followed by similar patterns

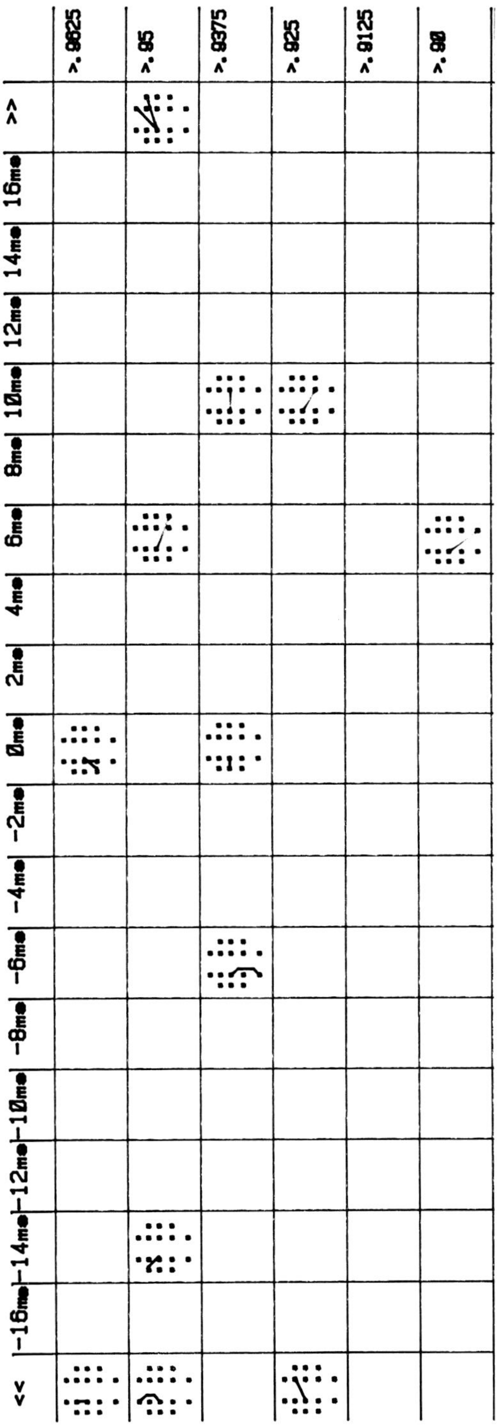

The Use of Cross-Correlation in the Display of Paroxysmal Events in the EEG

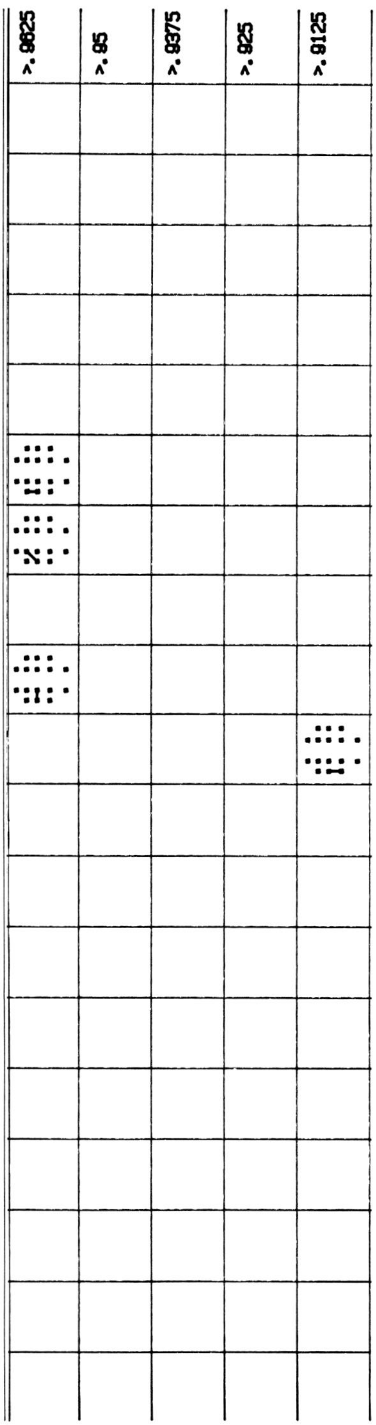

Figs. 1 and 2. Patient 1 (*top*), patient 2 (*bottom*): maximal correlation coefficient and corresponding time delay (in ms) mapped in a matrix. *Horizontal axis*, time delay; *vertical axis*, correlation coefficient

in T5 after a latent period of 6 ms. The third paroxysmal discharge which immediately follows the one described above, resembles the former one in many respects on visual analysis; however, computer assisted analysis reveals differences between the two patterns. The spike which now occurs at the same time in C3, P3, T3 and T5 is preceded by highly correlating patterns in the left frontal area, (F7, F3, FP1) and in occipital areas (02). Discharges spread to the contralateral side, with a latent period of 6 ms or 10 ms, but show opposite polarity there (see Fig. 1).

Unlike the spike, the following slow wave component appears only in the centrotemporal and parietal areas, quite similar to the second component of the paroxysmal event seen before.

Patient 2. One paroxysmal discharge was analyzed. Seizure activity here seems to appear almost simultaneously in all leads. Analysis of the first component (spike) shows that the discharges occur first in temporal areas and then, with latent periods of 2 ms, 6 ms and 8 ms, in central, frontal and anterotemporal areas respectively (Fig. 2). The second component (slow wave), on the other hand, seems to start in the left frontal area and, with a latent period of 10 ms, "spreads" to the contralateral side (FP2) or to other areas.

Patient 3. As far as visual examination of this generalized, very complex paroxysmal pattern was concerned, no statement about time differences could be made, since discharge seemed to appear synchronously at the various sites. Analyzing the first component (spike) and using as reference point the event in the right prefrontal area, one can see similar patterns (but with a high variability in correlation) at the same time in the left frontocentral, left parietal and right parietal or temporal areas (Fig. 3). These patterns are preceded by highly correlated events in the left prefrontal, right temporal and left temporal regions. The former set of events occur almost at the same time and show a high but varied correlation coefficient. After a short latent period (2 or 4 ms), activity spreads to the right central and right temporal areas. In contrast, the following slow wave shows only one similar pattern, in the left frontal area, which correlates highly with the reference point. It is preceded, by 6 or 8 ms, by similar patterns in the right frontal, right central and right parietal regions, and activity "spreads" to the right prefrontal, left central, left parietal and left anterotemporal regions, with latent periods of 4, 6 and 8 ms. Changing the reference point, the results remain the same.

In summary, regarding patient 1, the three paroxysmal events which were analyzed vary in the amount of simultaneously appearing graphic elements in different locations and in the nature of the preceding and following events. It is of some interest that the various compartments of one and the same paroxysmal pattern are of completely different character. As to patient 2, with this method a clear localized onset can be distinguished. This is also true for a second paroxysmal event later in the course of the EEG. In patient 3 the temporal clustering can be shown, but with variability between the appearing graphic elements. The compartments also differ in patients 2 and 3.

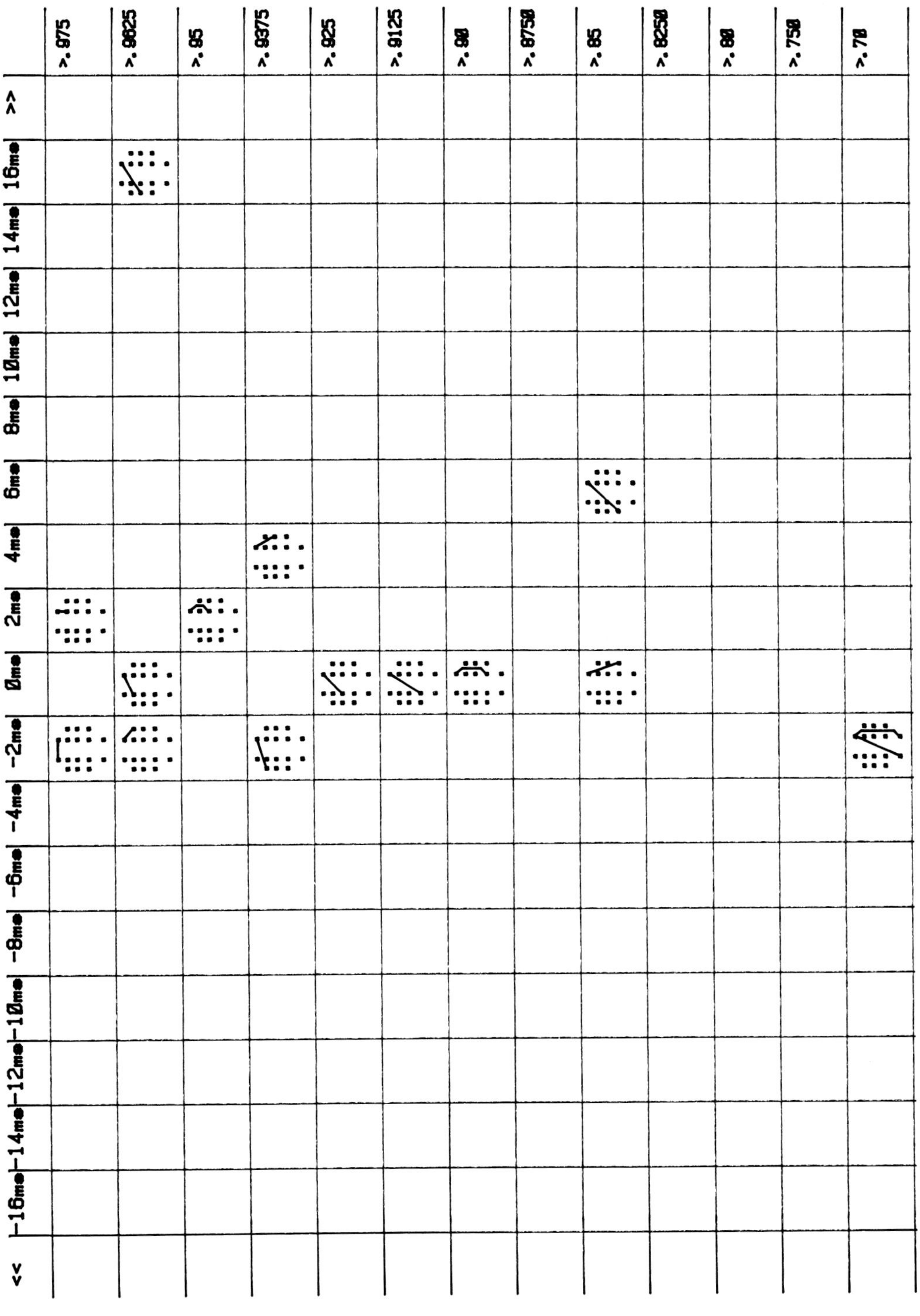

Fig. 3. Patient 3: maximal correlation coefficient and corresponding time delay (in ms) mapped in a matrix *Horizontal axis*, time delay; *vertical axis*, correlation coefficient

With the technique it might be possible to obtain more insight into the temporospatial dynamic appearance of paroxysmal events, not forgetting morphological criteria, the starting point of our analysis.

References

Bauer H (1984) Experimentelle Elektroenzephalographie. Huber, Bern
Brazier MAB (1972) Spread of seizure discharges in epilepsy: anatomical and electrophysiological considerations. Exp Neurol 36:263–272
Brazier MAB (1973) Electrical seizure discharges within the human brain: the problem of spread. In: Brazier MAB (ed) Epilepsy: its phenomenon in man. Academic, New York, pp 153–170
Cooper N, Osselton JW, Skar JG (1974) EEG technology, 2nd edn. Butterworth, London
Dummermuth G (1972) Elektroenzephalographie im Kindesalter. Thieme, Stuttgart
Gotman J (1981) Interhemispheric relations during bilateral spike and wave activity. Epilepsia 22:453–466
Gotman J (1983) Measurement of small time differences between EEG channels: method and application to epileptic seizure propagation. Electroencephalogr Clin Neurophysiol 56:501–514
Mars NJI (1982) Computer-augmented analysis of electroencephalograms in epilepsy. Doctoral Thesis, Technische Hogeschool Twente

Joint Studies of Event-Related Brain Potentials and ^{99m}Tc-Hexamethyl-propyleneamineoxime SPECT on Sensory-Guided Hand Tracking

W. LANG[1], M. LANG[2], I. PODREKA[1], E. SUESS[1], C. MÜLLER[1], M. STEINER[1], and L. DEECKE[1]

Introduction

In humans, measurements of regional cerebral blood flow (rCBF) and electrophysiological recordings offer the possibility of directly studying the neuronal activity of brain structures and of establishing functional-anatomical relations in behavioral tasks. Current trends in topographical studies of brain functions include the use of scalp-recorded slow negative potential shifts (SPs), which occur time-locked to the performance of cognitive or motor tasks. The reason for this is the physiolgical significance of slow, surface-negative cortical potential shifts as an indicator of cortical activation. The spatial resolution of scalp-recorded SPs is limited, but sufficient, for instance, to separate the neuronal activity of localized cortical structures which are involved when preparing motor performance of different parts of the body (Boschert and Deecke 1986). In the present experiments, various tasks on sensory-guided hand tracking have been investigated. There were two points of interest: (1) Are there modality-specific effects on performance-related potential shifts? (2) What are the effects on SPs when changing variables of motor output by establishing conflicting response selection paradigms? These questions have been investigated by measuring both SPs and rCBF.

Modality-Specific Effects on SPs

Sixteen right-handed students (14 male, two female, mean age 21 years) participated. During the experiment, the subjects fixed their gaze on a fixation point straight ahead of them (FIX; Fig. 1). They held a stylus in their right hand equipped with a pressure contact. By lowering then pen to the plate, a light spot in the left field of vision started moving, first for 1 s in a random direction, then for 1 s in another random direction. Thus, the time of the relevant sensory events, start of the stimulus and change in direction, were predictable, but direction was not. The subjects had to track the light spot that moved at a constant speed. Similarly, tactile stimuli were applied to the subject's left palm by a modified XY plotter and had to be tracked in a similar manner.

---

[1] Universität Wien, Neurologische Klinik, Lazarettgasse 14, 1097 Wien, Austria
[2] Universität Ulm, Neurologische Klinik, Steinhövelstr. 9, 7900 Ulm, Federal Republic of Germany

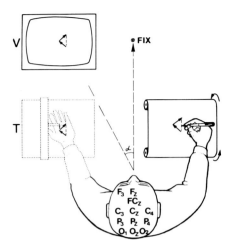

Fig. 1. Experimental set up. Subjects fixed their gaze at a point straight ahead and initiated the stimulus program by pressing down the stylus in the right hand. Stimuli were presented either in the left field of vision (visual tracking) or to the left palm (tactile tracking). Electrodes were positioned according to the 10/20 system; FCz was positioned halfway between Fz and Cz

Ag/AgCl electrodes were placed at positions as sketched in Fig. 1, linked ears serving for reference. Frequency band of amplification ranged between 0.066 and 70 Hz. Data were digitized at a sampling rate of 5.8 ms/point. Artifacts of eye movements were detected on line by monitoring the EOG and rejected from off-line averaging. A total of 128 artifact-free trials were averaged for each condition (for methods see Lang et al. 1984).

Modality-specific effects on performance-related SPs could be demonstrated by (a) comparing SPs recorded from corresponding sites of the two hemispheres and (b) comparing SPs between tactile and visual tracking for each recording. Figure 2 displays comparisons between hemispheres. Each sensory event, such as stimulus onset, change of stimulus direction and end of the stimulus program is preceded by SPs and followed by positive peaks. In order to quantify differences between hemispheres and conditions, the mean negativity within a 250-ms period preceding the change of stimulus direction ($t = 1$) was calculated. In the visual experiment, SPs differed significantly between the two hemispheres,

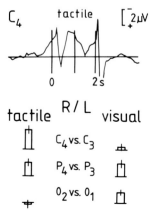

Fig. 2. Hemispheric asymmetry. *Top:* Event-related potentials in C4 in tactile tracking. *Vertical lines* indicate major events: voluntarily initiated onset of stimulus program at $t = 0$, change of stimulus direction at $t = 1$ s and the end of the stimulus program at $t = 2$ s. Note that these events are preceded by SPs and followed by positive P300-like deflections. *Bottom:* Mean negativities, calculated within a 250-ms period prior to $t = 1$, are compared between corresponding sites of the two hemispheres for central, parietal and occipital recordings. *Columns* above the horizontal line indicate larger amplitudes of negativity in recordings of the right hemisphere. Note that right hemispheric preponderance of negativity has a centroparietal distribution in tactile tracking but a parieto-occipital distribution in visual tracking. Double standard error is inserted in the columns

Fig. 3. Comparison between conditions. Amplitudes of the mean negativity as calculated within a 250-ms period preceding change of stimulus direction differ between conditions. Differences are displayed by columns in a topographical manner. *White columns* above the horizontal line indicate larger negativity in the tactile task than in the visual task; *hatched columns* below the horizontal line indicate larger negative amplitudes in the visual task. Double standard error is inserted in the columns

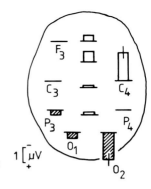

namely in parietal and to some degree in occipital recordings, with larger amplitudes over the right hemisphere. In the tactile task, hemispheric differences are found in central and parietal recordings (Fig. 2). This means that the right hemisphere, which primarily receives the sensory input, has larger amplitudes of SPs than the left hemisphere, which controls final mechanisms for movements of the right hand. This hemispheric asymmetry differs in topography when comparing visually and tactually guided movements. In the tactile experiments we have a centroparietal, in the visual experiment a parieto-occipital distribution of hemispheric asymmetry. As displayed in Fig. 3, SPs differ between tactile and visual tracking, with larger amplitudes of SPs in C4 in the tactile task, but larger amplitudes in O2 in the visual task.

Changes of SPs Related to Response Selection in a Conflicting Paradigm

The visual target had to be tracked by moving the right hand in different ways: In the learning task, tracking had to be performed in a mirrored manner, i.e., movements of the target to the right required hand moving to the left and vice versa, but movements up and down were not inverted. In the control task, the target had to be tracked in a normal, non-inverted fashion. Fourteen subjects participated in the experiment. The experimental arrangement was similar to the previous experiment, except that this time three successive random directions had to be tracked for 1.5 s and the position of the moving hand was displayed as a light spot on the screen. To perform well, subjects had to keep the light point within the target circle. The success of learning was calculated by relating the reduction of tracking error to the mean tracking error.

In the mirrored tracking task, performance-related SPs were significantly larger in frontal and central recordings (at F3, F4, Fz, FCz, C3, Cz, C4) than in the normal tracking control, with a maximum of difference at the frontocentral midline (FCz and Cz). In order to quantify the additional negativity, the

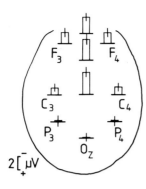

Fig. 4. Comparison between mirrored and normal tracking. Amplitudes of the performance-related SPs, as calculated by the mean negativity within the first 1.5 s of tracking, differ between the two tasks, with larger amplitudes in mirrored tracking in frontal and central recordings (*white columns* above the horizontal line)

mean negativity within the first 1.5 s of tracking was measured. The differences between the two conditions (dN) are displayed topographically in Fig. 4. In contrast to the learning-related additional negativity in frontal leads, there are no differences between the conditions in retrorolandic leads, namely, parietally and occipitally.

From these data we conclude that the frontal lobe may be critical for mechanisms of response selection in conflicting paradigms: On one side, the tendency of normal tracking had to be suppressed, on the other side, Ss had to transfer the concept of changing right and left into the tracking performance (Lang et al. 1983, 1986; Deecke et al. 1985).

Performance-related measurements of rCBF have been performed by the SPECT technique in order to substantiate these findings and to test concepts suggesting a functional significance of connections between frontal lobes and basal ganglia. 17 right-handed, male Ss were examined under both conditions, mirrored tracking and normal tracking. They continuously performed either the mirrored or the simple tracking over a 10-min period. Three minutes after the beginning of the task, the ^{99m}Tc-labeled lipophilic substance (hexamethylpropyleneamineoxime; HMPAO) was administered intravenously (for Methods see Podreka et al. 1987). From basic investigations, it is known that the tracer crosses the blood-brain barrier and is deposited in the cells within a period of 3–4 min after injection. It is distributed by the rCBF and remains trapped in the cells for several hours. Thus, there is enough time for equilibrium brain SPECT.

Compared to control values, visuomotor learning was associated with bihemispheric increases of the rCBF in the middle and inferior frontal gyri, basal ganglia (caudate nucleus and putamen), and frontomedial structures (including the supplementary motor area). High levels of significance (t test) were reached in the middle frontal gyri and in the frontomedial structures ($p<0.001$ and $p<0.005$ respectively; Lang et al. 1987).

References

Boschert J, Deecke L (1986) Cerebral potentials preceding voluntary toe, knee and hip movements and their vectors in human precentral gyrus. Brain Res 376:175–179

Deecke L, Kornhuber HH, Lang W, Lang M, Schreiber H (1985) Timing function of the frontal cortex in sequential motor and learning tasks. Hum Neurobiol 4:143–154

Lang W, Lang M, Kornhuber A, Deecke L, Kornhuber HH (1983) Human cerebral potentials and visuomotor learning. Pflugers Arch 399:342–344

Lang W, Lang M, Heise B, Deecke L, Kornhuber HH (1984) Brain potentials related to voluntary hand tracking: motivation and attention. Hum Neurobiol 3:235–240

Lang W, Lang M, Kornhuber A, Kornhuber HH (1986) Electrophysiological evidence for right frontal lobe dominance in spatial visuomotor learning. Arch Ital Biol 124:1–13

Lang W, Lang M, Podreka I, Suess E, Müller C, Steiner M, Deecke L (1987) Functional imaging (Tc 99m-HMPAO-SPECT) and movement related potentials in a joint study of human visuomotor learning. J Cereb Blood Flow Metab 7 (Suppl 1): S 314

Podreka I, Suess E, Goldenberg G, Steiner M, Brücke T, Müller C, Lang W, Neirinckx RD, Deecke L (1987) Initial experience with Tc-99m-hexamethylprophyleneamineoxime (Tc-99m-HM-PAO) brain SPECT. J Nucl Med 28:1657–1666

Section III Clinical Aspects

A Battery Approach to Clinical Utilisation of Topographic Brain Mapping

H.L. HAMBURGER[1]

Introduction

The introduction of commercially available personal computers has made topographic mapping of electrical brain fields easily accessible to the clinical neurophysiologist.

Untill recently the visual observation of paroxysmal EEG discharges has been preferred over computerised detection of paroxysmal events. However, spectral analysis using the fast Fourier transform (FFT) (Cooley and Tukey 1965) is far more accurate than subjective judgement in the detection of subtle asymmetries of EEG (Huffelen et al. 1984). The use of topographic mapping has made it possible to visualise elements that cannot be seen with the two above-mentioned methods (Duffy 1986).

Topographic mapping may also be used to analyse evoked potentials.

It has been suggested that only mapping can adequately display voltage distributions over the scalp of long-latency evoked potentials (Skrandies and Lehmann 1982; Lehmann and Skrandies 1984).

For every EP measurement 256 data points for all 21 channels are measured. Voltage distributions may be displayed in map form, and sequential display of all maps in time creates a cartoon. Consequently, information about time, space and voltage is available for inspection.

The use of computerised EEG and EP analysis makes it possible to compare patient data with a control group. Duffy and coworkers used the calculation of the z score to compare patient maps with a standard control file (Duffy et al. 1981) resulting in significance probability mapping (SPM). Also, group data can be compared to other groups using the t statistic. The advantage of using maps in conjunction with conventional EEG and EP is the simultaneous use of information on time, space and amplitudes of electrical brain fields. For this purpose, mapping has been done on a battery of FFT, EP and EEG data in our clinic since 1985. The aim of the present study was to find out whether or not mapping of EEG, FFT and EP offers significant advantages over conventional EEG analysis. Specifically: (1) Will a lesion be localised better using mapping techniques than in traditional EEG? (2) Is mapping superior to CT in delineating functional disturbances of the brain? We also wanted to study the advantages of mapping during patient follow-up.

---

[1] Municipal Hospital Slotervaart, Department of Neurology, Louwesweg 6, 1066 EC Amsterdam, The Netherlands

Materials and Methods

All studies were performed in a constantly lit sound-attenuated Faraday cage. EEG is recorded from 21 electrodes using the 10–20 system with addition of FpZ and OZ. Silver-silver chloride recording electrodes were attached to the scalp with collodion and filled with conductive jelly. Impedance of electrode skin contact was maintained below 2 kΩ. For all EEG recordings linked cheeks reference was used with a difference of impedance below 1 kΩ; for EPs the average reference was chosen (Lehmann and Skrandies 1980).

The electrical activity was filtered with bandpass of 0.5–35 Hz for EEG and 0.16–35 Hz for EP. Patient data were transferred from the scalp electrodes to a conventional EEG 21-channel polygraph. On-line analog signals were fed into a Biologic System Corp. Brain Atlas II computer. Sampling rate for all signals was 128 Hz per channel.

FFT was computed from 8–16 epochs of 2 s artefact-free EEG during eyes closed and eyes open conditions. Sessions were repeated for replicability.

Following the transformation of EEG data into the frequency domain, 64 two-dimensional colour maps were created, representing frequencies between 0 and 31.5 Hz, spaced 0.5 Hz apart. The display points were computed using a four-point linear interpolation algorithm. "Cold" colours represent low amplitudes and "warm" colours represent high amplitudes. Values are expressed in microvolts (root of mean square).

Flash visual evoked potential (VEP) is recorded for 21 channels during a 512-ms epoch, pattern reversal VEP samples during a 256-ms epoch. The flash VEP is always recorded with the patient alert, both eyes closed and the flash lamp 30 cm in front of his/her head. Pattern reversal VEP is recorded with the patient looking with both eyes at a checkerboard at the distance of 1 m, checksize 11 mm.

We use a slide projector and rotatable mirror method for stimulation. P300 is measured for a 1 024-ms epoch. Frequent stimuli consist of 1 000-Hz tone bursts for 30 ms, rise and fall time 5 ms at 75 dB. Target tones, given in a ratio of 1:5, consist of 2 000-Hz bursts for 30 ms, rise and fall time 5 ms at 75 dB.

Case Histories

Case 1

A 76-year-old man was referred to the outpatient neurological department because of suspected dementia.

The neurological examination suggested dressing and constructional apraxia. Furthermore, sensory dysphasia was found which explained his "dementia". No motor or sensory disturbances were present. A left parietal cerebral infarction was presumed. CT was inconclusive (Fig. 1) and EEG with topographic

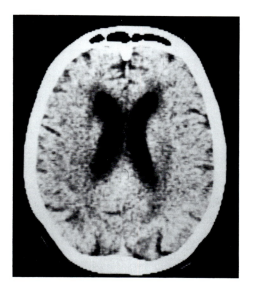

Fig. 1. Cage 1: CT scan. No focal changes can be seen. (All figures in this contribution were prepared using equipment from Biologic Systems Corporation, Mundelein, IL, USA)

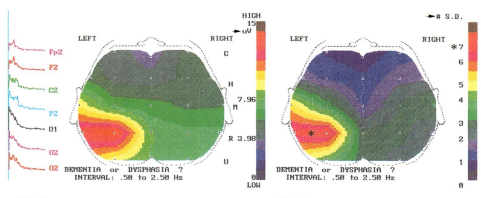

Fig. 2

Fig. 3

Fig. 2. Case 1: This frequency map shows the amplitudes between 0.5 and 2.5 Hz. A left-sided delta focus can be seen at T5 and P3. The red colour depicts the highest amplitude in the voltage distribution

Fig. 3. Case 1: The map here shows not frequencies, but number of standard deviations (SD) difference between the control group and the patient. The maximal difference is seen in the left parietotemporal region, but note that the right parietotemporal region also shows a 3–4 SD difference

mapping was performed. A left-sided delta and theta focus was found (Fig. 2). SPM shows more than 7 standard deviations (SD) difference between the patient and a control group in this frequency band (Fig. 3). Furthermore, a clear asymmetry of VEP P2 may be seen in which the left hemisphere is 28 ms slower than the right in showing maximum amplitude in the occipital area (Figs. 4, 5).

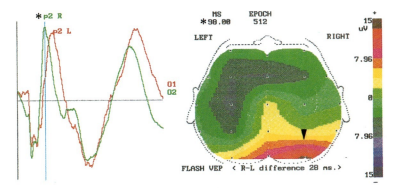

Fig. 4. Case 1: Latency map showing the amplitudes for the flash VEP at 98 ms. In this case the right occipital P2 is reached at a normal latency

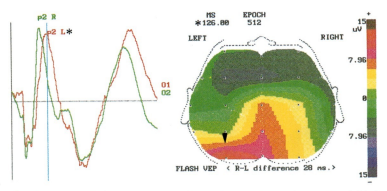

Fig. 5. Case 1: This latency map shows the amplitude for a P2 which is 28 ms later than for the right side at 126 ms. Amplitudes for both side are the same

Discussion. In this case the neurophysiological examination was more sensitive than the CT not only in showing the site of the lesion, but also in confirming the clinical diagnosis. This patient's disease was thought to be related to a vascular disorder, since the EEG, FFT and VEP data showed both cortical and subcortical disturbances. Two months later, follow-up CT after i.v. contrast showed diminished enhancement in the left parietal region.

Case 2

A 79-year-old woman was referred to the neurological department for transient attacks of paresis and numbness of the left arm and leg.

She was diagnosed to have TIAs and a CT scan was performed. Contrast enhancement did not reveal focal changes. Besides the attacks, which were also observed clinically, this patient showed no neurological disturbances.

EEG, FFT and EP revealed focal epileptic discharges in the right hemisphere (Figs. 6, 7). Traditional EEG also showed paroxysmal sharp and slow waves,

A Battery Approach to Clinical Utilisation of Topographic Brain Mapping 171

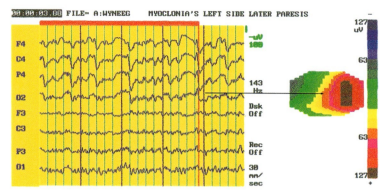

Fig. 6. Case 2: Momentary EEG amplitude MAP showing a right centrotemporal high amplitude distribution of a delta wave

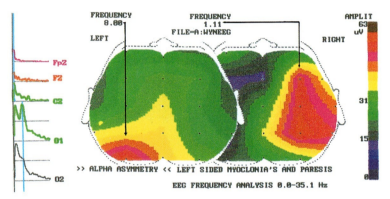

Fig. 7. Case 2: The frequency map of the data seen in Fig. 6 at 1 Hz. High amplitudes are seen in the right frontocentral region. Note the alpha asymmetry

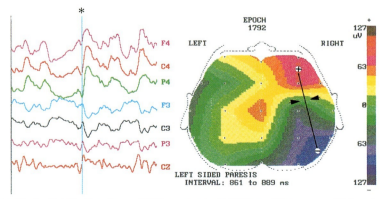

Fig. 8. Case 2: Amplitude distribution in an EEG segment of 1792 ms. The cursor (*) is set on a sharp wave; the focal aspect can be suspected from the wave shapes. The emergence of a "dipole" in the depth of the right central region (*arrow*) can be suspected

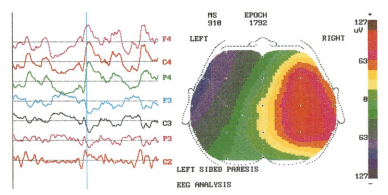

Fig. 9. Case 2: The momentary EEG map amplitude distribution for the delta wave following the sharp wave some 50 ms later than in Fig. 8

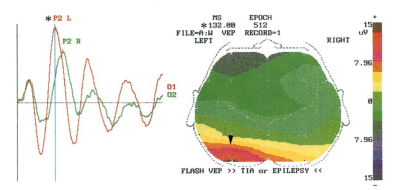

Fig. 10. Case 2: Flash EP shows an asymmetry for the P2. Latencies: 132 ms on left vs 162 ms on right

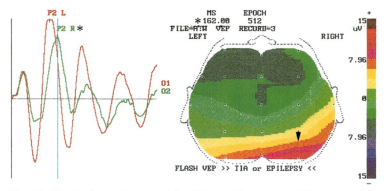

Fig. 11. Case 2: Same data as in Fig. 10 but with cursor at 160 ms

but on the basis of EEG alone, no exact localisation could be made. Raw EEG was stored on a magnetic device and spike segments were identified and averaged off line. In Fig. 8 a dipole can be suspected in the depth of the right hemisphere due to the sharp waves. The consequent delta wave is seen in Fig. 9.

VEPs also display an asymmetry, the right hemisphere showing the longest latencies (Figs. 10, 11).

Discussion. EEG and subsequent mapping were more useful than both CT and clinical neurological examination in understanding the pathophysiology of this case. A final diagnosis of epilepsy was established and the patient was treated accordingly. A different outcome would have resulted if only CT had been performed.

Case 3

A $1^1/_2$-year-old boy was admitted to the paediatric department of our hospital in September 1985. He suffered from a meningococcal septicaemia and was treated immediately with i.v. administered antibiotics. During recovery his parents noticed signs of visual disturbances. The little boy no longer looked at objects and familiar faces, although he still responded to familiar sounds. Ophthalmological examination showed no signs of ocular disease.

CT showed a small hypodense area in the left temporoparietal area which could not explain the visual disturbances (Fig. 12). EEG and VEPs were recorded in the tranditional way and with mapping. EEG and mapping showed high-amplitude, slow and sometimes sharp theta waves in the left temporoparietal area (Fig. 13).

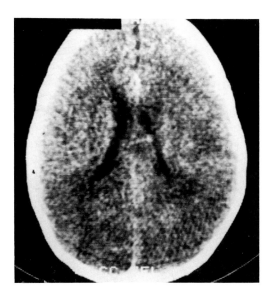

Fig. 12. Case 3: CT scan 1 month after meningococcal septicaemia. At that time the patient was not responding to visual stimuli

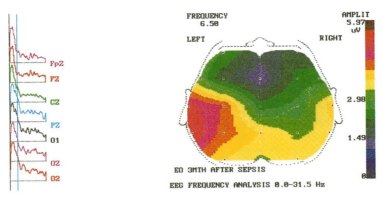

Fig. 13. Case 2: Frequency map at 6.5 Hz. Focal theta waves are seen in the left temporal area

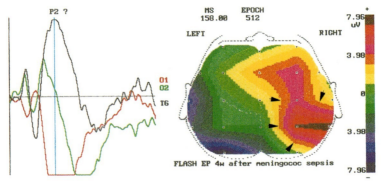

Fig. 14. Case 3: Momentary flash VEP map for P2 as is suggested from the amplitude distribution. Traditional wave shapes are shown on the left side for channels 01, 02 and T6. Decision on the latency for a P2 cannot be made on the basis of these data. The *arrows* indicate the site of the highest amplitude. The *question mark* expresses uncertainty whether this is the P2 distribution or not

Traditionally recorded VEPs were unequivocal. Flash VEP mapping showed no occipital activity. However, the map showed activity generated in the right centrotemporal area (Fig. 14).

The patient was discharged and returned in January 1986 for follow-up. EEG still showed slow and sharp theta waves on the left. VEP mapping showed a shorter P2 latency with a more parietal shift of the maximum amplitude on the right side and no recognizable P2 on the left (Fig. 15). Re-examination in May 1986 showed, for the first time, a right occipital activation in response to the flash (Fig. 16), the P2 latency being 120 ms on the right side and 220 ms on the left side.

Further testing in February 1987 did not show any focal theta. Flash VEP mapping now revealed a normal latency on the right side and a somewhat slower left occipital P2 (Fig. 17).

Our little patient does not show any signs of visual neglect, on the contrary, he has been manipulating various kinds of small objects in his new visual world.

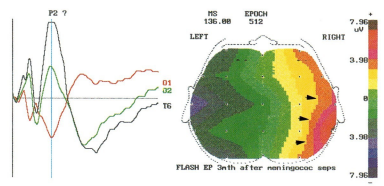

Fig. 15. Case 3: Flash VEP 3 months later is still equivocal. A P2 could not be suspected on the basis of the traditional wave shapes. The momentary map at maximal global field power is given

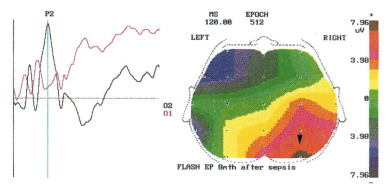

Fig. 16. Case 3: Flash VEP map 8 months after septicaemia shows normalised P2 amplitude distribution for the right hemisphere at 120 ms latency (*arrow*)

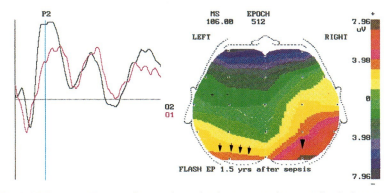

Fig. 17. Case 3: Flash VEP map 1.5 years after septicaemia shows a nearly normalised picture of traditional wave shapes as well as momentary map at 106 ms. The highest amplitudes on the left side were seen at 130 ms

Discussion. In this patient the follow-up of VEP mapping for over 1 year established the final diagnosis of reversible occipital blindness due to damage caused by meningococcal septicaemia. EEG and CT abnormalities were not sufficient to explain the clinical signs. The first VEP map results were also hard to interpret. Only the change of pattern noticed over the course of a year made it clear that an occipital disturbance was the primary cause for the blindness. Without mapping, this diagnosis would not have been as easily established.

Case 4

A 6-year-old boy was referred to the outpatient department because of learning difficulties. At school, more than at home, he was blinking his eyes excessively and was yawning all the time. Moreover, he was accused of deliberately ignoring his teachers. Examination by a school psychologist showed noticeable distractability and low attention span with periods of non-attentiveness.

Neurological examination showed no abnormalities and CT was completely normal (Fig. 18).

Topographic mapping of EEG spectra suggested a left-sided parieto-occipital slow theta focus during the eyes open and eyes closed conditions (Fig. 19). No paroxysmal signs were observed although the theta waves had a sharp segment.

VEP mapping was completely normal. P300 tests showed inconclusive results (Fig. 20). A centrotemporal voltage distribution is seen instead of the usual parietofrontal maximum and minimum.

Carbamazepine treatment was initiated, after which improvement was clinically evident and confirmed by neuropsychological examination. The patient's school performance improved as well and was within the normal range.

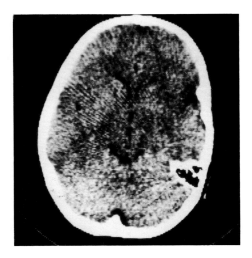

Fig. 18. Case 4: CT scan showing no abnormalities

A Battery Approach to Clinical Utilisation of Topographic Brain Mapping

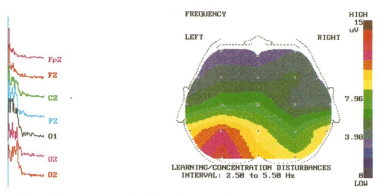

Fig. 19. Case 4: Focal slow theta waves in the left occipital region are seen in this frequency map in which the average amplitude is seen between 2.5 and 5.5 Hz

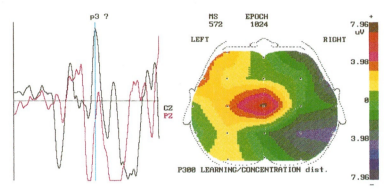

Fig. 20. Case 4: Momentary amplitude map at 572 ms for the P300 result of the target stimulus. The latency is rather large and the amplitude rather low with a maximum at Cz. The amplitude at Pz is low. The *question mark* indicates uncertainty about the precise latency of the P300

Follow-up study of EEG and FFT mapping 1 year later showed no asymmetries (Fig. 21). No abnormalities were present on the left. Again, VEP mapping for flash and pattern reversal were normal. P300 study now shows normal results in respect to latencies, but voltage distribution (Fig. 22) is still not normal.

Discussion. Serial evaluations have suggested that the first P300 measurement showed a pathological latency which recovered to normal limits following 1 year's administration of anti-epileptic drugs (post or propter?) However, voltage distribution was and still is pathological. The normalisation of the frequency pattern is seen quite often in follow-up studies of EEG. It remains to be seen whether or not this phenomenon is related to the above-mentioned pathophysiology.

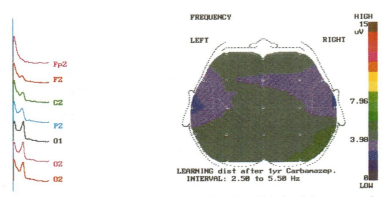

Fig. 21. Case 4: A frequency map 1 year later in which focal theta can no longer be seen

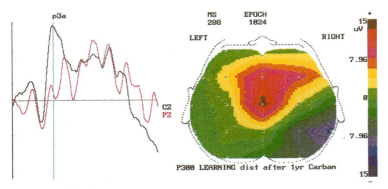

Fig. 22. Case 4: P300 latency has dropped after 1 year to 288 ms for the P3a; a P3b component is not clearly present. The amplitude map again shows a pathological centroparietal distribution. From the traditional curves at Cz and Pz no abnormality can be suspected. Only the amplitude map shows abnormal distribution

Case 5

A 21-year-old woman with no prior history of neurological disease suffered an epileptic fit, the day before she was referred to our outpatient department. Examination revealed no neurological deficit. The visual fields and visual acuity were normal.

One day later EEG was performed, showed only minor diffuse slowing and sharp theta waves during hyperventilation without specific localisation.

Mapping of FFT consistently showed a right occipital delta and theta focus (Fig. 23). Statistical comparison suggested a difference of 6 SD from the normal group (Fig. 24). Furthermore, the occipital alpha frequencies were 1.5 Hz slower on the right side than on the left side (Figs. 25, 26).

The visual evoked responses showed an occipital asymmetry in map amplitudes for left and right hemispheres (Fig. 27).

CT showed a large right occipital meningeoma, which was removed.

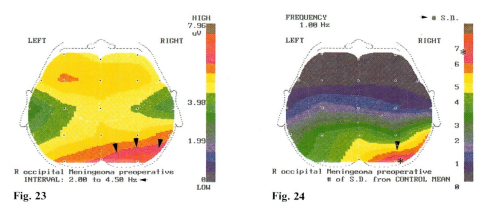

Fig. 23. Case 5: Focal delta waves appear in this frequency map at the site (*arrow*) where a meningeoma was later found

Fig. 24. Case 5: SPM for data seen in Fig. 23. A 6 SD difference between the patient and the control file can be seen. Note the 3–4 SD difference in the left occipital area

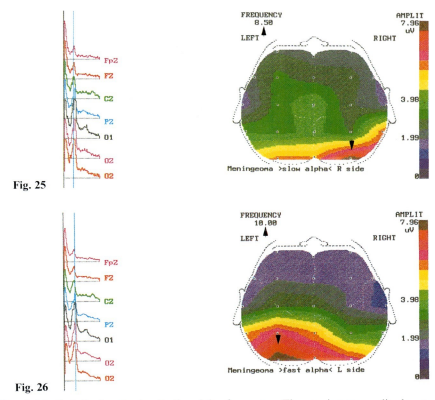

Figs. 25 and 26. Case 5: Asymmetry in the alpha frequency. The maximum amplitude on the right side is seen at 8.5 Hz (Fig. 25), while on the left side the maximal amplitude is seen at 10.0 Hz (Fig. 26)

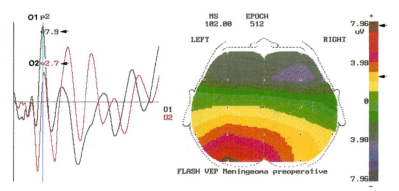

Fig. 27. Case 5: Flash VEP map for P2. An asymmetry is seen in which the amplitude at O2 is less than half the value measured at O1. The *arrows* at the left of the figure correspond to those at the right by the colour bar amplitude scale

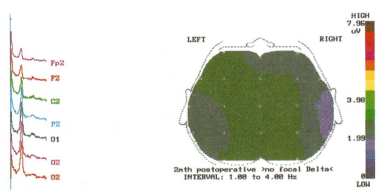

Fig. 28. Case 5: Focal delta is no longer seen 2 months after surgery in which the complete meningeoma was removed without doing structural damage to the cortex cerebri

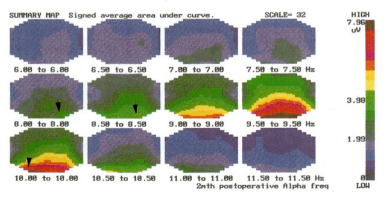

Fig. 29. Case 5: There is still an asymmetry in the alpha frequency band 2 months after operation. The asymmetry is still 0.5 Hz. The slower frequency maximum at O2, the faster at O1

A Battery Approach to Clinical Utilisation of Topographic Brain Mapping

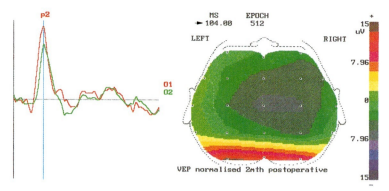

Fig. 30. Case 5: Flash VEP is normalised 2 months after removal of the meningeoma

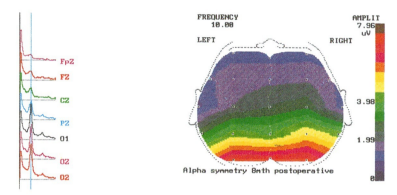

Fig. 31. Case 5: This frequency map shows normal alpha symmetry again at 10.0 Hz 8 months after operation

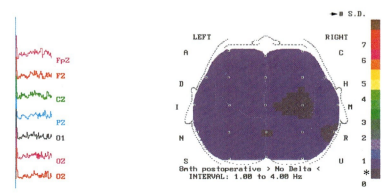

Fig. 32. Case 5: SPM data of FFT of case 5 at 8 months after operation. No more than 1 SD difference can be detected between this file and the control file

Two months later the patient returned for a neurological check-up, which showed no signs of neurological deficit. Again, EEG, FFT and VEP were performed. The right occipital delta and theta focus had disappeared (Fig. 28); alpha was still somewhat asymmetrical (Fig. 29). The VEP was normalised and symmetrical (Fig. 30). Eight months after operation a third neurophysiological check-up was performed. There were no pathological delta foci and no asymmetry of the alpha rhythm (Fig. 31), suggesting complete recovery (SPM data shown in Fig. 32).

Discussion. The initial right-sided lesion was obviously caused by the meningeoma and disappeared during the weeks following operation. The alpha rhythm and VEP needed a longer period to recover.

General Discussion

The use of quantitative EEG techniques has been suggested to be superior to traditional EEG assessment (van Huffelen et al. 1984). Recent developments enable us to produce topographic maps of electrical brain fields, serving as a new tool for more sophisticated analysis of EEG. Not only is background EEG measured, but also real-time EEG is studied for paroxysmally occurring events.

The results of this study show that mapping of FFT data is superior to visual EEG assessment of background activity. Traditional quantitative EEG results in long lists of numbers. As an aid to the examiner's eye these spectra can be displayed graphically. Consequently the localisation of a pathological finding is made in the clinical neurophysiologist's mind. However, the distinct advantage of mapping is that it provides the examiner with data that are ordered in frequency, in amplitude, and in space. With this tool one can recognize patterns in the EEG that could not be detected with traditional EEG spectral analysis alone (Duffy 1986; Hamburger 1987a).

For the identification of pathological states information from all 21 channels is weighted equally. This can only be achieved by using the spatial configuration of frequency maps as unbiased information for assessment of a global brain state (Lehmann 1986; Lehmann et al. 1987). The use of multimodality mapping allows us to form a more dynamic impression of brain function. Modern computer instrumentation makes it possible to interchange quickly between EEG, FFT and EP data and to perform these three measurements quickly and efficiently. Our cases show that a better and more adequate diagnosis can be reached on the basis of spatial information conveyed by these data. In addition, the time factor in follow-up allows us to get a better insight into the localisation of cerebral dysfunction.

Comparison with normative data is one of the methods used to decide whether or not results correspond to normal. This could never be done with traditional "paper" EEG.

SPM mapping can only be applied to show large differences between a patient and a control group. For the detection of more subtle changes this method is too coarse.

The vast quantity of data generated by mapping gives rise to more questions than answers, making new methods of interpretation necessary.

The use of spatial principal component analysis can be a great help in localizing maximal voltage differences in EP or spontaneous EEG maps. Moreover, global field power is a one-number statement for all electrodes, and the actual location of the Map's peaks and troughs (Lehmann and Skrandies 1980).

In analyzing frequency spectra there is no computation of a single overall statement for deciding the frequency and amplitude distribution that shows the largest abnormality. One should look through the whole range of frequency maps on the colour monitor to detect small shifts in the alpha rhythm and/or foci of high amplitude in the other frequency bands.

In many cases an asymmetrical slowing of alpha rhythm of 0.5 Hz is the only sign of pathology present in the EEG. A lesion might remain undetected or not precisely localised even with our highly sensitive methods of measurement. Mapping equipment should therefore never produce four or six summary maps of frequency bands. In our case 5 the right-left asymmetry would not have been detected if only summary maps of delta, theta, alpha and beta had been used.

However, it should be stated that EEG or mapping cannot replace CT for localisation of anatomical lesions. What mapping can be used for is the screening of patients with functional disorders, thus eliminating the high cost of performing too many screening CT scans. Clinical neurophysiological examination is superior to CT for measuring functional disturbances in brain disease. Furthermore, many patients have functional brain disorders without evident anatomical changes. This is the case in epilepsy, dyslexia and most dementias. In these patients CT or magnetic resonance imaging will give inconclusive results for diagnosis, whereas mapping of EEG, FFT and EP will most likely show severe disturbances (Hamburger 1986; Hamburger 1987b).

References

Cooley JW, Tukey JW (1965) An algorithm for the machine calculation of complex Fourier series. Math Comp 19:297–301

Duffy FH (1986) Brain electrical activity mapping. Issues and answers. In: Duffy FH (ed) Topographic mapping of brain electrical activity. Butterworths, Boston

Duffy FH, Bartels PH, Burchfield JL (1981) Significance probability mapping. An aid in the topographic analysis of brain electrical activity. Electroencephalogr Clin Neurophysiol 51:455–462

Hamburger HL (1986) Visual evoked potentials and brain electrical activity mapping. In: Gallai V (ed) Maturation of the CNS and evoked potentials. Elsevier, Amsterdam, pp 27–31

Hamburger HL (1987a) Psychophysiological function testing and topographic brain mapping. Clin Neurol Neurosurg 89(2):93

Hamburger HL (1987b) Brain mapping in patients with epilepsy. Clin Neurol Neurosurg 89(2):105

Huffelen AC van, Poortvliet DCJ, Wulp CJM van der (1984) Quantitative electro-encephalography in cerebral ischemia. Detection of abnormalities in normal EEG's. In: Pfurtscheller G, Jonkman EJ, Lopes da Silva FH (eds) Brain ischemia: quantitative EEG and imaging techniques. Elsevier, Amsterdam, pp 3–28

Lehmann D (1986) Spatial analysis of EEG and evoked potential data. In: Duffy FH (ed) Topographic mapping of brain electrical activity. Butterworths, Boston

Lehmann D, Skrandies W (1980) Reference-free identification of the components of checkerboard-evoked multichannel potential fields. Electroencephalogr Clin Neurophysiol 48:609–621

Lehmann D, Skrandies W (1984) Spatial analysis of evoked potentials in man. A review. Progr Neurobiol 23:227–250

Lehmann D, Ozaki H, Pal I (1987) EEG alpha map series-brain microstates by space oriented adaptive segmentation. Electroencephalogr Clin Neurophysiol 67:271–288

Skrandies W, Lehmann D (1982) Spatial principal components of multichannel maps evoked by lateral visual halffield stimuli. Electroencephalogr Clin Neurophysiol 54:662–667

Topography of Background EEG Rhythms in Normal Subjects and in Patients with Cerebrovascular Disorders

D. SAMSON-DOLLFUS, C. DELMER, Y. VASCHALDE, E. DREANO, and D. FODIL[1]

Introduction

The purpose of this work is to demonstrate that it is useful to study very carefully EEG mapping of background alpha, delta, theta and beta rhythms in patients with supratentorial ischemia and with a normal or subnormal EEG on visual assessment. In normal populations, there is now general agreement that the differences between young and healthy elderly people are very slight. These small differences can be expressed by various methods: multivariate analysis (John 1981; Kopruner and Pfurtscheller 1984; Jonkman et al. 1985; Senant et al. 1966a, b) and topographic EEG mapping (Duffy 1984) are now the most commonly used. To compare normal subjects and patients with brain ischemia, we have chosen to use brain electrical activity mapping. Jonkman et al. (1985), Kopruna and Pfurtscheller (1984), Van Huffelen et al. (1984), Pfurtscheller et al. (1981) and Tolonen et al. (1981) used quantitative EEG in patients with cerebrovascular diseases, but did not at that time use mapping to express their results.

Material and Methods

Twenty-nine normal subjects aged 22–82 years and 22 patients (42–75 years) with asymptomatic stenosis ($n=4$), transient ischemic attack (TIA; $n=8$) or ischemic cerebral vascular attacks (ICVA; $n=11$) were recorded. All of them had a *de visu* normal EEG, as did the subjects studied by Van Huffelen et al. (1984). The normal group was divided in two samples under ($n=15$) and over ($n=14$) 40 years of age. EEG brain mapping (Alvar Cartovar) was obtained from 16 active electrodes (10/20 system). The common reference was linked ears for normal subjects and either average common reference, linked ears or chin reference for patients (depending on the symptomatology and the suspected topography of the lesion).

Artifact-free 10-s or 30-s EEG samples were processed on a microcomputer. Fast Fourier Transformation was computed on successive 2-s samples. These power spectra (PS) were averaged. The data were recorded at rest with eyes closed and at rest with eyes open. EEG topographic display was decided from the listing of the values of each frequency PS between 1 and 30 Hz (0.5-Hz

---

[1] Laboratoire d'Explorations Neurologiques, Centre Hospitalier Universitaire, Pavillon Félix-Dévé, 76031 Rouen Cedex, France

steps). Most often, beta rhythms above 25 Hz were not displayed because of muscle artifacts; very often, delta rhythms were computed between 2 and 3.5 Hz to avoid eye artifacts.

Results

Normal Groups

There was no differences in the *delta band* between the younger and older control subjects: in both groups the delta band had a very small power spectrum, concentrated on central regions with the eyes closed, with very little increase when the eyes opened, if no eye-movement artifacts intervened.

In the *theta band*, the topography was the same, with a tendency to be more powerful in younger people and less powerful in the older group when the eyes were open.

On average, peak *alpha* frequency was the same (10 Hz) but the *bandwidth* was different: in younger people, occipital rhythms reacting to opening of the eyes were between 9 and 12.5 Hz. The 8-Hz band was much more diffuse. In the older group the alpha band was narrower and slower, 8.5–11 Hz; above 11 Hz these frequencies began to be parietal instead of occipital.

In young people, *beta 1 and beta 2 rhythms* were localized in the occipital regions and reacted when the eyes opened. In the older group, beta 1 and beta 2 rhythms were centroparietal, and were much more abundant, as already stated in 1967 by Matousek et al. They diminished when eyes open.

In summary, there were no differences in the slower rhythms (under 8 Hz) between younger and older controls, but differences in the topography of the alpha and beta rhythms were observed. Moreover, beta rhythms were much more powerful in older than in younger people. Table 1 shows the number of EEG mappings with "particularities" in each group. Particularities – for instance too much theta or delta, high asymmetry in alpha or poor visual reactivity – were more frequent in the older group than in the younger.

Table 1. Number of particularities found in normal controls

	n	Particularities					
		0	1	2	3	4	5
Group 1[a]	15	10	3	2	0	0	0
Group 2[b]	14	1	8	2	3	0	0

n, number of particularities observed on the map and number of subjects in each group

[a] Group 1: 23–40 years
[b] Group 2: 41–82 years

Patient Groups

The results from the patients compared to those from the age-matched older control group. Though the EEG seemed normal *de visu*, mapping detected abnormalities (called "particularities" in controls in power, topography and reactivity in the delta, theta, alpha and beta bands. One or two isolated particularities were observed more often in older than in younger normal subjects (Table 1). For that reason, we insisted that more than two abnormalities be present in a patient for him/her to be considered as having abnormal cerebral electrogenesis.

Theta and Delta Bands. The most evident pathological abnormalities in the slow theta and delta rhythms were an asymmetric PS increase and an occipital localization even if the lesion was more anterior.

Alpha Rhythms. The most striking abnormalities of alpha rhythms were in their localization and reactivity. In these patients, alpha was often localized in the centroparietal instead of the occipital region. The reactivity to opening of the eyes was quite often very poor.

Beta Rhythms. Beta rhythms were not abundant, particularly when asymmetry existed between the two hemispheres. In this case, it was abnormal to have fewer beta rhythms on the pathological side.

Conclusions

Significant abnormalities were more frequent in *TIA* due to carotid stenosis, three of every four patients), than in other etiologies (one in every four patients) (Table 2).

Table 2. Transient ischemic attacks

Patient no.	Side	Delay[a]	Number of abnormalities	
			Homolateral	Contralateral
Carotid stenosis				
1	Right	4 months	2	1
2	Right[b]	3 months	3	1
3	Right	6 days	4	0
4	Left	1 month	1	0
Cardiac embolism				
5	Left	8 days	0	0
6	Right	1 day	1	0
7	Left	1 day	3	0
Coagulation disease				
8	Left	3 days	1	0

[a] Delay between clinical symptomatology and EEG mapping
[b] Asymptomatic contralateral lesion

Table 3. Asymptomatic carotid stenosis

Patient no.	Side	Number of abnormalities	
		Homolateral	Contralateral
9	Left[a]	3	1
10	Right[a]	0	0
11	Right	3	0
12	Left	3	2

[a] Another stenosis existed on the other carotid

Table 4. Ischemic cerebral vascular attacks

Patient no.	Side	Delay[a]	Number of abnormalities	
			Homolateral	Contralateral
Carotid stenosis				
13	Right	3 months	3	0
14	Left[b]	8 days	0	1
15	Left	2 days	2	0
16	Right	2 days	3	1
17	Right[b]	3 weeks	1	3
17[c]	Right	7 weeks	1	3
18	Left	2 months	0	0
Middle cerebral ant. stenosis				
19	Left	10 days	2	0
Cardiac embolism				
20	Left	2 months	3	1
21	Left	5 days	6	0
Coagulation disease				
22	Left	10 days	4	1

[a] Delay between the first symptom and EEG mapping
[b] Asymptomatic contralateral lesion
[c] Between the two EEG mappings, this patient had a vertebrobasilar TIA

Three of the four patients with clinical *asymptomatic stenosis* had abnormal EEG mapping (Table 3).

Only four of the 11 patients with ICVA (Table 4) had a normal EEG mapping.

No relation was found to the date of the initial accident (Tables 2, 4).

Finally, it was very rare, but possible, to observe *bilateral abnormalities* even in strictly unilateral lesions (Tables 2, 4).

Discussion

We have chosen patients with ischemic brain disease or asymptomatic carotid stenosis, in both cases with a visually normal EEG. It is quite interesting that even in these cases, EEG brain mapping of the background ryhthms yielded better information than the rough EEG.

We were not as systematic as Koerner et al. (this volume) or Jonkman et al. (1985) in following the EEG evolution after the first manifestation of disease. However, we found no correlation between the age of the ischemic insult and the EEG findings (Tables 2, 4).

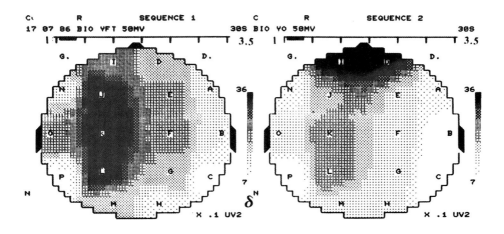

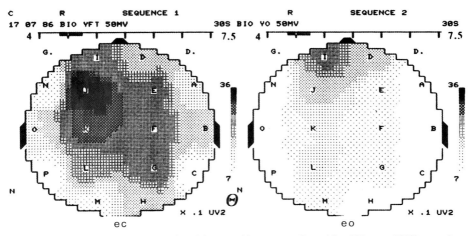

Fig. 1. Complete left sylvian stroke in a 74-year-old man, confirmed by CT scan. EEG mapping shows an obvious abnormality at the same location, 10 days after the stroke. *EC*, eyes closed; *EO*, eyes open. With eyes open there are eye artifacts in the delta band. *Upper maps*, delta band; *lower maps*, theta band

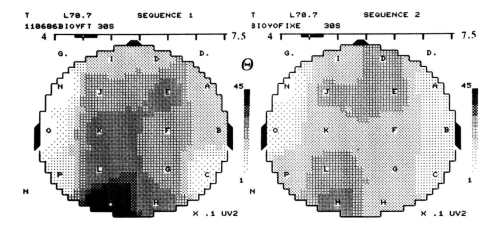

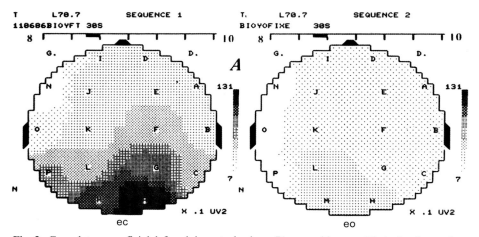

Fig. 2. Complete superficial left sylvian stroke in a 71-year-old man. Theta is observed on the left occipital area, which is very abnormal (*upper maps*). Alpha rhythms are normal on the right side (*lower maps*). *ec*, Eyes closed; *eo*, eyes open

The older control subjects have more particularities than the younger ones. This is certainly normal. Three of our normal older controls might possibly have had asymptomatic carotid stenosis: we did not perform Doppler examination of the carotids in our normal subjects.

The abnormalities appeared to be localized either exactly on the lesion (Fig. 1), or on the same side as the lesion but in different position (Fig. 2). In the latter cases, the EEG abnormality may be only functional and not anatomical.

Finally, since EEG mapping seems more powerful than rough EEG, and since it revealed different abnormalities than the CT scan, it would appear to be a very useful tool to follow up patients with vascular disorders, whether the etiology is vascular stenosis or cardiac embolism.

References

Duffy FH, Albert MS, McAnulty G, Garvez AJ (1984) Age-related differences in brain electrical activity of healthy subjects. Ann Neurol 16:430–438

John ER (1981) Neurometric evaluation of brain dysfunction related to learning disorders. Acta Neurol Scand [Suppl] 64(89):87–100

Jonkman EJ, Poortvliet DCJ, Veering MM, De Weerd AW, John ER (1985) The use of neurometrics in the study of patients with cerebral ischemia. Electroencephalogr Clin Neurophysiol 61:333–341

Kopruner V, Pfurtscheller G (1984) Multiparametric asymmetry score (MAS) – distinction between normal and ischaemic brains. Electroencephalogr Clin Neurophysiol 57:343–346

Matousek J, Volavka J, Roubicek, Roth Z (1967) EEG frequency analysis related to age in normal adults. Electroencephalogr clin Neurophysiol 23:162–167

Pfurtscheller G, Sager W, Wege W (1981) Correlations between CT scan and sensorimotor EEG rhythms in patients with cerebrovascular disorders. Electroencephalogr Clin Neurophysiol 52:473–485

Senant J, Delapierre G, Samson-Dollfus D, Tsouria Z, Bertoldi I (1986a) Analyse spectrale de l'électroencéphalogramme au cours du vieillissement. Evolution de différents paramètres. In: Court L, Trocherie S, Doucet C (eds) Le traitement du signal en électrophysiologie expérimentale et clinique du système nerveux central. Imprimerie Lefranc, Candé, pp 210–219

Senant J, Samson-Dollfus D, Delapierre G, Menard JF, Bertoldi-Lefever I (1986b) Analyse automatique de l'électroencéphalogramme et vieillissement chez des subjets normaux et vasculaires. Sem Hôp Paris 62:3505–3509

Tolonen U, Ahonen A, Sulg IA, Kuikka J, Kallanrata T, Koskinen M, Hokkanen E (1981) Serial measurements of quantitative EEG and cerebral blood flow and circulation time after brain infarction. Acta Neurol Scand 63:145–155

Van Huffelen AC, Poortvliet DCJ, van der Wulp CJM (1984) Quantitative electroencephalography in cerebral ischemia. Detection of abnormalities in "normal" EEGs. In: Pfurtscheller G, Jonkman EJ, Lopez DA, Silva FH (eds) Quantitative EEG and imaging techniques. Brain ischemia. Elsevier, Amsterdam, pp 3–28

P300 and Coma

B.M. Reuter and D.B. Linke[1]

Introduction

There can be no doubt about the importance of the early and middle latency components of the evoked potentials for the practice of clinical neurology and neurosurgery (for review, see Halliday 1981; Stöhr et al. 1982). Up to now, however, the late components of the evoked potentials have not been given much attention in intensive care medicine and neurology. We want to show that the late components may also be of clinical importance because the level of consciousness, which has to be evaluated in intensive care medicine, can correlate to them.

The best-known endogenous component of the evoked potential is P300 (Sutton et al. 1965; for review, see Rockstroh et al. 1982; Hillyard and Kutas 1983). The aim of our study was to investigate the correlation between the P300 (or P3) component of the evoked potential and the state, as well as the outcome of coma, of patients with severe head injury. Furthermore, we wanted to determine whether simple cognition – as expressed by P300 – occurs in stages of reduced consciousness.

P300 is generally accepted to be a measure for the stimulus discrimination ability in sequential information processing involving short-term memory (Tueting 1978; Hillyard and Woods 1979). It is a well-known fact, demonstrated by Squires et al. (1975), Courchesne (1978) and others, that there are two components, one in more frontal areas (the so-called P3a) and the other in the parietal areas (the so-called P3b). The P3a is correlated more with the orienting response, whereas the P3b is more cognitive and categorizing in nature (see Fig. 1).

P300 with a more frontal characteristic can be elicited in normal test persons in a state of passive attention in which they are asked to ignore stimuli. If the P3 complex can be elicited without directed attention it should be possible to perform this investigation in comatose patients.

It is of great theoretical and practical interest to see how the reduction of consciousness in different states of coma correlates to P300. As far as the theoretical interest is concerned, it is important to understand whether simple cognition can be processed without consciousness. Practical interest in P300 lies mainly in the need for better methods of evaluating the state of consciousness, of possibly reaching a prognosis and of gathering information about the involvement of the reticular formation (Desmedt 1980), the thalamus (Yingling and Hosobuchi 1984), the hippocampus (Squires 1983; Halgren et al. 1980) and the frontal and parietal cortex.

---

[1] Neurochirurgische Universitätsklinik, Sigmund-Freud-Str. 25, 5300 Bonn 1, Federal Republic of Germany

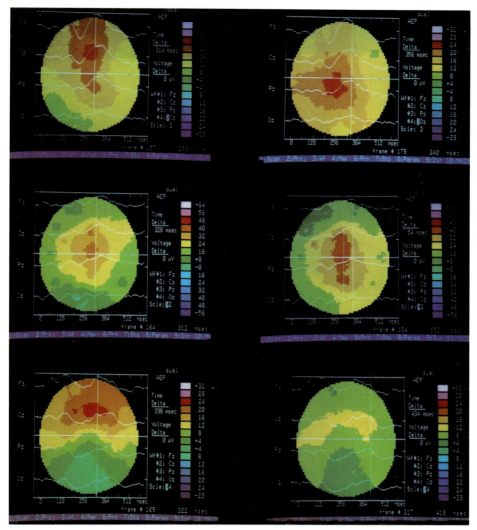

Fig. 1. P300 in different stages of consciousness. *Top:* P300 in a normal test person with directed attention (counting condition: P3a, P3b). *Middle:* P300 in a normal subject with non-directed attention (ignoring condition: P3a, P3b). *Bottom:* P300 in a comatose, non-rousable patient (Glasgow Coma Scale 7). The frontal P3a and the parietal P3b could be measured

Methods

Thirty-one comatose patients with closed head injuries were investigated using the P300 paradigm. We chose to use alternating tone bursts with high and low pitch tones intermingled at a ratio of 1:10. The burst frequencies were

1000 and 1500 Hz. The loudness was 85 dB SPL for both. We used monopolar recordings from Fz, Cz, Pz with linked mastoids, or a 28-channel brain electrical activity mapping technique. We chose a long interstimulus interval (ISI) of 2.3 s because we expected the occurrence of very late components.

Normal brainstem auditory evoked potentials and auditory evoked potentials of middle latency demonstrated the functional integrity of the auditory pathways. In some experiments a pretrigger of 400 ms was used as a baseline. The level of consciousness in our patients was ranked according to the Glasgow Coma Scale (Teasdale and Jennett 1974). In addition more extensive clinical neurological examinations were carried out regularly.

Results

In 13 patients we found no late components at all. In a further 11 patients the late components did not differ significantly from baseline recording. In three other patients we were able to record late latencies, for example P2, but failed to show the P3 wave.

Finally a group of four patients remained where P3 occurred as reaction to the infrequent stimuli. All these patients had a coma score of 7 on the Glasgow Coma Scale. These patients were not rousable, but showed coordinated reactions to pain stimuli. The averaged potentials after high and low pitch stimulation showed significant differences as calculated by the t test ($p<0.001$).

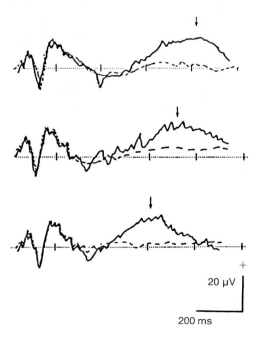

Fig. 2. P300 in coma. The P3 latency (in Cz) reduces with the improvement in the level of consciousness

The peak of the P3 wave was extended and occurred much later than 300 ms. For example, in the case of a 20-year-old male patient with closed head injury and diffuse brain edema, the peak of P3 occurred at 800 ms (Fig. 2). This was registered for the first time 8 days after the trauma with the patient being scored 7 on the Glasgow Coma Scale. In the following days the P3 latencies reduced continuously, improving parallel with his clinical condition. In the state of drowsiness P3 was still delayed, showing a latency of 600 ms. P3 was preceded by a broad negativity which is known as mismatch negativity (Näatänen et al. 1980; Ford and Hillyard 1981) and corresponds to the orienting response.

In the early stages of coma the P1 and P2 components had already returned to the normal range, whereas the P3 wave was still delayed and thus proved to be a sensitive parameter for assessing depth of coma.

Figure 1 (bottom) shows a delayed P300 in another comatose patient, also with a score of 7 on the Glasgow Coma Scale. All of the four patients showing the P3 phenomenon survived their closed head injury and showed only minor deficiencies according to the Glasgow Outcome Scale (Jennett and Bond 1975) 6 months after the trauma.

Discussion

The cognitive correlate of P3 in our setting remains to be determined. Does it have the quality of a nonspecific orienting response (see Squires 1975), or must it be correlated to higher cognition, as suggested by several authors in the discussion of P300 (see Tueting 1978; Donchin 1979, 1980; Desmedt 1980)?

The answer to this question is difficult because both phenomena generate a P3 wave, which can be differentiated only by topographic recording and habituation. In addition, the comparison between P3 of normal persons and comatose patients is difficult because of their different attentive states. Normal subjects are requested to actively ignore stimuli by for example reading a book, whereas comatose patients are passively – and without instruction – exposed to the paradigm. Reduced vigilance in coma and active switch of attention to another channel are different types of processing. Therefore one has to be very careful when comparing comatose patients with normal subjects.

In view of this, topography seems to be the most reliable method, showing the orienting response to be preferably distributed over the frontal areas. This corresponds to the P3a wave of Squires et al. (1975). In our findings the P3 wave was also seen in parietal areas. This resembles much more the normal distribution of P300. Usually P300 is associated with cognitive processing, and based on our findings we would like to suggest that elementary forms of cognition are possible even in some states of reduced consciousness.

References

Courchesne E (1978) Changes in P3 waves with event repetition: long term effects on scalp distribution and amplitude. Electroencephalogr Clin Neurophysiol 45:754–766

Desmedt J (1980) P300 in serial tasks; an essential post-decision closure mechanism. In: Kornhuber HH, Deecke L (eds) Motivation, motor and sensory processes of the brain. Electrical potentials, behavior and clinical use. Elsevier, Amsterdam, pp 682–688

Donchin E (1979) Event related brain potentials: a tool in the study of human information processing. In: Begleiter H (ed) Evoked brain potentials and behavior. Plenum, New York, pp 13–88

Donchin E, Israel JB (1980) Event related potentials and psychological theory. In: Kornhuber HH, Deecke L (eds) Motivation, motor and sensory processes of the brain. Electrical potentials, behavior and clinical use. Elsevier, Amsterdam, pp 697–716

Ford JM, Hillyard SA (1981) ERPs to interruptions of a steady rhythm. Psychophysiology 18:322–330

Halgren E, Squires NK, Wilson CL, Rohrbaugh JW, Babb TL, Crandall PH (1980) Endogenous potentials generated in the human hippocampal-formation by infrequent events. Science 210:803–805

Halliday AM (1981) Evoked potentials in clinical testing. Churchill Livingstone, London

Hillyard SA, Kutas M (1983) Electrophysiology of cognitive processing. Annu Rev Psychol 34:33–61

Hillyard SA, Woods D (1979) Electrophysiological analysis of human brain function. In: Gazzaniga M (ed) Handbook of behavioral neurobiology, vol 2. Plenum, New York, pp 345–378

Jennett B, Bond MR (1975) Assessment of outcome after severe brain damage. Lancet 1:480–481

Näätänen R, Gaillard AWK, Mäntysalo S (1980) Brain potential correlates of voluntary and involuntary attention. In: Kornhuber HH, Deecke L (eds) Motivation, motor and sensory processes of the brain. Electrical potentials, behavior and clinical use. Elsevier, Amsterdam, pp 343–348

Rockstroh B, Elbert T, Birbaumer N, Lutzenberger W (1982) Slow brain potentials and behavior. Urban and Schwarzenberg, Baltimore, pp 1–38

Squires NK (1983) Human endogenous limbic potentials: cross-modality and depth/surface comparisons in epileptic subjects. In: Gaillard AWK, Ritter W (eds) Tutorials in ERP research: endogenous components. North Holland, Amsterdam

Squires NK, Squires KC, Hillyard SA (1975) Two varieties of long-latency positive waves evoked by unpredictable auditory stimuli in man. Electroencephalogr Clin Neurophysiol 38:387–401

Stöhr M, Dichgans J, Diener HC, Buettner UW (1982) Evozierte Potentiale. Springer, Berlin Heidelberg New York Tokyo

Sutton S, Braren M, John ER, Zubin J (1965) Evoked potential correlates of stimulus uncertainty. Science 150:1187–1188

Teasdale G, Jennet B (1974) Assessment of coma and impaired consciousness: a practical scale. Lancet 2:81–84

Tueting P (1978) Event related potentials, cognitive events, and information processing: a summary of issues and discussion. In: Otto DA (ed) Multidisciplinary perspectives in event related brain potential research. US Environmental Protection Agency, Washington, pp 159–169

Yingling CD, Hosobuchi Y (1984) A subcortical correlate of P300 in man. Electroencephalogr Clin Neurophysiol 59:72–76

Structure Differences of Topographical EEG Mappings

R.H. JINDRA and R. VOLLMER[1]

Introduction

In recent years great efforts have been undertaken to compute two-dimensional mappings from EEG recordings. The algorithms have been taken from applied theory of stochastic processes or from electrodynamics. Regarding the first method, namely the computation of the second-order moments, the correlation function, or its integral transform the power spectra, are extended to vector-valued processes, including some additional features like cross-correlation, cross-spectra or coherency. It must be noted, however, that due to the registration procedure the signals are taken as potential differences between a local electrode and a reference point, including their statistical inferences. In such cases the correlation functions or their equivalent transforms are meaningless and therefore produce erroneous and misleading results. Methods based on electrodynamics, on the other hand, compute mappings by relaxation methods. The raw material is obtained by digital fourier transform (DFT) and means, physically, power. The mathematical background to this computation is Laplace's equation, which is not valid in the case of charges existing in the region of interest. A comprehensive study including various techniques based on the above principles was reported by Duffy (1986).

To meet these difficulties, the present authors introduced a new principle into topographical mapping (Jindra and Vollmer 1986), i.e., computation of the structure function. This quantity is not limited by mathematical or physical constraints such as those which limit the procedures described above. Additional features are discussed below. In a further computation procedure, confidence limits for the values of the structure function are used to detect differences in the structure projection of the brain's electrical activity onto the scalp.

Methods

The structure function is defined as the average squared difference between the actual point and the point where the difference is to be taken:

$$s(x_i) = \overline{(x_i - x_0)^2} \qquad (1)$$

---

[1] Ludwig-Boltzmann-Institut für Klinische Neurobiologie, Krankenhaus Wien-Lainz, Wolkersbergenstraße 1, 1130 Wien, Austria

Obviously, this value is easily obtained at the electrode positions. To compute values at points between the electrodes a linear combination of already available values is used:

$$s(x) = \sum_i a_i \cdot s(x_i) \tag{2}$$

The sole constraint imposed on the coefficients is the demand for minimum variance. Under this assumption the coefficients are the unknown variables in a system of N equations (N = number of electrodes) which is obtained by means of Lagrangian multipliers:

$$\sum_j a_j \cdot \overline{(x_j, x_i)} = \overline{(x, x_i)} \tag{3}$$

Since the values of the structure functions are random variables, confidence limits are computed. Assuming normal distribution, the variance of each value must be estimated. This is achieved by computation of the variance v^2 of a weighted sum of random variables:

$$v^2 = \sum_i a_i^2 \cdot \overline{(x_i, x_i)} + \sum_{i>j} 2 \cdot a_i \cdot a_j \cdot \overline{(x_i, x_j)} \tag{14}$$

The structure function is defined to differ at some point if the confidence limits (obtained by means of Student's t distribution) do not coincide. The electrodes on the scalp form disjunct trapezoids or rectangles. For each field the function was calculated at 10×10 points, including therefore the solution of a 16×16 equation system 800 times. The structure function is normed to 1 and encoded graphically in the shading of a quadrate: higher values of the structure function are represented by a greater extent of shading.

Results

To demonstrate the potential of the method two computations were performed. At the left and right of Fig. 1 two structure functions are shown. They represent 60 s of the scalp's potential differences before and after acupuncture respectively. The idea of this demonstration was to guarantee a defined time point where a change in the electrical activity may take place. Although the function values are individually normed to 1 and cannot be compared directly, the structural difference, which may be guessed at after inspection of the left and right pictures, is verified by the central picture. A shaded quadrate demonstrates a statistically significant difference at this point ($p < 0.01$), whereas in the case of nonshaded quadrates no difference may be assumed.

The same computation procedure was performed using two EEG samples (again of 60 s duration) from another proband. The time difference between

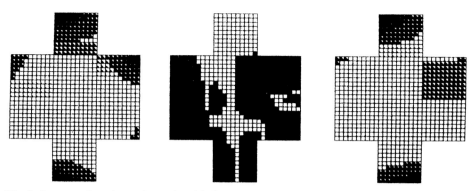

Fig. 1. Structure functions of a proband before and after acupuncture (left and right respectively). Registration was performed using the 10/20 system with Pz as reference electrode. The structure functions are computed for a bandwidth from 0.5 to 32 cps. Significant structure differences ($p<0.01$) are shown in the center (shaded)

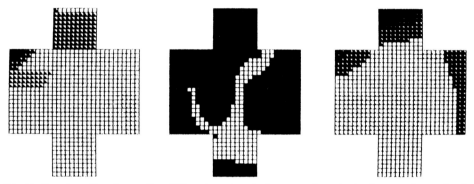

Fig. 2. Structure functions of a different proband: two samples obtained at an interval of 10 min. For conditions of registration, arrangement of structure functions and structural differences, see Fig. 1

the two samples was 10 min and there was no external influence on the proband. Significant differences may be recognized.

Such results demand great caution in establishing differences, since it seems to be very difficult to differentiate between physiological and other variables, even when using common statistical methods.

Discussion

The structure function offers a computation of topographical mapping of the EEG which is not restricted by constraints that are difficult to remove and which, in addition, can be used in computations of fields built up by differences.

Moreover, the construction of interior points (points between the electrodes) is advantageous in that not only spatial influences but also time-dependent influences of the function values obtained at the electrodes contribute to the computed value. The structure function is also consistent in that the estimated values at the electrode positions coincide with the computed values. Structure differences are related to both functional and morphological differences. This means that beside clinical investigations, pharmacologically induced changes in the electrical activity may also be verified. Moreover, the structure function prevents investigators from overinterpreting their results.

References

Duffy FH (1986) Topographic mapping of brain electrical activity. Butterworth, London

Jindra RH, Vollmer R (1986) Topographische Darstellung von EEG-Potentialen. In: Reisner T, Binder H, Deisenhammer E (eds) Advances in neuroimaging. Verlag der Wiener Medizinischen Akademie, Vienna, pp 290–292

Topographic Brain Mapping and Conventional Evoked Potential to Checkerboard Reversal and Semantic Visual Stimulation in a Dyslexic Boy with Amblyopia

D. WENZEL[1], U. BRANDL[1], and E. KRAUS-MACKIW[2]

Introduction

Amblyopia is defined as a loss of visual acuity caused by visual form deprivation and/or abnormal binocular interaction, for which no organic cause can be detected by the physical examination of the eye. As pointed out previously (Kraus-Mackiw et al. 1980), poor sensory binocularity with intermittent alternating central scotoma, as for example in amblyopia, can produce dyslexia, especially when the whole-word method is applied in learning to read and write. It is generally accepted that the end of the sensitive period for orthoptic management in amblyopia is about 8 years of age (von Noorden 1977), a time when dyslexia normally first becomes evident. Evoked potential (EP) measurement together with brain mapping is one direct method of studying cortical responses to different visual stimuli in amblyopia as well as in dyslexia and may help as a diagnostic tool in children to localize function and monitor therapy (Levi and Harwerth 1978, Duffy 1980).

We present the electrophysiological results over a $3^1/_2$ year period of a 12-year-old dyslexic boy with amblyopia whose combined orthoptic/pleoptic therapy started late, at $9^9/_{12}$ years, i.e., well after the so-called critical period of visual development, and whose vision normalized after 2 years' treatment from the clinical as well as the electrophysiological point of view.

Material and Methods

We present a normally developed 12-year-old boy without neurological disturbances. All tests and investigations as well as visual functions were normal. The ophthalmological diagnosis was primarily constant unilateral convergent strabismus of the left eye with amblyopia and dysharmonic anomalous retinal correspondence. Furthermore, despite very good intellectual performance, he was a disabled reader and poor writer. The first electrophysiological investigations were carried out at the age of $8^1/_2$ years. After 2 years of orthoptic/pleoptic therapy with foveolar training programs, starting at the age of $9^9/_{12}$ years, visual acuity and binocularity became normal. Regarding his reading and writing abilities, a good standard in high school has now been achieved.

---

[1] Universitäts-Kinderklinik Erlangen, Loschgestr. 15, 8520 Erlangen, Federal Republic of Germany
[2] Universitäts-Augenklinik Heidelberg, Bergheimerstr. 20, 6900 Heidelberg, Federal Republic of Germany

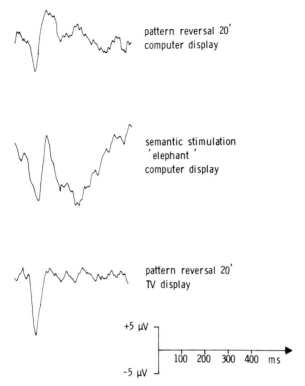

Fig. 1. VEPs to checkerboard reversal and semantic visual stimulation on CRT computer or TV display. Note the small P100 prolongation and pronounced late positive component (P200 wave) after foveal "elephant" stimulation constructed on a computer display (middle line)

Visual evoked potentials (VEPs) were recorded over the occipital region in a conventional manner and averaged to flash, different-sized checkerboard pattern reversal and semantic visual stimulation. Semantic pictures within a 3°–4° visual field – a house, a family, an elephant, a fish, words and so on – were constructed on a computer and reversed against split bars and points of the same overall luminance, simulating a "pattern reversal" effect. In fact, the evoked responses are comparable to classic pattern reversal stimulation by checks but show longer P100 latencies and clearly enhanced late positive components (P200) (Fig. 1). Brain maps were recorded first on a commercial brain mapping system (Neuroscience), later on our own mapping system constructed on a personal computer.

Results

Figure 2 shows the "typical" response to monocular checkerboard reversal to three different-sized visual checkerboard reversal stimuli at the age of $8^1/_2$ years. Using large patterns – stimulating predominantly extrafoveal regions – no differ-

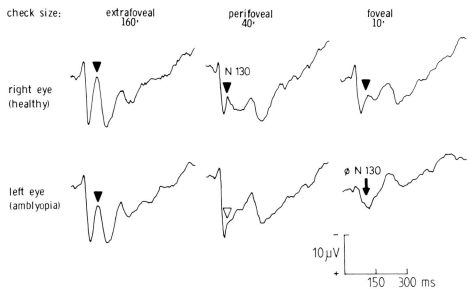

Fig. 2. Checkerboard reversal EP to three different check sizes (160, 40, 10 min of arc) in a $8^{1}/_{2}$ year-old dyslexic boy with strabismic amblyopia (left eye). The *closed triangle* points to the second positive component (N130). Using 40 min of arc the N130 component diminishes in the amblyopic eye (*open triangle*) and is lost using small "foveal" checksizes (10 min of arc). Using large checksizes (160 min of arc), no difference between the healthy right eye and amblyopic left eye is seen

ence between the healthy right and amblyopic left eye can be detected. A medium-sized pattern (40 min of arc) – corresponding to perifoveal retinal locus – again shows identical P100 latencies, but a diminished N130 component; if small patterns (10 min of arc) are used for stimulation – foveal retinal locus – the amplitude reduction, P100 latency increase and loss of N130 component in the amblyopic eye become evident (negative spatial tuning effect).

Using binocular vs monocular stimulation to check the electrophysiological amplitude summation (Fig. 3), no enhancement to binocular stimulation is seen before therapy started, but the summative effect becomes and remains positive after continuous visual therapy. The latency time of N130 becomes measurable in binocular stimulation and stays within normal limits as well as the N130 component to right-left monocular stimulation.

Regarding brain map recordings to foveal semantic "elephant" stimulation at the beginning of the visual training, the P100 and the P200 component stimulating the healthy right eye, are seen to display fairly symmetrical amplitude and activity distribution, but they are grossly asymmetrical when the amblyopic left eye is stimulated, with diminished amplitudes in the left temporal and parietal leads (Fig. 4a).

After $1^{1}/_{2}$ years of treatment, the control maps now show symmetrical activity distribution for right as well as for left monocular foveal semantic visual

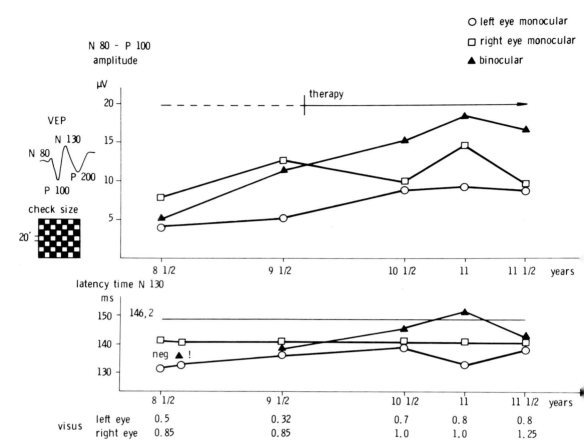

Fig. 3. Electrophysiological amplitude summation (N80-P100) and N130 latency time before and after visual therapy. Before initiation of therapy no binocular amplitude summation (*closed triangle*) is seen; after the beginning of visual training ($9^{9}/_{12}$ years of age) the amplitude summation effect progressively becomes positive. *Bottom:* the N130 latencies for binocular and monocular VEPs remain within normal limits (up to 146.2 ms)

stimulation (Fig. 4b). Binocularity, visual acuity and reading ability are almost normalized.

The effects of orthoptic management with bifoveolar training, programs with regard to binocularity, as shown by hemispheric differences of brain activities, are summarized in Fig. 5. With flash stimulation (Fig. 5a), amplitudes of late positive components (P200) in left parieto-occipital regions were lower before therapy ($9^{1}/_{2}$ years) and gradually became larger as treatment progressed ($10^{1}/_{2}$, $11^{1}/_{2}$ years).

When checkerboard reversal with large checksizes is offered (80 min of arc), the effect is the same as in flash stimulation, but more pronounced. Using the small "foveal" pattern reversal check stimulation, the hemispheric amplitude ratio inverted only $1^{9}/_{12}$ years after initiation of therapy. At that time, the

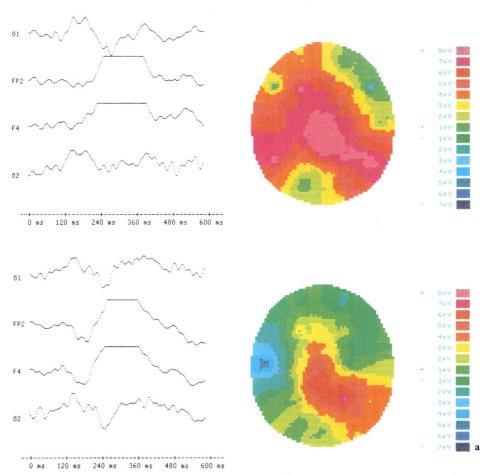

Fig. 4a, b. Brain maps of late positive components (P200) at the beginning (**a**) and after $1^1/_2$ years of visual training (**b**) due to semantic (elephant) visual stimulation. Note the amplitude differences stimulating the left amblyopic eye (*lower part*) at the beginning (**a**) and the symmetrical amplitude distribution after the visual training (**b**)

corresponding brain mapping activities showed a symmetrical distribution in dynamic brain mapping processes in both temporoparieto-occipital regions (see also Fig. 4b).

Discussion

Our results seem interesting from different points of view:

1. Objective normalization of the "typical" electrophysiological VEP findings in amblyopia (amplitude reduction, latency prolongation, negative spatial

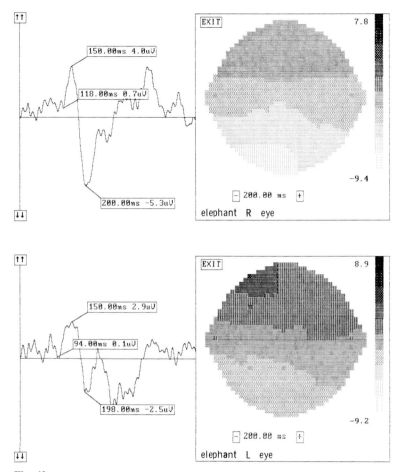

Fig. 4b

tuning effect) is possible even *after* the so-called critical or sensitive phase of the visual system, i.e., after 8 years of age. Thus, therapeutic efforts should be also made in older children with visual functional problems objectively monitored by VEP when small patterns are used (Wenzel 1987).

2. Our results – corresponding to the known data of EP and map studies (Conners 1971; Preston 1974; Duffy 1980; Simmons et al. 1986) – show diminished left temporoparieto-occipital activity in dyslexia (that is brain regions ordinarily involved in speech and reading). This electrophysiological asymmetry disappears after sophisticated foveolar training programs together with pleoptic-orthoptic management (Otto 1983; Schumacher 1985).

3. Our electrophysiological results demonstrate the complex brain plasticity in childhood, again *after* the sensitive phase, not only for the visual system (as seen from EP results) but also for other cortical regions (as demonstrated by brain mapping procedures).

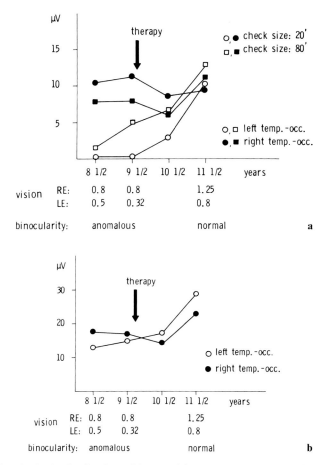

Fig. 5a, b. Temporo-occipital hemispheric distribution of late positive components (P200) in flash (**a**) and in checkerboard reversal (**b**) visual evoked responses. Before therapy ($8^{1}/_{2}$, $9^{1}/_{2}$ years of age) the P200 amplitude is pronounced in the right temporo-occipital region, but after visual training is initiated at $9^{9}/_{12}$ years of age P200 increases in the left temporo-occipital region ($10^{1}/_{2}$, $11^{1}/_{2}$ years of age). The effect is more pronounced for small checks (*circles*) than for larger ones (*rectangles*) (**b**). Clinically, visual acuity and binocularity normalize during the course of late-treated amblyopia

4. The clinical improvement of visual as well as electrophysiological functions do not prove that these are related directly to amblyopia-induced dyslexia, but argues strongly in favor of their influence on reading disability, at least from the therapeutic point of view. Further combined neurophysiological and clinical studies in dyslexia without amblyopia and in amblyopia without dyslexia are therefore in progress.

References

Conners CK (1971) Cortical visual evoked response in children with learning disorders. Psychophysiology 7:418–428

Duffy FH, Denckla MB, Bartels PH, Sandini G (1980) Dyslexia: regional differences in brain electrical activity by topographic mapping. Ann Neurol 7:412–420

Kraus-Mackiw E, Müller-Küppers M, Rabetge G (1980) Binocularity in 10- to 12-year-old children with poor writing and reading ability. Metabolic and pediatric ophthalmology, vol 4. Pergamon, New York, pp 93–96

Levi DM, Harwerth RS (1978) A sensory mechanism for amblyopia: electrophysiological studies. Am J Optom Physiol Opt 55:163–171

Otto J (1983) Optomotorische Reizmethode nach Otto und Rabetge. In: Francois J, Hollwich F (eds) Augenheilkunde in Klinik und Praxis, vol 3(1). Thieme, Stuttgart, pp 34–38

Preston MS, Guthrie JT, Childs B (1974) Visual evoked responses (VERs) in normal and disabled readers. Psychophysiology 11:452–457

Schuhmacher H (1985) Diagnostik und Therapie von visuellen Störfaktoren bei Kindern mit isolierter Lese-Rechtschreibschwäche. Ergebnisse eines Therapieprogrammes mit Okklusion. Thesis, Ruprecht-Karls-Universität, Heidelberg

Simmons JH, Languis ME, Drake ME (1986) Group difference in the P 300-wave between dyslexics and normals. Electroencephalogr Clin Neurophysiol 64:42–44

von Noorden GK (1977) Mechanisms of amblyopia. Adv Ophthalmol 34:93–115

Wenzel D, Kraus-Mackiw E (1987) Verlauf muster-evozierter Potentiale unterschiedlicher Ortsfrequenz bei spätbehandelter Amblyopie. Ophthalmology 129 (2–3):146–147

EEG Mapping in Patients with Transient Ischemic Attacks: A Follow-Up Study

E. KOERNER[1], E. OTT[1], P. KAISERFELD[1], G. PFURTSCHELLER[2], R. WOLF[1], G. LINDINGER[2], and H. LECHNER[1]

Introduction

The use of electroencephalography (EEG) as a diagnostic tool is based largely on a concept of human EEG normality defined by descriptive criteria, of which the alpha rhythm is the principal electrical activity (Berger 1929). One of the features of this activity is its tendency to be reduced in amplitude or to be blocked by either internal or external stimuli to the brain (Berger 1930). This event-related desynchronization (ERD) of the EEG may be used as a highly sensitive parameter in detecting even slight functional disturbances of the cortical activity (Pfurtscheller and Aranibar 1977), provided that analytic methods of quantify these blocking reactions are available.

The computerized analysis of EEG signals represented by topographic displays of EEG spectra gives information about the distribution of the cortical steady-state bioelectrical activity in the form of EEG maps (Duffy et al. 1978; Buchsbaum et al. 1982). Similarly, the percent changes of the power density following external stimuli may be displayed in their topographical localization and thus be termed ERD maps (Pfurtscheller and Aranibar 1977).

The aim of the present study was to investigate functional disorders of the cortex following cerebral transient ischemic attacks (TIAs) using computerized analysis of the EEG and to compare these data to investigations performed in follow-up situations.

Patients and Methods

In 11 patients (seven males, four females; age 53.3 ± 18.3 years, mean $\pm$ SD) with transient ischemic episodes in the middle cerebral artery (MCA) territories, EEG recordings were performed within 24 h following the acute event. Thereafter control measurements were carried out on the 7th and 30th days. The transient focal neurological deficit involved the left MCA territory in eight and the right MCA territory in three patients. The standard EEG evaluated by descriptive visual analysis was normal in six patients. Five patients showed slight focal alterations, coinciding in four of them with the hemisphere affected by the cerebrovascular episode. The recordings were performed with the pa-

---
[1] Universität Graz, Abteilung für Neurologie, Auenbruggerplatz 22, 8036 Graz, Austria
[2] Technische Universität Graz, Abteilung für medizinische Informatik, Intitut für Elektro- und Biomedizinische Technik, Inffeldgasse 18, 8010 Graz, Austria

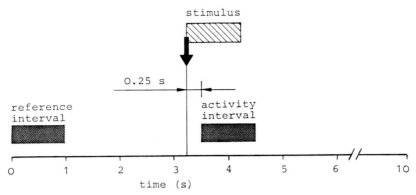

Fig. 1. The ERD was calculated as percent decrease in power of the activity period (starting 250 ms after onset of the stimulus) compared to the reference interval. Each map was displayed following performance of 60 10-s EEG sections

tient's eyes closed. Registrations with fluctuations of alertness showing a decrease of the EEG power density, appearance of sleep rhythms and EEG registrations not distinctly free of artifacts were excluded from the data analyses.

Each measurement consisted of four steps: (1) EEG during rest; (2) recordings during a vibration stimulus of the right and (3) recordings during a vibration stimulus of the left middle finger; (4) EEG registration during light stimulation. Since an impairment of attention was noted during step 4 in five patients, the evaluation of this part was excluded in their further calculation.

The duration of each step of the investigation amounted to 10 min; stimuli lasting 1 s were offered 60 times at 10-s intervals.

EEG maps presenting power and frequency distributions within a chosen bandwidth were calculated during rest. In addition, ERD maps for the different stimuli inputs were computed, displaying the percent differences from the reference period in the power spectra of the activity. The reference period corresponded to the first second of each 10-s EEG trace. The activity period was defined as a 1-s section of the EEG starting 250 ms after onset of the stimulus, wich was triggered within the fourth second (Fig. 1).

All investigations were carried out using the Beckman electrode cap. Additionally to the 10–20 system, four electrodes were placed over the precentral region and four over the postcentral region. However, the frontal electrodes (FP1 and FP2) were not included in the evaluation in order to avoid eye-movement artifacts. Bipolar registrations in a transverse configuration were analyzed (19 channels). All EEG signals were recorded with a time constant of 0.15 s and a low-pass filter cutoff frequency of 30 Hz. The sampling rate was 64/s for each channel and the computer (PDP 11/73) checked for artifacts, excluding all segments containing an A/D converter overflow.

In the present paper the blocking reaction, expressed as percent decrease in power density, was calculated in the regions of interest over the cortex (vibration stimuli: Cz-C3, Cz-C4; light stimuli: T6-P4, P3-T5).

Each measurement was compared to a healthy control group ($n=15$; 11 males, 4 females; age 32 ± 8 years). Particular attention was paid to the individual basic EEG rhythm both in normals and in the patients' group and only those presenting a clear alpha activity selected by visual analysis were used for evaluation.

Statistical analyses were performed using Student's t test and differences were considered significant at a level of 5% ($p<0.05$).

Results

ERD in Patients with TIAs Compared to Normals

The cortical ERD was distinctly reduced within the hemisphere affected by the cerebrovascular deficit, compared to controls (Table 1). These functional disorders were noted following vibration stimuli as well as following light application during the first measurement within 24 h after the appearance of the transient focal neurological episode.

Table 1. Event-related desynchronization (%)

	VR/VA	VL/VNA	Diff.	LR/LA	LL/LNA	Diff.
Normals	42 (14)*	36 (20)	6 (19)	42 (16)**	39 (19)	3 (1)*
TIAs	30 (19)	42 (17)	13 (14)	19 (19)	37 (25)	18 (16)

Standard deviation in parentheses
VR/VL, vibration: right/left (normals); VA/VNA, vibration: affected/non-affected hemisphere; LR/LF, light: right/left (normals); LA/LNA, light: affected and non-affected hemisphere; Diff., Difference right/left in normals, affected/non-affected hemisphere in TIAs
* $p<0.05$; ** $p<0.01$

ERD in Patients with TIAs at Follow-Up

Vibration Stimuli. The ERD, expressed as percent decrease of EEG power following vibration stimuli, showed clear asymmetry when compared to the blocking reaction of both the affected and the healthy hemisphere (Fig. 2). Within the first 24 h following the acute event, the difference amounted to 13% (affected hemisphere 29.6%, nonaffected hemisphere 42.3%) and even increased to 18% 7 days later. One month following the ischemic attack the difference of the desynchronization effect induced by vibration stimuli amounted to that seen in the control group.

Light Stimulation. The activation pattern following light stimulation (Fig. 3) showed a similar asymmetric desynchronization with a difference of 18% over the corresponding regions during the first measurement (ischemic hemisphere 19%, healthy hemisphere 37%). This presumed functional deficit persisted dur-

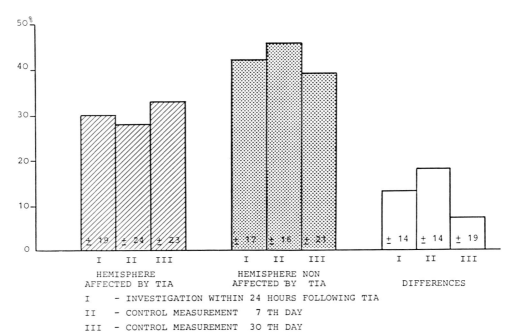

Fig. 2. Follow-up of the ERD (%) within the two hemispheres following vibration stimuli of the middle finger in patients with TIAs. For details see text. $+/-$, standard deviation

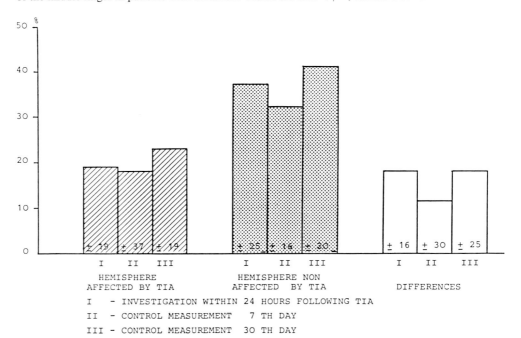

Fig. 3. Follow-up of the ERD (%) following light stimulation within the two hemispheres in patients with TIAs. For details see text. $+/-$, standard deviation

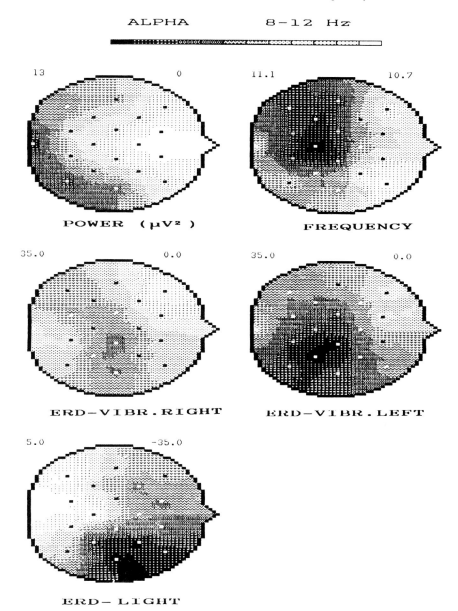

Fig. 4. Topographic displays of EEG activity during rest (left and right at *top*) and ERD maps following external stimuli (ERD expressed as percent power decrease) in eight patients with TIAs localized within the left MCA territory. Investigation performed during the first 24 h following the cerebrovascular episode. The numbers above each map correspond to the minimal (*right*) and maximal (*left*) values related to the scale

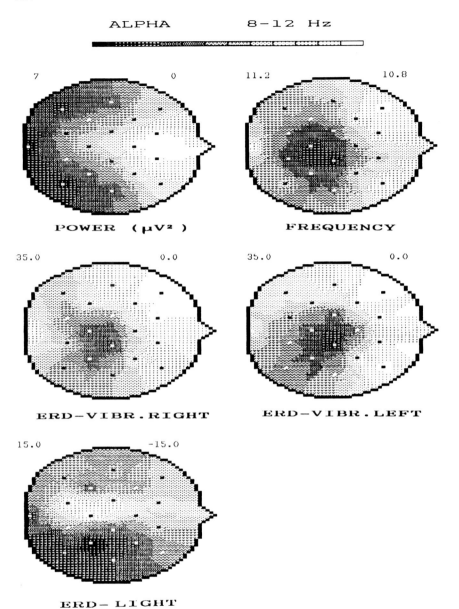

Fig. 5. Topographic displays of EEG and ERD maps derived 7 days following transient ischemic episodes. For details see Fig. 4 legend

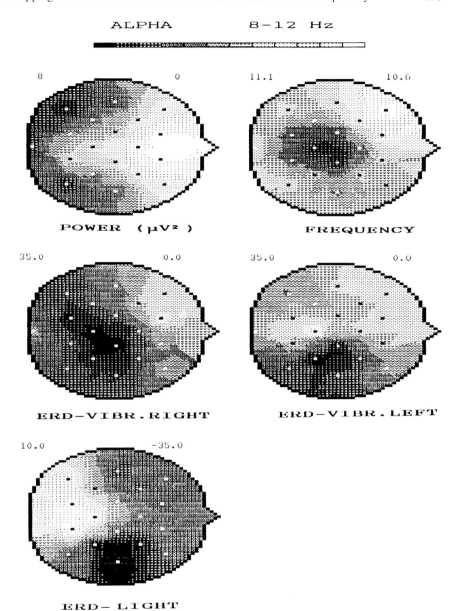

Fig. 6. Topographic displays of EEG and ERD maps derived 1 month following transient ischemic episodes. For details see Fig. 4 legend

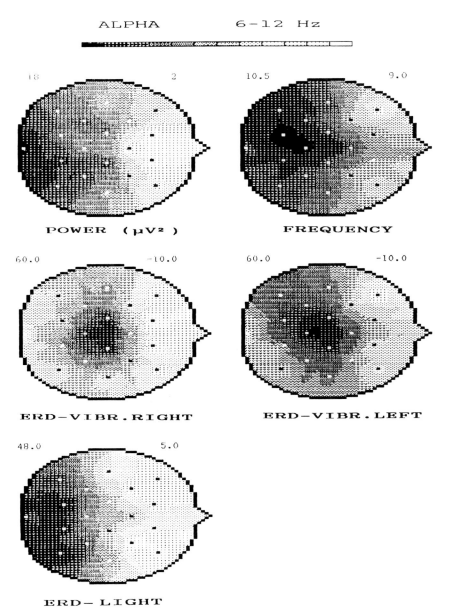

Fig. 7. Topographic displays of EEG and ERD maps in a 43-year-old healthy man. For details see Fig. 4 legend

ing the total observation period and was thus clearly, though not significantly, greater than in the controls.

Topographic Display. The topographic displays of the three measurements in the eight patients with TIAs involving the left hemisphere are shown in Figs. 4–6.

As can be seen from Fig. 4, both a clear power deficit and, simultaneously, an increase of the alpha frequency were found over the left (affected) hemisphere during rest. While the ERD was diminished after the vibration stimulus of the right hand, a distinct blocking reaction was observed following left side stimulation. No activation pattern in the affected hemisphere was seen during light stimulation.

After a time interval of 7 days the asymmetric pattern of the power and the frequency distribution had disappeared (Fig. 5). Likewise, the ERD evoked by vibration stimuli did not show any differences between the two hemispheres. However, the asymmetric desynchronization pattern following light stimulation was still evident.

Similar results were obtained in the investigation 30 days after the TIA (Fig. 6). The desynchronization following vibration stimuli was apparently restored, but a clear dysfunction was present within the hemisphere involved following light stimuli. For comparison to identical measurements in control subjects, the symmetric reactions to the stimuli administered are shown in a representative sample in Fig. 7.

Discussion

The importance of computerized EEG analysis in ischemic conditions of the brain was stressed by van Huffelen et al. (1980). Recently, the use of multichannel spectral analysis has been proposed, this technique showing the clear superiority of computerized evaluation over routine visual assessment in patients with minor cerebral ischemia. Additional topographic displays of the data provide an overview of the distribution of the different EEG parameters within a given frequency range (Jonkman et al. 1986). In this respect particular interest can be directed toward somatosensory activation patterns in patients affected by ischemia of the MCA territory. The degree of severity of the resulting cerebral dysfunction may be derived from these stimulation arrangements, and the amount of restitution may be quantified by the performance at follow-up studies, as shown in our patient sample.

A difficulty of interpretation may arise from the large number of different EEG spectral parameters, each of them available within variable frequency bands. In the present paper the impact of the conventional alpha frequency band, of its distribution at rest and of its activation by external stimuli has been investigated. Thus, a quantity of other interesting parameters have had to be neglected, but particular attention will have to be paid to definition of EEG variables representative for certain physiological and pathophysiological functions of cortical activity.

Data confined to the alpha frequency band showed a clear asymmetric distribution of both power and frequency. With respect to the stimulation procedures, the ERD was reduced within the affected hemisphere following vibration input as well as following light stimulation on the 1st day after the episode compared to normals. Control investigations of the patient group revealed an enhancement of power and frequency distribution and of the blocking reaction to vibration stimuli; however, a presumed functional disorder derived from the results following light stimulation was still noted at the end of the observation period.

Correlation studies with other functional investigation techniques such as SPECT or PET, ultrasound and nuclear magnetic imaging should support the interpretation of the different alterations of EEG parameters. This method not only offers the possibility of studying pathophysiological functional parameters, but may also provide information on a variety of cognitive processes in the human brain.

References

Berger H (1929) Über das Elektrenkephalogramm des Menschen. Arch Psychiat Nervenkr 87:527–570. English translation by Gloor P (1969) Hans Berger on the electroencephalogram of man. Electroencephalogr Clin Neurophysiol [Suppl] 28:37–73

Berger H (1930) Über das Elektrenkephalogramm des Menschen. J Physiol Neurol 40:160–179. English translation by Gloor P (1969) Hans Berger on the electroencephalogram of man. Electroencephalogr Clin Neurophysiol [Suppl] 28:75–93

Buchsbaum MS, Rigal F, Coppola R, Cappelletti J, King C, Johnson J (1982) A new system for grey-level surface distribution maps of electrical activity. Electroencephalogr Clin Neurophysiol 53:237–242

Duffy FH, Burchfiel JL, Lombroso CT (1978) Brain electrical activity mapping (BEAM): a method for extending the clinical utility of EEG and evoked potential data. Ann Neurol 5:309–321

Jonkman EJ, van Huffelen AG, Pfurtscheller G (1986) Quantitative EEG in cerebral ischemia. In: Lopes da Silva FH, Strom van Leeuwen W, Remond A (eds) Clinical applications of computer analysis of EEG and other neurophysiological signals. Elsevier, Amsterdam, pp 205–237 (Handbook of electroencephalography and clinical neurophysiology, vol 2)

Pfurtscheller G, Aranibar A (1977) Event-related cortical desynchronization detected by power measurements of scalp EEG. Electroencephalogr Clin Neurophysiol 42:817–826

Van Huffelen AC, Poortvliet DCJ, van der Wulp CJM, Magnus O (1980) Quantitative EEG in cerebral ischemia. A. Parameters for the detection of abnormalities in "normal" EEGs in patients with acute unilateral cerebral ischemia (A.U.C.I.). In: Lechner H, Aranibar A (eds) EEG and Clinical Neurophysiology. Excerpta Medica, Amsterdam, pp 125–130

EEG Mapping in Pathological Aging and Dementia: Utility for Diagnosis and Therapeutic Evaluation

B. Gueguen[1], P. Etevenon[1], D. Plancon[1], J. Gaches[1], J. De Recondo[2], and P. Rondot[2]

Introduction

Quantified EEG (Remond 1961; Drohocki 1968; Walter and Brazier 1968; Dolce and Kunkel 1975; Etevenon 1977) and mapping (Lehmann 1971; Ragot and Remond 1978; Duffy et al. 1981; Buchsbaum et al. 1982) have allowed more precise and reliable EEG analysis than visual methods. However, while the place of these methods in daily clinical practice is being debated they are giving rise to an excess of pictorial and numerical data. Much work has been published concerning aging and dementia (Duffy et al. 1984a, b; Coben et al. 1985; Penttila et al. 1985; Gueguen et al. 1986; Senant et al. 1986), but only a few studies in the past 2 years have really used EEG as a tool for diagnosis or for therapeutic evaluation (Cutler et al. 1985; Little et al. 1985; Bruno et al. 1986; Delwaïde et al. 1986; Partanen et al. 1986; Schwartz and Kolstaedt 1986). EEG changes occur early in dementia and are well correlated with the stage of cognitive impairment (Coben et al. 1985; Penttila et al. 1985). We report here preliminary results concerning the usefulness of quantified EEG methods in diagnosis and treatment of pathological aging.

Methods

Subjects

To avoid false data we applied very strict criteria for the selection of demented subjects. Curable dementia was excluded on the basis of blood cell count, sedimentation rate, serum levels of thyroid hormones and vitamins, syphilis serology, CT scan and cervical vascular echography. Hachinski's score was always 0 or 1. Demented patients were almost all at the same stage, namely stage 5, of Reisberg's global deterioration scale (Reisberg et al. 1982). Hamilton's scale for depression, mini mental state of Folstein, disability score and neuropsychological testing were also used for assessment of dementia. More than 25 demented people were recorded, but only eight could be included in the study to be sure as possible that the features observed would be characteristics of degenerative dementia. These patients were divided into two groups: presenile (below 65, years, $n=4$) and senile (above 65, $n=4$). Normal controls were living

---

[1] Department of Clinical Neurophysiology, [2] Department of Neurology, Sainte-Anne Hospital, 1rue Cabanis, 75674 Paris Cedex 14, France

at home with no past history of vascular or systemic disease and with no treatment. This explains the low number of normals: three subjects above 65 and three below 65 (range 50–65). Seven young volunteers (aged 20–45 years) were also recorded to detect possible modifications with physiological aging.

Recording

A 16-channel EEG mapping system (Cartovar) was used. Electrodes were disposed according to the modified 10–20 International System (no electrodes on the midline). An averaged mean reference was used (Lehmann 1971). Recordings were made with the subjects at rest, in a sound-attenuated room, in a semireclining position. Both hemispheres were recorded simultaneously, first with the subject's eyes closed and then with eyes open. Data acquisition was made during 6-s epochs, allowing accurate rejection of EEG samples with artifacts. Five of these 6-s epochs were then averaged. The studied spectral bands were: delta (0.5–3 Hz), theta (3.5–7.5 Hz), alpha (8–13 Hz) and beta (14–30 Hz). Many parameters were studied using absolute amplitude (in μV^2) or relative amplitude (in percentage of the global spectrum power). Three of these parameters appeared to be the most discriminant: (1) The alpha/theta ratio was shown to be disturbed very early in dementia (Penttila et al. 1985). This ratio gives a nice topographic picture of alpha dominant posterior activity and avoids contamination by ocular and myographic artifacts. (2) Alpha reactivity expressed as alpha power residual value after the eyes are opened and corresponding to the ratio of alpha power value during the eyes open situation

Table 1. Quantified EEG parameters commonly used for diagnosis and therapeutic evaluation in dementia

---

Non-dynamic parameters
  Alpha/theta ratio on the posterior areas
  Mean frequency in the coupled theta + alpha bands
  Right vs left asymmetry
  Spatialization index (anteroposterior gradient)

Dynamic parameters
  Alpha reactivity on the posterior areas
  Responses to physiological activation (photic stimulation, hyperventilation)
  Responses to functional activation (motor, cognitive, etc)

Fig. 1 a–f. Normal subjects. In normal young people alpha/theta ratio values are high (maximum = 2.82) (**a**), with clear predominance on the posterior areas. Alpha activity is thus the dominant background posterior activity. The dominant mean frequency is 9.6 Hz (**e**) and the reactivity on the same posterior areas is near 60% (**c**). In old people (over 65 years) EEG parameters are quite similar. Alpha/theta ratios confirm a high predominance of alpha activity with a well-preserved posterior topography (**b**). Mean frequency in the alpha band is near 9 Hz (**d**) and the reactivity is not very different from that in young people (**f**). *EO*, eyes open; *EC*, eyes closed

EEG Mapping in Pathological Aging and Dementia 221

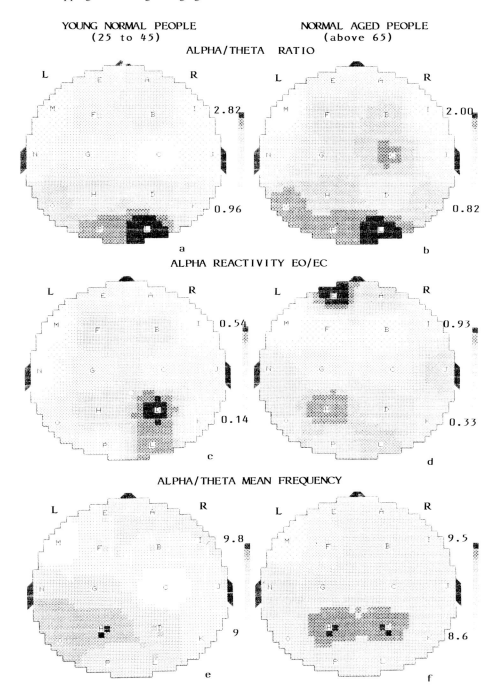

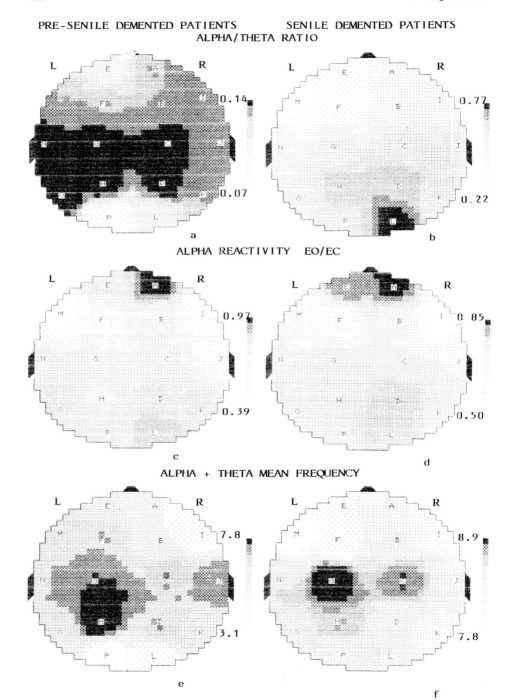

to alpha power value with eyes closed. (3) Mean centroid frequency, calculated here for the associated spectral band theta + alpha. This allows a nice visualization of the slowing of the dominant activity on the posterior areas of the scalp with a shift into the theta band. Some other parameters are commonly used and are shown in Table 1.

Asymmetry and spatialization are particularly changed in arteriopathic dementia. As for dynamic parameters, response to photic stimulation is absent very early in dementia of the presenile type. Responses to cognitive activations are still under assessment.

Results

Results are expressed with mean maps of each group and are clearly exposed in Fig. 1 for normal young and old people, and in Fig. 2 for presenile and senile demented patients.

Discussion

Two main points arise from this study. First, EEG in normal old people is not very different from that in normal young subjects. This is in accordance with the findings of Hughes and Cayaffa (1977), Matecjek (1979) and Duffy et al. (1984), and allows precise definition of the potential usefulness of this method in the diagnosis of dementias:
- Differentiation of pathological and normal aging
- Early detection of dementias and cognitive disturbances in older people
- Differentiation of subgroups: vascular and degenerative dementias, senile vs presenile, evolutive and neuropsychological aspects

Selection of a control population in clinical study of aging should now involve quantified EEG or mapping to ensure inclusion of normal subjects only. The therapeutic utility of quantified EEG or mapping is based on this capacity for accurate selection and categorization of subjects. The clear distinction between presenile and senile dementia demonstrated in this study is in accordance with biochemical and neuropsychological data (Bondareff 1983; Rossor et al. 1984) showing a greater impairment in presenile than in senile

Fig. 2a–f. Demented people. Presenile demented patients show a breakdown in alpha/theta ratio values, between 0.14 and 0.07 with a maximum on the posterior areas. Alpha activity has almost disappeared (**a**). Alpha reactivity is almost zero (**c**). The mean dominant posterior frequency is very low near 7 Hz (**e**). In senile demented people, disturbances of EEG parameters are less pronounced. The alpha/theta ratio maximum is 0.77 on posterior areas with a relative preservation of the posterior portion of the residual alpha activity (**b**). Reactivity is weaker than in normals (**d**). The mean dominant posterior frequency is near 8 Hz (**f**). *EO*, eyes open; *EC*, eyes closed

dementia. The main application of these methods could be in therapeutic evaluation. EEG is a known method in psychopharmacology (Fink 1974; Itil 1974; Matejcek 1979) but drug effects on brain are not easy to visualize in dementias. Indeed, the correlations between EEG abnormalities and the biochemical modifications observed in these diseases remain unclear, as do many other questions: Are EEG modifications reversible? From which structural cellular changes do these abnormalities come? Is regression of EEG slowing conceivable? Or are we dealing only with a lack of aggravation of EEG with time in a demented treated group in comparison with a control non-treated group, as suggested by Partanen et al. (1986)? We hope a more extensive study currently under way in our department will help answer these questions.

References

Bondareff W (1983) Age and Alzheimer's disease. Lancet 1447

Bruno G, Mohr E, Gillespie M, Fedio P, Chase TN (1986) Muscarinic agonist therapy in Alzheimer's disease. Arch Neurol 43:659–661

Buchsbaum MS, Rigal F, Coppola R, Cappeletti J, King C, Johnson J (1982) A new system for gray-level surface distribution maps of electrical activity. Electroencephalogr Clin Neurophysiol 53:237–242

Coben AL, Danziger W, Storandt M (1985) A longitudinal EEG study of mild senile dementia of Alzheimer type: changes at 1 year and at 2.5 years. Electroencephalogr Clin Neurophysiol 61:101–112

Cutler NR, Haxby J, Kay AD, Narang PK, Lesko LJ, Costa JL, Ninos M, Linnoila M, Potter WZ, Renfrew JW, Moore AM (1985) Evaluation of Zimeldine in Alzheimer's disease. Arch Neurol 42:744–748

Delwaide PJ, Gyselynck-Mambourg AM, Hurlet A, Ylieff M (1986) Double-blind randomized controlled study of phosphatidylserine in senile demented patients. Acta Neurol Scand 73:136–140

Dolce G, Kunkel H (1975) CEAN-Computerized EEG Analysis. Fischer, Stuttgart

Drohocki Z (1968) Quantitative electroencephalography: history, methods, applications. Electroencephalogr Clin Neurophysiol 25:303

Duffy FH, Bartels P, Burchfield JL (1981) Significance probability mapping: an aid in the topographic analysis of brain electrical activity. Electroencephalogr Clin Neurophysiol 51:455–462

Duffy FH, Albert MS, McAnulty G, Garvery J (1984a) Age related differences in brain electrical activity in healthy subjects. Ann Neurol 16:430–438

Duffy FH, Albert MS, McAnulty G (1984b) Brain electrical activity in patients with presenile and senile dementia of the Alzheimer type. Ann Neurol 16:439–448

Etevenon P (1977) Electroencephalographie sur ordinateur (analyse quantitative et statistique). Thèse de Doctorat, Factulté des Sciences, Paris.

Fink M (1974) EEG application in psychopharmacology. Psychopharmacol Agents 111: pp 159–174

Gueguen B, Kobrzynska E, Rondot P, Etevenon P, De Recondo J, Gaches J (1986) EEG cartography as an aid for early detection of dementia in the elderly. In: Senile dementias: early detection. Bes A, Cahn J, Cahn R, Hoyer S, Marc-Vergnes JP, Wisniewski HM (eds) Libbey, Paris, pp 165–170

Hughes JR, Cayaffa JJ (1977) The EEG in patients at different ages without organic cerebral disease. Electroencephalogr Clin Neurophysiol 42:776–784

Itil TM (1974) Quantitative pharmaco-electroencephalography. Mod Probl Pharmacopsychiatry 8:43–75

Lehmann D (1971) Multichannel topography of human alpha EEG fields. Electroencephalogr Clin Neurophysiol 31:439–449

Little A, Levy R, Chuaqui-Kidd P, Hand D (1985) A double-blind, placebo controlled trial of high-dose lecithin in Alzheimer's disease. J Neurol Neurosurg Psychiatry 48:736–742

Matejcez M (1979) Pharmaco-encephalography: the value of quantified EEG. Psychopharmacol Pharmacopsychiatr 12:126–136

Partanen JV, Soininen H, Riekkinen PJ (1986) Does an ACTH derivative (org 2766) prevent deterioration of EEG in Alzheimer's disease? Electroencephalogr Clin Neurophysiol 63:547–551

Penttila M, Partanen JW, Soininen H, Riekkinen PJ (1985) Quantitative analysis of occipital EEG in different stages of Alzheimer's disease. Electroencephalogr Clin Neurophysiol 60:1–6

Ragot RA, Remond A (1978) EEG field mapping. Electroencephalogr Clin Neurophysiol 45:417–421

Reisberg B, Ferris SH, De Leon MJ, Crook TH (1982) The global deterioration scale for assessment of primary degenerative dementia. Am J Psychiatry 139(9):1136–1139

Remond A (1961) Integrated and topological analysis of the EEG. Electroencephalogr Clin Neurophysiol [Suppl] 20:64–67

Rossor MN, Juersen LL, Reynolds GP, Mountjoy CQ, Roth M (1984) Neurochemical characteristics of early and late onset Alzheimer's disease. Br Med J [Clin Res] 288:961–1064

Schwartz SA, Kohlstaedt EV (1986) Physostigmine effects in Alzheimer's disease. Relationship to dementia severity. Life Sci 38:1021–1028

Senant J, Samson-Dollfus D, Delapierre G, Menard JF, Bertoldi-Lefever I (1986) Analyse automatique de l'EEG et vieillissement chez les sujets normaux et vasculaires. Sem Hop Paris 44:3505–3509

Walter DO, Brazier AB (1968) Advances in EEG analysis. Electroencephalogr Clin Neurophysiol [Suppl] 27:1–75

Topographic Characteristics of EEG During a Saturation Dive to a 31 ATA Helium-Oxygen Environment with Specific Reference to Fmθ or FIRDA*

S. Matsuoka[1], C. Kadoya[1], S. Okuda[1], S. Wada[1], and M. Mori[2]

Introduction

There are many electrophysiological studies concerning saturation excursion dives in hyperbaric environments, that reveal an increase in the theta wave (Procter et al. 1972; Bennett et al. 1982; Naquet et al. 1984). However, in traditional electroencephalography (EEG), no detailed analyses have been done to clarify the nature of the theta wave in this situation because of the restrictions imposed by the environment and the limitations associated with the induction electrode. Therefore, it is necessary to adopt a multielectrode induction recording system. Using the 16-channel recording system we developed (Ueno and Matsuoka 1975), a topographic display of the EEG has been employed to conduct underwater experiments in an attempt to establish the changes occurring in the EEG (in all frequency bands) at different sea depths and to establish a correlation between the regions in which these changes occur.

Materials and Methods

Sixteen divers participated in the saturation excursion dives to 300 m, all healthy experienced divers, highly motivated and very cooperative. The experimental hyperbaric environment was a 31 ATA simulation for 1 month in the human diving simulator Seadragon VI at the Japan Marine Science and Technology Center, Yokosuka, during the period 1982–1985. Hyperbaric helium-oxygen dives to 31 ATA took place according to the schedule shown in Fig. 1.

The computer display system of the EEG consists of two parts (Ueno et al. 1975). One derives the equivalent potential for extraction of specific EEG activities superimposed on the background activities. The other part of the computer display system involves computation for mapping. Potential fields of EEG frequency bands are printed out on a line printer as shown in the topographic maps. The electrodes of the 10–20 system are rearranged on a two-dimensional plane. The 16 channels of the EEG are recorded by a monopolar montage

---

* This investigation was supported by a special grant from the Japanese Ministry of Labor for Studies of Industrial Ecological Sciences

[1] Department of Neurosurgery, University of Occupational and Environmental Health, Kitakyushu 807, Japan
[2] Japan Marine Science and Technology Center, Tokosuka 237, Japan

Topographic Characteristics of EEG During a Saturation Dive

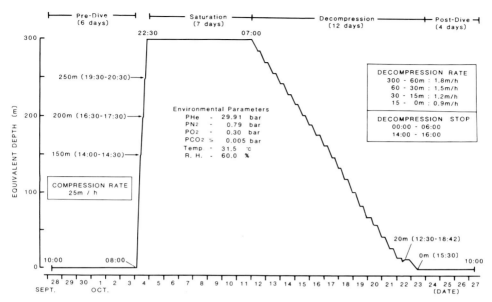

Fig. 1. Dive profile at Seadragon VI

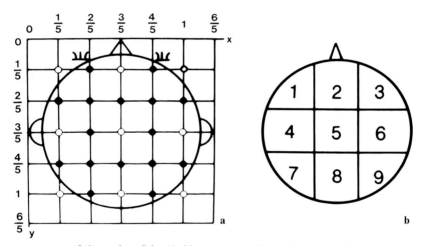

Fig. 2. a Rearrangement of electrodes of the 10–20 system on a dimensional plane for mapping. *Black circles* show measured electrodes; unmeasured electrodes at nine grid points, marked with *white circles*, are assumed beforehand in order to utilize the interpolation function. **b** Edited location of EEG

with a common reference electrode on the ear. Unmeasured potentials are estimated from neighboring potentials. The potentials between grid points are approximated by a two-variable sampling function. The interpolated values are quantified to 11 levels, and finally, potential fields are mapped on color cathode ray tubes (CRT) (Fig. 2a). On the basis of the potentials in 25 locations, two-dimensionally displayed with a computerized topographic EEG scanner, a division is made into nine blocks to determine the average value for each block, and the data are analyzed using a distribution technique (Fig. 2b) (Matsuoka et al. 1984).

Results

We analyzed the data using our distribution technique and obtained a distribution analysis table (Table 1). From the results, it was ascertained that a depth-related effect and a location-related effect do exist. The EEG pattern changed depending on depth and location.

We have tried to establish how the EEG pattern for each location changes with depth. For example, regarding the theta wave, Table 2 presents linear equations, applicable when the changes in the data for the different positions of the theta wave have been fitted into a straight line, and the corresponding correlation coefficients. The relationship between the linear equations and the

Table 1. Results of analysis of variance of EEG data

Factors	Sum square	Degrees of freedom	Mean squares	F value	f
Theta					
Depth	128.1226	6	21.3538	34.2866	<0.01
Location of EEG	114.6523	8	14.3315	23.0114	<0.01
Error	29.8945	48	0.6228		
Total	272.6694	62			
Alpha					
Depth	131.0352	6	20.8392	8.6910	<0.01
Location of EEG	2112.7031	8	264.0879	105.0946	<0.01
Error	120.6172	48	2.5192		
Total	2364.3555	62			

Table 2. The variation of EEG (theta wave) and the location

Block	1	2	3	4	5	6	7	8	9
Mean	13.1250	12.7813	11.1938	9.5875	11.2813	8.6813	11.7525	11.0688	9.1813
Standard deviation	2.0554	1.6489	1.4808	1.2909	2.0462	1.0245	2.0947	1.1487	1.2438
r	−0.5612[a]	−0.7303[b]	−0.6797[b]	−0.7183[b]	−0.7716[b]	−0.7677[b]	−0.5264[a]	−0.7170[b]	−0.2411
a	−0.0110	−0.0116	−0.0097	−0.0089	−0.0151	−0.0075	−0.0106	−0.0079	−0.0029
b	11.4559	11.0146	9.7172	8.2272	8.9650	7.5274	10.1448	9.8604	8.7413

r, coefficient of correlation; a, b, regression coefficients
[a] $p<0.05$; [b] $p<0.01$

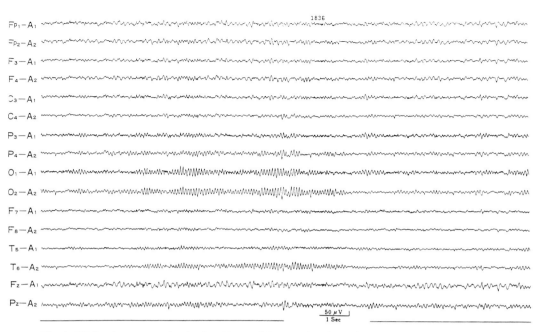

Fig. 3. EEG: theta waves in the Fz, Fp$_1$ and Fp$_2$ at the time of laughter greater than 250 m below sea level

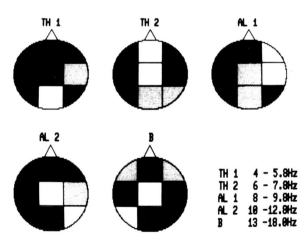

TH 1	4 - 5.8Hz
TH 2	6 - 7.8Hz
AL 1	8 - 9.8Hz
AL 2	10 -12.8Hz
B	13 -18.8Hz

Fig. 4. The plot corresponding to the EEG in Fig. 3, relating to the different locations of the brain. *White square:* $\geq x+SD$, *dotted square:* $<X-SD$. X, averaged value of power spectra

correlation coefficients can be expressed as: $y=aX+b$, where x is the depth and y, the brain potential. The sign preceding a (i.e., denoting the slope of the straight line) is minus in all cases (e.g., theta) (Table 2). This means that with increasing depth, the potential will increase. Let us next take the correlation

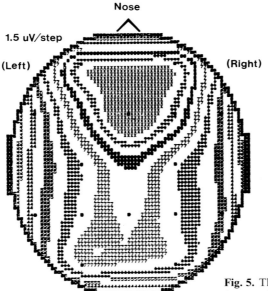

Fig. 5. The spectra numerical printout of the topographic map of the theta wave in the EEG in Fig. 3

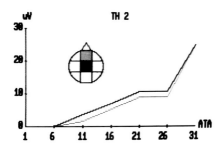

Fig. 6. Correlation between EEG and pressure (ATA). *Heavy line:* high potential of Th_1; *light line:* lower potential of Th_2

coefficient and try to establish whether this straight line is meaningful or not. It becomes clear that the alpha wave shows significant variations to the frontal prominence, and the theta wave to the midline frontal region (Fig. 3). Figure 4 reveals the corresponding plots relating to the different locations of the brain by a microcomputer display. Figure 5 shows the characteristic pattern of the theta wave (Fmθ) at depths greater than 250 m below sea level; the wave is strongest at f_z in the frontal midline which was similar to Fmθ (Yamaguchi 1981). Figure 6 illustrates the correlation between EEG and pressure.

All the divers answered a questionnaire and kept a personal log of their signs and symptoms of high pressure nervous syndrome (HPNS), and characteristic features were noted in the emotional and mental status, for example a transient episode of laughter or euphoric status at a depth greater than 21 ATA. At the same time, topographic EEG revealed a type of frontal midline theta wave which was associated with the diffuse alpha wave. Thus, an intimate correlation between frontal midline theta wave and laughter or euphoric status was also observed during the compression and decompression processes in the saturation dive. The divers became accustomed to this environment after 24 h, 32 h and 80 h on the bottom. These results show that there are significant individual variations in susceptibility to subjective signs and symptoms.

Discussions and Conclusion

A two-dimensional display of the EEG developed by us was applied to recordings from divers during the compression period of a 31 ATA saturation dive. Significant correlations between dive depth and EEG potential were observed at individual mapping locations (the alpha wave showed a significant variation in type of diffuse alpha, and the theta wave, for the frontal midline region) which were developed paroxysmally in relatively brief bursts supplanting or intermixing in the normal background rhythms. In addition, to elucidate the development mechanism of the theta wave, we compared the frontal intermittent rhythmic delta activity (FIRDA) (Daly 1975) and the frontal midline theta wave (Fmθ). Fmθ was mostly seen at Fz with the maximum amplitude, whereas FIRDA was located anterior to Fz (Matsuoka et al. 1987). FIRDA abnormal rhythms result from the deranged functions not of cortical neurons, but of subcortical pacemakers driving cortical neurons. Although its mechanism of origin is uncertain, the midline theta rhythm appears to represent a nonspecific variant of theta activity that can occur in a mixed group of patients with various diagnoses (Westmoreland and Klass 1986), in normal EEG, or be related to certain mental activities (Yamaguchi 1981). In our cases, the theta wave, topographically similar to Fmθ, was associated mostly with some characteristic features of HPNS, such as a transient episode of laughter or euphoric status at a depth greater than 21 ATA. An intimate correlation between Fmθ and laughter was also observed during compression and decompression processes of a saturation dive in a helium-oxygen environment. Therefore, Fmθ may be related not to the mental performance but to the affective phenomena induced by helium under high pressure.

Acknowledgements. The authors thank Mr. Ishikawa for technical assistance and Mr. Yamamoto for statistical analysis.

References

Bennett PB, Coggin R, Mcleod M (1982) Effect of compression rate on use of trimix to ameliorate HPNS in man to 686 m (2250 ft) Undersea Biomed Res 9:335–351

Daly DD (1975) Genesis of abnormal activity. In: Antorne R (ed) Handbook of electroencephalography and clinical neurophysiology, vol 14/C. Elsevier, Amsterdam, pp 5–10

Matsuoka S, Tokuda H, Ishikawa T (1984) The idea of computer topographic display of EEG for clinical assessment of EEG and evoked potential data. In: Matsumoto K (ed) Topographic electroencephalography in clinical testing. Neuron-sha, Tokyo, pp 23–33 (in Japanese)

Matsuoka S, Okuda S, Wada S, Kadoya C, Ishikawa T, Yamamoto S, Mori M (1987) Topographic characteristics of EEG during a saturation dive to 31 ATA helium-oxygen environment. Clin Encephalogr 29:584–593 (in Japanese)

Naquet R, Lemaire C, Rostain JC (1984) High pressure nervous syndrome: psychometric and clinico-electrophysiological correlations. Philos Trans R Soc Lond [Biol] 304:95–102

Procter LD, Carey CR, Lee RM et al. (1972) Electroencephalographic changes during saturation excursion dives to a simulated sea water depth of 1000 feet. Aerospace Med 43(8):867–877

Ueno S, Matsuoka S (1975) Topographic display of slow wave types of EEG abnormality in patients with brain lesions. Jpn J Med Electronics Biol Eng 14:118–124 (in Japanese)

Ueno S, Matsuoka S, Mizoguchi T et al. (1975) Topographic computer display of abnormal EEG activities in patients with CNS diseases. Memoirs of the Faculty of Eng, Kyushu Univ 34:195–209

Westmoreland BF, Klass DW (1986) Midline theta rhythm. Arch Neurolog 43:139–141

Yamaguchi Y (1981) Frontal midline theta activity. In: Yamaguchi N, Fujisawa K, (eds). Recent advances in EEG and EMG data processing. Elsevier/North-Holland, Amsterdam, pp 391–396

Spectral and Frequency Analysis of the Central EEG Activity in Parkinson's Disease Patients with Alzheimer's Disease: The Development During Nootropic Therapy

E.W. FÜNFGELD[1]

The goal of the present investigation is to answer the following questions: What is the meaning of high EEG amplitudes in the frontal and central regions, the so-called anteriorization? Can any clarification be achieved by means of advanced EEG techniques?

Material and Technique

The investigation was based on the EEG findings in 1101 patients with Parkinson's disease. Using the conventional technique, definitely normal EEGs were found in only one-third (360) of these patients. In 456 Parkinson's patients with different stages of senile dementia of the Alzheimer type we were able to derive EEG controls, either after 4–8 weeks' therapy or later on the occasion of the second or third admission up to 24 months after the first EEG. Of these 456 patients, 112 (24.5%) showed a so-called anteriorization of power. We divided these patients into three subgroups according to stage of anteriorization:
1. Alpha anteriorization in cases with normal or borderline EEG results. Of 189 cases in this group 38 (20%) displayed anteriorization.
2. Slight to moderate or medium generalized slowing in conventional EEG. Of 252 patients in this group 69 (27%) showed slight a alpha but more expressed theta anteriorization.
3. Severe slowing of the curves. Of the 15 patients in this group, five had theta and delta anteriorization, sometimes with alpha waves superimposed (33%).

Results

Examples will be presented of the different techniques and montages used.

Picker-Schwarzer Spectral Analysis

Case Report. A 76-year-old female Parkinsonian patient had slight signs of senile dementia of Alzheimer's type (SDAT). Her EEG at first showed high

---

[1] Schloßberg-Klinik Wittgenstein, Schloßstraße 40, 5928 Bad Laasphe, Federal Republic of Germany and Medizinische Fakultät, Universität Marburg, Baldingerstr., 3550 Marburg, Federal Republic of Germany

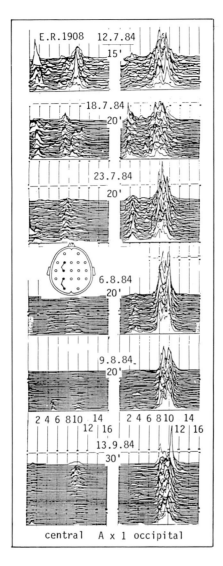

Fig. 1. Case 1: spectral analysis

theta amplitudes in the left central region, occipital slowed alpha and some theta waves (our stage 2). Between July 12 and July 18, five infusions of 250 ml protein-free blood extract together with 12 g piracetam were given. Before the next EEG control (July 23) a further five infusions were administered, each accompanied by 3.98 mg ergoloidmesylates orally. During this time the high central EEG activity was markedly reduced and the occipital waves were faster. Then, until August 6, the daily medication was only 600 mg pyritinol, and from then until the last EEG on September 13 the patient received 1 g pyritinol, 2.4 g piracetam and antiparkinsonian drugs. Apart from some artifacts the central activity disappeared step by step and the occipital waves became faster

Spectral and Frequency Analysis of the Central EEG Activity

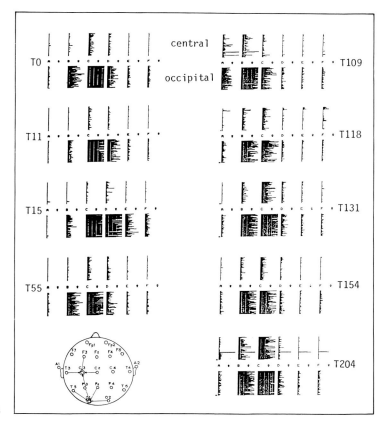

Fig. 2. Case 2: frequency analysis

at the same time, with the result that anteriorization was abolished. As shown in Fig. 1, we used a longitudinal montage with two channels deriving from the left central and left occipital region.

Picker-Schwarzer Trend Monitor

A newer system of frequency analysis, the Picker-Schwarzer Trend Monitor, System ETM 2002, Modell 2264, for fast Fourier analysis gives more informations. We have been using this system since July 1985. An EEG follow-up study is given (Fig. 2) as an example of the results achieved with this method.

Case Report. A 69-year-old patient had suffered from severe Parkinson's disease for many years. At the time of his admission he needed total help, even with eating. He stayed in our hospital for more than 6 months, during which time we recorded 20 EEGs, nine of which are shown in Fig. 2. As montage we used the source derivation (Hjorth 1975). At time 0 – before the beginning of the nootropic treatment – in the *central region* there were theta waves from 6 to

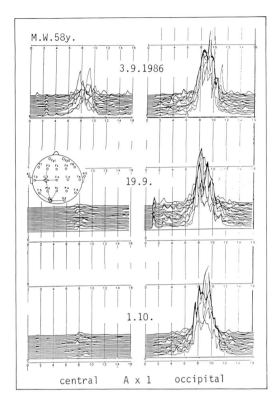

Fig. 3. Case 3: spectral analysis

8 cycles/s in band C and a small amount of slow alpha waves, 8–9 cycles/s, in band D. In the *occipital region* there were mostly theta waves from 6 to 8 cycles/s and slower theta waves from 3 to 6 cycles/s (in bands C and B); the alpha activity was quite poor (our stage 2). At the 11th day and, even more markedly, at the 15th day the central activity was diminished. Occipitally we found fewer waves from 3 to 6 cycles/s and many more waves from 8 to 9 cycles/s and from 9 to 10 cycles/s, even a few waves from 10 to 12 cycles/s. The appearance of faster waves is attributed to the infusion therapy, consisting of a protein-free blood extract and infusions with amantadine sulfate. Clinically the patient was more lively and interested in his surroundings and in TV. However, after 3 weeks he got very severe pneumonia with several relapses in the following weeks, during which time we observed very high levels of blood lipids. After 3 months the frequency analysis on day 109 showed nearly pure delta and theta waves centrally and occipitally. The following analysis revealed a diminution of the delta waves but the central theta activity was even more increased (stage 3). Clinically the patient had deteriorated markedly: severe generalized rigidity, total lack of spontaneity and drive, very few reactions to external stimuli, no verbal reactions but a telling glance, vertical paralysis of eye movements. Our final diagnosis: subcortical arteriosclerotic encephalopathy (Binswanger's disease).

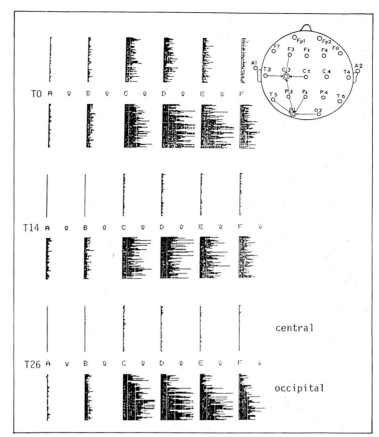

Fig. 4. Case 3: frequency analysis

The Brain Mapping and Imaging Technique

In the 6 months up to the time of writing, the System Beta site, brain mapping and imaging technique developed by Prof. T. Itil, Department of Biological Psychiatry, New York Medical College and the HZI Research Center, Tarrytown, New York was used. We were able to compare this technique with the two previous techniques in the same patient.

Case Report. A 58-year-old woman with a history of rapidly progressing Parkinson's disease and psychic disturbances was admitted to our hospital. Fifteen months earlier she had been diagnosed in the neurological department of the Max Planck Institute at Cologne as having slight parkinsonism and SDAT with slowed EEG, and positron emission tomography showed reduced glucose metabolism, bilateral in the parietotemporo-occipital region and in the insular anterotemporal region more marked on the left side. CT showed some slight hypodensities near the ventricles. Over a period of 26 days we administered

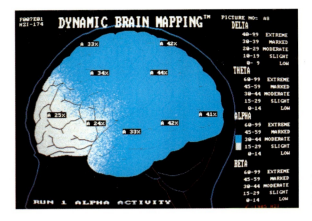

Fig. 5. Case 3: brain mapping, left side. Distribution of alpha waves before therapy

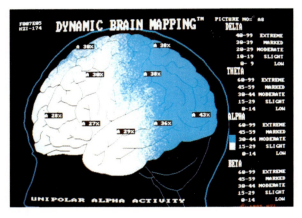

Fig. 6. Case 3: brain mapping, left side. Distribution of alpha waves after 26 days' therapy

300 mg phosphatidylserine daily and recorded EEG weekly using the conventional and the three computer techniques.

Spectral analyses before the treatment and on day 14 (September 19) and day 26 (October 1) showed a marked reduction of central theta and alpha activity (Fig. 3).

Frequency analyses showed the same findings, but on day 26 we observed a slight increase of the alpha frequencies 10–12 cycles/s in the occipital region (band F; see Fig. 4).

Brain mapping and imaging technique: From the multiple possibilities of this technique – each montage gives 27 different colored pictures on the monitor and finally a summarizing printout with statistical data – only the changes of the alpha waves are given. On September 3 (Fig. 5) a high percentage of alpha was observed in the frontal, central and temporal regions, a typical anteriorization. On October 1 this status was changed: the differences between the same regions ranged from +3% to −6% (Fig. 6). Result: The anteriorization was slightly diminished.

Clinically the patient's movements were slightly faster, but the main changes were observed in her psychic status: improvement in mood; more drive and concentration; a diminution from 45 to 22 points in the Sandoz Geriatric Rating Scale.

Discussion

Differences of EEG findings in normal aging and in dementia were extensively described by Obrist (1979) and Visser (1985). Some correlations between the slowed EEG and psychological tests were reported. Concerning rehabilitation, the prognosis in elderly patients with diffuse slowed EEG activity was significantly poorer than in patients with purely focal abnormalities. In parkinsonian patients Lücking and Berger (1984) first published a description of a slowed background activity. This activity was "frequently associated" with a pathological spread of these waves to the frontal region. In our experience not all patients with a diffuse slowed EEG and SDAT showed such anteriorization of some frequencies – alpha anteriorization, as Herrmann and Schärer (1986) described – or of all frequency bands as we have reported in this paper. In our patient group nearly 25% showed this phenomenon; it seems not to be linked with an alteration of vigilance, as Herrmann and Schärer (1986) pointed out. If we take in account that technical and other conditions (nearly all EEG records were taken before noon) were stable, the anteriorization might have other reasons and other sources than vigilance alone. It seems that the phenomenon of anteriorization is linked with some special subcortical generators in certain particular aging or vascular processes, as we showed in our case with Binswanger's disease for theta and delta waves.

Pedley and Miller (1983) and Visser (1985) published EEG traces of a patient with Creutzfeldt-Jakob disease and with a state of dementia; the recordings showed anteriorization of delta waves corresponding to our stage 3.

In some patients the anteriorization was diminished/abolished by nootropics. It might be that the montage used, mainly the source derivation after Hjorth, allows registration of the anteriorization more clearly than other montages. Recently a montage was used which included the midline electrode F_z to T_3 or T_4; this gives even better results than the source derivation.

We hope that the new techniques with brain mapping and imaging method will enlarge our knowledge of this phenomenon and of the influences of nootropic drugs.

Summary

In Parkinson's disease patients with SDAT the diffuse high frontal and central brain wave activity – compared to parietal or occipital regions – may have some diagnostic value. The phenomenon of anteriorisation, classified into three stages, has to be differentiated from hypersynchronic wave activity, which is also sometimes observed in these cases. Nootropic drugs – for instance a protein-free blood extract, piracetam, pyritinol and phosphatidylserine – were able to diminish or abolish this phenomenon, which can be shown much more clearly by using special montages and computer-assisted EEG methods such as Fourier spectral and/or frequency analysis. Undoubtedly the brain mapping and imaging system will be the preferred method in the future.

Further studies using modern imaging systems may help to yield detailed information about the underlaying processes.

References

Herrmann WM, Schärer E (1986) Pharmakoelektroencephalographie und gerontologische Forschung. In: Lauter H, Möller HJ, Zimmer R (eds) Untersuchungs- und Behandlungsverfahren in der Gerontopsychiatrie. Springer, Berlin Heidelberg New York Tokyo, pp 137–150

Hjorth B (1975) An one-line transformation of EEG scalp potentials into orthogonal source derivations. Electroencephalogr Clin Neurophysiol 39:526–530

Itil TM, Shapiro DM, Eralp E, Akman A, Itil K, Garbizu C (1985) A new brain function diagnostic unit, including the dynamic brain mapping of computer analysed EEG, evoked potentials and sleep. New Trends Exp Clin Psychiatr 1–2:107–177

Lücking CH, Berger W (1984) EEG-Befunde bei Parkinsonkranken. In: Fischer PA (ed) Parkinson plus. Springer, Berlin Heidelberg New York Tokyo, pp 101–109

Obrist WD (1979) Electroencephalographic changes in normal aging and dementia. In: Hoffmeister F, Müller C (eds) Brain function in old age. Springer, Berlin Heidelberg New York, pp 102–111

Pedley TA, Miller JA (1983) Clinical neurophysiology of aging and dementia. Adv Neurol 38:31–49

Visser SL (1985) EEG and evoked potentials in the diagnosis of dementias. In: Traber J, Gipsen WH (eds) Senile dementia of Alzheimer type. Springer, Berlin Heidelberg New York Tokyo, pp 102–116

EEG and EP Mapping in Patients with Senile Dementia of Alzheimer Type Before and After Treatment with Pyritinol

R. Ihl[1], K. Maurer[1], T. Dierks[1], and W. Wannenmacher[2]

Introduction

The electroencephalogram (EEG) and evoked potentials (EP) show changes in electrical brain activity both in physiological aging and in senile dementia of the Alzheimer type (SDAT). In physiological aging there is slowing of the main alpha frequency in the order of 0.5–1 Hz (Visser 1985). In addition, an increase of beta activity from 12% in young adults to 24% in aged persons and an increase of slow activity from 7% to 15% can be observed. In SDAT the slowing of the alpha rhythm can be in the range of 1–3 Hz, so that an alpha frequency of 8 Hz and less is achieved. The amount of theta and delta activity can rise considerably (Gordon and Sim 1967). Focal lesions are not common in SDAT but are frequent findings in dementia due to multiple infarction (MID).

Alterations of EP are observed with increasing age but are less pronounced than the EEG changes. Maurer et al. (in this volume) describe changes of auditory EP (AEP) and especially of the acoustically elicited P300.

The first article describing the use of brain electrical activity mapping (BEAM) in patients with SDAT appeared in 1984 (Duffy et al. 1984). The aims of the study reported here were (a) to delineate the topographic distribution of the four main EEG frequencies (delta, theta, alpha and beta) in an aged control group and in patients suffering from SDAT, and (b) to demonstrate the effects of the nootropic substance pyritinol on EEG parameters in SDAT patients.

Subjects

We investigated six geriatric controls (mean age 74.2 years) and six patients with SDAT diagnosed and treated in the Department of Psychiatry, University of Würzburg. All SDAT patients showed well-defined EEG alterations after administration of a single dose of 600 mg pyritinol. The mean age of the patients was 70.8 years. The diagnosis of SDAT was based upon DSM-III and ICD-9 criteria. The Hachinski-Score modified according to Rosen et al. (1980) was

---

[1] Department of Psychiatry, University of Würzburg, Füchsleinstr. 15, 8700 Würzburg, Federal Republic of Germany
[2] Institute of Psychology, University of Technology, 6100 Darmstadt 1, Federal Republic of Germany

applied to differentiate between MID and SDAT and only those patients with scores less than 2 were considered for further analysis. For rating the cognitive state of the patient the Brief Cognitive Rating Scale (BCRS) according to Reisberg et al. (1983) was used. Only patients in stages 3–5 (moderate severity) were included. The EEG measurements were performed before administration of a single dose of 600 mg pyritinol and 2 and 4 h after drug ingestion.

Methods

The procedure used is described in detail by Dierks et al. in this volume. Nineteen electrodes were applied to the scalp according to the 10–20 system. The linked mastoids served as reference. The electrical activity of the brain was fed into a mapping system (Brain Atlas III, Bio-logic Systems Corp.). The EEG was recorded only in the eyes closed alert (EC) state. The 0–31.5 Hz segment was divided for further analysis into the following four frequency bands: delta (0–3.5 Hz), theta (4–7.5 Hz), alpha (8–11.5 Hz) and beta (12–15.5 Hz). The data analysis comprised the calculation of group means and variances for each point. For comparison between geriatric normals and SDAT patients, calculations according to Student's t test were performed. Differences in the main α-frequency between the two groups were tested for statistical significance using a Mann Whitney U-test.

Results

Figure 1 a, b shows the topography of the main four frequency ranges investigated in this study for the geriatric control group and for SDAT patients. There was a considerable increase in delta and theta activity in the SDAT group. This could be confirmed by the t value maps (Fig. 2, critical values for all t-maps: $n=16$; $df=14$; $P<0.05$ for $t>2.15$; $P<0.01$ for $t>2.98$) with maximal difference between the groups at points T3, P3, P4 and T6 for the delta and point Cz for the theta activity (Fig. 3).

The alpha activity diminished and disintegrated in the SDAT group. However, differences failed to reach significance (Fig. 4). The slow beta activity showed a similar tendency as alpha with a decrease pattern shown in Fig. 1b.

Most remarkable were findings of a slowing of the alpha rhythm, which exhibited its maximal power between 10.5 and 11 Hz in the geriatric control group (Fig. 5a) and between 7 and 9 Hz in the SDAT group (Fig. 5b); $U=8$, $P<0.005$).

Four hours after administration of a single dose of 600 mg pyritinol the EEG of the SDAT group underwent considerable changes, which are shown in Fig. 6. Delta and theta activity decreased, whereas alpha increased, especially in the parietal area, where under pyritinol higher power values were obtained

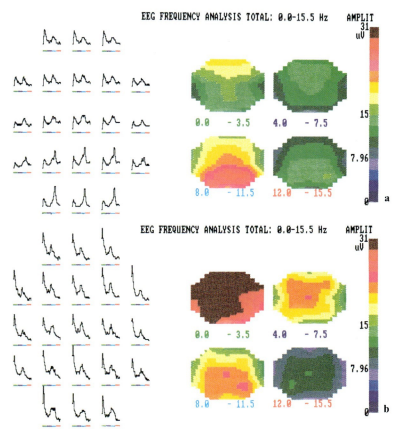

Fig. 1a, b. EEG topography in geriatric controls (**a**) and SDAT patients (**b**). Increase of delta and theta and decrease of alpha and beta in the SDAT group. (All figures in this contribution were prepared using equipment from Bio-logic Systems Corporation, Mundelein, IL, USA)

than in the geriatric control group. A similar tendency could be observed for slow beta activity. The corresponding t value maps are shown in Figs. 7 and 8, with negative t values for the delta and theta and positive t values for the alpha activity.

Discussion

The most consistent finding in untreated SDAT patients compared to an age-matched geriatric control group was an increase of slow activity (delta and theta) and a decrease of alpha and beta. These are well-known phenomena and have already been described by Letemendia and Pampeglione (1958) and Gordon and Sim (1967). New information, however, could be yielded by our

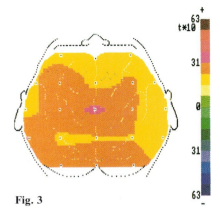
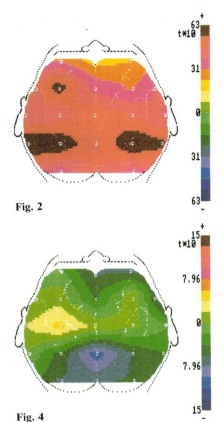

Fig. 2. These *t* value map exhibit the difference in delta activity between the control and SDAT groups. *Red* indicates an increase of slow activity. Maximal delta occurred at points T5, P3, P4 and T6

Fig. 3. A *t* value map for theta activity. The difference was maximal in central and left temporoparietal areas

Fig. 4. A *t* value map for alpha activity, with indication of a parietal decrease (Pz) in the SDAT group

topographic display of the EEG activity. The alpha rhythm lost its typical parieto-occipital presence and showed signs of disintegration and anterior displacement. At the same time a decrease of the main alpha frequency could be observed in the range of about 2–3 Hz. Delta and theta increased considerably, with temporoparieto-occipital predominance. This EEG phenomenon cannot be explained solely by a selective loss of cholinergic neurones in the hippocampus (Bowen et al. 1977; Davies and Maloney 1976), because "dead cells tell no tales" (Roth 1979). Sims et al. (1980) found reduced acetylcholine synthesis in their study of glucose metabolism and acetylcholine synthesis in relation to neuronal activity in Alzheimer's disease. The hypothesis of an abnormal cholinergic system is also supported by studies showing that anticholinergic drugs such as atropine produce a slowing in the EEG. The contrary occurred after administration of physostigmine, a cholinesterase inhibitor, which brought about a decrease of slow activity and a stabilization of alpha.

Besides a disturbance of cholinergic activity, we have to take into consideration a more structural lesion in cortical areas. One major observation in our study was that in addition to the anterior shift of the main alpha frequency, an accentuation of slowing occurred in parietotemporo-occipital regions. This

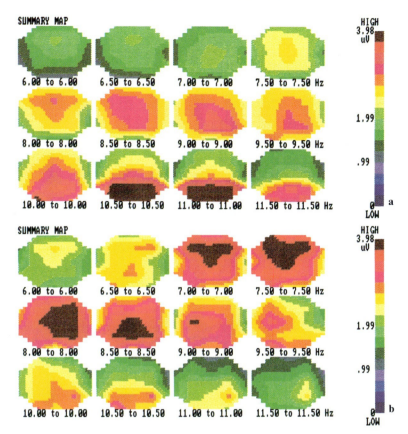

Fig. 5a, b. EEG maps covering a frequency range between 6 and 11.5 Hz in **a** geriatric controls and **b** SDAT patients. In SDAT patients a slowing of main alpha to values between 7 and 9 Hz took place

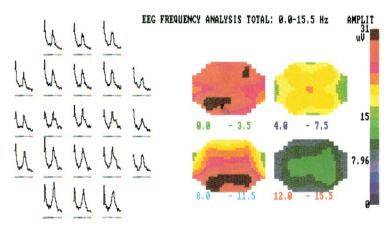

Fig. 6. EEG topography in the frequency ranges delta, theta, alpha and beta after administration of pyritinol

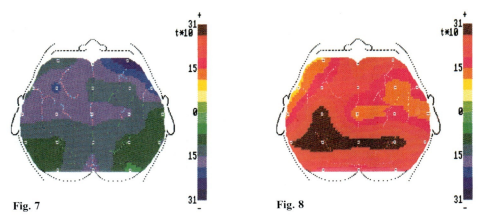

Fig. 7. A *t* value map comparing delta activity before and after administration of pyritinol. Decrease of delta is indicated by negative *t* values

Fig. 8. A *t* value map comparing alpha activity before and after administration of pyritinol. An increase and a stabilization of alpha is visible (*red:* positive *t* values), especially in parietal areas

is clearly shown in Fig. 2, where *t* values of 3.2 were achieved in the delta activity at T3, P3, P4 and T6, indicating a significant slowing in these areas. This pattern points to a cortical lesion on both hemispheres with temporoparietal accentuation and frontal preservation. A similar pattern with a preserved frontal field was observed by Maurer et al. (this volume) using their P300 topography in SDAT patients. This pattern may be consistent with the "hyperfrontality" described by Stigsby et al. (1981). They found a decrease of blood flow postcentrally and an increase precentrally. Noteworthy in this context are measurements of glucose metabolism by means of PET in SDAT patients. Friedland et al. (1983) and Forster et al. (1984) found a relative frontal increase and temporoparietal decrease of the metabolic rate of glucose. Brun and Gustavson (1976) did a postmortem study on seven patients with SDAT and found a neural degeneration affecting temporoparieto-occipital areas most severely. By means of structural and functional imaging procedures it was therefore possible to delineate a lesion pattern which pointed to predominant temporoparieto-occipital cortical involvement sparing frontal structures.

In our investigation the onset, duration and severity of the SDAT disease has been documented. One of our patients with late onset, 5 years duration of disease and a very severe course exhibited, in contrast to others, additional involvement of the frontal lobe. This finding points to spreading of the degenerative process also towards frontal structures in severe stages of the disease.

The above-mentioned generalized slowing in the delta and theta range and a destabilization of alpha in combination with an anterior shift was a consistent finding in untreated SDAT patients. After a single dose of 600 mg pyritinol, these alterations underwent an obvious change in all cases: Alpha exhibited a posterior shift and an acceleration of its main frequency, delta and theta decreased markedly (Fig. 6). Similar findings were described by Kuenkel and Westphal (1970), Herrmann et al. (1986), and Saletu et al. (this volume) indicating an activating vigilance-raising effect of pyritinol. Described for the first time here is the topographic aspect of the EEG alterations induced by pyritinol: in SDAT patients under therapy the EEG pattern approached that observed in an age-matched geriatric control group.

No interpretation of the effect of pyritinol upon central nervous structures in SDAT patients can be given considering solely the irreversible loss of cholinergic neurons projecting to the hippocampus and cortex, but successful interpretation may be possible using the fluid-mosaic model of the membrane, which may explain in part the reversibility of some EEG features under therapy. With increasing age the membrane becomes increasingly rigid. Concomitantly the Na/K ATPase undergoes a decrease of activity in the order of 20%–25%. Both the dopamine uptake and the release of acetylcholine show a decrement. These morphological and biochemical signs of physiological aging are combined with only slight alteration of EEG (Fig. 1a). In patients with SDAT, however, the EEG changes were much more obvious, permitting the assumption that the above-mentioned partly reversible phenomena are so pronounced that a clinically obvious stage of the demential process is reached, with signs of severe intellectual deterioration including memory disturbances and marked reduction in cognitive abilities. It was shown in our study that the electrophysiological concomitants of the demential process due to pathomechanisms within the fluid-mosaic model of the membrane can be improved by administration of a single dose of 600 mg pyritinol. This permits the prediction that with chronic application of the substance the restoring effect might be maintained and might also lead to an amelioration of cognitive function and behavior in SDAT patients. A study of the effects of chronic treatment over a period of 12 weeks is currently under way and will be completed soon.

References

Bowen DM, Smith DB, White P, Flack RHA, Carrasco LH, Gedye Jl, Davison AN (1977) Chemical pathology of the organic dementias. Brain 100:427–453

Brun A, Gustavson L (1976) Distribution of cerebral degeneration in Alzheimer's disease. Arch Psychiatr Nervenkr 223:15–33

Davies P, Malony AJF (1976) Selective loss of central cholinergic neurons in Alzheimer's disease. Lancet 2:1403

Duffy FH, Albert SM, McAnulty G (1984) Brain electrical activity in patients with presenile and senile dementia of Alzheimer type. Ann Neurol 16:439–448

Foster NL, Chase TN, Mansi L, Brooks R, Fedio P, Petronas NJ, di Chiro G (1984) Cortical abnormalities in Alzheimer's disease. Ann Neurol 16:649–654

Friedland RP, Buddinger TF, Ganz E, Yano Y, Mathis CA, Koss B, Ober BA, Huesman RH, Derenzo SE (1983) Regional cerebral metabolic alterations in dementia of the Alzheimer type: positron emission topography with Fluorodeoxyglucose. J Comput Assist Tomogr 7:590–598

Gordon EB, Sim M (1967) The EEG in presenile dementia. J Neurol Neurosurg Psychiatry 30:285–291

Herrmann WM, Kern U, Röhmel J (1986) Contributions to the search for vigilance indicative EEG variables. Pharmacopsychiatry 19:75–83

Kuenkel H, Westphal M (1970) Quantitative EEG analysis of pyrithioxine action. Pharmaco psychiatry 1:41–49

Letemendia F, Pampligione G (1958) Clinical and electroencephalographic observations in Alzheimer's disease. J Neurol Neurosurg Psychiatry 21:167–172

Reisberg B, London E, Ferris SH, Borenstein J, Scheier L, de Leon MJ (1983) The brief cognitive rating scale: language, motoric and mood, concomitants in primary degenerative dementia (PDD). Psychopharmacol Bull 19:702–708

Rosen WG, Mohs RC, Davis KL (1984) A new rating scale for Alzheimer's desease. Am J Psychiatry 14:1356–1364

Roth M (1979) The early diagnosis of Alzheimer's disease-summary. In: Glenn AIM, Whalley LJ (eds) Alzheimer's disease. Churchill-Livingstone, Edinburgh, pp 133–136

Sims NR, Bowen DM, Smith CCT, Flack RHA, Davison AN, Snowden JS, Neary D (1980) Glucose metabolism and acetylcholine synthesis in relation to neuronal activity in Alzheimer's disease. Lancet 1:333–336

Stigsby B, Johansson G, Ingvar DH (1981) Regional EEG analysis and regional cerebral blood flow in Alzheimer's and Pick's disease. Electroencephalogr Clin Neurophysiol 51:537–547

Visser SL (1985) EEG and evoked potentials in the diagnosis of dementia. In: Traber J, Gispen WH (eds) Senile dementia of the Alzheimer type. Springer, Berlin Heidelberg New York Tokyo, pp 102–116

EEG Mapping in Epilepsy

J. GACHES and B. GUEGUEN[1]

Introduction

Despite the fact that using Fast Fourier transforms (FFT) to non-stationary signals is somewhat questionable, we have applied this method since 1982 (Etevenon et al. 1982; Gueguen and Gaches 1986) in cases of epilepsy.

Methodology and Patients

We used a 16-channels recording system (Cartovar 2000), the distribution of the electrodes closely resembling that in the international 10/20 system. Maps were obtained from sequential segments of records lasting 6 s or a multiple thereof, with the patient in different conditions (relaxed, eyes closed then open; during hyperventilation; during photic stimulation). Examination included simultaneous conventional EEG tracing.

Seventy-eight epileptic patients were selected on the basis of an accurate clinical assessment including CT scan and conventional EEGs. The 37 women and 41 men, aged between 11 and 79 years, were divided into two groups according to the CT data: abnormal (lesional) or normal. Epilepsies were classified, according to their clinical characteristics into generalized (GS), simple partial (SPS) and complex partial (CPS) seizures. We separated conventional EEG data into diffuse discharges, localized discharges or normal, and EEG mapping data into permanent, intermittent or topographically variable abnormalities, or normal. Qualities of the main background activity, i.e., postero-anterior diffusion, reactivity and possible asymmetry of the alpha rhythm (Gaches and Gueguen 1986), were evaluated, as well as the morphology of power spectra.

Results

The usual expression of the interictal abnormalities on the maps, whether CT scan is abnormal or normal, consists of a localized hyperdensity (corresponding to excessive power) in a segment of the total EEG frequency band. This localized hyperdensity usually concerns a segment overlapping parts of the delta and

---

[1] Service d'Exploration Fonctionnelle du Système Nerveux, Centre Hospitalier Sainte Anne, 1 rue Cabanis, 75674 Paris Cedex, France

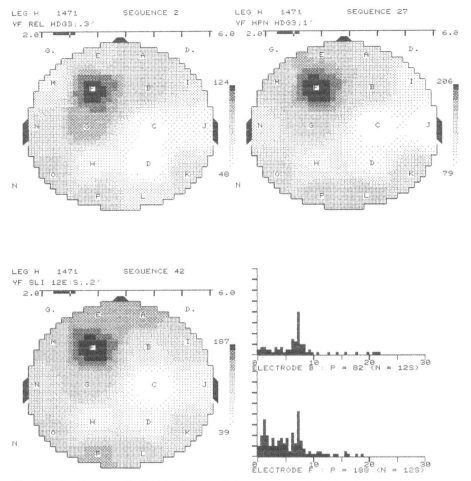

Fig. 1. Male, 31 years old, CPS for 3 years. CT scan: non-evolutive left frontal oligodendroglioma with internal and posterior location. All the sequential EEG maps show on the scalp an area with hyperdensity for the frequency segment 2–7 Hz, here reduced to 2–6 Hz in order to avoid sub-alpha expression and see the focus more clearly. Note: the stable and permanent location of the abnormal area; the increase of the power values during hyperventilation (sequence 27, *upper right*: 206 µV^2) and during photic stimulation (sequence 42, *lower left*: 187 µV^2), compared to the initial values at rest (sequence 2, *upper left*: 124 µV^2); the "comb" aspect of the spectrum corresponding to the F electrode; and the difference in power values between F (left side) and B (right side of scalp): 188 vs 82 µV^2

theta bands (Gaches et al. 1986; Gueguen and Gaches 1986), for instance 2–6 Hz (Fig. 1). In some cases, this segment extends into the alpha band (Fig. 2, left), or even into the beta band. In a few cases, only the beta band is involved (Fig. 2, right). More often, beta hyperdensity is close to the delta-theta area.

This abnormal area is either permanent (present on all the sequential maps), or intermittent (present on some maps only, but always at the same location).

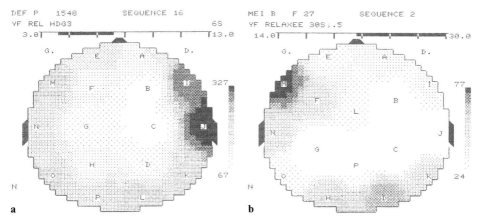

Fig. 2a, b. EEG mapping in two cases of epilepsy with CPS and normal CT scan. **a** Male, 34 years old, possible neonatal anoxia, GS appearing in infancy, then occasional CPS. Map expresses a permanent hyperdensity area on the right temporal region for the frequency segment 3–13 Hz. Normal conventional EEG. **b** Female, 27 years old, CPS (and occasional GS) for 15 years. An anterior left temporal focus appears only with fast frequencies (beta band: 14–30 Hz). Part of the "alpha" activity (corresponding to 14 Hz) is seen upon the occipital areas, higher on the right hemiscalp (opposite to the focus)

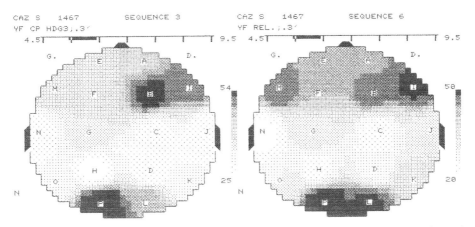

Fig. 3. Displacement of the power peak into the limits of the abnormal area on the scalp. Male, 18 years old, CPS for 3 years. Normal CT scan. Sequential maps: 18 s duration. Permanent hyperdensity area located on the right anterior temporal and posterior frontal regions. Within the limits of this area, the peak of maximum density varies in location, sometimes appearing at electrode B (frontal, sequence 3), sometimes at electrode I (temporal, sequence 6). Such a displacement occurred continuously on the 30 sequences recorded under identical conditions for this patient. Note: the abnormal frequency segment is 4.5–9.5 Hz, including part of the alpha band; alpha rhythm appears on the maps with a normal location on the occipital areas, but higher on the left (opposite hemiscalp to the focus); power values are comparable for all sequences under the same conditions (here 50–58 μV^2)

Table 1. Forty-one cases of epilepsy with lesional CT scan

	Generalized seizures	Simple partial seizures	Complex partial seizures	Total
Conventional EEG				
Focalized	7	9	10	26
Diffuse	3	2	2	7
Normal	–	3	5	8
EEG mapping				
Permanent focus	9	12	13	34
Intermittent focus	1	1	2	4
Variable foci	–	–	2	2
Normal	–	1	–	1
Total	10	14	17	41

Table 2. Thirty-seven cases of epilepsy with normal CT scan

	Generalised seizures	Simple partial seizures	Complex partial seizures	Total
Conventional EEG				
Focalized	1	1	14	16
Diffuse	5	1	8	14
Normal	2	–	5	7
EEG mapping				
Permanent focus	4	2	21	27
Intermittent focus	3	–	2	5
Variable foci	1	–	2	3
Normal	–	–	2	2
Total	8	2	27	37

In a few cases, hyperdensities vary topographically from map to map: these cases correspond to more severe forms of the disease. The limits of the abnormal area extend around a peak of maximum power. The position of this peak varies somewhat from map to map within these spatial limits (Fig. 3). The power values remain similar throughout the abnormal area in the same condition of the patient (at rest). They increase greatly during fits and also increase, usually to a lesser degree, during hyperventilation and photic stimulation (Fig. 1).

In cases with abnormal CT scan, localization on the maps and on the computerized X-ray imaging is always similar, with good approximation (Fig. 1). CT scan and EEG mapping show the best superposable imaging when the lesion is close to the cortex. However, EEG mapping was normal in a patient suffering a congenital subarachnoïd cyst with occasional SPS (the only normal map in this series).

Table 1 summarizes the results in the 41 cases with lesional CT scan.

The fact that such a localization exists on maps in subjects with proved focal lesions lends value to the results obtained when the CT scan remains normal. Figure 2 shows two examples of CPS with permanent focus on EEG mapping but normal CT scan.

Table 2 summarizes the results in the 37 cases with normal CT scan.

Discussion

We will not discuss the application of FFT algorithms to non-stationary signals: this point has been covered extensively elsewhere (Remond 1986). However, we underline that our research deals above all with interictal recordings and uses rather long sequence durations (18–60 s), such that EEG signals are quasi-stationary. We believe that under these conditions EEG mapping, in cases of epilepsy, expresses the regional or local impairment of the part of the brain concerned with the release of discharges. Finally, we leave the discharges themselves and concentrate on the local abnormalities of the EEG background activity to ascertain whether they are permanent or present only around the time of a discharge. This could explain why a localization is seen on the maps while diffuse discharges are observed on conventional EEG records. Comparable interictal EEG mapping has been also reported by Valmier et al. (1986), and correlated with decreased regional cerebral blood flow. Results obtained with other procedures, such as those of Japanese authors mapping the spike itself (Kowada and Yoneya 1983; Shichijo et al. 1983; Takahashi et al. 1983), are coherent with our findings.

Another of our results concerns the morphology of the power spectra. In no case can EEG mapping alone yield data about the morphology of the EEG abnormalities, so important for characterization of epileptic tracings. This difficulty is overcome by comparing the sequential maps to the corresponding segments of the simultaneously recorded conventional tracing. However, we noticed that the spectra take on a more or less regular "comb" appearance in the case of epilepsy. This special feature may exist spontaneously or may appear only during photic stimulation (Fig. 4). It is more marked in the localized abnormal area on the scalp (Fig. 1). However, this phenomenon is of value only when the epoch duration is over 18 s; with a shorter epoch it could be an artifact of the FFT algorithm. With epoch duration reaching 30 s, we did not observe the "comb" in non-epileptic lesions in our series. The mathematical theory of "chaos" could perhaps explain this phenomenon.

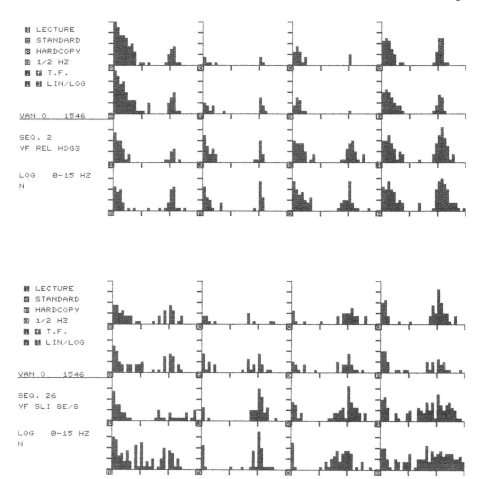

Fig. 4. Morphological aspect of the spectra. Female, 57 years old, occasional CPS with some secondary generalization for 2 years. Normal CT scan. EEG mapping: permanent hyperdensity area in the 4-6 Hz frequency segment upon the left anterior temporal region of the scalp (electrode *m*). The figure presents power spectra between 0 and 15 Hz obtained simultaneously from the 16 electrodes. *Top:* patient at rest; *bottom:* during photic stimulation (eight flashes per second). Photic stimulation conferred a "comb" morphology on the spectrum, more marked for electrode *m*. Duration of the sequences is the same in both conditions (24 s)

Conclusions

The pragmatic application of EEG mapping to cases of epilepsy, above all epilepsy characterized by CPS, shows that the method is able to define localized abnormalities even when CT scan is normal and conventional EEG expresses only diffuse discharges or remains normal. EEG mapping thus appears to be an interesting method for the clinical and fundamental investigation of epilepsy.

References

Etevenon P, Peron-Magnan P, Verdeaux G, Gaches J, Deniker P (1982) Electroencéphalographie quantitative en neurologie et psychiatrie: images topographiques d'EEG, effets d'agents psychotropes, typologie de la schizophrénie. In: Colloque National de Génie Biologique et Médical. Documents analytiques. Paule, Toulouse, 473A 43

Gaches J, Gueguen B (1986) EEG computerized analysis and cartography. In: Bes A, Cahn J, Cahn R, Hoyer S, Marc-Vergnes JP, Wisniewski HM (eds) Current problems in senile dementias. John Libbey-Eurotext, London Paris, pp 134–143

Gaches J, Gueguen B, Etevenon P (1986) Application de la cartographie EEG à la pratique neurologique. In: Court L, Trocherie S, Doucet J (eds) Le traitement du signal en électrophysiologie expérimentale et clinique du système nerveux central. Actes du Congrés International, 11–15 December 1984, Paris, part 1, pp 192–209. Available from Commissariat à l'Energie Atomique Dpt Protection Sanitaire Service Documentation BP 6 F-92265 Fontenay-aux-Roses Cedex

Gueguen B, Gaches J (1986) La cartographie EEG dans les epilepsies à crises partielles. Rev Electroencephalogr Neurophysiol Clin 16:217–228

Kowada M, Yoneya M (1983) Twenty-five channels color topography of the spike. Proceedings of Second Japanese Conference of Topographic Electroencephalography, pp 121–130

Remond A (1986) Computer analysis of EEG and other neurophysiological signals. In: Lopes da Silva FH, Storm van Leuwen W, Remond A (eds) Handbook of Electroencephalography and clinical Neurophysiology revised series, vol 2. Elsevier-North-Holland, Amsterdam

Shichijo F, Masuda T, Matsumoto K (1983) Sequential analysis of epileptic spikes with dynamic topography. In: Proceedings of Second Japanese Conference of Topographic Electroencephalography, pp 115–120

Takahashi H, Yasue M, Ishijima B (1983) The scalp topography and its dynamic display of spikes and spikes-waves in patients with epileptic disorders. In: Topographic electroencephalography in clinical testing: proceedings of Second Japanese Conference of Topographic Electroencephalography. pp 173–180

Valmier J, Touchon J, Baldy-Moulinier M (1986) Etude des débits sanguins régionaux dans les epilepsies partielles complexes lésionnelles et non lésionnelles. Rev Electroencephalogr Neurophysiol Clin 16:229–237

Topographic Representation of Brainstem Lesions: Brainstem Auditory Evoked Potentials Compared with Nuclear Magnetic Resonance Imaging in Multiple Sclerosis*

K. Baum[1], W. Scheuler[2], U. Hegerl[3], W. Girke[1], and W. Schörner[4]

Introduction

The high resolution capacity of nuclear magnetic resonance (NMR) imaging provides a sensitive tool for the detection of demyelinating plaques in the brainstem (Baum et al. 1986, Runge et al. 1984). The comparison of NMR and brainstem auditory evoked potentials (BAEPs) is aimed at clarifying the topographical informativeness of BAEPs (Kjaer 1980).

Material and Methods

Forty-six inpatients with multiple sclerosis were examined. Responses to 1 500 monaural rectangular clicks (intensity 70 or 75 dB SL, stimulation rate 9.3 or 11.1 Hz, duration 0.1 ms) were averaged with a Pathfinder II (Nicolet Biomedical), bandpass filter 150–3 000 Hz. The absolute latencies of the earliest abnormal brainstem potentials, marking the most caudal level of the neurophysiological disturbance (Maurer et al. 1980), were used for the topographical comparison.

NMR imaging was performed with a 0.35- or 0.5-tesla magnetome (Siemens) in two spin echo (SE) sequences (SE 1600/35 + 70 ms) in axial planes with slice thicknesses of 10 mm. The atlas of Kretschmann and Weinrich (1984) was used as a reference for the localization of lesions in the brainstem auditory pathways.

Results

Lesions in the brainstem auditory pathways were verified in 43.5% of the patients by BAEPs and in 39.1% by NMR. Concerning brainstem levels, in 16 (72.7%) of 22 patients with abnormalities at least one lesion detected by NMR matched the BAEP findings (Fig. 1). There were only a few minor deviations from the neurophysiologically assumed functional levels. The concordance be-

---

* Supported by the Bundesministerium für Forschung und Technologie, Bonn, project no. 01 VF 142.

[1] Abteilungen für Neurologie, [2] Neurophysiologie, [3] Psychiatrie, [4] Radiologie des Universitäts-Klinikums Charlottenburg der Freien Universität Berlin, Eschenallee 3, 1000 Berlin 19, Federal Republic of Germany

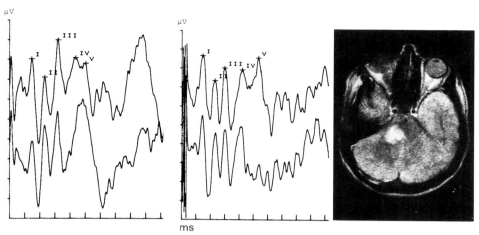

Fig. 1. Multiple sclerosis patient, 30 years old, second exacerbation. BAEPs (ipsilateral recordings): *left*, left ear with normal findings; *middle*, right ear with abnormal delay of wave V. *Right:* NMR: large lesion in the rostral pons with emphasis on the left side

tween BAEPs and NMR was significant (χ^2 test, $p \leq 0.01$) for the whole patient group.

Unilaterally emphasized BAEP findings were compatible in only 33.3% of cases with ipsilateral brainstem lesions verified by NMR. Progressively lengthened absolute latencies which have been interpreted as polytopic lesions in the longitudinal direction (Maurer 1983) did not correspond with multiple lesions in the brainstem auditory pathways as shown by NMR.

Discussion

This study confirms the topographical informativeness of BAEPs regarding the level of brainstem lesions. In only a few patients did the neurophysiologically assumed brainstem levels of the abnormalities show minor deviations from the morphologically detected lesions. The fact that the BAEP and NMR findings did not match completely might be due partly to the limited spatial resolution of NMR and partly to the complex functional mechanisms in the auditory brainstem system, where neuronal structures are simultaneously and successively excited in longitudinal and transverse planes. The view that there is preponderant ipsilateral generation of BAEPs is not supported by this study.

References

Baum K, Girke W, Bräu H, Schörner W, Felix R (1986) Erstmanifestation der Encephalomyelitis disseminata: MRT-Vergleichsstudie gegenüber gesicherter Encephalomyelitis disseminata. Nervenarzt 57:455–460

Kjaer M (1980) Localizing brain stem lesions with brain stem auditory evoked potentials. Acta Neurol Scand 61:265–274

Kretschmann HJ, Weinrich W (1984) Neuroanatomie der kraniellen Computertomographie: Grundlagen und klinische Anwendung. Thieme, Stuttgart

Maurer K, Schäfer E, Hopf HC, Leitner H (1980) The location by early auditory evoked potentials (EAEP) of acoustic nerve and brainstem demyelination in multiple sclerosis (MS). J Neurol 223:43–58

Maurer K (1983) Akustisch evozierte Potentiale. In: Lowitzsch K, Maurer K, Hopf HC (eds) Evozierte Potentiale in der klinischen Diagnostik. Thieme, Stuttgart

Runge VM, Price AC, Kirshner HS, Allen JH, Partain CL, James AE Jr (1984) Magnetic resonance imaging of multiple sclerosis: a study of pulse technique efficacy. AJR 143:1015–1026

Topographic EEG Features During Deep Isoflurane Anesthesia in Patients with Major Depressive Disorders

G. CARL[1], T. DIERKS[1], W. ENGELHARDT[2], and K. MAURER[1]

Introduction

After electrically induced grand mal seizures during electroconvulsive therapy (ECT), a brief period of electrocerebral silence can be seen in the EEG. According to a recent hypothesis (Langer et al. 1985) this EEG pattern is necessary for the success of ECT in depressive patients. Isoflurane is the only volatile anesthetic known that in concentrations above 2 MAC (minimal anesthetic concentration) leads to burst-suppression or isoelectric EEG waveforms. At these concentrations severe or lasting adverse effects do not occur. Patients of the category who did not respond to antidepressive drugs and would normally have been treated with ECT in our department were given isoflurane anesthetics. The topographic distribution of cerebral electrical activity during anesthesia was recorded using the brain mapping method of EEG.

Patients and Methods

Seven patients (three male, four female) between 21 and 60 years of age with major depressive disorders (DSM-III) were treated. After adequate antidepressive drug treatment had failed, informed consent was obtained from the patients. Following a further thorough clinical and laboratory examination the patients were anesthetized every other day up to a total of six sessions. Two days before the first anesthesia all antidepressive drugs and neuroleptics were discontinued. Benzodiazepines were administered throughout. In the unpremedicated patients anesthesia was induced after a precurarizing dose of alcuronium with thiopental. Intubation of the trachea was facilitated with succinylcholine. Subsequently anesthesia was maintained with increasing isoflurane concentrations up to 4% volume in nitrous oxide/oxygen. After the burst-suppression EEG appeared, the inspiratory isoflurane concentration was reduced in steps to zero. Suppression patterns, briefly interrupted by burst, lasted approximately 4–8 min. EEG, blood pressure, ECG, heart rate, end-tidal carbon dioxide and isoflurane concentrations were continuously registered. EEG was continuously recorded with a 19-channel Brain Atlas III (Bio-logic Systems Corp.). Off-line frequency analysis was done for the segment 0–31.5 Hz. The frequency spectra at different concentrations of alveolar isoflurane were compared.

---

[1] Department of Psychiatry, University of Würzburg, Füchsleinstr. 15, 8700 Würzburg, Federal Republic of Germany
[2] Department of Anesthesiology, University of Würzburg, Josef-Schneider-Straße 10, 8700 Würzburg, Federal Republic of Germany

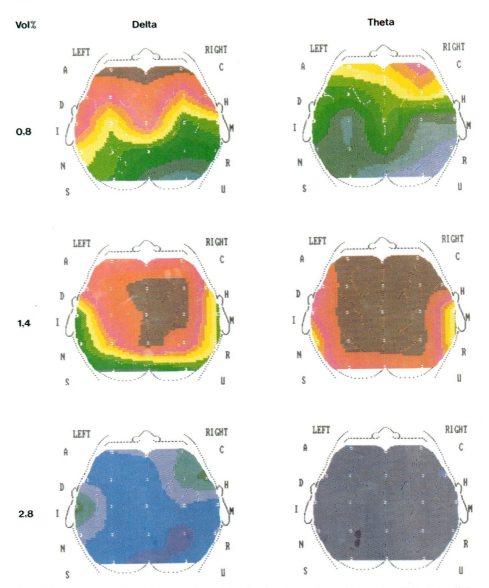

Fig. 1. Brain electrical activity mapping of the delta (0–3.5 Hz), theta (4.0–7.5 Hz), alpha (8.0–11.5 Hz) and beta$_1$ (12–15.5 Hz) bands during 0.8%, 1.4% and 2.8% volume isoflurane anesthesia in a 47-year-old female patient

Topographic EEG Features During Deep Isoflurane Anesthesia in Patients 261

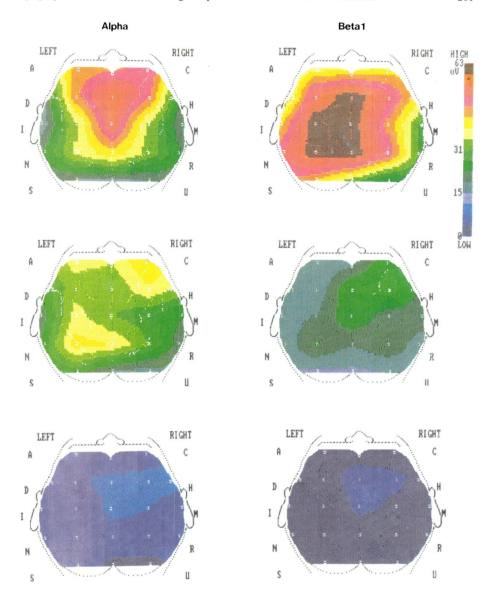

Results

At approximately 0.4% volume isoflurane (end-expiratory) the first changes in EEG frequencies and EEG topography became visible. The influence upon the EEG of the thiopental injection was minimal. With increasing isoflurane concentrations the slow-wave activity in the delta and theta range augmented considerably. At 0.8% volume isoflurane delta and theta waves were restricted mainly to frontal areas (Fig. 1). Concomitant with an increase to 1.4% volume the delta and theta activity became more widespread, appearing also in central, parietal and occipital areas (Fig. 1). The alpha activity, which shifted from occipital to frontal structures with increasing concentration of the anesthetic up to 0.8% volume, decreased when a concentration of 1.4% volume was attained (Fig. 1).

The beta activity, which was primarily located in frontal and central areas, decreased rapidly when a concentration of 1.4% volume was reached. At higher concentrations (above 1.4% volume) delta and theta waves appeared over almost the entire cortex, accompanied by a rapid decrease of alpha and beta waves (Fig. 1). At 2.8% volume the electrical activity of the brain indicated no further activity across the entire spectrum, except for artifacts in the delta band which were probably due to breathing.

The burst-suppression EEG appeared on average at 3% volume isoflurane. At even higher concentrations of the anesthesia (more than 3.2% volume) an isoelectric EEG appeared which was no longer interrupted by bursts. At this concentration of anesthesia four patients had dilated pupils and three patients miosis without reaction to light. Eyelid and corneal reflexes were extinguished.

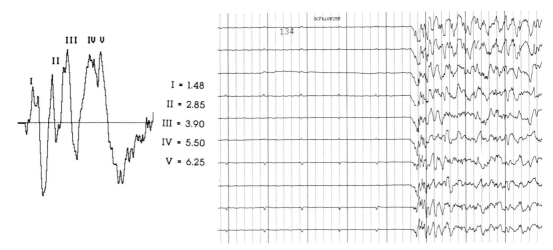

Fig. 2. EAEP during burst-suppression EEG induced by 2.8% volume isoflurane anesthesia. Same patient as in Fig. 1. (Prepared using equipment from Bio-logic Systems Corporation, Mundelein, IL, USA)

The shape of the early auditory evoked potentials (EAEP) remained stable (Fig. 2), but latencies of wave V became prolonged to values up to 6.1 ms (normal: 5.75 ± 0.18 ms).

The narcosis lasted approximately 45 min. The patients were awake immediately after the extubation and were able to answer simple questions. No disturbances in orientation or memory were observed.

Discussion

In concentrations less than 2 MAC an increase of delta and theta activity and a decrease and frontal shift of alpha activity could be observed. In addition, a temporary increase of beta occurred in an early stage of narcosis. Such EEG changes are known with other volatile anesthetics, for instance halothane (Eger 1981; Pichlmayr et al. 1983). It can be assumed that under anesthesia, activity of deeper cortical structures is obtained when the concentration is augmented (Pichlmayr et al. 1983).

By means of topographic display of EEG data we were now able to delineate the topographic changes in the four main frequency bands. In this way it could be demonstrated that a burst-suppression EEG was reached in nontoxic concentrations over the whole head.

Usually the extinction of the electrical activity of the cortex coincides with a severe depression of the brainstem with vegetative dysregulation (maximally wide pupils nonreactive to light). Contrary to halothane, an evoked response cannot be elicited during deep isoflurane anesthesia using the somatosensory modality (Peterson et al. 1986). We therefore applied the EAEP, which confirmed the dysregulation of the brainstem by showing delayed midbrain components (wave V).

Newberg and Michenfelder (1983) observed a cerebroprotective effect of isoflurane under hypoxaemic and ischaemic conditions. One reason may be the suppression of mainly cortical structures, which was shown by our EEG maps, and only a slight involvement (Schmidt and Chraemmer-Jorgensen 1986) of the brainstem, where EAEP exhibited a latency delay of midbrain structures but no decay of the waves originating in medullary or pontine brainstem areas.

One reason for the possible antidepressive effect of isoflurane narcosis may be the above-described pathophysiological mechanism. We cannot, however, profitably discuss the supposed psychotropic effect of isoflurane narcotherapy before comparative studies with ECT have been performed. Another benefit of the study is the knowledge of the topography of the electrical activity of the brain under various concentrations of isoflurane. The data may be useful for EEG monitoring under isoflurane anesthesia during surgery, especially in conditions where cerebral blood flow is decreased (carotid surgery).

References

Eger E (1981) Isoflurane: a review. Anesthesiology 55:559–576
Langer G, Neumark J, Koining G, Graf M, Schönbeck G (1985) Rapid psychotherapeutic effects with isoflurane (ES narcotherapy) in treatment-refactory depressed patients. Neuropsychobiology 14:118–120
Newberg L, Michenfelder J (1983) Cerebral protection by isoflurane during hypoxemia or ischemia. Anesthesiology 59:29–35
Peterson D, Drummond J, Todd M (1986) Effects of halothane and isoflurane on somatosensory evoked potentials in man. Anesthesiology 61:344–346
Pichlmayr I, Lips U, Künkel H (eds) (1983) Das Elektroencephalogramm in der Anästhesie. Springer, Berlin Heidelberg New York
Schmidt J, Chraemmer-Jorgensen B (1986) Auditory evoked potentials during isoflurane anaesthesia. Acta Anaesthesiol Scand 30:378–380

Flash Visual Evoked Potential Topographic Mapping: Normative and Clinical Data

E.J. Hammond[1], C.P. Barber[1], and B.J. Wilder[1, 2]

Introduction

Little is known about the neural sources of various components of the flash-evoked potential. Although the anatomy and physiology of human striate and peristriate cortex have been well studied, there is a paucity of information about visual projections to areas outside the occipital lobe (Von Essen 1979). Anatomical (Kuypers et al. 1965; Pandya and Kuypers 1969) and physiological (Bignall and Imbert 1969; Boyd et al. 1971) studies have indicated cortico-cortical connections from visual association areas to the parietal lobe, premotor cortex, prefrontal cortex and middle and inferior temporal gyri. Depth recordings in humans (Walter and Walter 1949; Brazier 1964) have shown visual evoked potentials in frontal and temporal regions. Little is known, however, about the functional relationship between these areas. Accordingly, we performed a prospective mapping study in a series of normal subjects and patients with focal cerebral lesions.

Methods

Recordings were made in a control group comprised of 40 neurologically normal subjects (ages 20–45 years, mean 30.1 years), mostly hospital staff. Patients ($n = 40$) with cerebral lesions verified by computed tomography were selected in a prospective manner. Lesions included infarction, tumor, arteriovenous malformation, encephalomalacia, and lobectomy. Patients gave informed consent.

The stimulus was a white stroboscopic xenon flash (Grass Intruments PS22, intensity setting of 1). All stimuli were presented binocularly. The audible click caused by the xenon flash was masked. Stimuli were presented with a variable repetition rate, interstimulus intervals ranging from 600 ms to 5 s. Stimuli were presented with the subjects' eyes open. All recordings were made on a 16-channel averager (Cadwell 8400). Amplifier bandpass was 1–100 Hz. At least two trials were run of each stimulus condition; 100 epochs comprised each averaged response. Electrodes were applied according to the international 10–20 system, and electrode impedances were maintained at less than 5 kΩ. Linked earlobes served as reference.

---

[1] Neurology and [2] Medical Research Services, Veterans Administration Medical Center, Gainesville, FL 32602, USA

Results

Normal Subjects

A topographically complex series of waves (Fig. 1) different from both the pattern reversal and red LED stimuli (see Hammond et al., this volume) was seen. Usually an anterior N12–15, P40–50, N45–50, N60–70 complex reflecting various components of the electroretinogram (Allison et al. 1977), followed by a series of waves with high intersubject variability, usually an N90–100, P160–180, and a broad negativity peaking at around 250–300 ms could be recorded. An occipital P80–100, N105–115, P180 complex and a central P80–100, N110, P180 are also prominent. Four subjects showed poorly defined "simplified" potentials. Figure 2 shows typical waveform variability across normal subjects.

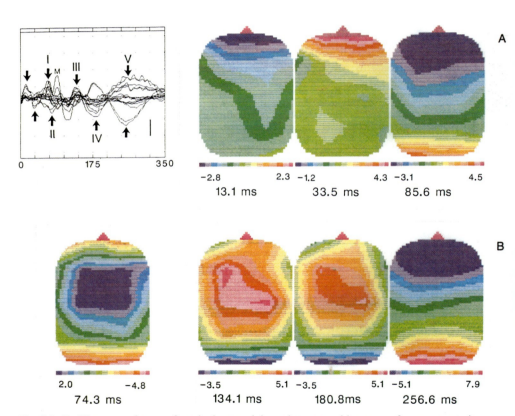

Fig. 1A, B. Time waveforms of evoked potentials and topographic maps of components in a normal subject. Roman numeral nomenclature follows classification of Ciganek (described in text); *first two arrows* signify electroretinogram a-wave and b-wave; M signifies an inconsistently recorded unilateral myogenic component. All stimuli were presented binocularly with full-field stimulation. In this and in all other figures, positivity is plotted *downward* in waveform plots and in *red* in topographic maps. Amplitude calibration, 5 µV

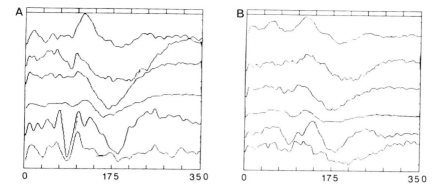

Fig. 2 A, B. Variability of white flash-evoked potentials in six normal subjects. Note variability in amplitude and latency across subjects for most components. **A** Occipital, **B** central white flash VEP

The Roman numeral nomenclature used by Ciganek (1961) and Kooi and Marshall (1979) is useful to describe these various components, although not all subjects have all components. Wave I appears as a widespread negative potential with a latency of 40–60 ms. The small amplitude of this component (around 3 µV) makes maps of its topographic distribution very susceptible to changes in the baseline. Wave II is an occipital-parietal surface positivity with a latency of 60–80 ms and an amplitude twice that of wave I. Wave III is an occipital-parietal temporal negativity at 80–120 ms. Wave IV is an occipital positive potential, latency 100–140 ms. Wave V is the largest component, latency 130–160 ms. It appears as a large negative component in the occipital and temporal regions. Wave VI, latency 160–220 ms, usually has a parietal maximum. Five components are recorded in a restricted frontal region. A large N140–200 seen in some subjects is probably the same as the "F wave" described by Kooi et al. (1968). A P130 seen in some subjects is probably myogenic in origin (Allison et al. 1977).

Effects of Intensity

Not all subjects are able to fixate on a xenon flash stimulus, as produced by a standard laboratory stimulator, without blinking. Normative data in the eyes closed condition is therefore imperative. Figure 3 shows the effects of changing stimulus intensity and also the effects of eye closure. It can be seen that suitable potentials can be recorded at a low intensity setting (with eyes open), but eye closure tends to abolish waves prior to 150 ms post-stimulus. Maximal intensity does little to bring out these early components if the eyes are closed and actually increases the latency of later components, presumably due to retinal saturation.

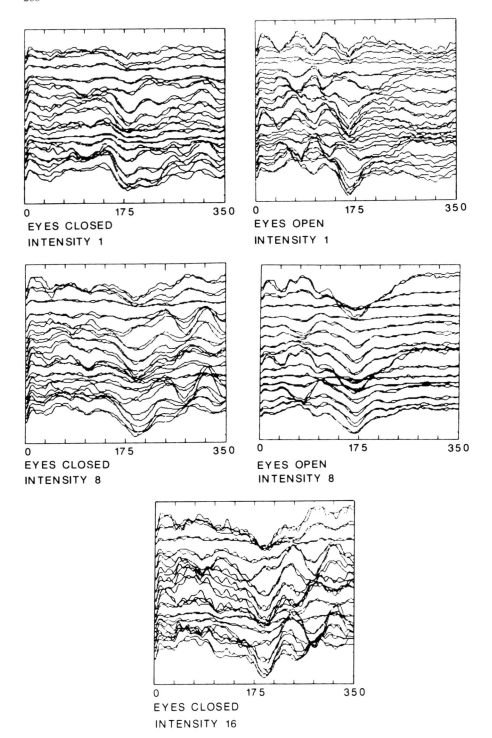

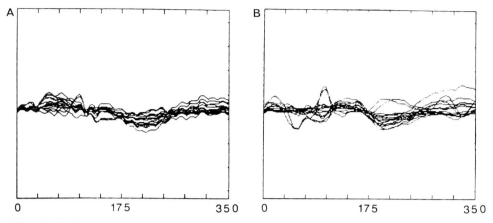

Fig. 4A, B. Comparison of chin reference with linked earlobe reference; 16-channel recording. **A** Chin ref., **B** linked earlobe ref.

Effects of Reference Electrode Location

We found the linked earlobe reference to be most suitable and reliable for routine clinical work. Figure 4 compares a chin reference with linked earlobes and it can be seen that the full complement of waves occurs only with the earlobe derivation. A neck reference proved noisy in several normal subjects and patients.

Patients

Patients generally showed the same number of components and scalp topography as normals. As discussed below, certain focal lesions could cause either a diminution or apparent enhancement in amplitude.

Discussion

Pattern reversal, red LED goggles and white xenon flash evoke potentials with differing waveforms and scalp distributions. The complex distribution of flash-evoked potentials suggests that many cortical regions will be susceptible to

◁──

Fig. 3. Evoked potential waveforms as a function of stimulus intensity in a normal subject. Closing the eyes has a significant effect on recording potentials of less than 150 ms latency. Electrode montage, from top to bottom: FP1, F7, T3, T5, O1, P3, C3, F3, FP2, F8, T4, T6, O2, P4, C4, F4

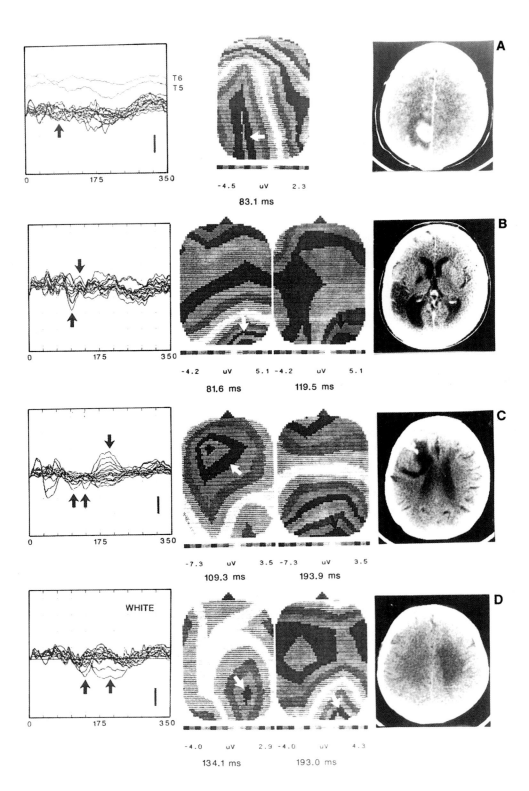

physiological analysis using visual evoked potential (VEP) topographic mapping.

Examination of typical waveforms of flash-evoked potentials shown in Fig. 2 shows considerable intersubject variability in time waveform that would indicate poor clinical applicability in comparison, for example, to pattern reversal stimulation, a stimulus with relatively low intersubject response variability. This would be the case for single-channel recording, but multiple-channel recording provides for assessment of hemispheric asymmetries within a given patient (see Fig. 5).

Clearly, a unilateral absence of a particular component (assuming equal stimulation of each eye with a full-field stimulus) is suggestive of a focal lesion. Kooi and Marshall (1979) reported amplitude asymmetries of up to 50% in normals. We have not seen consistent asymmetries this large in our healthy normal subjects, although such asymmetries might be encountered in a larger sample size.

The present results indicate that topographic mapping of VEPs can provide data on the location of lesions remote from the occipital area. All patients with occipital lesions showed at least one abnormal component; usually several (but not all) components evoked by either pattern reversal, red LED or white xenon flash stimulus were asymmetric. Two types of abnormalities were seen: one in which a component was depressed over the site of a cerebral lesion and one in which the component appeared to be enhanced (see Fig. 5). A similar enhancement was also noted in the extensive studies of Kooi and Marshall (1979). Although this might be due to some hyperexcitability of neurons, an alternative explanation might be that this is a paradoxical lateralization phenomenon (Blumhardt and Halliday 1979) whereby potentials are best recorded over the hemisphere contralateral to the actual generator site due to the orientation of a dipole source. Thus, a lesion affecting cells on the right would affect a potential recorded on the left. Normally functioning cells on the left would generate a normal potential on the right, thus giving the appearance of a paradoxical enhancement over the affected hemisphere. Whether or not this is the explanation for the paradoxical enhancement will require further study.

Particularly interesting is the complex topography of flash-evoked potentials and how certain components can be affected by central, temporal, premotor and prefrontal cerebral lesions. It is our impression, from our clinical material, that it is necessary for one or more of the occipital-temporal or occipital-frontal projection pathways to be affected in order to affect a non-occipital visual evoked potential. Further topographic mapping of VEPs in patients with discrete cortical lesions will be necessary to elucidate the functional neuroanatomy of the human visual system.

◁───

Fig. 5 A–D. Flash-evoked potential topograms, time waveforms, and computed tomography scans in patients with focal lesions. *Black arrows* on topograms signify negative components, *white arrows* signify positive components. **A** Forty-year-old man with falx meningioma; temporal component is enhanced over hemisphere with tumor. **B** Fifty-nine-year-old man with left temporal tumor: components ipsilateral to lesion are diminished. **C** Thirty-two-year-old woman with left frontal glioblastoma; frontal component is enhanced over lesion. **D** Fifty-year-old man with right parietal tumor

Acknowledgement. The authors are grateful to Janet Wootten and Anne Crawford for manuscript preparation.

References

Allison T, Matsumiya Y, Goff GD, Goff WR (1977) The scalp topography of human visual evoked potentials. Electroencephalogr Clin Neurophysiol 42:185–197

Bignall KE, Imbert M (1969) Polysensory and cortico-cortical projections to frontal lobe of squirrel and rhesus monkeys. Electroencephalogr Clin Neurophysiol 26:206–215

Blumhardt LD, Halliday AM (1979) Hemisphere contributions to the composition of the pattern evoked potential waveform. Exp Brain Res 36:59–69

Boyd EH, Pandya DN, Bignall KE (1971) Homotopic and nonhomotopic interhemispheric cortical projections in the squirrel monkey. Exp Neurol 32:256–274

Brazier MAB (1964) Evoked responses recorded from the depths of human brain. Ann NY Acad Sci 112:33–59

Ciganek L (1961) The EEG response (evoked potential) to light stimulus in man. Electroencephalogr Clin Neurophysiol 13:165–172

Kooi KA, Marshall RE (1979) Visual evoked potentials in central disorders of the visual system. Harper and Row, Cambridge, MA

Kooi KA, Shafii M, Richey ET (1968) Differentiation between visually evoked F and V potentials. Electroencephalogr Clin Neurophysiol 24:482–485

Kuypers HGJM, Szwarcbart MK, Mishkin M, Rosvold HE (1965) Occipitotemporal corticocortical connections in the rhesus monkey. Exp Neurol 11:245–262

Pandya DN, Kuypers HGJM (1969) Cortico-cortical connections in the rhesus monkey. Brain Res 13:13–36

Van Essen DC (1979) Visual areas of the mammalian cerebral cortex. Annu Rev Neurosci 2:227–263

Walter VJ, Walter WG (1949) The central effects of rhythmic sensory stimulation. Electroencephalogr Clin Neurophysiol 1:57–86

Event-Related Potentials in Patients with Brain Tumors and Traumatic Head Injuries

H.M. Olbrich[1], H.E. Nau[2], J. Fritze[1], and E. Lodemann[1]

Introduction

Research in cognitive psychophysiology has shown that event-related potentials (ERPs) reflect specific processes of human information processing (Gaillard and Ritter 1983). We have carried out ERP recording and neuropsychological testing in patients with brain tumors and traumatic head injuries in order to obtain some information about the neuroanatomical substrate of ERPs and about the utility of ERPs for the evaluation of cognitive impairment.

Methods

The findings reported here are based on three previous studies (Olbrich et al. 1986a, b, c) and were obtained from 21 patients with supratentorial brain tumors (mean age 55.8 years), 18 patients with severe head injuries (mean age 30.8 years) and two age-matched control groups. The trauma patients were tested during post-traumatic amnesia (PTA) and were retested after recovering from PTA. Auditory ERPs were recorded from F_z, C_z, P_z, C_3, C_4, T_3 and T_4 and the patients were administered five tests measuring cognitive functioning. A detailed description of patients and methods used is contained in our previous papers.

Findings and Discussion

Evoked potential waveforms from individual cases are shown in Figs. 1 and 2. Assuming that unilateral brain damage could be associated with unilateral loss of ERP generators resulting in reduction of component amplitudes predominantly over the lesioned hemisphere, ERP amplitudes from C_3 and C_4 electrode sites were compared with respect to the hemisphere affected in patients with unilateral cerebral involvement (Table 1). Statistical analysis revealed no significant group difference for N1, P2, or P3. This might, among various possible

---

[1] Psychiatrische Universitätsklinik, Hufelandstr. 55, 4300 Essen 1, Federal Republic of Germany
[2] Neurochirurgische Universitätsklinik, Hufelandstr. 55, 4300 Essen 1, Federal Republic of Germany

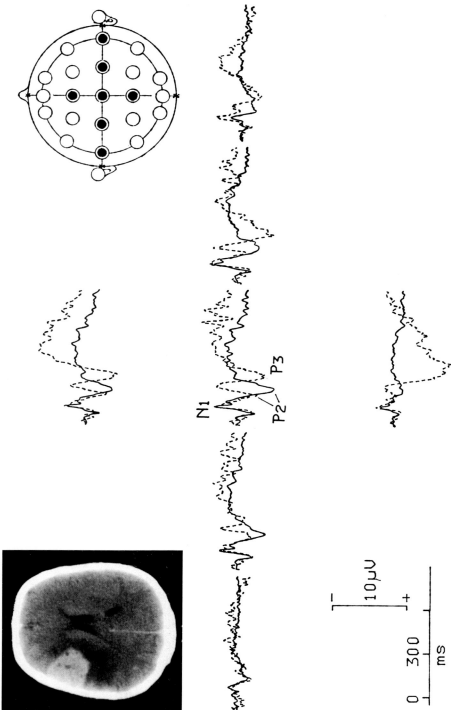

Fig. 1. Recordings from a patient with a left-sided meningioma, showing event-related responses to the frequent (——— 800 Hz) and rare (--- 1400 Hz) tones of an "oddball" detection paradigm. Note the marked decrease in P3 amplitude over the affected hemisphere. (From Olbrich et al. 1986c)

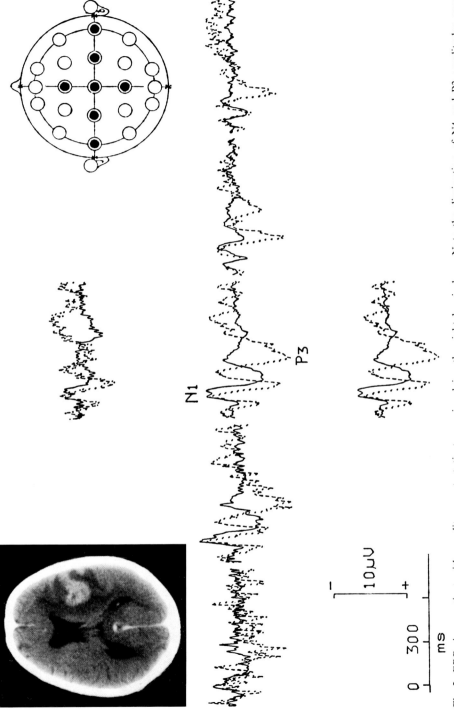

Fig. 2. ERPs in a patient with a solitary metastatic tumor involving the right hemisphere. Note the diminution of N1 and P3 amplitudes over the lesioned hemisphere compared to the contralateral side. (——— 800 Hz, --- 1400 Hz) (From Olbrich et al. 1986c)

Table 1. Amplitudes (µV) of event-related potentials over lesioned and intact hemisphere (mean, SD)

	Tumor group (n=15)		Trauma group (n=10)	
	Lesioned	Intact	Lesioned	Intact
N1	4.81 (2.02)	5.53 (1.97)	4.37 (2.49)	4.42 (1.68)
P2	3.01 (2.07)	3.44 (2.37)	2.46 (1.93)	2.63 (2.42)
P3	4.18 (3.90)	3.27 (3.23)	0.70 (2.74)	1.13 (4.30)

Table 2. Rates of tumor and trauma patients concordantly classified as normal or abnormal by P3 latency and psychological test scores (%)

	Mini mental state	Benton	Digit span	Retention of objects	D2 test	
					GZ	GZ-F
Tumor						
P3 latency	87	73	80	64	69	77
Trauma						
P3 latency at first test	87	87	47	77	40	60
P3 latency at second test	27	13	20	15	0	0

mechanisms, be caused by the fact that the tumors and focal brain injuries have sometimes not involved structures which contribute to the generation of the scalp-recorded ERPs and/or have caused remote effects on areas of the contralateral hemisphere where ERPs are generated or modulated. Like us, several other groups who performed ERP studies in patients with lesions of distinct brain regions have obtained no consistent results regarding the potential sources of ERP components (Wood et al. 1984).

For the tumor patients and trauma patients tested at early stages of injury the following results were obtained for N1, P2 (both evaluated from C_z waveform), P3 (from P_z waveform) and the psychometric variables. Both the tumor and the trauma group had significantly smaller N1 amplitudes, longer P3 latencies and, for all the cognitive measures used, significantly lower scores than the corresponding control group. In classifying individual patients as normal or abnormal in terms of P3 latency (abnormal: more than 2 SD above the mean of the control group) and psychological test scores (abnormal: more than 2 SD below the normal value) a strong concordance was found between P3 latency and the neuropsychological measures (Table 2, first two rows). P3 latency may provide a practical and useful measure of intellectual function in tumor and trauma patients, in whom neuropsychological testing is frequently limited due to handicaps of movement and linguistic skills.

For the trauma patients studied at follow-up no concordance between P3 latency and neuropsychological variables was found (Table 2), because psychometric measures had returned to normal values whereas P3 latency continued to be abnormally prolonged (383 ± 27.2 ms for the patient group compared with 323 ± 13.2 ms for the control group). The sensitivity of P3 latency in revealing subtle post-traumatic changes of brain function, as shown by these findings, may thus be clinically useful and deserves further research.

References

Gaillard AWK, Ritter W (eds) (1983) Tutorials in event related potential research: endogenous components. North-Holland, Amsterdam

Olbrich HM, Lanczos L, Lodemann E, Zerbin D, Engelmeier MP, Nau HE, Schmit-Neuerburg KP (1986a) Ereigniskorrelierte Hirnpotentiale und intellektuelle Beeinträchtigung – eine Untersuchung bei Patienten mit Hirntumor und Schädelhirntrauma. Fortschr Neurol Psychiatr 54:182–188

Olbrich HM, Nau HE, Lodemann E, Zerbin D, Schmit-Neuerburg KP (1986b) Evoked potential assessment of mental function during recovery from severe head injury. J Surg Neurol 26:112–118

Olbrich HM, Nau HE, Zerbin D, Lanczos L, Lodemann E, Engelmeier MP, Grote W (1986c) Clinical application of event related potentials in patients with brain tumours and traumatic head injuries. Acta Neurochirurgica 80:116–122

Wood CC, McCarthy G, Squires NK, Vaughan HG, Woods DL, McCallum WC (1984) Anatomical and physiological substrates of event-related potentials. Two case studies. Ann NY Acad Sci 425:681–721

Mapping of EEG in Patients with Intracranial Structural Lesions

H. Poimann[1], K. Maurer[2], and T. Dierks[2]

Introduction

Various imaging procedures help to elucidate abnormalities of brain structure and function. CT scan and NMR are excellent tools for studying anatomy, while PET scan and cerebral blood flow studies are two of the techniques capable of revealing brain function. Some of the latter methods suffer the disadvantage of being invasive. Thus, diagnosticians have turned again to the EEG, which has the advantage of being noninvasive and of analyzing functional states of short duration in the millisecond range. In 1979 Duffy et al. published the first report on clinical application of brain electrical activity mapping (BEAM). Since then there has been rapid growth in the literature on the use of the EEG mapping method for localization of brain lesions (Duffy et al. 1984; Nuwer 1986). In the present study we have examined the topographic distribution of EEG spectral energy in a group of patients with intracerebral tumors and malformations of different etiology.

Methods

EEG data were obtained from 19 electrodes placed on the scalp according to the 10–20 system. Spontaneous EEG was recorded in the resting condition with eyes closed. Special care was taken to minimize eye and muscle artifacts. For data collection the Brain Atlas III was used (Bio-logic Systems Corp.).

Raw EEG recordings were stored on magnetic disk for further off-line analysis. Twelve artifact-free 2-s epochs were chosen randomly from each EEG and transformed into frequency spectra using Fourier transforms. The values of the frequency spectra were then displayed on a computer monitor. The scalp areas around the original 19 electrodes were filled in by linear interpolation between the four nearest electrodes. Maps of the activity were constructed for eight frequency bands: delta (0–3.5 Hz), theta (4–7.5 Hz), alpha (8–11.5 Hz), $beta_1$ to $beta_5$ (12–31.5 Hz). Since cerebral lesions are characterized mainly by slow EEG activity, the main interest was focused on delta and theta activity.

For further evaluation, EEG topography and CT findings were compared.

---

[1] Department of Neurosurgery, University of Würzburg, Josef-Schneider-Straße 11, 8700 Würzburg, Federal Republic of Germany
[2] Department of Psychiatry, University of Würzburg, Füchsleinstr. 15, 8700 Würzburg, Federal Republic of Germany

Table 1. Demographics, diagnoses and results of CT and EEG mapping in 14 neurosurgical patients

Case	Age (years)	Sex	Diagnosis	Brain sectors (see Fig. 1)						
				1	2	3	4	5	6	
1.	25	M	Right frontoprecentral astrocytoma	+	+					EEG
				+	+					CT
2.	26	M	Left temporal hemangioma	+				+	+	EEG
								+	+	CT
3.	21	M	Epileptic seizures	+	+	+			+	EEG
										CT
4.	47	M	Bifrontal astrocytoma	+				+	+	EEG
				+				+	+	CT
5.	33	F	Right occipital ependymoma, left parietal tumor		+	+				EEG
					+	+		+		CT
6.	56	F	Right occipital metastasis		+	+				EEG
						+				CT
7.	23	F	Right epileptic focus	+	+	+			+	EEG
										CT
8.	57	F	Right frontotemporal glioblastoma	+	+					EEG
				+	+					CT
9.	64	F	Right frontal tumor	+	+					EEG
				+	+					CT
10.	48	F	Right occipital hemangioma	+	+	+				EEG
					+	+				CT
11.	22	F	Right cerebellar astrocytoma			+				EEG
						+	+			CT
12.	62	F	Right frontal falx meningioma	+	+				+	EEG
				+					+	CT
13.	64	F	Left frontolateral glioblastoma	+				+	+	EEG
				+				+	+	CT
14.	30	M	Left precentral astrocytoma					+	+	EEG
							+	+		CT

+, signs of brain lesion

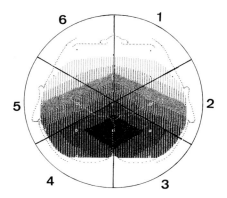

Fig. 1. Head format from above with the six brain sectors used in this study to achieve a statistical comparison between CT and EEG findings. Numbers correspond to the six brain sectors in Table 1.
(All figures in this contribution were prepared using equipment from Bio-logic Systems Corporation, Mundelein, IL, USA)

In order to apply an appropriate statistical procedure the scalp surface was divided into six sectors. Each hemisphere consisted of three sectors: a frontal sector, a central and temporal sector and a parietal and occipital sector (Fig. 1). Each sector was examined using CT and EEG mapping for change from normal conditions. The results of CT and EEG rating for the six sectors are shown in Table 1.

The sign test was used to check for statistically significant differences between CT findings and EEG maps in each sector in each of the 14 patients. Altogether, therefore, 84 sectors were evaluated.

Subjects

Sector evaluation of EEG maps and CT images was carried out in 14 unselected patients who sought treatment for previously diagnosed intracranial tumors, vascular malformation or epileptic seizures. Age, sex and diagnosis are shown in Table 1.

The patients were grouped according to CT and NMR as having:
A. Structural lesions in one region (patients 1, 2, 6, 8, 9, 10, 11, 14)
B. Multilocular structural lesions (patients 4, 5, 12, 13)
C. No structural lesion but functional disturbances (patients 3, 7).

Results

Group A

In the eight patients with one well-defined lesion in the CT, 44 of 48 brain sectors exhibited coincident CT and EEG mapping results. In the remaining four sectors the differences in topography were due to the EEG slowing covering a wider area than the circumscribed CT lesions. Two of the four sectors were

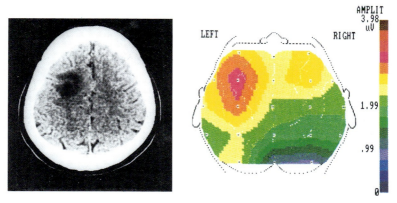

Fig. 2. Patient with a left precentral astrocytoma (case 14). *Left:* CT; *right:* EEG map with slow activity in the theta range (6 Hz), especially at point F3

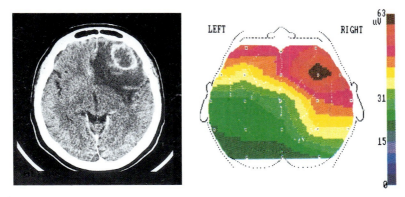

Fig. 3. Patient with a right frontotemporal glioblastoma (case 8). *Left:* CT; *right:* EEG map with slow activity in the delta band, especially at point F4

in patients with a vascular malfunction in the temporal and occipital area (cases 2, 10), and in these cases the EEG maps contained more information than the CT images.

Case Reports

Patient 14. A 30-year-old male showing no neurological deficit experienced an epileptic seizure beginning in the right arm. CT (Fig. 2) showed a hypodense zone over the left precentral area. The EEG map elucidated slow activity in the theta range in scalp area F3 corresponding to the hypodensity in the CT.

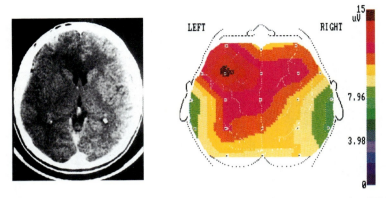

Fig. 4. Patient with a bifrontal astrocytoma (case 4). *Left:* CT; *right:* EEG map with slow activity in the theta band, especially at point F3

Patient 8. A 57-year-old female with a psychosyndrome developed an affective disorder and headaches. CT (Fig. 3) showed a right frontal glioblastoma with perifocal edema. The EEG maps verified the tumor and exhibited slow activity over the right frontal and temporal electrodes with a maximum at F4.

Group B

In the cases with multilocular lesions on CT (cases 4, 5, 12, 13), only two of 24 sectors exhibited significant differences between CT and EEG findings.

Case Report

Patient 4. A 47-year-old male with a previous history of seizures showed no neurological deficit. CT demonstrated a bifrontal astrocytoma. (WHO II) with growth predominantly on the left side (Fig. 4), while edema was observed with an accentuation in the right frontal lobe. The EEG map exhibited increased theta activity over the frontal lobes with a maximum over the F3 electrode.

Group C

Both patients without detectable structural damage on CT (cases 3, 7) had extensively altered and asymmetric EEG maps. These two patients with epileptic seizures underwent neurosurgery. These cases accounted for most of the inconsistencies between the structural and functional imaging methods.

Case Reports

Patient 3. A 21-year-old male had therapy-resistant focal seizures on the left side of the body. CT and angiography revealed no pathological findings. NMR

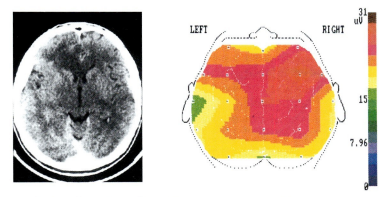

Fig. 5. Patient with epileptic seizures (case 7). CCT was normal, but EEG maps revealed a focus in the 2–4 Hz frequency band, especially at points F4 and F8

showed two areas with prolonged T1 and T2 relaxation times in the right precentral and sylvic region. EEG maps exhibited slow activity over the right hemisphere with an accentuation at cerebral points C4 and F4.

Patient 7. A 23-year-old female showed no neurological deficits. For 10 years she had been suffering from therapy-resistant seizures. CT and NMR were normal. Foramen ovale electrodes exhibited an epileptic focus in the right hippocampus. Conventional EEG showed no clear focal change in electrical activity. The EEG maps, however, revealed asymmetric activity in the theta range with a maximum at electrodes F4 and F8 over the right hemisphere (Fig. 5).

Discussion

Over 40% of intracranial tumors are still not diagnosed correctly, and it is often a relatively long time before patients are given adequate treatment (Diemath 1987). There is no doubt that EEG may be of dubious value or even unnecessary when CT or NMR scan already show a clear focal defect. Compared to routine EEG, however, topographic mapping of EEG provides information which is clinically more useful and is even able to localize tumors in cases where CT is not available.

All cases in this study showed slowing of EEG activity in the theta and delta band in the lesioned areas. The EEG maps exactly delineated regions of damaged cerebral activity. In 12 of 14 cases the findings of EEG mapping coincided with those of CT and NMR. In two patients (cases 3, 7), however, the topographic display of EEG data was superior to CT and NMR. These two patients had clinical seizures and no signs of structural damage on CT and NMR. Thus in some cases EEG mapping seems to be more sensitive to slight intracerebral damage than CT, NMR or even other functional test procedures such as PET and SPECT. Of special interest was the detection on EEG mapping of subtle structural changes depicted later or not at all by CT. This was the case in patient 5, where signs of an additional left parietal tumor were found on CT 2 months after the EEG had indicated a right occipital damage.

In summary our study demonstrated that EEG mapping is a valuable first diagnostic step, yielding topographic information of intracerebral damage. Its advantages over the imaging methods are noninvasiveness and extremely short analysis times, in the order of several milliseconds. This allows the topographic display of very short events, such as signs of an epileptiform activity like sharp waves and even spikes. This ability to detect spikes guarantees the superiority of EEG mapping over other imaging methods.

References

Diemath HP (1987) Gefahren unterlassener diagnostischer Maßnahmen. Gesamtverband Deutscher Nervenärzte 1987

Duffy FH, Albert MS, McAnulty G (1984) Brain electrical activity mapping in patients with presenile and senile dementia of the Alzheimer-type. Ann Neurol 16:439–448

Nuwer MR (1986) Identification of focal lesions in epileptics by computerized electroencephalogram and evoked potential. Ann Neurol 18:155–162

Topographic Brain Mapping and Neuroendocrine Parameters in a Patient with Addison's Disease and a Depressive Syndrome Before and After Treatment with Hydrocortisone

R. Rupprecht[1], T. Dierks[1], G. Reifschneider[1], F.v. Baumgarten[1], K. Maurer[1], and J. Pichl[2]

Introduction

Electroencephalographic alpha activity is reported to be reduced in Addison's disease (Christian 1982; Gibbs and Gibbs 1964). Investigations of the influence of adrenocorticotrophin (ACTH) and hydrocortisone on electroencephalographic activity have yielded conflicting results: some authors found an increase, others a decrease of alpha activity (Krump 1956; Thiébaut et al. 1958).

Patient and Methods

Patient

In order to determine the effect of parenteral application of 100 mg hydrocortisone on topographic brain mapping (BM) of EEG, a 73-year-old male patient with Addison's disease and a depressive syndrome (major depressive disorder with melancholia) was studied. Two metabolic crises had already occurred, and thus cortisol was substituted 25-15-5 mg daily in order to prevent further endocrinological crises.

Methods

We performed topographic brain mapping of EEG at 8 am the day before and at 8 am an hour after parenteral administration of 100 mg hydrocortisone at 7 am.

The EEG was recorded with an 18-channel Brain Atlas III machine (Biologic Systems Corp.). The electrodes were placed according to the 10–20 system. Linked mastoids were used as references. Eight 2000-ms samples were randomly selected from each EEG recording and checked for artifacts. Only the 0–31.5 Hz segment was analyzed, and a mean of each recording was calculated.

---

[1] Department of Psychiatry, University of Würzburg, Füchsleinstr. 15, 8700 Würzburg, Federal Republic of Germany
[2] Department of Internal Medicine, University of Erlangen, 8520 Erlangen, Federal Republic of Germany

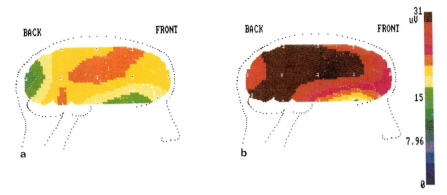

Fig. 1a, b. EEG maps of activity of alpha band (8–11.5 Hz) in right hemisphere. **a** At 8 am before hydrocortisone infusion. **b** At 8 am after hydrocortisone infusion. (Prepared using equipment from Bio-logic Systems Corporation, Mundelein, IL, USA)

Additionally, blood samples for determination of cortisol, prolactin and growth hormone were drawn at 8 am and 4 pm before and after hydrocortisone infusion, and Hamilton scores were obtained at 11 am.

Results

Comparison of the means showed an increase in alpha activity after infusion of hydrocortisone, with a maximum over the right hemisphere (Fig. 1) in connection with a strong rise of plasma cortisol an hour after hydrocortisone administration (Fig. 2). In the afternoon, however, the cortisol value was within the normal range. Prolactin showed a marked diurnal rhythm: the morning level after hydrocortisone infusion was lower than the day before. Hydrocortisone administration affected neither growth hormone levels nor severity of depression. The Hamilton score decreased only from 34 to 30 points.

Discussion

A rise in plasma cortisol was accompanied by an increase in alpha rhythm, supporting previous reports of reduced alpha activity in Addison's disease which might be due to hypoglycemic states (Christian 1982; Gibbs and Gibbs 1964). Among conflicting results concerning the effect of hydrocortisone on EEG activity (Krump 1956; Thiébaut et al. 1958), our results point to a regional stabilization of alpha activity in connection with a rise in cortisol but a decrease in prolactin levels.

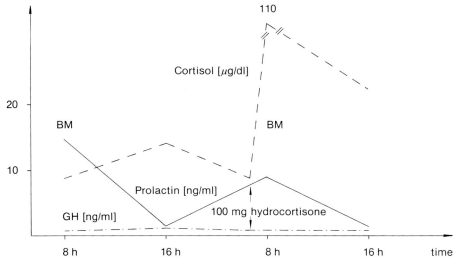

Fig. 2. Cortisol, prolactin and growth hormone (*GH*) levels before and after hydrocortisone infusion

References

Christian W (1982) Klinische Elektroenzephalographie. Thieme, Stuttgart
Gibbs FA, Gibbs EL (1964) Neurological and psychiatric disorders. Addison-Wesley, Reading, Mass. (Atlas of electroencephalography, vol 3)
Krump JE (1956) Die klinische Bedeutung des EEG bei Vergiftungen, Endotoxikosen und Endokrinopathien. VEB Verlag Volk und Gesundheit, Berlin
Thiébaut F, Rohmer F, Wackenheim A (1958) Contribution à l'étude electroencéphalographique des syndroms endocriniens. Electroenceph Clin Neurophysiol 10:1

Dexfenfluramine Profile in Quantitative EEG and Its Topographical Aspects

C. SEBBAN[1], K. LE ROCH[1], G. BENKEMOUN[1], C. DEBOUZY[1], and P. BAUD[2]

Introduction

Dexfenfluramine chlorhydrate (Isomeride) is a drug used for the treatment of obesity (Finer et al. 1985; Enzi et al. 1986). This compound reduces disorders of eating behavior, with a specific effect on diet selection, carbohydrate-rich meals being decreased while protein consumption is unaffected (Wurtman et al. 1985). Such a shift in diet selection can be produced experimentally by hypothalamic injection of serotonin (5-HT) (Blundell 1984; Leibowitz 1985). Dexfenfluramine is an indirect agonist of 5-HT, increasing its release and inhibiting its reuptake (Garattini et al. 1985). 5-HT terminals are widely distributed in the cerebral cortex, so dexfenfluramine could act on large brain areas. Such a general action can be studied by quantitative EEG (Q-EEG) and its brain mapping. The aim of this study is to describe the EEG variations induced by three different doses of dexfenfluramine in healthy young subjects.

Methods

Subjects

Three groups of nine subjects each were selected for this study. All were male, students, nonobese and proven healthy in an initial clinical, psychometric and neurological examination. Their mean age was 22 ± 2 years (range 19–26 years). None of the included subjects smoked or were caffeine abusers, and they had taken no medication for at least 3 months. All the subjects were informed about the purpose and the timing of the study and gave their written informed consent.

Treatment

The Q-EEG variations induced by 15, 30 and 60 mg of dexfenfluramine in single oral administrations were studied in three groups of selected subjects.

---

[1] Hôpital Charles Foix, Explorations Fonctionnelles, 7, Avenue de la République, 94205 Ivry/Seine, France
[2] Hôpital Henry Dunant, Red Cross Pain Center, 95, rue Michel Ange, 75016 Paris, France

Experimental Design

For each dosage, this was a double-blind cross-over study. Each subject was randomized to receive either dexfenfluramine or placebo, followed by the other after a 1-week washout period.

Each subject arrived at the laboratory at noon and a standardized meal was eaten. The EEG electrodes were placed at 12.30 p.m., after which the subject rested until 1 p.m. At 1 p.m. and 1.45 p.m. two EEG recordings were performed (baseline recordings). Treatment (dexfenfluramine or placebo) was taken at 2 p.m., then EEG recordings were monitored at hourly intervals until 8 p.m. (i.e. 1, 2, 3, 4, 5 and 6 h after treatment).

EEG Recordings

EEG signals were collected by scalp electrodes. The recordings were realized with the patient's eyes open and their total duration was 4 min.

After amplification and anti-aliasing filtering (32 Hz, 90 dB/octave), the 16 signals were digitized and submitted to a fast Fourier transform computed in real time from 1 to 30 Hz (Cartovar 2000, Alvar Electronic, France).

Data Analysis

For each subject and recording session, an average power spectrum was calculated for six scalp areas (prerolandic, rolandic, temporal, parietal, occipital, sagittal). The variations of these power spectra at each time after drug administration was then calculated relative to the predrug power spectra. This was done by dividing the power at each time after treatment by the power before administration. These ratios were calculated for each frequency component, scalp area and subject and were submitted to an analysis of variance (ANOVA). The Q-EEG profile of dexfenfluramine was determined for each time, scalp area and subject by the differences in time-related variations after drug and after placebo administration (drug effect minus placebo effect).

Results

EEG Profile of Dexfenfluramine

The average EEG profiles observed 6 h after treatment for the three dosages are shown in Fig. 1. These profiles are averages for all the scalp areas. At a low dose (15 mg), dexfenfluramine induces a decrease of low-frequency power, especially concerning the theta band and the slow alpha band. At 30 mg, the effect on low-frequency components intensifies, and the decrease in the 7.5–13 Hz range is larger. Moreover, an increase of power appears for the fast components – such an effect not being visible with 15 mg. At 60 mg, all the

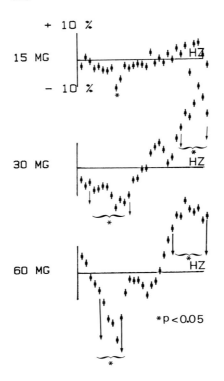

Fig. 1. Mean Q-EEG profile for the ensemble of all scalp areas for the three dosages. Each profile was determined by the difference in time-related variations after drug and after placebo administration (drug effect minus placebo effect). This difference was calculated for each Hz from 1 to 30 Hz. Each profile was averaged for the nine subjects tested at each dosage

effects accentuate considerably. The most important effect is the increase of beta components, which is more marked than with 30 mg.

Topographical Aspects of Q-EEG: Effects of Dexfenfluramine

For all the post-placebo recordings and for each dosage, an inter-subject average brain map of power variations was drawn for the 3.5–7 Hz, 7.5–10 Hz and 18–28 Hz components.

Figure 2 shows such maps for the 6th h after treatment administration for the 3.5–7 Hz components. With placebo, there was nearly no modification, the mean ratio 6th h/pretreatment being near to 1. With 15 mg, there was only a slight decrease of power in temporofrontal regions. With 30 mg, and even more markedly with 60 mg, the power decrease for these frequency components was more pronounced, essentially in central areas. These scalp-related differences were highly significant, as indicated by the ANOVA.

As can be seen in Fig. 3, the same phenomenon was observed for the frequency components from 7.5 to 13 Hz. The decrease of power with dexfenfluramine was dose-dependent and homogeneous on the scalp, except for the posterior sagittal lead where the decrease was significantly more important at 30 and 60 mg.

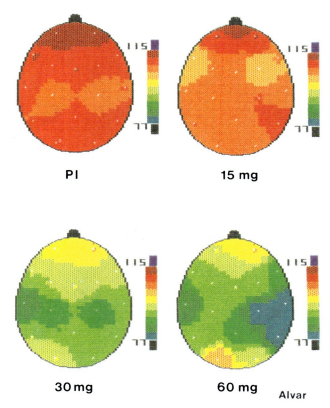

Fig. 2. Topographic brain mapping of power variations for the 3.0–7.5 Hz band 6 h after dexfenfluramine administration (15-30-60 mg). No variation is represented by the 100 value on the scale. The correspondence between value and color is linear. *Top left:* the power variations in 27 subjects in the placebo session

Figure 4 illustrates the effects on the 18–28 Hz components. Dexfenfluramine induced an increase of these power components which was highly specific in its distribution, limited to temporal regions. Again, these scalp differences were highly significant.

Time-Related Evolution of the Dexfenfluramine Effects on EEG Maps

Figure 5 shows an example of the evolution of the EEG effects of 60 mg dexfenfluramine according to time, for the frequency components from 18 to 28 Hz. The temporal increase of power clearly appeared 3 h after drug administration and was more pronounced at 4, 5 and 6 h afterwards.

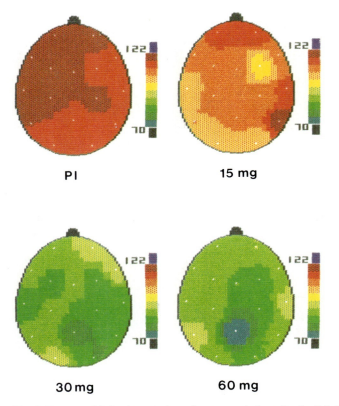

Fig. 3. Topographic brain mapping of power variations for the 7.5–10 Hz band 6 h after dexfenfluramine administration (15-30-60 mg). No variation is represented by the 100 value on the scale. The correspondence between value and color is linear. *Top left:* the power variations in 27 subjects in the placebo session

Discussion

The EEG profile of dexfenfluramine 6 h after drug administration is characterized by a decrease of theta and slow alpha powers and an increase of beta power. There was a high reliability of these power variations, as shown by the results observed for the three dosages, each studied in nine different subjects. Moreover, there was a clear increase of the power variations with increased dosage.

These effect are in keeping with the results of previous work by Fink et al. (1971). Using baseline cross-frequency band, the showed that fenfluramine (40 mg), the racemic compound, was characterized by increased beta activity and decreased delta activity. However, in healthy volunteers, administration of the 5-HT agonists fluoxetine (Saletu and Grünberger 1985), fluvoxamine

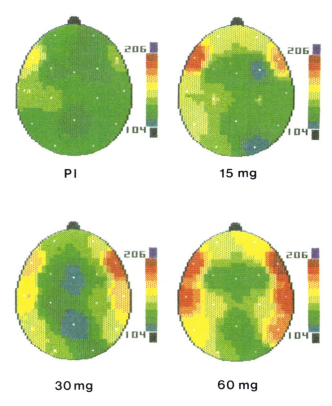

Fig. 4. Topographic brain mapping of power variations for the 18–28 Hz band 6 h after dexfenfluramine administration (15-30-60 mg). No variation is represented by the 100 value on the scale. The correspondence between value and color is linear. *Top left:* the power variations in 27 subjects in the placebo session

(Saletu et al. 1980) and zimelidine (Saletu et al. 1986) is associated with an increased alpha power and a decreased beta relative power. Such a profile is termed "desimipramine type." These results are not in accordance with our observations. Such discrepancies could have several explanations:

1. Fluoxetine, fluvoxamine and zimelidine act only as inhibitors of 5-HT reuptake with no effect on 5-HT release, whereas dexfenfluramine also enhances 5-HT release. This difference in neurochemical mechanism could account for the differences in EEG profile. In this regard, it could be interesting to compare the dexfenfluramine profile with that of a 5-HT direct agonist.
2. Previous reports on the EEG profiles of drugs inhibiting 5-HT reuptake describe the profiles using standard frequency bands. This could cancel out opposite power variations for different parts of these bands. This was illustrated in our study by the opposite variations observed for slow and fast alpha components.

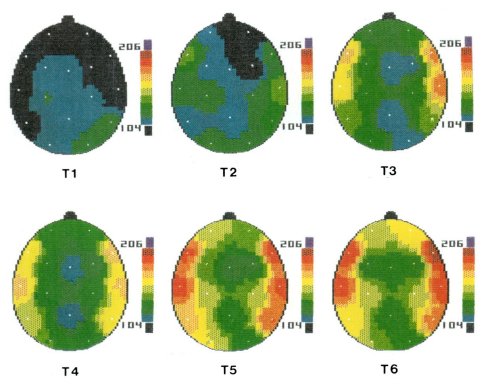

Fig. 5. Power variations from 1 to 6 h after drug administration for the 18–28 Hz components after 60 mg dexfenfluramine. *T1–T6*, 1, 2, 3, 4, 5 and 6 h after drug administration

3. Previous studies (Saletu et al. 1980, 1985, 1986) used bipolar leads, generally between occipital and vertex electrodes. In this condition, it may be possible that an unequal power decrease for the two locations will appear in the power spectrum of the bipolar lead as an increased power. Topographic brain mapping of dexfenfluramine EEG effects suggests that this could be the case. Indeed, for 7.5–10 Hz components, the power decrease was highly significant in all scalp areas but significantly higher in the posterior sagittal lead (i.e., near Cz).

The main interest of the brain mapping of EEG variations with dexfenfluramine appeared for the 18–28 Hz components. For the 15-mg dose, Fig. 4 shows some evidence of a topographic power increase, despite the lack of significant variations for the ensemble of scalp areas (Fig. 1). This was confirmed by a significant area × treatment ANOVA interaction. Moreover, the time-related variations of the power variations for the 18–28 Hz components were evident on brain mapping (Fig. 5). They are correlated with dexfenfluramine pharmacokinetics (Rowland and Carlton 1986).

Topographic brain mapping appears to be a useful tool for determining the CNS specificity of related pharmacological compounds.

References

Blundell JE (1984) Serotonin and appetite. Neuropharmacology 23:1537–1551

Enzi G, Crepaldi G et al. (1986) Efficacy and safety of dextrofenfluramine in obese patients: a multicenter study. 15th CLINP Congress, Puerto Rico, 14–17 Dec 1986

Finer N, Craddock D, Lavielle R, Keen H (1985) Dextrofenfluramine in the treatment of refractory obesity. Curr Ther Res 38:847–854

Fink M, Shapiro DM, Itil T (1971) EEG profiles of fenfluramine, amoborbitol nd dextroamphetamine in normal volunteers. Psychopharmacologia 22:369–383

Garattini S, Mennini T, Bendotti C, Invernizzi R, Samanin R (1985) Neurochemical mechanism of action of drugs which modify feedings via the serotoninergic system. Appetite 2 (Suppl):15–38

Leibowitz SF, Shor-Posner E (1986) Hypothalmic serotonin in control of eating behavior. In: Ferrari F, Brambilla F (eds) Disorders of eating behavior. Pergamon, Oxford, pp 343–352

Rowland NE, Carlton J (1986) Neurobiology of an anorectic drug: fenfluramine. Prog Neurobiol 27:13–62

Saletu B, Grünberger J (1985) Classification and determination of cerebral bioavailability of fluoxetine: pharmacokinetic, pharmaco-EEG and psychometric analysis. J Clin Psychiatry 46(3):45–52

Saletu B, Grünberger J, Rajna P., Karobath M (1980) Cloroxamine and fluvoxamine-2 biogenic amine re-uptake inhibiting anti-depressants. Quantitative EEG, psychometric and pharmacokinetic studies in man. J Neural Transm 49:63–86

Saletu B, Grünberger J, Linzmayer L (1986) On central effects of serotonin re-uptake inhibitors: quantitative EEG and psychometric studies with sectroline and zimelidine. J Neural Transm 67:241–266

Wurtman J, Wurtman R, Mark S, Tsay R, Gilbert W, Growden J (1985) D-Fenfluramine selectively suppresses carbohydrate snacking by obese subjects. Int J Eating Disorders 4:89–99

Synchrony (Measured by Cross-Correlation) in Children with Cognitive Impairments

G. SPIEL[1,2], F. BENNINGER[2], and M. FEUCHT[2]

Introduction

Neuropsychiatrists specializing in children's disturbances are often confronted with the problem of differential diagnosis in the field of performance disorders concerning schoolchildren. At present there is no accepted system of diseases or syndromes in this field. Various descriptions of syndromes have been published. In principle, from a clinical point of view, a distinction is made between the hyperkinetic-inattention syndrome and the group of specific learning disabilities, e.g. dyslexia. Various synonyms and partly overlapping terms, such as minimal brain damage (MBD) and minimal cerebral dysfunction (MCD), are used to denote children with disorders in conduct and performance. As far as the hyperkinetic-inattention syndrome is concerned, guidelines are given in ICD-9 (WHO 1978) and in DSM-III (Spitzer et al. 1982). Relevant symptoms are hyperactivity, inattention, distractability, lack of concentration, irritability, and low frustration threshold. These are often the underlying reasons for problems in school and abnormal social relations (e.g., Steinhausen 1985); however, there are also a large number of children whose learning disabilities are not observed in conjunction with hyperkinesis.

In 1932, Berger observed a reduction in amplitude and frequency of alpha rhythm among severely retarded children (Gloor 1969). Later, Kreezer (1939) did not find the usual correlation between mental age and the alpha index in retarded non-Down's syndrome subjects, compared with a group of Down's syndrome patients. In the intervening years many studies have been carried out under the hypothesis that there are correlations between mental abilities and alpha activity. Often, not only clinical estimation of the degree of retarded mental functions, but also intelligence tests were used, in particular the Wechsler Intelligence Scale for Children (WISC). Regarding mental abilities, two approaches can be distinguished: on the one hand, disease entity studies, and on the other, studies comparing EEG parameters with achievement tests, especially scores of intelligence tests.

There is not doubt that a variety of information about CNS functions can be detected in the EEG, and that different components and parameters of the EEG are more or less relevant for studying possible relations between the neurophysiological data and the degree of various cognitive abilities.

Since Binet's empirical approach towards the phenomenon of intelligence

---

[1] Neurologische Universitätsklinik Wien, Lazarettgasse 14, 1090 Wien, Austria
[2] Universitätsklinik für Neuropsychiatrie des Kindes- und Jugendalters, Währinger Gürtel 18–20, 1090 Wien, Austria

(Binet and Simon 1908), discussions on this topic revolve around the question of whether intelligence is one general dimension (Spearman 1927), or whether it has an inherent structure, possibly of hierarchical nature (beginning with Thurston in 1938).

From the point of view of neurology, which concerns itself with localized brain activity and not only with mass actions, the ideas of Vernon (1960) and Thomson (1939) are of special significance. Vernon's concept differentiated a group of intelligence factors called "verbal-educational" from a "practical-mechanical" factor. More generally, Thomson suggested that intellectual function could be thought of as a group of many single capabilities in various degrees of association with each other.

Factor analysis is an instrument to obtain information about the dependencies in a given data structure. This multivariate statistical analysis was often used regarding intelligence measurements. The results obtained with this factor-analytic approach have been instrumental in shaping theories on the concept "intelligence." The most popular intelligence measures used for children between the ages of 7 and 10 years are the Hamburg-Wechsler Intelligence Scales for Children (HAWIK) – quite similar to WISC – which provide a global intelligence score and also scores from ten subtests. These measures are not independent. With factor analysis, Schubert and Berlach (1982) showed that the subtests can be grouped according to two factors. This study was done on a group clinically comparable to yet diagnostically different from our sample. Schubert and Berlach extracted two factors. The subtest "*Allgemeines Wissen*" (AW; "Information" in the WISC) loaded maximally in factor 1, which is best determined by subtests where verbal abilities are necessary. The subtest "*Figuren Legen*" (FL; Object assembly" in the WISC), on the other hand, loaded maximally in factor 2, which resembles intelligence measurements without obvious language involvement and where constructive processes are often dependent on the analysis of spatial relations.

This study deals with the question of performance disorders concerning children of public school age who are grouped according to test results in the HAWIK intelligence scale, especially regarding the subtests AW and FL. Do these children show specific differences in patterns of coherence in the resting EEG between various topological areas?

Subjects

The sample consisted of 51 children aged 7–10 years, primarily heterogeneous with respect to diagnosis, who were referred because of learning disabilities and performance disorders. The diagnosis showed a severe hyperactive-inattention syndrome in five of them, while the others complained of specific or general learning disorders. All the children's parents were thoroughly interviewed. Both the neurosocial and psychiatric examinations of the children were carried out by the same physician. To check intelligence, the HAWIK was administered. The following diagnoses led to exclusion from the sample: IQ less than 95, manifest cerebral kinetic disorders, perception disorders, epilepsy. In no case had drugs been administered to the children; especially no CNS-stimulating drugs.

Design of Study, Method of EEG Analysis

Covariance is a measure used to detect the similarity of two signals, but it is also dependent on the respective amplitudes of the signals. Thus, two signals can have a large covariance either because they are similar or simply because they both have large amplitudes. To make the covariance independent of the signal amplitudes it is divided by the square root of the product of the variance of each of the two signals. This normalized covariance becomes the correlation coefficient. If the two signals are of identical patterns the correlation coefficient is $+1$, even though the signals may be of different amplitudes. If the signals are identical but of opposite polarity, the correlation coefficient is -1. Any other degree of similarity will fall between $+1$ and -1. In the case of unsystematic linear relations between two signals, a correlation coefficient near 0 can be expected.

With the correlation coefficient the similarity between two EEG epochs can be determined. By stepwise shift of one of the signals at regular intervals along the time axis (lag), correlation analyses can be calculated between this leading displaced signal and the other original one lagging behind. The relation between them ascertained in this way – calculating correlation coefficients and measuring the increase in time delay – is expressed in the correlation function. With this strategy can be distinguished not only the maximum possible similarity between two EEG epochs, but also the time delay – number of lags – between them.

The EEG data (routine examination, approximately 30 min, patient awake with eyes closed, 10/20 system, bipolar derivation, Beckmann Accu-trace 16, low-frequency filter 0.3 s, high-frequency filter 70 Hz) are digitalized every 8 ms and stored on magnetic tape to be analyzed off line (HP1000 computer system, 2250 M&C processing system, 7912 disk, 7945 disk, 7970b digital tape unit, 2631 printer, 2645 terminal, 2623 terminal, 9278 plotter).

Twenty-four samples of 2-s epochs, visually artifact-free in longitudinal EEG derivation, were taken for further analysis with these cross-correlation techniques (see above).

Each derivation was analyzed in comparison with all others with respect to their similarity. Altogether, 120 comparisons were calculated. The mean value of the 24 correlation coefficients regarding each comparison between two channels was taken as the measure of similarity.

The population was grouped according to performance level in the HAWIK subtests AW (information) and FL (object assembly) (group 1: 1–9; group 2: 10–11; group 3: 12–13; group 4: ≥ 14). Possible relationships between performance level and correlation coefficient were tested using analysis of variance.

Synchrony (Measured by Cross-Correlation) in Children with Cognitive Impairments 299

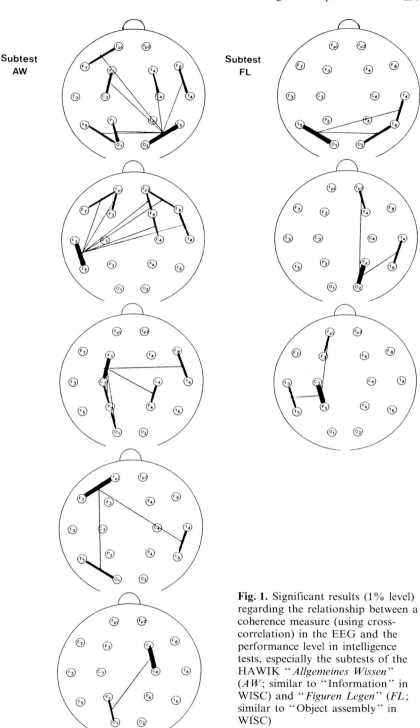

Fig. 1. Significant results (1% level) regarding the relationship between a coherence measure (using cross-correlation) in the EEG and the performance level in intelligence tests, especially the subtests of the HAWIK "*Allgemeines Wissen*" (*AW*; similar to "Information" in WISC) and "*Figuren Legen*" (*FL*; similar to "Object assembly" in WISC)

Results

Only those results reaching the $p<0.01$ level regarding the relation between the synchrony in different derivations and the performance level in the subtests AW and FL of the HAWIK intelligence scale will be discussed (see Table 1).

There are generally more coherence patterns if the relations to the scores in AW are examined (five types regarding AW; three regarding FL). The coherence patterns regarding AW show intra- and interhemispheric relations in four cases and only interhemispheric relations only in one. On the other hand regarding FL only one pattern shows an interhemispheric relation, the other two are strictly intrahemispheric.

It is of some interest that three coherence patterns regarding AW show relations between left hemispheric bipolar derivations and others of the ipsi- and contralateral side. Only one pattern shows a relation between the derivation occipitotemporal on the right side and various other derivations. In interpreting this result, the particular kind of relations have to be taken into consideration individually. The result obtained between F4-C4/P3-O1 does not lend itself to easy interpretation.

Taking the FL scores as criterion, one strictly right hemispheric relationship can be found.

In essence, linear relations of a positive nature are observed. Only the relation between the coherence measure intrahemispheric on the right side of the brain and performance in FL shows negative dependencies, and one pattern of an unsystematic relationship.

Non-linear relations with both criteria can be shown between the occipitoparietal, occipitotemporal and temporal regions if both the coherence and performance measures have undercut the $p<0.1$ level.

References

Binet A, Simon T (1908) Le developpement de l'intelligence chez les enfants. Ann Psychol 14:1–94

Gloor P (1969) Hans Berger on the electroencephalogram of man. Electroencephalogr Clin Neurophysiol 28:649

Kreezer G (1939) Intelligence level and occipital alpha rhythm in the mongolian type of mental deficiency. Am J Psychol 52:503–532

Schubert MT, Berlach G (1982) Neue Richtlinien zur Integration des Hamburg-Wechsler-Intelligenztests für Kinder (HAWIK). Z Klin Psychol Psychopathol Psychother 11:253–279

Spearman C (1927) The abilities of man. McMillan, London

Spitzer R (ed) (1982) Diagnostic and Statistical Manual of Mental Disorders, 3rd edn. Am Psychiatr Assoc, Washington

Steinhausen B (1985) Das hyperaktiv aufmerksamkeitsgestörte Kind. Kohlmann, Bad Lauterberg

Thomson GH (1939) The factorial analysis of human ability. University of London Press

Thurston L (1938) Primary mental abilities. University of Chicago Press

Vernon P (1960) Intelligence and attainment tests. University of London Press

World Health Organization (1978) ICD 9th Revision: mental disorders. Glossary and guide to their classification in accordance with 9th revision of the international classification of disease. WHO, Geneva

Section IV Psychophysiological Aspects

Cortical Activation Pattern During Reading and Recognition of Words Studied with Dynamic Event-Related Desynchronization Mapping*

G. Pfurtscheller[1] and W. Klimesch[2]

Introduction

It has been known since the publication of work by Berger (1933), Jasper and Andrews (1938) and Jasper and Penfield (1949) that in conscious human subjects sensory perception or motor behavior results in a localized and transient blocking of rhythmic alpha and/or beta band activity. Voluntary movement serves for blocking the central intrinsic rhythm in a manner similar to the blocking of the occipital alpha rhythm with visual stimulation or opening of the eyes. The blocking occurs before the actual initiation of a movement and thus seems to be closely related to the mechanism of attention or readiness to respond and associated with preparation for movement (Chatrian et al. 1959). Event-related blocking of alpha rhythm during visual stimulation is maximal over occipital regions (Grünewald et al. 1980; Pfurtscheller and Aranibar 1978).

Because such a blocking or amplitude attenuation of rhythmic alpha and beta band activity is closely linked to an internally or externally paced event (stimulus, movement, speech etc.), it was termed event-related desynchronization (ERD) (Pfurtscheller and Aranibar 1977, 1979).

This paper reports aspects of the spatiotemporal pattern of cortical ERD during a reading and recognition task. The dynamic ERD mapping was used for analyzing and displaying the pattern of cortical desynchronization.

Materials and Methods

Subjects

A sample of nine right-handed male students served as subjects in the present study. Their mean age was 26 years. Handedness was controlled by a questionnaire. All subjects were paid for their participation in the experiment.

---

* This research work was supported by the Fonds zur Förderung der wissenschaftlichen Forschung in Österreich, project 5240, and the Bundesministerium für Wissenschaft und Forschung.

[1] Abteilung für medizinische Informatik, Institut für Elektro- und biomedizinische Technik, Technische Universität Graz, and Ludwig Boltzmann-Institut für medizinische Informatik, A8010 Graz

[2] Abteilung für physiologische Psychologie, Institut für Psychologie, Universität Salzburg, A5020 Salzburg, Austria

Experimental Paradigm

When studying the cortical activation during cognitive processes, the most important requirement is to separate the cognitive from the sensory components of a task. In the experiments reported below, this is done by holding sensory components constant and varying only the instruction for the tasks. Two different tasks, a reading and a recognition task, were used in the present study. In the reading task, 48 concrete works, denoting animals or tools, were presented on a computer-controlled video terminal with an interstimulus interval of 5 s. Exposure time was 250 ms. A warning signal appeared 1 s before the presentation of a word. The subjects were instructed to read each word attentively.

After the reading task a recognition task was performed. The same set of 48 words served as targets, and a different but semantically related set of 48 words was used as distractors. The 48 targets and the 48 distractors were presented in a randomized order. The subjects' task was to distinguish between words already presented in the reading task and words which had not been presented before, responding verbally with "old" or "new" respectively. Reaction time was measured from stimulus onset to speech onset. Speech onset was detected by a microphone. As in the reading task, all words were exposed for 250 ms and presented via a computer-controlled video terminal. A warning signal appeared 1 s before stimulus presentation. The interstimulus interval was 6 s. An extensive describtion of these experiments can be found in Klimesch et al. (1986).

Data Acquisition and Processing

A modified "electro-cap" with 30 electrodes was used for the acquisition of EEG signals. Of those 30 electrodes, 21 were placed according to the international 10–20 system, while nine electrodes were additionally assigned to posterior, premotor and Broca's areas. The signals were amplified by a 30-channel biosignal isolation amplifier (frequency response 1.5–30 Hz). The output was linked to an anti-aliasing filter bank (cutoff 30 Hz, 120 dB/octave) and furthermore to a 32-channel analog-to-digital converter of a PDP 11/73 computer.

The EEG data were digitized at a rate of 64 samples/s, using epochs of 4 s for the reading task and 5 s for the recognition task. For the on-line control of the experiment, the 30 stimulus-synchronous EEG trials were displayed continuously on a high-resolution color monitor and stored on disk. The individual EEG epochs were processed according to the methods described elsewhere (Pfurtscheller and Aranibar 1977, 1979). After digital band-pass filtering, squaring of the samples and averaging over all epochs, band power values were obtained. In order to reduce the variance, eight consecutive power values were averaged and power values were obtained at intervals of 125 ms for each channel. The first second of each trial was chosen as a reference interval and the percentage alpha power decrease (or increase), as a measure of ERD (Pfurtscheller and Aranibar 1979), was calculated for each 125-ms time interval.

Map Computation and Display

A four-nearest-neighbor interpolation algorithm (Buchsbaum et al. 1982) was chosen to compute ERD images from 30 channels at intervals of 125 ms. Six or 20 maps were displayed on a color display with 56×56 matrices using a scale with 20 different colors. Hard copies were made photographically as well as on a black-and-white matrix printer.

Results

Two different types of results must be distinguished – the topographical pattern of desynchronization and the time course of desynchronization, which was computed at intervals of 125 s. All of the results reported below are based on those 48 words which were presented in the reading as well as in the recognition task. Since each subject had to perform both tasks and stimulus conditions were held constant, any change of cortical activation between the two tasks can be attributed to cognitive but not to sensory processes.

ERD maps averaged over all nine subjects are shown in Fig. 1. The first (maps 1375) represent the time 625 ms before word presentation, the last (maps 3500) were calculated 1500 ms after word presentation. The upper row of each panel in Fig. 1 represents the averaged data from the reading task and the lower row the data from the recognition task.

Topographical results are also shown in Table 1. Here, for all nine subjects, those regions of maximal desynchronization are displayed which occurred within 625 ms after stimulus presentation in the reading and recognition tasks. The reason for this procedure was to separate cognitive from motor processes. Because the average reaction time for a verbal response in the recognition task was 1169 ms, we considered the analyzed interval from 0 to 625 ms as short enough not to be confounded with the onset of motor processes. The data displayed in Fig. 1 demonstrate three characteristic features: (1) the magnitude, size and localization of the ERD maximum differs between the reading and recognition task; (2) the duration and time course of the ERD differs between the two tasks; (3) the ERD is present before word presentation.

Magnitude, Size and Localization of ERD Maximum

For the reading task the topographical results exhibit a pattern which is typical for visual perception: For all nine subjects an ERD focus was found over the occipital region. Furthermore, six of the nine subjects showed a more widespread activation, including parieto-occipital regions. The map 2500 in Fig. 1b displays occipitally localized ERD maxima at about 500 ms after world presentation. The reading task and the recognition task revealed somewhat different patterns of cortical activation. In the latter, the ERD was more widespread and maximal desynchronization shifted from occipital to parietal regions (com-

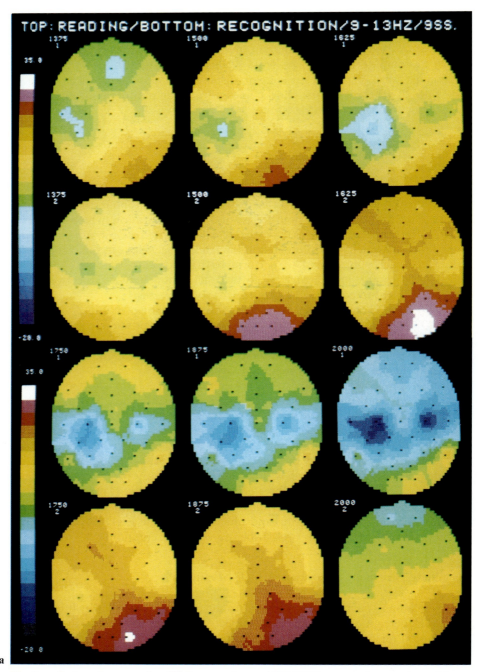

Fig. 1. a Series of consecutive ERD maps (maps 1375–2000) averaged over nine subjects: *upper row*, data from reading experiment; *lower row*, data from recognition experiment. The numbers mark the time in milliseconds from beginning of EEG sampling. Word presentation was at 2000–2125 ms. The *color scale* on the left indicates a change of the alpha power (ERD)

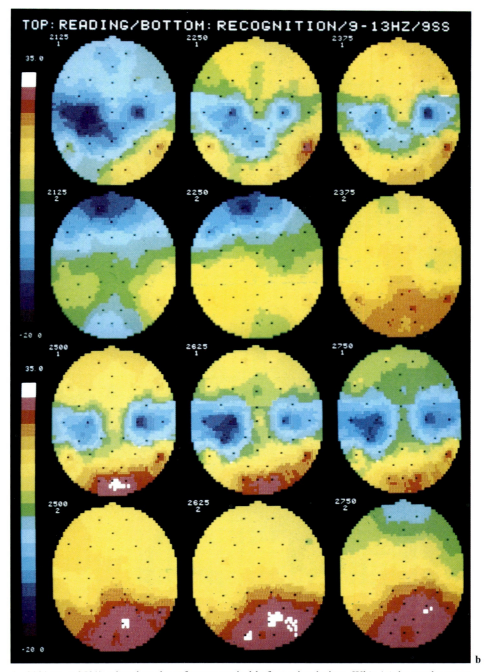

(−20% to +35%) related to the reference period before stimulation. *White/violet* marks areas with maximal ERD, followed by *yellow*, *green* and *light-blue*. *Dark-blue* marks areas with slightly enhanced alpha power. **b** Maps 2125–2750. **c** Maps 2875–3500

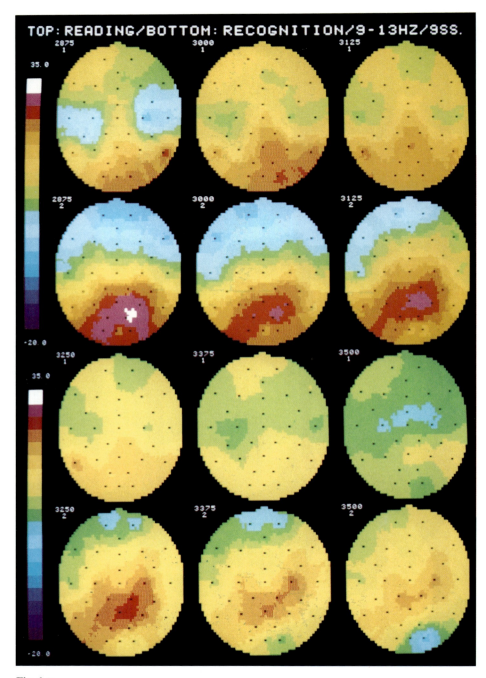

Fig. 1 c

Table 1. Regions with maximal ERD in reading and recognition tasks

Subject no.	Reading				Recognition			
	F	P	P/O	O	F	P	P/O	O
1	×	×		×		×	×	×
2	×			×		×	×	×
3				×	×	×	×	×
4			×	×		×	×	
5			×	×	×	×	×	
6			×	×		×	×	×
7			×	×				
8			×	×		×	×	×
9	×		×	×	×			

F, frontal; P, parietal; P/O, parieto-occipital; O, occipital

pare maps 2500 and 2750 in Fig. 1b). Analysis of the results of statistical tests (McNemar tests for the significance of changes) shows that a significant change in the pattern of cortical activation occurred for parietal regions ($p < 0.02$, two-tailed test) only, not for occipital, parieto-occipital or frontal regions.

Duration and Time Course of ERD

Inspection of the maps in Fig. 1 shows that in the reading task the maximal ERD (white in the maps) is present 500 ms after stimulus (word) onset (map 2500). In the recognition task, maximal ERD is found 500–875 ms after stimulus onset (maps 2500–2875) and is present much longer than in the reading task. In the recognition task the ERD drops between 1125 and 1250 ms after stimulus onset (Fig. 1c, maps 3125 and 3250), and this fits the average reaction time of 1169 ms. Thus, the results demonstrate good correspondence between a behavioral variable (reaction time) and a physiological measure (offset of desynchronization).

Time of Appearance of ERD

As can be seen in Fig. 1a, the ERD in the reading task starts immediately after the warning signal and reaches its maximum 500 ms before stimulus onset (map 1500). In the recognition task the ERD is more widespread, larger in magnitude and reaches its maximum 375 ms before stimulus onset (map 1625). In contrast to the reading task, the ERD is present up to the time of word presentation. In both tasks the topographical ERD pattern in the interstimulus interval is similar to the pattern obtained after reading and recognition respectively.

Discussion

The type of desynchronization studied in this paper is event-related, phasic, i.e., short-lasting, and regional and has been termed "event-related desynchronization" or ERD. In earlier studies, this ERD was studied extensively during voluntary, self-paced thumb or hand movement using a transverse montage along central areas and across the vertex (Pfurtscheller and Aranibar 1979, 1980). The voluntary movement ERD is phasic, bilaterally symmetrical and occurs immediately before, during and after a movement. The strict localization of the ERD in the sensorimotor cortex was demonstrated by the ERD mapping technique (Pfurtscheller et al. 1984). This confirms the findings of Jasper and Penfield (1949), Chatrian (1976) and Kuhlman (1978) on the functional reactivity of sensorimotor or mu rhythms.

In contrast to voluntary movement, 1-s light stimulation results also in a short-lasting ERD divided into an "on" and an "off" effect (Pfurtscheller and Aranibar 1978), clearly more pronounced over the occipital than over the central region. Therefore it is not surprising that the reading of words results in a maximal ERD over occipital areas in all investigated subjects. This localized desynchronization of occipital alpha rhythm during neutral light stimulation or reading of words represents stimulus-related phasic alpha power attenuation and is clearly different from a reduction of occipital alpha rhythm found during reading a text (Creutzfeldt et al. 1969).

This phasic desynchronization must be considered in close relationship to visual afferences and visual information processing. The longer-lasting desynchronization (over minutes) reported by Creutzfeldt et al. 1969 and others probably reflects more diffuse and less modality-specific brain mechanism.

It is very unlikely to assume that the short-lasting alpha blocking is related to visuo-oculomotor activity (Mulholland 1969) because during the 1-s light stimulation the subjects had their eyes closed and during the reading task one word was presented after the other at intervals of 5 s or more and the subjects were instructed to keep their eyes constant during the data acquisition periods. In an eye blink-controlled experiment, Grünewald et al. (1980) found also a phasic alpha attenuation after light stimulation which was maximal over the occipital region.

Although words were presented for a period of 250 ms only, the ERD lasted about 1 s over occipital areas (see Fig. 1). This is quite surprising, because no further instruction was given and no response was required in the reading task. Because subjects may not have felt any time pressure in the reading task and because of the long duration of the interstimulus interval (5 s), subjects had time for additional cognitive processes for which they were not instructed. Presumably, subjects began to make associations or to imagine the object denoted by the word.

The ERD is therefore a phenomenon related not only to the interruption of thalamic and thalamocortical mechanisms responsible for the generation of rhythmic alpha band activity during externally paced stimulation (Pfurtscheller and Aranibar 1977) or to the internally paced planning of a voluntary movement

(Pfurtscheller and Aranibar 1979), but also to the modality-specific processing of information.

During the recognition of words the ERD was more widespread, of larger magnitude, and embraced not only occipital and parieto-occipital but also, in particular, parietal regions. On the basis of this result it may be assumed that parietal regions play an important role in processes of memorization and retrieval of visual information. This interpretation is in good agreement with the results of a regional cerebral blood flow study carried out by Maximillian et al. (1978), who reported an increase of blood flow in occipital and parieto-occipital regions during a visual memory task.

A major problem in measuring and topographically displaying the ERD is represented by the fact that the amount of alpha band power in the reference interval – the ERD is measured by the alpha power decrease in relation to the power in a 1-s reference interval before each stimulation – is not always the same. This means that the general amount of alpha activity depends on the degree of activation, arousal, attention, interest and engagement, which can change in one subject during an experimental session and also differs from subject to subject. When there is no alpha rhythm, no desynchronization can be detected either. With respect to these considerations, it is interesting to note that 11% of normal and relaxed adults show little or no alpha activity (Gibbs et al. 1943); in such subjects alpha activity may even be enhanced due to light stimulation (Morrell 1966). These differing reactions – alpha reduction, alpha enhancement – depend more on individual differences (Creutzfeldt et al. 1969) than on the type of task. In this study we have made no attempt to select subjects according to their amount of alpha rhythm, but this could be a criterion for further studies.

Another problem in topographic mapping, not specific to the ERD but of general interest in all types of mapping, is the choice of the type of derivation (unipolar, bipolar, common average reference, Laplacian etc.). An extensive discussion of this problem can be found in Pfurtscheller (1988). In the present study a linked earlobe reference was used. Calculation of transverse bipolar derivations using the referential recording resulted in slightly modified maps where the ERD seems to be more pronounced and localized. Comparison of maps using different types of derivations will be the subject of another study.

An interesting document is provided by the maps 1500 to 1875 in Fig. 1, lower row. These maps demonstrate quite clearly that the ERD can be observed not only after but also before the presentation of a word. The ERD over wide frontal areas probably reflects a more diffuse mechanism of selective attention, readiness or expectancy, while the occipital ERD most likely shows specific anticipational processes. Thus, it is tempting to assume that those brain areas which are subsequently used to perform the task are "preactivated" shortly before the stimulus is presented, similar as found during the process of planning a voluntary movement (Pfurtscheller and Aranibar 1979; Pfurtscheller et al. 1986), where activation of central areas starts about 1 s before the onset of the motor action.

Comparison of contingent negative variation (CNV) and "alpha attenuation response" (AAR) – another measurement of ERD – during a tone-light response paradigm showed some similar functional reactivity during the interstimulus interval but with different spatiotemporal characteristics (Grünewald et al. 1980). However, it is of interest to note that in Grünewald's study the maximal attenuation response did not occur immediately before the visual stimulus but about 625–750 ms after the warning signal. A similar result was obtained in the reading task, where the ERD maximum was also short-lasting and occurred 375–500 ms after the warning signal.

The new method of dynamic ERD mapping is a promising tool for the analysis of spatiotemporal aspects of cortical activation pattern not only during self-paced movements and sensory stimulation, but also during cognitive processes. The current status of dynamic ERD mapping, however, still evinces a number of problems – choice of reference interval, type of derivation, number of electrodes, selection of frequency bands etc. To resolve some of these problems, further research must be carried out.

References

Berger H (1933) Über das Elektrenkephalogramm des Menschen. Arch Psychiatr Nervenkr 100:301–320

Buchsbaum MS, Rigal F, Coppola R, Capelletti J, King C, Johnson J (1982) A new system for gray-level surface distribution maps of electrical activity. Electroencephalogr Clin Neurophysiol 53:237–242

Chatrian GE (1976) The mu rhythm. In: Remond A (ed) Handbook of electroencephalography and clinical neurophysiology, vol 6. Elsevier, Amsterdam, 46–49

Chatrian GE, Petersen MC, Lazarre JA (1959) The blocking of the rolandic wicket rhythm and some central changes related to movement. Electroencephalogr Clin Neurophysiol 11:497–510

Creutzfeldt O, Grünewald G, Simonova O, Schmitz H (1969) Changes of the basic rhythms of the EEG during the performance of mental and visuomotor tasks. In: Evans CR, Mulholland B (eds) Attention in neurophysiology. Butterworth, London, pp 148–168

Gibbs FA, Gibbs EL, Lennox WG (1943) Electroencephalographic classification of epileptic patients and control subjects. Arch Neurol Psychiatr 50:111–128

Grünewald G, Grünewald-Zuberbier E, Netz J (1980) Event-related changes of EEG alpha activity in relation to slow potential shifts. Dev Neurosci 10:235–248

Jasper H, Andrews HL (1938) Electroencephalography III. Normal differentiations of occipital and precentral regions in man. Arch Neurol Psychiatr 39:96–115

Jasper H, Penfield W (1949) Electrocorticograms in man: effect of voluntary movement upon the electrical activity of the precentral gyrus. Arch Psychiatr Z Neurol 183:163–174

Klimesch W, Pfurtscheller G, Lindinger G (1986) Das kortikale Aktivierungsmuster bei verbalen Gedächtnisaufgaben. Sprache und Kognition 3:140–154

Kuhlman WM (1978) Functional topography of the human mu rhythm. Electroencephalogr Clin Neurophysiol 44:83–93

Maximilian VA, Prohovnik I, Risberg J, Haakonsson K (1978) Regional blood flow changes in the left cerebral hemisphere during word pair learning and recall. Brain Lang 6:22–31

Morrell LK (1966) Some characteristics of stimulus provoked alpha activity. Electroencephalogr Clin Neurophysiol 21:552–561

Mulholland TB (1969) The concept of attention and the electroencephalographic alpha rhythm. In: Evans CR, Mulholland TB (eds) Attention in Neurophysiology. Butterworth, London, pp 100–127

Pfurtscheller G (1988) Mapping of event-related desynchronization and type of derivation Electroencephalogr Clin Neurophysiol 70:190–193

Pfurtscheller G, Aranibar A (1977) Event-related cortical desynchronization detected by power measurements of scalp EEG. Electroencephalogr Clin Neurophysiol 42:817–826

Pfurtscheller G, Aranibar A (1978) On and off effects in the background EEG activity during one-second photic stimulation. Electroencephalogr Clin Neurophysiol 44:307–316

Pfurtscheller G, Aranibar A (1979) Evaluation of event-related desynchronization (ERD) preceding and following self-paced movement. Electroencephalogr Clin Neurophysiol 46:138–147

Pfurtscheller G, Aranibar A (1980) Voluntary movement ERD: normative studies. In: Pfurtscheller G, Buser P, Lopes da Silva FH, Petsche H (eds) Rhythmic EEG activities and cortical functioning. Elsevier, Amsterdam, pp 151–177

Pfurtscheller G, Ladurner G, Maresch H, Vollmer R (1984) In: Pfurtscheller G, Jonkman J, Lopes da Silva FH (eds) Brain ischemia – quantitative EEG and imaging techniques. Elsevier, Amsterdam, pp 287–302

Pfurtscheller G, Lindinger G, Klimesch W (1986) Dynamisches EEG Mapping – bildgebendes Verfahren für die Untersuchung perzeptiver motorischer und kognitiver Hirnleistungen. Z EEG-EMG 17:113–116

Topography of Preparation- and Performance-Related Slow Negative Potential Shifts in Verbal and Spatial Tasks

F. UHL[1], W. LANG[1], M. LANG[2], A. KORNHUBER[2], and L. DEECKE[1]

Introduction

It is well established that a simple voluntary movement is preceded by a slow negative cortical potential shift. This preparatory negative wave was first reported by Kornhuber and Deecke (1965) and called *Bereitschaftspotential* (BP) or readiness potential. In subsequent investigations performed by Lang et al. (1984, this volume), the method of movement-related potential recording was extended to more complex actions: a simple voluntary movement triggered the onset of sensory-guided movements of the hand. This experimental design was suitable for the investigation of anticipatory adjustments directed toward the forthcoming sensorimotor task. In the BP preceding the task, electrophysiological signs of attention directed toward the presentation of the sensory cues could be demonstrated.

In the present paradigm, a voluntary movement initiated the presentation of verbal or spatial stimuli which were relevant to the subsequent action. The experimental aim was to examine how the verbal or spatial quality of the stimulus would affect the topography of slow negative potential shifts generated when preparing as well as when performing the task.

Methods

Experiments were carried out in 15 healthy right-handed students aged between 18 and 24 years. Subjects initiated the tachistoscopic presentation of slides lasting 100 ms by pressing a stylus with their right or left hand (Fig. 1).

The slides contained either verbal or spatial material which had immediately to be reproduced either by writing or by drawing. The verbal material consisted of abstract words, the spatial material of stereogeometric figures. Visual stimuli were projected in either the left or the right hemifield of vision and had to be reproduced by either the left hand or by the right one. Thus, the experiment included three factors – hemifield of vision, performing hand, and material – the combinations of which resulted in eight different tasks. These tasks were performed in blocks. The subjects had knowledge of the characteristics (hemi-

---

[1] Neurologische Klinik, Universität Wien, Lazarettgasse 14, 1090 Wien, Austria
[2] Abteilung für Neurologie, Universität Ulm, Steinhövelstr. 9, 7900 Ulm, Federal Republic of Germany

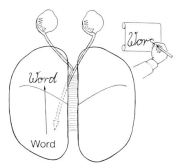

Fig. 1. Experimental arrangement in the VRR condition (verbal material, right visual hemifield, right hand

field of vision, material) of the forthcoming stimulus when initiating the trial. Thus, they were able to use anticipatory, stimulus-bound adjustments.

In each task, 64 artifact-free trials of cerebral potentials were averaged time-locked to the voluntarily initiated stimulus presentation. Cortical potentials in F3, F4, FCz (midway between Fz and Cz), C3, Cz, C4, P3, P4, O1, and O2, referred to linked earlobes, and the EOG (medial upper vs lateral lower right orbital rim) were recorded using Ag/AgCl surface electrodes and AC amplifiers with a time constant of 2.8 s and an upper cutoff at 70 Hz. Trials which were contaminated by eye movement artifacts were rejected from averaging. Data were digitized at a sampling rate of 1 count/5.86 ms and analyzed within a period of 6 s, 4 s of which was pre-trigger.

In order to quantify brain potentials related to the preparation of the task, the mean amplitude of the BP in the last 150 ms preceding the self-paced stimulus initiation (N-BP) was calculated. The mean negativity within an interval of 750–1750 ms after stimulus onset (N-P) was measured to describe brain potentials reflecting performance, either writing or drawing.

The effects of the variables material, hemifield of vision and performing hand on preparation-related (N-BP) and on performance-related potentials (N-P) were tested by means of analysis of variance.

Results and Discussion

In the period of preparation for the task, only the factor "performing hand" had a significant influence on N-BP: performance of the left hand led to an increase of N-BP in C4 ($p<0.005$). Stimulus characteristics (material, hemifield of vision) had no significant effect on N-BP. There were, however, some minor effects, which should be noted although their significance could not be proven in the global tests which were applied: If *verbal* material was projected in the

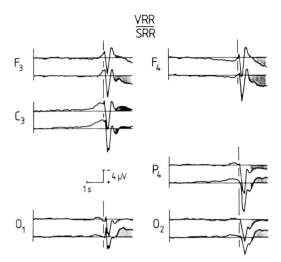

Fig. 2. Grand averages across 15 subjects for those electrodes which showed material-specific effects on performance-related potentials. Negativity up. The *vertical* line indicates stimulus onset. Two conditions are compared: VRR (verbal material, right hemifield of vision, right hand) in the *upper rows*, SRR (analogous to VRR except that material was spatial) in the *lower rows*. N-P was measured within the *dotted area*

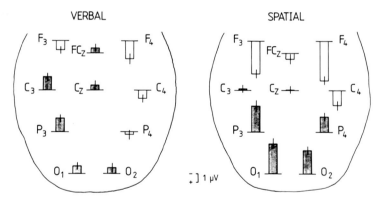

Fig. 3. *Left:* mean amplitudes of N-P averaged across the four verbal tasks. *Right:* N-P amplitudes across the four spatial tasks. SEM inserted. *Hatched columns* above the horizontal line indicate negative amplitudes of N-P

*r*ight hemifield of vision and the *r*ight hand performed the movement (condition VRR, see Fig. 2 upper lines), there was almost no BP in recordings of the right hemisphere. In contrast, the presentation of *s*patial material in the otherwise analogous situation (SRR) was accompanied by a significant BP in P4, which may be taken as a sign of anticipatory adjustment to the subsequent information processing of spatial material.

Clear results were obtained in the period of performance. Performance-related potentials (N-P) varied significantly as a function of the material. This was true for F3 ($p<0.001$), F4 ($p<0.007$), and C3 ($p<0.02$) on one side and for P4 ($p<0.009$), O1 ($p<0.002$), and O2 ($p<0.01$) on the other side. In F3, F4, and C3, N-P were more negative during writing than they were during drawing. The contrary effect was found in P4, O1, and O2: amplitudes of N-P were more negative when drawing than when writing (Fig. 2). Averages of N-P across either the four verbal or the four spatial tasks are displayed in Fig. 3. In the verbal tasks there is hemispheric asymmetry with larger amplitudes of N-P in recordings of the left hemisphere. In the spatial tasks, the figure visualizes the enhancement of performance-related negativity in parieto-occipital regions and its decrease in frontocentral ones. It is concluded that in the present task stimulus-bound preparatory mechanisms are either not present or have not been recordable. Slow negative potential shifts associated with information processing and reproduction are sensitive to material-specific effects.

References

Kornhuber HH, Deecke L (1965) Hirnpotentialänderungen bei Willkürbewegungen und passiven Bewegungen des Menschen: Bereitschaftspotential und reafferente Potentiale. Pflügers Arch 284:1–17

Lang W, Lang M, Heise B, Deecke L, Kornhuber HH (1984) Brain potentials related to voluntary hand tracking, motivation and attention. Hum Neurobiol 3:235–240

Topographic Brain Mapping of Transient Visual Attention

A. TAGHAVY, C.F.A. KÜGLER, and H. LÖSSLEIN[1]

Introduction

Longitudinal studies of patients with multiple sclerosis require not only determination of the well-known P100 in the context of pattern visual evoked potentials, but also an analysis of potentials being related to cognitive processes (Sutton et al. 1965). We therefore developed the visually elicited P300 by using two different kinds of checkerboard stimuli (A and B) which were randomly flashed to the subjects out of the gray background of a TV screen (Taghavy and Kügler 1985, 1986a, b). Systematic analysis of the PFP300 complexes revealed the following results: The PFP300 complexes are composed of a clearly recognizable negative wave peaking at about 250 ms (N250) followed by a sharp positive potential rise (PFP300) which is terminated by a negative potential decay (N400). Since the latencies of those peaks were closely related to different stages of information processing, we called the preceding negativity (N250) the "differentiating potential," PFP300 the "processing potential" and N400 the "terminating potential." We also found marked changes of the PFP300 amplitudes. These were in general about 3 times higher in the PFP300 complexes elicited by the rare, task-relevant B stimuli than in those elicited by the frequent, task-irrelevant A stimuli (Taghavy and Kügler 1986a). These amplitude variations were caused mainly by differing degrees of attention toward the eliciting stimuli. The subjects, who had to keep a running total in their heads of the infrequent B stimuli only, had to stay alert for the appearance of the rare B stimuli throughout the experiment in order to perform the task selectively ("sustained attention"). In contrast the degree of attention paid to A stimuli had only to be sufficient to differentiate them from the B stimuli ("floating attention").

In the present study we want to report third condition of attention, i.e., "transient attention," which lies between the floating and sustained attention levels.

Method

The 13 healthy male subjects ranged between 21 and 35 years of age. They sat in darkness in a Faraday box 1.5 m in front of a TV screen onto which two different kinds of checkerboard stimuli, A and B (A:B=80:20), were

[1] Neurologische Klinik der Universität, Schwabachanlage 6, 8520 Erlangen, Federal Republic of Germany

flashed (flash duration 120 ms) at a rate varying randomly between 0.6 and 1.3 Hz. The subjects did not know when the randomly presented rare (20%) (B stimuli (checksize 12.5' visual angle) would interrupt the sequence of the frequently (80%) flashed A stimuli (checksize 50' visual angle). The potentials were derived from right and left hemispheres against linked mastoid electrodes by a 16-channel Nic EEG 1A97 (time constant, TC=0.1; filter, Flt=30 Hz; sensitivity, SN=100 µV) and a Nic Pathfinder II (analysis time, AT=750 ms; number of averages, NA=150). Sixteen PFP300 potentials were obtained for each of the 13 subjects. The latencies of N250, P300 and N400 as well as the PFP300 amplitudes were measured. These data were averaged over all subjects for each of the 16 electrode locations and further evaluated statistically by t-difference tests. Furthermore, we calculated a grand average of the 16 PFP300 potentials of the 13 subjects and performed various brain mapping procedures on these mean potentials.

Results

The latencies of the PFP300 were shortest in the region of Fz and Ps (see also Fig. 1, middle image), where it first reached its highest amplitude level. This can be seen by increment mapping procedures.

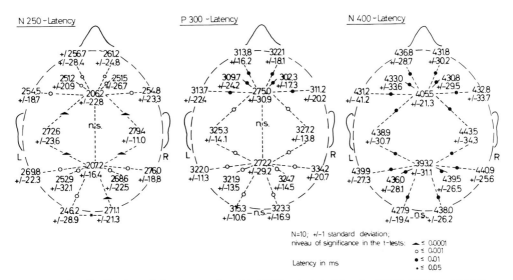

Fig. 1. The distribution of the mean values (± 1 SD) calculated for the N250, P300 and N400 latencies of the PFP300 complex (from left to right) over the scalp according to the corresponding electrode locations of the 10–20 system (Fp1, Fp2, F7, F8, F3, F4, Fz, Pz, C3, C4, T5, T6, P3, P4, O1 and O2 against linked mastoid electrodes). The lines between the mean values (± 1 SD) indicate that t-difference tests were performed between the single values of the PFP300 parameters obtained at the corresponding electrode locations

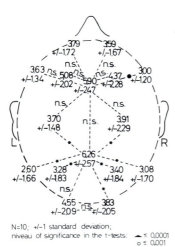

Fig. 2. The distribution of the mean values (±1 SD) of the ascending PFP300 amplitudes (measured from N250 to PFP300a) over the scalp according to the electrode locations described in Fig. 1. *t*-Difference tests were performed in the same manner as in Fig. 1

N=10; +/−1 standard deviation;
niveau of significance in the t-tests:
▲ ≤ 0,0001
○ ≤ 0,001
● ≤ 0,01
∗ ≤ 0,05

Amplitudes in µV

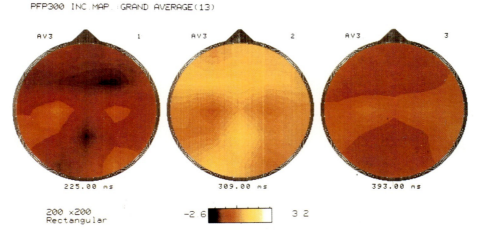

Fig. 3. The average (n = 13) distribution of N250 (image *1*), PFP300 (image *2*) and N400 (image *3*) over the scalp in the condition of surprise (= transient attention). *AV3*, the "image file" of the mean PFP300 potentials obtained in the condition of surprise; *200 × 200 Rectangular*, selected size of the mapping matrix with rectangular interpolation specification

The same was found for N250 and N400, which also rose at first at these midline locations (Fig. 1, left and right images).

The PFP300 was most prominent in bilateral frontal and left occipital locations (Fig. 3, middle image). In contrast to the images obtained by topographic mapping, the calculated mean values of the PFP300 amplitudes (Fig. 2) were highest over Fz, Pz and O1. This is because the peak-to-peak PFP300 amplitude measurements were made wherever each peak reached its maximum value, whereas the mapped images were taken from one point in time.

The N250 and N400 were distributed similarly (Fig. 3).

Discussion

At least one great advantage of electrical brain mapping is its capacity for multichannel evoked potential recording (Lehmann and Skandries 1980). This enabled us to study the distribution of the PFP300 complex, which we had previously been able to derive only between Oz and Fz with Cz as ground. At present we are engaged in studying the PFP300 components as the underlying brain electrical activity of well-defined psychological or cognitive processes. From a philosophical point of view, a reductionalistic approach to this topic is inevitable: relation of "reduced" mental states to "reduced" electrical brain states in order to possibly bridge the gap between microneuroscience and higher psychological levels. Electrical brain mapping holds such promise (Duffy et al. 1979).

Consciousness by a wakeful subject is distinct from awareness. Awareness in the context of our experiments, however, comprises floating attention, surprise or transient attention and sustained attention. These three attention states can be subjected to experimentation in the framework of electrophysiological recording. Whatever else happens in detail in the stream of consciousness with regard to content lies beyond the reach of this technique. Therefore we attempted only to relate these clear-cut psychological states to possible changes in the PFP300 complex: The higher the degree of attention toward the stimuli, the larger the ascending PFP300 amplitudes (Taghavy and Kügler 1986a). We had already studied the topographic mapping of these endogenous potentials in the condition of selective sustained attention (Taghavy et al. 1987): PFP300 was most pronounced in bilateral frontal and left occipital locations N250 and N400 behaved similarly. This study of the effects of transient visual attention on the PFP300 complex revealed similarly distributed but attenuated PFP300, N250 and N400 components. A more elaborate comparison between the two conditions is needed, however, and such a study is in preparation.

References

Duffy FH, Burchfield JL, Lombrosco CT (1979) Brain electrical activity mapping (BEAM): a method for extending the clinical utility of EEG and evoked potentials. Data Ann Neurol 5:308–321

Lehmann D, Skandries W (1980) Reference-free identification of components of checkerboard-evoked multichannel potential fields. Electroencephalogr Clin Neurophysiol 48:609–621

Sutton S, Braren M, Zubin J (1965) Evoked-potential correlates of stimulus uncertainty. Science 150:1187–1188

Taghavy A, Kügler CFA (1985) The influence of different visual discrimination tasks on the pattern flash elicited P300-complex. Pflügers Arch 405(2):66

Taghavy A, Kügler CFA (1986a) The effect of selective versus floating attention on the visually elicited P300-complex. Int Neurosci 29(3, 4):190–191

Taghavy A, Kügler CFA (1986b) Die durch aufleuchtende Schachbrettmuster evozierten Komponenten des P300-Komplexes sind wiederholungszuverlässig und geschlechtsunabhängig. Z EEG – EMG 17:168

Taghavy A, Kügler CFA, Lösslein H, Schwind M (1987) Increment mapping of the visual P300-complex supplemented by multichannel amplitude and latency measurements. Neurology 37 [Suppl 1]:377

Patterns of Event-Related Brain Potentials in Paired Associative Learning Tasks: Learning and Directed Attention

M. Lang[1], W. Lang[2], F. Uhl[2], and A. Kornhuber[1]

Methods

Subjects

The 18 subjects (mean age 22 years) voluntarily initiated each trial by pressing two buttons simultaneously. At the same time a verbal stimulus (S1) was projected in the subjects' central field of vision, followed 2.2 s later by a second stimulus S2 which the subjects had to associate to S1. Visual verbal stimuli in four paired verbal associative learning tasks differed in their semantic content: meaningful (S+; e.g., hill, valley) or meaningless (S−; e.g., mugö, atej). Well-established associations (of two S+ stimuli with contrary meaning or of S− stimuli, which were also overtrained in advance) did not require learning. They served as control conditions (L−) and were compared to learning tasks (L+), where new word pairs were associated (Fig. 1). The instruction was to memorize (M) S+ material by finding a semantic context (pair: "master" − "hill" → association: "the master is sitting on top of the hill"); the S− material had to be memorized by iteration. The subjects also had to reproduce the learned material in a cued recall (R) paradigm. An imperative visual stimulus (Si) 2.2 s after S2 required a motor response, whether the projected S1-S2 combination was right or wrong.

Recording. Frontal, central, temporal and parietal electrodes (10/20 system); FCz mid-frontocentral; electrooculogram and electromyogram.

Reference. Linked ears; impedance differences were balanced.

Average of Slow Surface Negative Potentials (SPs). Sixty-four artifact-free trials per condition and subject.

Learning. Error scores in the recall conditions.

Dependent measurements and statistics. N-S2 (mean negativity N during the epoch of 1 s duration prior to S2); N-E (N during encoding, 1.5 s to 2.5 s after S2); N-IS (N 1 s prior to Si); lateralization.

---

[1] Abteilung für Neurologie, Universität Ulm, Steinhövelstr. 9, 7900 Ulm, Federal Republic of Germany
[2] Neurologische Klinik, Universität Wien, Lazarettgasse 14, 1090 Wien, Austria

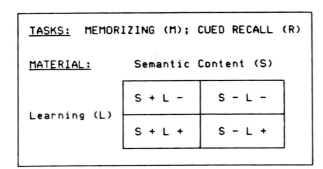

Fig. 1. Tasks and material of the learning experiment

Analysis of Variance. This included the factors of semantic content (S) and learning (L).

Results

The average curve shows characteristic components: the *Bereitschaftspotential* (BP; readiness potential) prior to the voluntary task initiation; a contingent negative variation (CNV) in the S1 and S2 interval; memorizing-related negativity (in M) or a CNV prior to Si after S2 (in R).

The most important results of the memorizing tasks were as follows: (a) The N-S2 amplitude (S+ and S−) was significantly influenced by the factor L at parietal leads. N-S2 was enhanced in L+ compared to L−. (b) Left frontocentral N-E and frontal lateralization were significantly influenced by the factor L. N-E was enhanced and more to the left during L+ than during L− (Fig. 2).

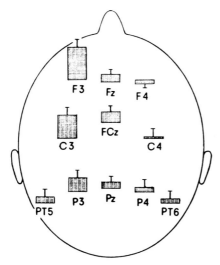

Fig. 2. Topography of differences between increased N-E in the learning tasks (L+) and N-E in the control tasks (L−); here S+ material. Left frontocentral differences were significant ($p < 0.01$). The *bars* show 2 SE. F3 difference: 2.2 µV

Lateralization to the left was also found for N-IS prior to R and for N-S2 in the L+ tasks during R (to a lesser extent; not significant and not significantly influenced by the factor L). Again this is a local frontocentral phenomenon.

SPs during our learning epochs were not influenced by the semantic content of the stimulus, although lateralization was stronger in the S+ condition than in the S− condition.

Discussion

We interpret the cortical activity (negativity), which is enhanced during learning and dominant over the left (verbal) frontocentral region, as an electrophysiological sign of mechanisms for verbal cognitive processing, for associative learning and memorizing. A difference in frontal lobe activity between encoding and retrieval systems is suggested, since the factor L influenced the frontal and central SPs during M but not during R. Cortical activity seems to be stronger during memorizing (building up new associations) and less expressed in the recall tasks, in which the subjects created a hypothesis after S1 which they checked after presentation of S2.

Verbal deficits are well known after left frontal lobe damage; however, the presence of a cognitive learning performance requiring conceptual abilities, seems to be critical for differentiation of the two tasks L+ and L−, which were both verbal (see also Deecke et al. 1985; Lang et al. 1987). Parietal N-S2 in the memorizing task reflects directed attention (see Mountcastle et al. 1975) toward relevant external stimuli. In contrast to the L− control task, the S2 stimulus, as expected, could not be anticipated in the L+ task.

References

Deecke L, Kornhuber HH, Lang W, Lang M, Schreiber H (1985) Timing function of the frontal cortex in sequential motor and learning tasks. Hum Neurobiol 4:143–154

Lang M, Lang W, Uhl F, Kornhuber A, Deecke L, Kornhuber HH (1987) Slow negative potential shifts indicating verbal cognitive learning in a concept formation task. Hum Neurobiol 6:183–190

Mountcastle VB, Lynch JC, Georgopoulos A, Sakata H, Acuna C (1975) Posterior parietal association cortex of the monkey: command functions for operations within the extrapersonal space. J Neurophysiol 43:118–136

Brain Lateralization in Stress Reactions

D.B. LINKE, B.M. REUTER, and M. KURTHEN[1]

Lateralization Factors for Cognitive Function

There is a vast amount of literature on the lateralization of brain functions in relation to cognitive processing and psychological features of mental activity. The lateralization of cognitive functions is not only genetically and ontogenetically fixed and determined, but can also shift depending on the information to be processed. EEG alpha asymmetries have been recorded in relation to the kind of information being processed in reading, in such a way that more imaginative reading contents cause more desynchronization in the right hemisphere, whereas more logical information content is correlated to an activation of the left hemisphere. Thus there exists an interactive situation as far as the structure of the brain and the information to be handled are concerned. This interaction can become very dynamic in nature, such that sometimes information may be processed by one hemisphere although it is more appropriate for the other hemisphere. This sticking to one hemisphere instead of shifting all the time is an economic method of information processing and is a form of mental disposition (Durwen and Linke 1985). Many psychological parameters have been worked out which show a relation of cognitive information processing to general biological parameters, such as sex and age. Of special interest is the concept of Geschwind and Galaburda (1985a, b), who showed that the cognitive factors may correlate with endocrinological and immunological factors. On this basis a convergence of neuropsychological research and stress research is possible. Many biological parameters have been shown to correlate with stress reactions. Thus the immunological system does interact with the endocrinological stress system. Therefore it is possible that the great problem of stress research, the specification of personality factors in individually different stress reactions, may be solved by a neuropsychological approach in which psychological parameters are correlated to hemispheric dominance and via this missing link to the stress reaction. In such a conception the vegetative functions would be seen in an intimate connection with cognitive functions, as demonstrated, for instance, by galvanic skin response studies, in which lateralizations of the response occurred in relation to the kind of information being processed (Hugdahl et al. 1983). Information about hemisphere asymmetries does exist from different starting points of investigation (Biersack et al. 1987; Kurthen et al. 1988). The aim of our study was to look for asymmetries in hemispheric function due to stress activity.

---

[1] Neurochirurgische Universitätsklinik, Sigmund-Freud-Str. 25, 5300 Bonn 1, Federal Republic of Germany

Experiments and Results

In 28 right-handed persons we studied the activity pattern of the cerebral hemispheres by the brain electrical activity mapping (BEAM) technique in a structured stress experiment. The normal test persons had to perform cognitive processes (manipulation of a keyboard for a computer car driving game) under different degrees of stress (game difficulty and car noise). The manipulation of the keyboard had to be performed bimanually to avoid hemispheric shifts by motor asymmetry. The BEAM technique was used to show the frequency and amplitude distribution, which displayed more desynchronizations in the right hemisphere (Fig. 1).

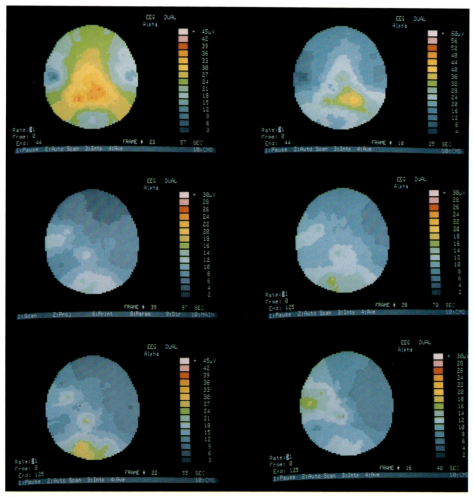

Fig. 1. BEAM demonstration of absence of lateralization in relaxation (*upper* images) but clear lateralization in stress reactions

Toward a Neuropsychological Model of the Interaction of Stress Reactions and Cognitive Processes

On the basis of our findings a closer relation has to be recognized between cognitive functions and the system responsible for stress reactions. Two principal types of interaction are possible. (1) The perception of stress may be lateralized in respect to hemispheric activity because stress factors are more global and unspecific in nature than other kinds of cognitive information. Due to this, lateralization of brain activity as demonstrated by the BEAM technique may occur and one may wonder whether stress could be counteracted by a more cognitive left hemispheric disposition, the unspecific information being processed more consciously. (2) The other possible type of interaction is related to the disposing nature of the stress reactions for right hemispheric activation. It is thought that the stress reactions running through the brainstem have different effects on the two hemispheres of the telencephalon.

References

Biersack HJ, Linke DB et al. (1987) Brain SPECT with 99m Tc-HMPAO before and during Wada test – case reports. J Nucl Med 28:1763–1767

Durwen HF, Linke DB (1985) Electromyographic mirror activity as indicator of mental disposition? World Congress of Neurology, Hamburg, 1–6 Sept. 1985

Geschwind A, Galaburda AM (1985a) Cerebral lateralization. Biological mechanisms, associations and pathology: I. A hypothesis and a program for research. Arch Neurol 42:428–459

Geschwind A, Galaburda M (1985b) Cerebral lateralization. Biologial mechanisms, associations and pathology: III. A hypothesis and a program for research. Arch Neurol 42:634–654

Hugdahl K, Broman JE, Franzon M (1983) Effect of stimulus content and brain lateralization on the habituation of the electrodermal orienting reaction (OR). Biol Psychol 17:153–168

Kurthen M, Biersack HJ, Linke DB (1988) Präoperative Diagnostik: Wada-Test mit SPECT-Kontrolle zur Hirnfunktionslokalisation bei therapieresistenter Epilepsie. Neurochirurgia (Stuttg) 31 (1988) 96–98

EEG Dynamic Cartography of Wakefulness, Sleep and Dreams: A Movie

P. ETEVENON[1]

Introduction

The time-course variability of spontaneous EEG activity over the scalp is particularly well displayed in the form of a movie showing the rapid topographic waxing and waning of electrical power. However, two problems arise. First, it is difficult to conduct a real-time experiment which involves spectral protocols for recording EEG topography changes over the scalp. The second difficulty is in providing enough successive EEG maps which may become successive frames for a specially made research movie.

In 1971, Lehmann in Zürich made a first experimental movie of 3 min showing the EEG spontaneous electrical changes that took place over 2 s, recording instantaneous EEG activity simultaneously in 64 EEG channels at 750 Hz sampling frequency per channel. After computing the isopotential curves, the movie was made using frames of 8 ms interval, 20 alpha waves representing 400 images. The back- and -white movie camera was then synchronized at 8 frames/s. Later, Duffy presented a "cartoon" display of successive BEAM (brain electrical activity mapping) successive EEG power maps expressed on a fast, color display, high-resolution monitor. A display of 125 successive maps in 25 s was presented in real time for a speed on the color display monitor of 5 frames/s. Coppola (personal communication, 1986), produced an experimental short movie of one night of sleep as recorded using EEG where each frame was an EEG power map. In 1984, at a meeting of the French EEG Society in Tours, Gaches presented a 6-min black-and-white movie called Cartographie du sommeil lent d'après-midi, where each EEG power map was projected for 2 s before being replaced by the next. At the same meeting, Etevenon (1985a) presented a first black-and-white movie of 11 min showing 236 frames of successive EEG power maps (absolute root mean square (RMS) amplitude between 0 and 30 Hz) representing the first (80 min) and the second (114 min) sleep cycles of a specially recorded night of sleep. Two different sequences were presented: a fast accelerated sequence where each EEG map was shown (in 0.16 s or 4 frames/s) for four images only, and a second lower sequence where each EEG map was displayed and filmed for about one half second (0.48 s) for 12 successive similar images (12 frames/s).

Further improvement was made by computing, publishing (Etevenon and Guillou 1986; Etevenon 1987) and presenting in a new didactic movie (Etevenon 1985b) the typical EEG power maps corresponding to each state of wakefulness

---
[1] Chargé de recherche INSERM, Centre Esquirol, CHU Côte de Nacre, 14033-Caen Cedex, France

(eyes open, eyes closed) and sleep (I, II, III, IV, paradoxical sleep). However, this was still not satisfactory because of the "jumps" between the chosen experimental EEG power maps.

For this reason we produced, in 1986, special programs (analogous to those of Perrin et al. 1987a, b) allowing double interpolation in space and time, enabling us to make EEG dynamic cartography of wakefulness, sleep and dream stages, which were checked together with dream content obtained after provoked awakenings during the recorded night, followed by dream recalls and reports (Etevenon and Guillou 1986; Etevenon 1987). These programs will be described in detail in forthcoming reports of industrial research and development (through INSERM and ANVAR).

Methods

Protocol of Pilot Longitudinal Sleep Study

The detailed protocol of this longitudinal study has already been published (Etevenon and Guillou 1986). A bilateral montage of 16 electrodes over the scalp was chosen with common average reference. Two devices were used simultaneously: a 16-channel EEG recorder (Reega 2000 Alvar) coupled with an 8-channel EEG used for polygraphy. The subject was a normal female volunteer of 55 years with a university background presenting a high alpha amplitude, eyes closed, well accustomed to EEG laboratory conditions and a very good at dream recall. On 4 December 1984 she spent a night in the EEG laboratory. She was awakened three times at the end of the first sleep cycles and was asked to recall her dreams following drowsy sleep (stage I; first awakening) and REM stages (paradoxical sleep: second and third awakenings).

EEG Mapping

The 16 EEGs were submitted on line to spectral EEG analysis for periods of 6 s, 30 s or 1 min (Cartovar 2 Alvar). Spectral data were recorded on floppy disks, allowing later editing of EEG maps for the raw EEG amplitude values and three broad frequency band amplitude values (0–7, 8–12, 13–30 Hz). Spectral values were also fed into a Hewlett-Packard minicomputer (HP 1000, 21 MXF) for further averaging and statistical comparisons and later editing before filming the color power maps on a fast-screen high-resolution graphic terminal monitor.

Sleep stages were also scored separately by two experienced electroencephalographers and later the artifact-free EEG maps were classified and averaged according to sleep stages. The contents of the three dream reports were also analyzed in terms of sensory and perceptual activation (hearing, vision, touch and movement) for further understanding of the EEG maps preceding the provoked awakenings (Etevenon and Guillou 1986).

EEG Mapping Computations

Two controlled states of vigilance during wakefulness were obtained: active wakefulness with eyes open, followed by quiet wakefulness with eyes closed (Etevenon and Guillou 1986). This was followed by 500 epochs spectrally analyzed during the night, providing 500 raw EEG mean RMS amplitude maps, 500 delta and theta mean amplitude EEG maps, 500 alpha mean amplitude EEG maps and 500 delta mean amplitude EEG maps.

After a drastic selection of maps, typical EEG maps for each state of vigilance and sleep were computed together with correlations between the maximal amplitude values of these typical maps (Etevenon and Guillou 1986). It was observed that the raw EEG power maps (between 0 and 30 Hz) were the most descriptive maps of the wakefulness (alpha correlations) and sleep stages, and the movies were then compiled exclusively from these maps.

Results

Typical colored maps of the two states of wakefulness (active and quiet) and of the main stages of sleep (I, II, III, IV, paradoxical) are presented in Fig. 1. Each EEG mean amplitude map is made of 10 colors, between light-red for the minimal amplitude value, representing the highest activated location on the scalp (we have previously defined local EEG activation by decreased mean amplitude and increased mean frequency), and the deepest blue for the maximal amplitude value, representing the lowest activated location on the scalp (the most deactivated spot). For each map this highest mean amplitude value was also represented on the right as a vertical bar increasing or decreasing between the bottom (fixed at 10 µV minimal RMS amplitude value) and the top (fixed at 250 µV maximal RMS amplitude value) of the column. Each EEG map was optimized and showed red (activated) and blue (deactivated) locations. Thus the vertical blue bar on the right depicted the global activation of the EEG maps: low maximal amplitudes for active wakefulness eyes open, stage I and REM, high maximal amplitudes for stages III and IV of slow wave sleep.

The typical EEG maps present structured topographical patterns according to the observed states and stages. The red activated spots of active wakefulness, stage I and REM are mostly located on the left temporal and central areas, together, at times, with the right parietal area. In quiet wakefulness, eyes closed, the red activated areas extend from the temporocentral areas to the frontal areas, characteristic of the diffuse global attention process. Stage II EEG maps are characterized by two blue deactivated areas: one on the prefrontal, premotor area, probably related mainly to the sleep spindles reflecting possible inactivation of motor programs, the other on the posterior occipital pole. Stages III and IV of sleep were characterized by more blue areas than red areas, located symmetrically over the anterior, frontal and posterior-occipital poles. Moreover, the EEG dynamic cartography movie has revealed a slowly oscillating process of 10–20 s for maximal delta waves (highly correlated with raw EEG maximal

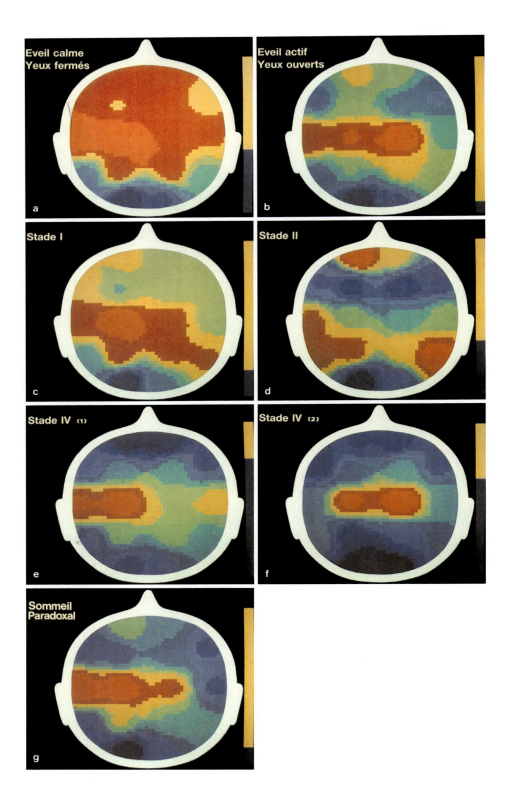

amplitude blue areas on the successive maps), shifting slowly between anterior and posterior areas.

Finally, we were interested by the activated red spot areas and their topographic shifts as well as time changes, during the periods of stage I and REM preceding the provoked awakenings with dream recalls and dream reports. It appears that the red spots change very quickly, mostly over the temporal (auditory) and central (somatosensory and motor primary) areas. One of the most interesting finding was obtained during the first REM period, when appeared a red activated spot located over the left central area (suggesting, right hand active projection). The 11-min REM period was accelerated sixfold in the movie, which ended at the time of provoked awakening when the subject reported an auditory, visual and kinesthesic dream of carrying luggage in the right hand before taking a train in the Gare de Lyon railway station in Paris.

EEG dynamic cartography enables us to speed up the real-time events scanned by EEG mean amplitude mappings. The time course variability of changes of topographic activated and deactivated areas, can then be displayed in such a way that new events may be seen as oscillating slow waves, in stages III and IV, or as activated spots (over primary sensory and motor areas) which may correspond to spontaneous physiological electrical activities concomittant with the subjective psychological events of dreams. This last aspect has been discussed already (Etevenon and Guillou 1986; Etevenon 1987), and two new movies have been realized (Etevenon 1986a, b) showing the unique value of the new EEG dynamic cartography as a way of understanding, exploring and probing normal (and pathological) brain function during waking, sleeping and dreaming states.

Nevertheless, the present methodology and special programming for dynamic EEG cartography, arrived at after 2 years minute study of a pilot recording of a first night of sleep, must be confirmed by follow-up studies and by work in other EEG cartography laboratories.

Acknowledgements. We are grateful to Miss S. Guillou, Mrs. M. Toussaint and M. Saddi for programming assistance and to Professor Bisconte for high-resolution and high-speed color image treatment. We also wish to express our thanks to CNRS-Audiovisuel, INSERM, Laboratoires Specia and Biocom for coproducing our two most recent movies.

◁───

Fig. 1 a–g. Typical EEG mean amplitude maps (between 0 and 30 Hz) for two states of wakefulness – active wakefulness, eyes open (*éveil actif yeux ouverts*) and quiet wakefulness, eyes closed (*éveil calme yeux fermés*) – and five stages of sleep – stage (*Stade*) I; stage II; two successive epochs, (1) and (2), of stage IV; paradoxical sleep or REM stage (*sommeil paradoxal*). Each typical EEG map is made up of a spectrum of 10 colors between light-red (lowest EEG mean amplitude of the map for the most "activated" area) and deep-blue (highest EEG mean amplitude of the map for the most "deactivated" area). The vertical *blue bar* on the *right* of each map indicates the highest EEG amplitude of the map (from 10 µV at the bottom to 250 µV at the top of the column). This blue bar is an index of global activation (or deactivation) of the EEG map. See text for further comments

References

Etevenon P (1985a) Cartographie d'une nuit de sommeil. Communication avec film produit par le CNRS-Audiovisuel. 4 Juin 1985: Société d'EEG et de Neurophysiologie clinique, Tours, "Sommeil humain normal et pathologique"

Etevenon P (1985b) Le cerveau à la carte (Film). Laboratoires Specia

Etevenon P (1986a) La caverne de Platon ou cartographie d'une nuit de sommeil et de rêve. (16-mm color movie, optic sound, 26 min coproduced by CNRS-Audiovisuel, INSERM, Laboratoires Specia, Biocom)

Etevenon P (1986b) Cartographie EEG dynamique de l'éveil, du sommeil et du rêve. (16-mm color movie 7 min, coproduced by CNRS-Audiovisuel, INSERM, Laboratoires Specia, Biocom)

Etevenon P (1987) Du rêve à l'éveil. Bases physiologiques du sommeil. Chapitre V: "Cartographie d'une nuit de sommeil et de rêve". Albin Michel, Paris

Etevenon P, Guillou S (1986) EEG cartography of a night of sleep and dreams. A longitudinal study with provoked awakenings. Neuropsychobiology 16(2–3):146–151

Perrin F, Pernier J, Bertrand O, Giard MH, Echallier JF (1987a) Mapping of scalp potentials by a surface spline interpolation. Electroenceph clin Neurophysiol 66:75–81

Perrin F, Bertrand O, Pernier J (1987b) Scalp current density mapping: value and estimation from potential data. IEEE-BME 34(4):283–288

Section V Evoked Potential Mapping

Visual Evoked Potential Topography: Physiological and Cognitive Components

W. SKRANDIES[1]

Topographical Principles

Electrical brain activity as recorded from the intact scalp of man constitutes an electrical field whose configuration varies over time. Intracranial neuronal generator populations produce potential changes which are recorded by conventional EEG machines as voltages. Such potential difference waveforms reflect the difference in electrical potential or the potential gradient along a line between the locations of two scalp electrodes which are connected to an amplifier channel. Potential waveforms are ambiguous, since their shape and configuration depend both on the electrode locations and the choice of the reference electrode. When only nine scalp electrodes are used for recording, 72 different waveshapes may be obtained. We also note that none of the electrode locations could serve better than the others as reference electrode since no inactive point is available (see Nunez 1981), and any of the nine electrodes may be selected to serve as recording reference. Thus, from nine recording electrodes are obtained nine different sets consisting of eight potential waveshapes each – all of which look different (for illustration of such a data set refer to Skrandies 1987, Fig. 4). It is impossible to evaluate such extensive data sets which contain redundant information by simple inspection or by waveshape comparisons, and thus, the analysis of electrical activity must not deal with reference-dependent potential waveshapes (Lehmann and Skrandies 1984; Skrandies 1986, 1987).

On the other hand, topographical analysis aims at directly assessing the electrical fields of the brain whose spatial configurations do not depend on electrode locations or reference sites (Skrandies 1986). The correct interpretation of electrical brain activity data rests on the use of unambiguous recording and data analysis techniques in order that one may arrive at physiologically meaningful interpretations of the electrical data recorded. Such topographical analysis techniques treat electrical brain activity as potential fields, and topographical methods have been developed for both spontaneous and event-related activity during recent years (Lehmann 1972; Lehmann and Skrandies 1980, 1984; Skrandies and Lehmann 1982a, b).

Topographical analysis is used primarily in order to detect covariations between certain features of the scalp potential fields and experimental conditions manipulated by the investigator. Measures derived from such data are used as unambiguous descriptors of the electrical brain activity, and they have been employed successfully to study visual information processing in man (e.g.,

---

[1] Max-Planck-Institut für Physiologische und Klinische Forschung, Parkstraße 1, 6350 Bad Nauheim, Federal Republic of Germany

Skrandies 1987). The aim of evoked potential studies is to detect subsets or so-called components of electrical brain activity that are defined in terms of latency (with respect to some external or internal event) and topographical scalp distribution patterns. It appears reasonable to define component latency as the occurrence time of maximal activity in the electrical field reflecting synchronous activation of a maximal number of intracranial neuronal elements. In order to quantify the amount of activity in a given scalp potential field we have proposed a measure of 'global field power' that is computed as the mean of all possible potential differences in the field corresponding to the standard deviation of all recording electrodes with respect to the average reference (see review by Lehmann and Skrandies 1984). Scalp potential fields with steep gradients and pronounced peaks and throughs will result in high global field power, while global field power is low in electrical fields with only shallow gradients that have a flat appearance. Thus, the maximum in a plot of global field power over time determines component latency. In a second step the features of the scalp potential field are analyzed at these component latencies. Derived measures like location of potential maxima and minima, and steepness and orientation of gradients in the field are by definition independent of the reference electrode, and they will give an adequate description of the electrical brain activity.

It is important to note that mapping of electrical activity does not allow us directly to draw conclusions on the exact neuroanatomical locations of the intracranial sources. Neuronal mass activity produces electrical fields which spread via volume conduction throughout the brain and can be recorded at locations distant from the generating source. This has been shown in a study on various stages of the cat visual system, where single-unit activity and field potentials were compared (Skrandies et al. 1978). Thus, model dipole computations always have to rest on certain explicit (and sometimes implicit) assumptions concerning the number, location and spatial extent of the dipole as well as the homogeneity and geometry of the intracranial media in order to arrive at physiologically meaningful solutions (e.g., Kavanagh et al. 1978; Sidman et al. 1978). It is also obvious that the "inverse problem" of how to determine the sources of potentials in a conductive medium when the scalp potential field is given has no unique solution (von Helmholtz 1853). The computation of equivalent dipoles thus must be regarded as a further step of data reduction. The multidimensional scalp data space consisting of potential measurements from many electrode locations may be explained or modelled by an equivalent dipole data space with typically fewer dimensions. It is also evident that such a data reduction has to be performed for each post-stimulus time point separately.

Irrespective of whether the exact intracranial generator populations can be determined, the evaluation of scalp potential data combined with the knowledge on the anatomy and physiology of the human visual system may allow useful physiological interpretations. Scalp topography is a means of characterizing electrical brain activity unambiguously in terms of latency and scalp location. Comparison of scalp potential fields obtained in different experimental conditions (e.g., different physical stimulus parameters, different subjective, psychological states, or normal vs pathological neurophysiological traits) may be used to test hypotheses on the identity or nonidentity of the neuronal populations activated by these stimulus and subject conditions. Identical scalp potential fields may or may not be generated by identical neuronal populations, while nonidentical potential fields must be caused by different intracranial generator mechanisms. Thus, all we can study is a systematic variation of the electrical brain activity, and we are interested in variations of scalp potential fields caused by the manipulation of independent experimental stimulus parameters.

Mapping of electrical brain activity in itself does not constitute an analysis of the recorded data but it is a prerequisite for unambiguous extraction of quantitative features of the scalp recorded electrical data. In a second step of data analysis such derived topographical measures must be used to test differences between experimental conditions statistically. The aim of the present chapter is to illustrate how visually evoked brain activity is quantitatively analyzed, revealing fundamental steps in visual information processing of the human nervous system.

Visual Evoked Potential Topography and Localized Stimuli

Visual stimuli are processed at the cortical level in several different sensory projection areas, most of which display an orderly retinotopic organization (van Essen 1985). Various areas investigated with single-cell recordings appear to be involved in different aspects of visual information processing, and already primary areas of the visual cortex may show functional differences as reflected by the local distribution and densities of physiologically different cell types like simple, complex and hypercomplex cells.

Human visual evoked brain activity recorded from the intact scalp is influenced by physical stimulus parameters like luminance, contrast, or pattern size as well as by the location of the stimulus on the retina. This section will describe how the retinotopic organization of the human visual cortex is reflected by visual evoked potential (VEP) topography. I will illustrate how upper and lower or left and right hemiretinal stimuli affect the scalp topography of visually evoked brain activity in a systematic way.

When responses elicited by stimuli presented to the upper or lower retinal half are compared, differences between stimulus conditions in terms of component latency and component location become obvious. Figure 1 illustrates map series obtained with a checkerboard reversal stimulus presented to the upper (Fig. 1A) or to the lower (Fig. 1B) hemiretina. In both map series an occipital positivity gradually develops around 100 ms latency and reaches a maximum surrounded by steep gradients. At later times this occipital positivity is replaced by a relative negativity. It is obvious from Fig. 1 that upper retinal stimuli are followed by electrical brain activity with shorter component latencies than lower hemiretinal stimuli as indicated by the occurrence times of maximal global field power (asterisks, in Fig. 1A, B). Upper retinal stimuli evoke an occipital positivity starting at 80 ms which reaches its maximum between 92 and 98 ms

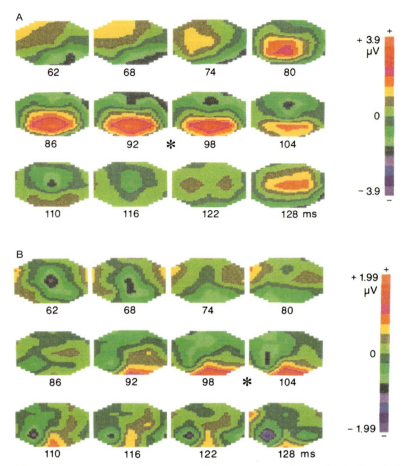

Fig. 1 A, B. Series of scalp potential fields obtained with a checkerboard reversal stimulus presented to the upper (**A**) or lower (**B**) hemiretina. Each map presents the mean activity computed over successive time points ranging from 62 to 128 ms at 6 ms intervals. (Circular stimulus field of 16° diameter, 50′ checks, 96% contrast, two reversals per second.) Potential values are color-coded as shown on the voltage scales on the *right* (relative positivity in *red*, relative negativity in *blue*, all referred to the average reference). Note different scales for potential fields evoked by upper and by lower retinal stimuli. Maximal global field power, denoted by *asterisks*, occurs for the upper retina earlier than for the lower retina. Evoked activity was recorded from an array of 21 electrodes as shown in head schema in Fig. 2. (Data were collected with a Biologic Brain Atlas III; courtesy M. Capaul and D. Lehmann)

and has disappeared after 104 ms (see Fig. 1 A). On the other hand, with lower retinal stimuli the occipital positive component begins to develop only at 92 ms and can be seen throughout the analysis time intervals presented in Fig. 1 B. Such a latency difference appeared as a systematic feature in various studies (e.g., Lehmann et al. 1977; Lehmann and Skrandies 1979a) and has been shown to be correlated with neuroanatomical and physiological differences and with

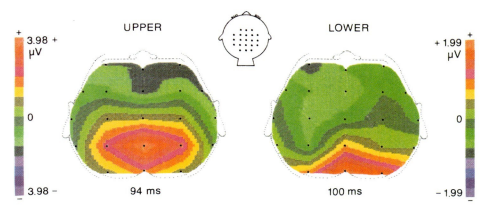

Fig. 2. Scalp potential fields evoked by upper or lower retinal checkerboard reversal stimuli at times of maximal global field power (94 ms for upper, 100 ms for lower retinal stimuli). Both potential fields are dominated by an occipital positivity at component latency, but the scalp locations of the extreme values and of potential gradients are different. Components evoked by upper retinal stimuli are located on the scalp anteriorly to those evoked by lower retinal stimuli. For electrode array and voltage scales see *inset*; same convention as in Fig. 1. (Data were collected with a Biologic Brain Atlas III; courtesy M. Capaul and D. Lehmann)

a functional superiority of the upper over the lower hemiretina in various species (for an extensive review of neurophysiological, electrophysiological and psychophysical studies see Skrandies 1987).

It is also obvious from Fig. 1 that stimuli presented to the lower retina yield smaller amplitudes in the evoked scalp potential fields, reflected by the fewer number of field lines and the smaller potential gradients in the fields evoked by lower retinal stimuli (note the different voltage scales when comparing Fig. 1 A and Fig. 1 B). The position of the potential maxima in the fields is also different in the two stimulus conditions: upper retinal stimuli produce field maxima located anteriorly to those evoked by lower retinal stimuli. This becomes obvious when we compare the scalp potential fields obtained at times of maximal global field power. Figure 2 (left) illustrates the potential field evoked by upper retinal stimuli at 94 ms, and Figure 2 (right) shows the corresponding map following lower retinal stimuli at component latency (100 ms). The difference in scalp location of the occipital positive component in the anterior-posterior direction is consistent with the neurophysiological knowledge on the retinotopic representation of the visual field in the primary visual cortex of man. Stimulus information presented to upper retinal areas is routed to cortical regions above the calcarine fissure, while lower retinal stimuli are represented in areas below the calcarine fissure. In terms of scalp topography of the potential fields this pattern of retinotopic projections is expected to result in a more posterior scalp location for components evoked by lower retinal stimuli presented at the same horizontal eccentricity.

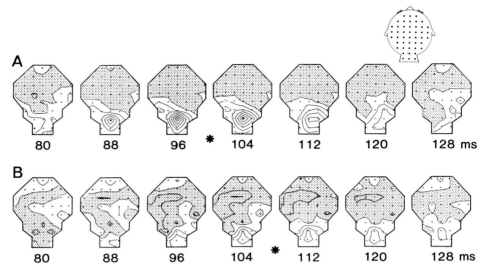

Fig. 3A, B. Topographical map series from 80 to 128 ms recorded from 45 channels evoked by upper (**A**) and lower (**B**) hemiretinal checkerboard reversal stimulation. Note differences in latency and scalp location of the evoked components (100 ms vs 108 ms; see *asterisks*). The electrode array covers the whole head as shown in the *inset; circled electrode* at inion; equipotential lines in steps of 1.0 µV; *dotted areas* negative with respect to the average reference

Additional topographical data obtained from another subject are illustrated in Fig. 3 showing potential fields as map series between 80 and 128 ms recorded from an array of 45 electrodes (see inset). The stimulus presented to the upper retina yields an occurrence time of maximal global field power of 100 ms, while the brain component evoked by the lower retinal stimulus has a latency of 108 ms (asterisks in Fig. 3).

Component location differences in the anterior-posterior direction can also be seen in Fig. 3. Thus, the influence of retinal stimulus location reflected in the evoked scalp potential field configurations is consistent with the neurophysiologically determined visual field representation in the primary visual cortex of man. In addition, such location differences could be confirmed in a study where intracranial and surface multichannel potential fields were recorded simultaneously in human patients (Lehmann et al. 1982).

The knowledge on latency differences between upper and lower hemiretinal stimuli revealed by measurements of global field power has some direct practical implications. A major clinical application of VEP measurements is the establishment of damage to the optic nerve, where no other symptomatic quantification is possible. Prolongation of VEP latency of only a few milliseconds may result in a pathological classification. In a study on 325 patients suspected of multiple sclerosis, Skrandies (1987) has shown that the existing physiological differences between upper and lower retinal areas may be accompanied by a dramatic increase of false-negative classifications (i.e., pathological cases become classified as normal).

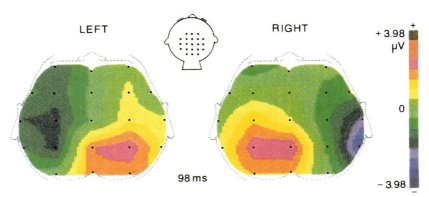

Fig. 4. Scalp potential fields evoked by lateralized checkerboard reversal stimuli at time of component latency (98 ms). (Circular stimulus field of 16° diameter, 50' checks, 96% contrast, two reversals per second.) Lateral hemiretinal stimulation yields potential fields with potential maxima over the hemisphere contralateral to the hemiretina stimulated. Note mirror-image distribution patterns for left and right hemiretinal stimuli. For electrode array and voltage scale see *inset;* same convention as in Fig. 1. (Data were collected with a Biologic Brain Atlas III; courtesy M. Capaul and D. Lehmann)

Stimuli in the left and right visual half-fields are routed to the visual cortex of the contralateral hemisphere. Thus, with lateral hemiretinal stimulation one would expect a lateralization of the electrical brain activity toward the hemisphere ipsilateral to the hemiretina stimulated. However, with checkerboard reversal stimuli a so-called paradoxical lateralization of the evoked potential activity has been described repeatedly (Barrett et al. 1976; Lehmann and Skrandies 1979b; Skrandies 1981). Asymmetrical occipital scalp field distributions are elicited by lateralized hemiretinal checkerboard reversal stimuli as illustrated in Fig. 4. This figure displays scalp potential fields at times of maximal global field power evoked by left (Fig. 4 left) or right (Fig. 4, right) hemiretinal checkerboard reversal stimuli. Stimulation of the left hemiretinal areas is followed by a P100 component with a potential field maximum over the right occiput, while right hemiretinal stimuli produce electrical brain activity lateralized over the left hemisphere as illustrated in Fig. 4 for the potential fields at the times of maximal global field power. We also note that an identical component latency of 98 ms results for both left and right hemiretinal visual stimuli. The equipotential lines in the field distributions are oriented in such a way that potential gradients result which are steepest over the hemisphere ipsilateral to the hemiretina stimulated. The scalp distributions evoked by left and right hemiretinal stimulation appear to be symmetrical to each other with respect to the midline. When potential gradients, and not potential maxima, in the scalp fields are assumed to be indicative of the localization of intracerebral neuronal generators, then these scalp potential distributions are consistent with the interpretation of a correct intracerebral lateralization of the electrical brain activity. Model dipole computations on multichannel (45 channels) evoked potential fields obtained in a population of six healthy subjects as well as intracerebral recordings in human patients confirmed that the neuronal generators were most likely located in the occipital areas of the hemisphere ipsilateral to the hemiretina stimulated (Lehmann et al. 1982).

In addition, we could show that the degree of lateralization depends on the lateral extension of the visual stimulus on the retina. Scalp potential fields of a subject population recorded from 45 electrodes elicited by lateralized large (26° arc diameter) or small (13° arc diameter) checkerboard reversal stimuli were decomposed by a spatial principle components analysis (spatial PCA, see Skrandies and Lehmann 1982b). This spatial PCA yielded three basic scalp potential field distributions which accounted for 93.4% of the variance in the data. This means that the original 45-channel recordings may be reconstructed with an error of less than 7% by using only three components which were defined by the spatial PCA as basic field distributions. One of these components displayed a lateralized potential field configuration, and it was related to retinal stimulus location. The contribution of this laterality component to the potential fields showed a systematic and statistically significant covariation with the size and eccentricity of the visual target. With smaller stimuli the amount of lateralization was smaller than with large stimuli which showed a paradoxical lateralization. Thus, potential field maxima at component latencies around 100 ms tended to be located close to the sagittal midline with 13° arc stimuli, while with larger stimuli we observed a lateralization towards the hemisphere contralateral to the hemiretina stimulated. In this study we also demonstrated that with visual stimuli presented in the center the component score on the laterality component was near zero, supporting the notion that this component reflects retinal stimulus lateralization (Skrandies and Lehmann 1982b).

Such more detailed topographical analyses show that the features of the electrical scalp field configurations are consistent with the neuroanatomical projection of the retina onto the primary visual cortex. Lateralized stimuli near to the midline activate neural structures close to the occipital pole of the hemisphere, while peripheral visual stimuli also activate medial parts of the calcarine fissure. With the net activity of neuronal generator populations oriented toward the contralateral hemisphere, one would expect a more pronounced paradoxical lateralization of potential field maxima for large than for small visual targets. This confirms that our scalp potential field data (Skrandies and Lehmann 1982b), as well as the above-mentioned intracerebral recordings (Lehmann et al. 1982), are in good agreement with the neurophysiological representation of the visual field in the primary visual cortex of man.

Topographical Correlates of Stimulus Characteristics: Presentation Mode

Changes of physical stimulus parameters also have some effect on the features of evoked electrical brain activity. In earlier studies we have described scalp

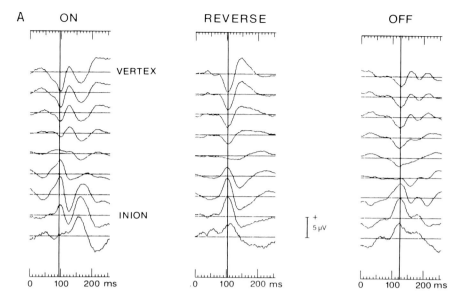
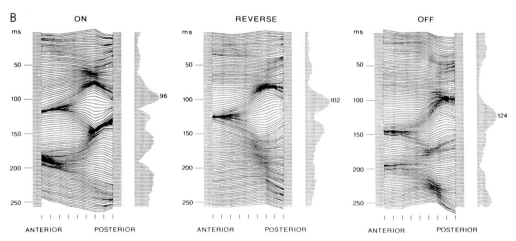

Fig. 5. **A** Potential waveshapes recorded from a row of nine electrodes along the midline between the vertex (*first trace*) and 7% below the inion. A checkerboard pattern with 30′ checks was presented as onset, reversal, or offset stimulus. Average reference data. Time of maximal global field power denoted by *vertical lines*. **B** Data of **A** shown topographically as a series of potential profiles constructed between 5 and 255 ms after stimulation (*time runs from top to bottom*). Global field power is plotted adjacent to each profile series. Note topographical differences between presentation modes and different occurrence times of maximal global field power. For further discussion of these data refer to Skrandies (1987)

potential fields elicited by different presentation modes of the identical visual stimulus (Skrandies et al. 1980; Skrandies 1984b, 1987) or by dynamic random-dot patterns containing horizontal disparities (Skrandies and Vomberg 1985). When a checkerboard pattern is presented as a pattern onset (appearance), pattern offset (disappearance) or contrast reversal stimulus without any temporal mean luminance changes in these three conditions, the electrical brain activity shows interesting differences in both latency and scalp location of the evoked components. By computing cross-correlation functions of multichannel waveshape patterns referred to the average reference, Skrandies (1987) found that the features of pattern reversal evoked activity cannot be predicted on the basis of onset and offset activity. The cross-correlation functions illustrated that the onset and offset activity were both more similar to the computed mean response [(onset + offset)/2] than was the reversal activity (see Table 3 of Skrandies 1987). This indicates that contrast reversal activity is not simply the summation of local onset and offset activity. Further analysis of scalp distribution data as series of potential profiles along the sagittal midline revealed additional differences between the brain activity elicited by the different presentation modes.

Figure 5A illustrates potential waveshapes evoked by the onset, offset or contrast reversal of the identical checkerboard pattern (8.7 by 11.4° arc test field; 30' arc checksize; 62% contrast) presented at a constant mean luminance of 13.6 cd/m^2. The major component for all stimulus presentation modes in Fig. 5 is an occipital positivity which occurs at about 100 ms after stimulation, and there appear systematic differences in component latency (see vertical lines drawn at times of maximal global field power). This finding is also reflected by the plots of global field power as a function of time in Fig. 5B, which displays the same data as series of potential profiles. Potential profiles were constructed at each time point by entering each potential value at the respective electrode position. Thus, this data display presents the scalp potential fields as a function of successive post-stimulus time points. Time runs from top to bottom in Fig. 5B while scalp location runs from right to left.

The major features of the scalp potential fields elicited by various stimulus presentation modes appeared to be very similar (Fig. 5B). In the profile series one can see that during the first 50 ms flat potential distributions prevail, and then a positivity surrounded by steep gradients develops, reaching its maximum at 96 ms for onset, at 102 ms for reversal, and at 124 ms for offset stimuli. The amount of electrical activity at each instant was computed as global field power, which is plotted adjacent to each profile series, and reaches its maximum at different times. Such differences in component latency between presentation modes are a consistent finding. Statistically significant differences in component latency were found in a population of 13 adults with onset stimuli yielding shorter values (mean over 13 subjects 94.2 ms) than reversal stimuli (mean over 13 subjects 108.1 ms) or offset stimuli (mean over 13 subjects 124.0 ms). We also note that the latency difference between reversal and offset achieved statistical significance. In addition, significantly smaller component latencies for upper than lower retinal stimuli were obtained for all presentation modes (see Skrandies 1987 for a complete discussion of the data). These findings indicate that the above-mentioned physiological and functional difference between upper

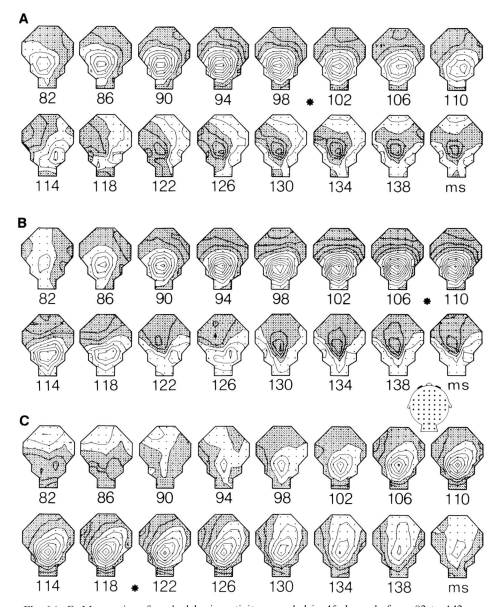

Fig. 6A–C. Map series of evoked brain activity recorded in 45 channels from 82 to 142 ms. Different presentation modes of an identical checkerboard pattern yield different occurrence times of maximal global field power as denoted by *asterisks* (**A** onset, 98 ms component latency; **B** contrast reversal, 106 ms component latency; **C** offset presentation mode, 118 ms component latency). The electrode array covers the whole head as shown in *inset*, circled electrode at inion; equipotential lines in steps of 1.0 μV; *dotted areas* negative with respect to the average reference

and lower retinal areas is a global result independent of stimulus presentation mode.

Although the same major features are present in each profile series, there are distinct differences in component location, which changes with presentation mode. In Fig. 5B one may see that the potential maximum for onset is anterior to that evoked by reversal or offset stimuli. Such differences were again statistically confirmed in a population of 13 subjects, and all component locations were shown to be significantly different from each other (Skrandies 1987). Onset produced components located most anteriorly on the scalp (mean over 13 subjects 5.14 cm above the inion), followed by reversal components (mean over 13 subjects 2.05 cm above the inion), while offset components were located at the inion. All of the component location differences were statistically significant (see Table 2 of Skrandies 1987 for details).

Further support for the notion that different neuronal generating mechanisms are activated by different presentation modes stems from additional experiments. Complete scalp potential fields evoked by different presentation modes are illustrated in Fig. 6. Evoked brain activity was recorded from 45 electrodes, and is shown as map series of scalp potential fields from 82 to 142 ms. Checkerboard pattern onset (Fig. 6A), reversal (Fig. 6B) and offset (Fig. 6C) yield comparable scalp distributions with an occipital positivity occurring around 100 ms. Global field power reaches its maximum (denoted by asterisks in Fig. 6) at different times after stimulation, and differences in component latency similar to those described above can be seen in these maps illustrating the complete scalp potential fields (onset 98 ms; reversal 106 ms; offset 118 ms).

These electrophysiological data suggest that differently located or oriented neuronal generator populations are activated when the same visual stimulus occurs in different presentation modes. The latency differences between onset and offset stimuli are in line with earlier psychophysical studies which demonstrated significantly shorter motor reaction times to onset than to offset stimuli (e.g., Bartlett et al. 1968).

Topographical Correlates of Stimulus Characteristics: Spatial Frequency

Visual stimuli of different spatial frequencies are believed to be analyzed in parallel channels of the human visual system (e.g., Blakemore and Campbell 1969). Experiments on the functional morphology of the cat visual cortex showed that there is a regular arrangement of assemblies of neurones selectively tuned to different spatial frequencies (Tootell et al. 1981) similar to the well-known ocularity and orientation columns of the visual cortex described by Hubel and Wiesel (1959, 1962). Selective activation of different neuronal structures may result in different spatial patterns of scalp potential distributions, and electrical brain activity elicited by grating stimuli of different spatial frequency and orientation was studied in detail. Figure 7 presents a series of topographical maps between 90 and 126 ms after the time of contrast reversal evoked by vertical gratings of different spatial frequencies. The general feature in the map series is an occipital positivity occurring around 100 ms latency. Times of maximal global field power (denoted by asterisks in Fig. 7) appear to change systematically with increasing spatial frequency. Gratings with a spatial frequency of 1.15 cycles/degree (c/d) and 2.3 c/d (Fig. 7A, B) have a component latency of 100 ms, while stimuli of higher spatial frequency yield larger component latencies. With 4.6 c/d a latency of 112 ms results (Fig. 7C), and with a stimulus of 9.2 c/d latency increases to 116 ms (Fig. 7D). This change of component latency with changing spatial frequency was a consistent finding in a population of 12 subjects studied in detail (Skrandies 1984a). With low spatial frequencies of 1.15 c/d and 2.3 c/d the latency values were the shortest and were comparable. All other statistical comparisons testing the latency increase caused by higher spatial frequencies were highly significant.

The scalp potential fields showed also some changes with different spatial frequencies: With increasing spatial frequency the strength of the evoked brain response decreased significantly. When comparing the maps obtained at times of maximal global field power in Fig. 7 it is obvious that the packing density of the equipotential lines is different. With low spatial frequencies (1.15 c/d and 2.3 c/d) the maps display a potential range of 6.75 µV in the potential field, while a spatial frequency of 4.6 c/d produces only 5.25 µV, and with the highest spatial frequency, potential fields with only 3.0 µV potential range result.

On the other hand, there appear no differences in component location in the map series shown in Fig. 7A–D. The occipital potential maximum occurs for all stimulus conditions at the same electrode in the midline, concentrically surrounded by steep, negative, potential gradients. This was a common finding in a population of 12 subjects (see Skrandies 1984a for details).

The scalp recorded data thus suggest that the topography of the evoked electrical brain component does not change with variation of spatial frequency. This negative result may be explained by data from animal experiments. As is known from the morphological study by Tootell et al. (1981), spatial frequency columns in the cat visual cortex are only about 1 mm wide, and scalp recordings might simply not be sensitive enough to detect such subtle differences. In addition, each part of the visual field must be analyzed by functional modules of cortical neurones simultaneously in various spatial frequency channels. Thus, the recording of mass activity must not be expected to allow the distinction of separate subunits within these small functional neuronal modules.

The data presented showed effects of spatial frequency mainly on component latency, which increased with increasing spatial frequency of a grating stimulus. This finding is in agreement with psychophysical studies by Breitmeyer (1975) and Lupp et al. (1976), who reported that motor reaction time also depends on the spatial frequency of a visual stimulus. In addition, contrast sensitivity measured psychophysically also decreases with increasing spatial frequency (cf. Skrandies 1985). Larger component latencies and a decrease in global field power appear to be the electrophysiological reflection of a reduced efficiency in processing visual stimuli of high spatial frequency.

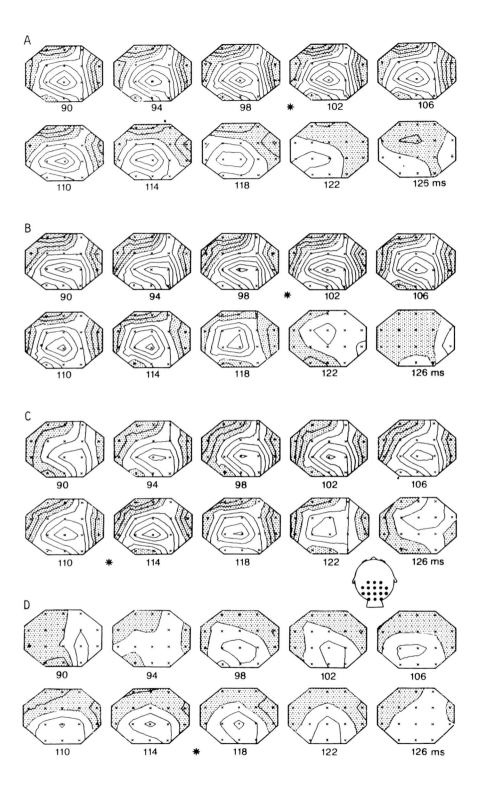

Topographical Correlates of Stimulus Characteristics: Stereoscopic Stimuli

The half-field data given in the section on the effect of stimulus location suggest that the P100 component of the VEP is of cortical origin. Those scalp distributions displayed covariations with stimulus field size which are consistent with the anatomical geometry of the cortical representation of different retinal areas.

Studies using visual stimuli which must be processed at the level of the visual cortex further support the notion of a cortical origin of the P100 component. With dynamic random-dot stereograms (RDS) a visual target can only be perceived when the two monocular RDS stimuli are binocularly fused. The only stimulus information is contained in the horizontal disparity of the input to the two eyes. This binocular fusion of horizontally disparate stimuli crucial for depth perception takes place only at the level of the visual cortex (cf. Julesz 1971), and Skrandies and Vomberg (1985) showed that similar electrical brain activity was elicited by dynamic RDS stimuli and binocular stimuli containing contrast borders. The evoked potential data presented in Fig. 8A and B prove that the RDS stimuli exclusively activate neuronal structures concerned with depth perception. When the stimulus is viewed binocularly, the horizontal disparity information is processed in such a way that a stereoscopic percept results. This is accompanied by the stimulus time locked electrical brain activity shown in Fig. 8A. Under monocular viewing conditions the subject perceives only dynamic random noise, and changes in horizontal disparity which occur at time 0 do not produce evoked potential activity (Fig. 8B). Further support for interpreting the evoked brain activity of Fig. 8A as a neuronal correlate of depth perception stems from a study on patients with pathologically reduced stereovision. In an earlier study we demonstrated that the perceptual reduction of stereoscopic vision is paralleled by changes in the evoked electrical brain activity (Vomberg and Skrandies 1985), and disparity perception thresholds determined psychophysically correlated highly with those determined by electrophysiological recordings.

The neuronal processing of horizontal disparity information depends on intact binocularity and the activation of cortical detectors of disparate retinal images. It appears of major interest to know whether binocular processing and perception of depth is performed by the same or by different neuronal generator populations. In order to test this question we compared scalp potential fields evoked by dynamic RDS stimuli (containing only disparity information) with those evoked by binocular stimuli which contain contrast borders. The size

---

Fig. 7 A–D. Scalp potential fields between 90 and 126 ms evoked by vertical grating stimuli of different spatial frequencies (**A** 1.15 c/d; **B** 2.3 c/d; **C** 4.6 c/d; **D** 9.2 c/d). Occurrence times of evoked components are marked by *asterisks*, and latency changes with different spatial frequencies are apparent. Recordings from 16 scalp electrodes referred to the average reference (see *head schema*); equipotential lines in steps of 0.75 µV; *dotted areas* negative with respect to the average reference. For further discussion of these data refer to Skrandies (1984a)

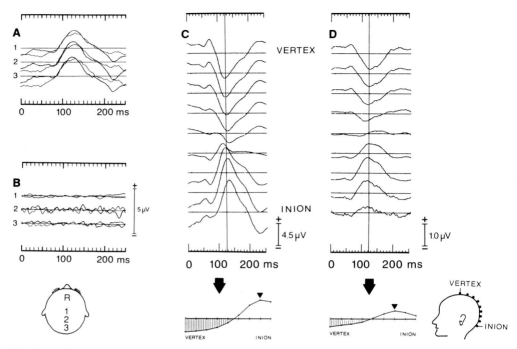

Fig. 8. A Electrical brain activity recorded from three occipital electrodes in the midline referred to a frontal reference electrode (see *head schema below*). Dynamic RDS stimuli were modulated in depth, and a binocular viewing condition repeatedly evokes an occipital component (compare *superimposed traces*). **B** Same recording and stimulus condition as in **A**, but with monocular stimulation, illustrating that the dynamic RDS stimulus contains no monocular cues (no stimulus-related activity can be recorded). **C** Grand mean potential waveshapes of 15 subjects evoked by a binocular checkerboard stimulus containing contrast borders. *Vertical line* at the time of maximal global field power; the corresponding potential profile at component latency is shown *below*. Average reference data were recorded from a midline row of nine electrodes equidistantly spaced between the vertex and 5 mm above the inion (see *head schema on the right*). **D** Grand mean potential waveshapes of 15 subjects evoked by a stereoscopic checkerboard stimulus displayed as dynamic RDS stimulus. *Vertical line*, time of maximal global field power; the corresponding potential profile at component latency is shown *below*. Average reference data were recorded from a midline row of nine electrodes equidistantly spaced between the vertex and 5 mm above the inion (see *head schema on the right*)

as well as the mean luminance of the stimuli was identical for both recording conditions. In a population of 15 healthy volunteers we recorded electrical brain activity elicited either by a checkerboard pattern reversing in depth or by the contrast reversal of a comparable binocularly viewed checkerboard pattern. Both stimulus conditions yielded, as a major feature, occipital positive components with similar latencies. However, with stereoscopic stimuli component amplitudes were much smaller than with conventional binocular contrast stimuli, as illustrated by the grand mean data in Fig. 8C and D. This difference in amplitude was statistically significant in the subject population (0.74 µV vs 3.32 µV; $t = 8.14$, $p < 0.0005$). The result suggests that in the human visual cortex

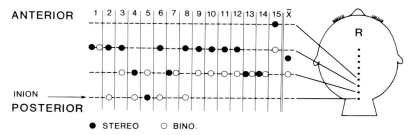

Fig. 9. Scalp locations in the anterior-posterior direction on the scalp of components evoked by binocular contrast stimuli (*open circles*) or by comparable stereoscopic stimuli (*dots*). Individual data of 15 subjects and mean locations are given

fewer neurones are activated synchronously by the stereoscopic stimulus, which displays only horizontal disparity information, than by a comparable stimulus consisting of contrast borders.

The scalp topography of the stereoscopically evoked brain activity showed some interesting features. Both RDS stimuli and binocular contrast stimuli were followed by an occipital positivity around 100 ms latency. There were, however, small but statistically significant differences in component location which are obvious in the potential profiles contructed at the times of maximal global field power (Fig. 8C, D). In most of the 15 subjects the potential maximum evoked by stereoscopic stimuli was located further anterior than that evoked in the binocular contrast condition. Figure 9 summarizes the component locations at individual times of maximal global field power, giving for both stimulus conditions the maximum location along the sagittal midline for each of the 15 subjects. The occipital positivity for stereoscopic stimuli was located further anterior on the scalp (mean 4.25 cm above the inion) than that elicited in the binocular contrast condition (mean 2.45 cm above the inion). A mean difference of 1.80 cm resulted which was statistically significant ($t = 3.59$, $p < 0.0025$). Further analysis of the data revealed that differences in component location were not restricted to the occurrence times of the components. The scalp locations of potential maxima and minima were analyzed in detail over the whole recording epoch (Skrandies 1986). Significant differences in scalp location of the potential maxima and minima between stereoscopic and contrast evoked electrical brain activity were established by computing paired t tests. The results suggest that the time course of the neuronal activation patterns is similar in both conditions while their topography is different: both potential maxima and minima have significantly different locations over longer time periods (Skrandies 1986). These data indicate that the complete neuronal activation cycle is different in the two experimental conditions, suggesting sustained differences in the activation of nonidentical neuronal generator populations.

The differences in scalp topography prove that differently located (or oriented) neuronal generator populations are activated by dynamic RDS stimuli. Such a result is consistent with single-unit recordings in the visual cortex of monkeys, where neurones were found which were activated by horizontal disparities. Hubel and Wiesel (1970) and von der Heydt et al. (1981) reported that the visual area 18 contained more neurons which were depth-sensitive than the primary visual cortex (area 17). In man, area 18 lies anterior to area 17, and our results are in line with the interpretation that also in man, area 18 is more involved in depth perception than the primary visual cortex when visual stimuli with horizontal disparity are viewed binocularly.

Higher Visual Information Processing: Topography of Cognitive Components

With more demanding tasks, cognitive processes may be investigated using event-related electrical activity. Endogenous components of evoked activity are defined by their covariation with internal stimulus-processing mechanisms (Donchin et al. 1978). Such components of electrical brain activity may be related to aspects of perceptual and cognitive events which must be defined by strictly controlled behavioral tasks.

Topographical analysis techniques have been used to relate evoked components to aspects of higher visual information processing (Skrandies 1983; Skrandies et al. 1984). Evoked potential data were collected in 16 channels during the performance of a visual information processing task, and components were related to factors such as attention, relevance of the stimulus, and the probability of occurrence of a task-relevant stimulus. Chapman et al. (1979) and Skrandies (1983) give a detailed description of the basic experimental design. Each stimulus was made task-relevant or task-irrelevant by instruction, and visual stimuli were presented randomly and independently in different retinal locations. Scalp potential fields evoked by expected, task-relevant stimuli are illustrated in Fig. 10 as map series from 16 ms before stimulus presentation to 688 ms after stimulus presentation. The relevant stimulus occurred either in the center (Fig. 10B) or on the left (Fig. 10A) or on the right (Fig. 10C) hemiretina. Early times at or before stimulus presentation show potential field configurations with negative extreme values. Such a component reflects a contingent negative variation (Walter et al. 1964) indexing expectancy, and it is not evoked by unexpected irrelevant stimuli (Skrandies 1983). Latencies corresponding to the P100 activity show scalp potential fields which are lateralized when task-relevant stimuli were presented to the left or right hemiretina (Note that at 112 ms latency maps are mirror images in Fig. 10A and C). At later times, beyond

Fig. 10A–C. Series of scalp fields evoked by task-relevant visual stimuli presented in the center (**B**), or on the left (**A**) and right (**C**) hemiretina between between 16 ms before and 688 ms after stimulus presentation. Times before and at stimulus presentation display CNV activity; late times are dominated by positive components. Note changes in field configurations with different retinal stimulus locations. Recordings in 16 channels referred to the average reference (see *head schema*); equipotential lines in steps of 1.0 µV; *dotted areas* negative with respect to the average reference. *Negative numbers* refer to times before stimulus presentation, *positive numbers* give latencies after stimulus occurrence (both in milliseconds)

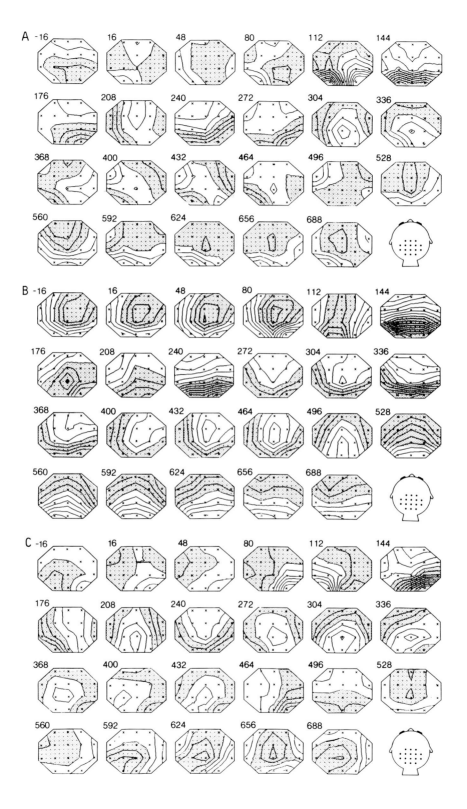

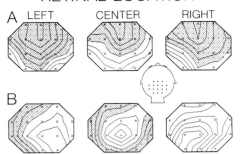

Fig. 11 A, B. Scalp field distributions of a P300 component identified by a principle components analysis. Values in the fields refer to component scores related to different experimental conditions

300 ms, the scalp fields are dominated by relative positivities. These late positive components are evoked only by task-relevant stimuli which had to be discriminated and categorized by the subjects. The behavior of the late positive components across experimental conditions was consistent with the data on P300 and "slow wave" components reported in the literature (see Skrandies 1983 for a detailed discussion).

Among other components, the P300 component was also derived from a PCA performed on the raw data consisting of 3072 evoked potentials. The scalp distributions of its component scores elicited in six different experimental conditions are illustrated in Fig. 11. It is obvious that visual stimuli which were irrelevant for the task, and thus presumably were ignored by the subject, are not followed by a P300 component (Fig. 11 A). On the other hand, with task-relevant, attended to stimuli a potential field results with a maximal positivity over parietal areas (Fig. 11 B). A surprising finding of these experiments was that the topographic distribution of the P300 component was influenced by the retinal location of the stimulus. Figure 11 illustrates the potential fields for stimuli presented in the center and on the left or right retina. Relevant central stimuli yield a positive, concentric parietal distribution while relevant, lateralized stimuli also produce peaks in the midline but there are hemispheric differences with a relative positivity over the hemisphere contralateral to the hemiretina stimulated (Fig. 11 B). The potential gradients are steeper toward the ipsilateral hemisphere, as is plain when comparing the distributions in Fig. 11 B. We also note that the lateralization of the P300 component scores derived from a PCA is in very good agreement with the original potential fields shown in Fig. 10. The P300 activity occurs in Fig. 10 with latencies of 336 and 368 ms. The potential fields evoked by lateralized task-relevant stimuli of Fig. 10 show the same topographical features as the component scores.

These findings on the topography of P300 do not support the general notion that this component is independent of the physical stimulus parameters. Due to the retinotopic representation of the visual field at several cortical processing areas (van Essen 1985), high-level visual information processing is also influenced by the location of the stimulus on the retina, and it appears conceivable that the P300 component does not exclusively index specific task-related information processing.

Summary and Conclusion

Visual stimuli are followed by electrical activity that can be recorded from the occipital areas overlying the visual cortex. The present paper illustrates how the scalp topography of VEPs is affected by various physical stimulus conditions as well as by higher processes related to visual information processing.

Half-field stimuli presented in the upper, lower, right or left visual field elicit electrical brain activity in different parts of the visual cortex consistent with predictions based on neuroanatomical knowledge. Conclusions derived from scalp topography could also be confirmed with intracranial recordings in human patients. In addition, comparison of component latencies evoked by upper or lower hemiretinal stimuli yields evidence of a functional superiority of the upper over the lower retinal system.

Analysis of VEP topography following the presentation of an identical checkerboard pattern as *pattern onset, pattern offset, or pattern reversal* gives some evidence that different neuronal generator structures are activated when different presentation modes are used. With grating stimuli of different *spatial frequency* the basic topographic pattern of the activity remains constant while there are significant effects on component latency and amplitude.

Stereoscopic random dot stimuli evoke electrical brain activity at the level of the visual cortex, and it is shown that the classical P100 component is of cortical origin. In addition, evidence is presented that neurones processing binocular disparity information form a distinct class which is different from contrast-sensitive cortical structures which are also activated binocularly.

Multichannel recordings obtained during the performance of an information-processing task illustrate the scalp topography of *cognitive evoked components* related to information processing. Late cognitive components can be influenced not only by internal steps in information processing but also by physical stimulus parameters such as the location of the stimulus on the retina.

The topographic analysis strategies described are transparent and easy to apply, and they yield directly quantitative measures on component latency (times of maximal global field power) and scalp topography. Measures like location of maxima and minima and location and orientation of potential gradients are reference-independent characteristics of the scalp field distributions. Such derived values can then be used to compare statistically electrical brain activitiy elicited by different experimental and subject conditions.

The combination of topographical information on electrical brain activity and knowledge on the physiological processing mechanisms of the human visual system is a powerful experimental tool in the study of visual perception of man.

References

Barrett G, Blumhardt L, Halliday, AM Halliday, E Kriss, A (1976) A paradox in the lateralization of the visual evoked response. Nature 261:253–255

Bartlett NR, Sticht TG, Pease VP (1968) Effects of wavelength and retinal locus on the reaction time to onset and offset stimulation. J Exp Psychol 78:699–701

Blakemore C, Campbell FW (1969) On the existence of neurones in the human visual system selectively sensitive to the orientation and size of retinal images. J Physiol (Lond) 203:237–260

Breitmeyer BG (1975) Simple reaction time as a measure of the temporal response properties of transient and sustained channels. Vision Res 15:1411–1412

Chapman RM, McCrary JW, Bragdon HR, Chapman JA (1979) Latent components of event-related potentials functionally related to information processing. In: Desmedt JE (ed) Progress in clinical neurophysiology, vol 6. Karger, Basel, pp 80–105

Donchin E, Ritter W, McCallum WC (1978) Cognitive psychophysiology: the endogenous components of the ERP. In: Callaway E, Tueting P, Koslow SH (eds) Event-related potentials in man. Academic, New York, pp 349–411

Hubel DH, Wiesel TN (1959) Receptive fields of single neurones in the cat's striate cortex. J Physiol (Lond) 148:574–591

Hubel DH, Wiesel TN (1962) Receptive fields, binocular interaction and functional architecture in the cat's visual cortex. J Physiol (Lond) 160:106–154

Hubel DH, Wiesel TN (1970) Cells sensitive to binocular depth in area 18 of the macaque monkey cortex. Nature 225:41–42

Julesz B (1971) Foundations of cyclopean perception. University of Chicago Press, Chicago, p 406

Kavanagh RN, Darcey TM, Lehmann D, Fender DH (1978) Evaluation of methods for three-dimensional localization of electrical sources in the human brain. IEEE Trans Biomed Eng 25:421–429

Lehmann D (1972) Human scalp EEG fields: evoked, alpha, sleep and spike-wave patterns. In: Petsche HH, Brazier MAB (eds) Synchronization of EEG activity in epilepsies. Springer, Wien, pp 307–325

Lehmann D, Skrandies W (1979a) Multichannel evoked potential fields show different properties of human upper and lower hemiretinal systems. Exp Brain Res 35:151–159

Lehmann D, Skrandies W (1979b) Multichannel mapping of spatial distributions of scalp potential fields evoked by checkerboard reversal to different retinal areas. In: Lehmann D, Callaway E (eds) Human evoked potentials: applications and problems. Plenum, New York, pp 201–214

Lehmann D, Skrandies W (1980) Reference-free identification of components of checkerboard – evoked multichannel potential fields. Electroencephalogr Clin Neurophysiol 48:609–621

Lehmann D, Skrandies W (1984) Spatial analysis of evoked potentials in man: a review. Prog Neurobiol 23:227–250

Lehmann D, Darcey TM, Skrandies W (1982) Intracerebral and scalp fields evoked by hemiretinal checkerboard reversal, and modelling of their dipole generators. In: Courjon J, Maugiere F, Revol M (eds) Clinical applications of evoked potentials in neurology. Raven, New York, pp 41–48

Lehmann G, Meles HP, Mir Z (1977) Average multichannel EEG potential fields evoked from upper and lower hemiretina: latency differences. Electroencephalogr Clin Neurophysiol 43:725–731

Lupp K, Hauske G, Wolf W (1976) Perceptual latencies to sinusoidal gratings. Vision Res 16:969–972

Nunez P (1981) Electric fields of the brain. Oxford University Press, New York

Sidman RD, Giambalvo V, Allison T, Bergey P (1978) A method for localization of sources of human cerebral potentials evoked by sensory stimuli. Sensory Proc 2:116–129

Skrandies W (1981) Latent components of potentials evoked by visual stimuli in different retinal locations. Int J Neurosci 14:77–84

Skrandies W (1983) Information processing and evoked potentials: topography of early and late components. Adv Biol Psychiatry 13:1–12

Skrandies W (1984a) Scalp potential fields evoked by grating stimuli: effects of spatial frequency and orientation. Electroencephalogr Clin Neurophysiol 58:325–332

Skrandies W (1984b) Differences of visual evoked potential latencies and topographies depending on retinal location and presentation mode. Pflügers Arch 400:31

Skrandies W (1985) Human contrast sensitivity: reginal retinal differences. Hum Neurobiol 4:95–97

Skrandies W (1986) Visual evoked potential topography: methods and results. In: Duffy FH (ed) Topographic mapping of brain electrical activity. Butterworths, Boston, pp 7–28

Skrandies W (1987) The upper and lower visual field of man: electrophysiological and functional differences. In: Ottoson D (ed) Progress in sensory physiology, vol 8. Springer, Berlin Heidelberg New York Tokyo, pp 1–93

Skrandies W, Lehmann D (1982a) Occurrence time and scalp location of components of evoked EEG potential fields. In: Herrmann WM (ed) Electroencephalography in drug research. Fischer, Stuttgart, pp 183–192

Skrandies W, Lehmann D (1982b) Spatial principal components of multichannel maps evoked by lateral visual half – field stimuli. Electroencephalogr Clin Neurophysiol 54:662–667

Skrandies W, Vomberg HE (1985) Stereoscopic stimuli activate different cortical neurones in man: electrophysiological evidence. Int J Psychophysiol 2:293–296

Skrandies W, Wässle H, Peichl L (1978) Are field potentials an appropriate method for demonstrating connections in the brain? Exp Neurol 60:509–521

Skrandies W, Richter M, Lehmann D (1980) Checkerboard evoked potentials: topography and latency for onset, offset, and reversal. Prog Brain Res 54:291–295

Skrandies W, Chapman RM, McCrary JW, Chapman JA (1984) Distribution of latent components related to information processing. Ann NY Acad Sci 425:271–277

Tootell RB, Silverman MS, De Valois RL (1981) Spatial frequency columns in primary visual cortex. Science 214:813–815

van Essen DC (1985) Functional organization of primate visual cortex. In: Peters A, Jones EG (eds) Cerebral cortex, vol 3. Plenum, New York, pp 259–329

Vomberg HE, Skrandies W (1985) Untersuchung des Stereosehens im Zufallspunktmuster-VECP: Normbefunde und klinische Anwendung. Klin Monatsbl Augenheilkd 187:205–208

von der Heydt R, Hänni P, Dürsteler M, Peterhans E (1981) Neuronal responses to stereoscopic stimuli in the alert monkey – a comparison between striate and prestriate cortex. Pflügers Arch 391:34

von Helmholtz H (1853) Über einige Gesetze der Vertheilung elektrischer Ströme in körperlichen Leitern, mit Anwendung auf die thierelektrischen Versuche. Ann Phys Chemie 29:211–233, 253–377

Walter WG, Cooper R, Aldridge VJ, McCallum WC, Winter AL (1964) Contingent negative variation: an electric sign of sensorimotor association and expectancy in the human brain. Nature 203:380–384

Localization of the Visually Evoked Response: The Pattern Appearance Response

B.W. VAN DIJK and H. SPEKREIJSE[1]

Introduction

It is not possible to find the sources of evoked potentials (EPs) or EEG activity unless it is known *how many sources* exist and what their *character* (e.g., monopoles or multipoles) might be. In this paper a method is described that determines the dimensionality of the response space and subsequently uses the spatial information contained by the distribution of the response components over the electrodes to obtain the positions and strengths of the generating sources.

We will use the visually evoked potential (VEP), in particular the pattern onset VEP, as an example to explain the method, which, however, is applicable to any set of responses (electrical or magnetical) recorded from the scalp.

Source Localization

Figure 1 shows the VEPs recorded at 24 scalp electrodes upon a pattern-onset stimulus. The electrodes were placed in horizontal rows, each row 3 cm apart; the distance between electrodes in each row was also 3 cm. A reference electrode was placed at the frontal midline. The responses were bandpass-filtered (0.3 and 70 Hz). The subject viewed a TV monitor with a mean illumination strength of 600 cd. m^{-2} subtending 8.4° × 8.4°. The pattern was a checkerboard which appeared and disappeared without illumination change in a 300/500 ms duty cycle. A time interval of 100 ms was selected from all 24 responses. The selected interval is depicted by the heavy lines in Fig. 1 and contains the first two dominant response peaks of the appearance response. The positive-negative-positive complex of the appearance response is generally described by three subsequent peaks denoted C_I, C_{II}, C_{III} respectively. From the figure it is, however, evident that the different peaks have different shapes and latencies at different electrodes, and therefore the activity cannot be described by a set of independent successive peaks and troughs. Our method aims to unravel the VEP in independent components which may be overlapping in space and time.

Principal Component Analysis

The first question to be answered is: "How many sources are minimally responsible for this set of 24 responses?" The answer to this question can be obtained

---

[1] The Netherlands Ophthalmic Research Institute PO Box 12141, 1100 AC Amsterdam-Zuidoost, The Netherlands

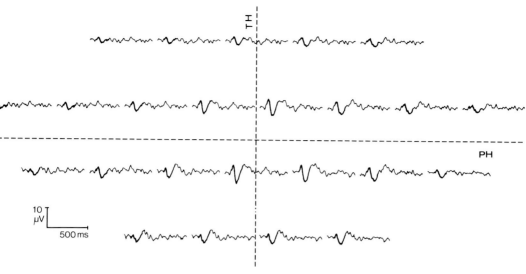

Fig. 1. Pattern appearance-disappearance responses from 24 electrode derivations represented topologically. The *heavy lines* indicate the time interval selected for analysis (79–179 ms). The axes represent the coordinate frame used in the contour plots of Figs. 3 and 4. The inion lies at phi = 0°, theta = −15°

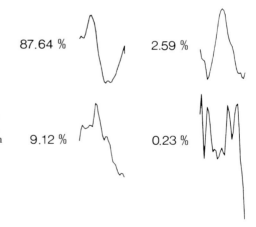

Fig. 2. The first four principal components found for the set of 24 responses of Fig. 1. The first two components suffice to explain more than 95% of the power as indicated by the numbers next to each component. Note that principal components are normalized time functions; as a result, the maximum amplitude of each principal component and its sign have no meaning

through principal component analysis (PCA). The outcome of PCA, a purely mathematical exercise, is a set of normalized time functions, a set of amplitude terms and a set of normalized distribution functions. The time functions are called principal components, the products of amplitude terms and distribution functions are called factor loadings. These sets have no meaning other than that they are the most efficient to represent the responses, i.e., the first n principal components explain at least as much of the power in the set of responses as any other set of n time functions and distributions. Since each EP recording necessarily contains noise, PCA immediately reveals how many principal components explain the significant variance.

Figure 2 shows the principal components found in our example, the numbers denoting the percentage of the power of the responses explained by the component. In this particular case the signal-to-noise ratio was approximately 19:1, so noise made up about 5% of the response power. Hence the first two principal components are sufficient to describe the response set; the others are buried in the noise. In other words PCA has shown that in our example we should look for at least two response components.

Dipole Distributions

The PCs found and their factor loadings do not necessarily represent these fundamental components. PCA has a mathematical rather than physiological basis.

In our method we obtain the underlying components using the spatial information in the set of responses, under the assumption that most cortical sources express themselves as mathematical point dipoles. De Munck and Spekreijse (this volume) have shown that such is true even if large cortical areas are activated.

If we succeed in finding linear combinations of the factor loading distributions of the principal components, which yield potential distributions that are in accordance with dipole sources, then we will have explained the significant power in the responses in terms of two dipole sources. In the time interval of the analysis the sources have a fixed position and orientation; their strength varies in time.

Figure 3 (left) depicts the factor loading distributions of the first two principal components in contour plots, as well as the best fitting dipole distributions. Two different combinations of these two distributions can be found that yield optimal fits to dipole distributions. With "optimal" we mean that the square deviation of each of the new factor loading distributions from a fitted dipolar potential distribution is minimal. These new distributions are depicted on the right of Fig. 3 together with the fitted dipole distributions.

The process of finding combinations of factor loadings is equivalent to performing a (non-rigid) body transformation, and we have termed it "rotation." Of course the time functions are also changed by the rotation process and a new set is obtained corresponding to the new set of distributions.

A detailed description of the mathematics involved can be found in Maier et al. (1987).

The Pattern Onset Response

We have applied the procedure described above to a set of pattern appearance/disappearance VEPs in order to test whether a given cortical area (e.g., primary

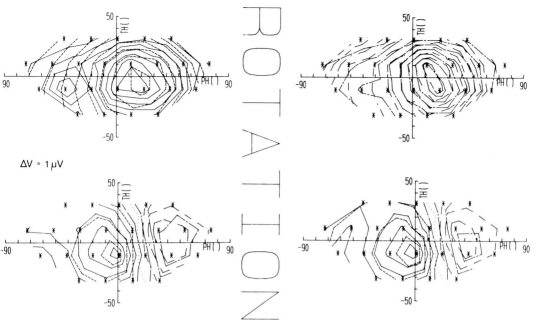

Fig. 3. *Left:* Contour plots of the factor loading distributions of the first (top) and the second (bottom) principal component. *Continuous lines* represent positive factor loading values, *dotted lines* zero values, and *dashed/dotted lines* negative values. Also shown are the best-fitting dipolar distributions, represented by *short dashed lines, long-short dashed lines* and *long dashed lines* for positive, zero, and negative potentials respectively. The distance between contours is 1 µV. *Right:* The contour plots of the two linear combinations of the factor loadings from Fig. 3 (left) that fitted mathematical dipole distributions. Details as in Fig. 3 (left)

visual cortex) contributes to the responses with the same expression regardless of eccentricity. The recording procedures are identical to those of the experiment in Fig. 1. The checkerboard pattern was restricted to the lower left quadrant of the visual field and covered the following range of eccentricities: 0°–1°, 1°–2°, 2°–4° and 4°–8°. The checksize was 12′ for the foveal stimulus and was adjusted in accordance with cortical magnification for the other eccentricities; the contrast was chosen such that the response amplitude was approximately 10 µV.

Figure 4 shows the results. For all eccentricities two components sufficed to describe the significant variance in the C_I–C_{II} interval. The time functions of the components are given by the inserts in the figure. For each eccentricity one component had a positive-negative shape while the other was negative only; we called them PC1 and PC2 respectively. The distributions over the electrodes of PC1 for the different eccentricities are depicted in the left column of Fig. 4, those of PC2 in the right column.

The distributions of the PC1 and PC2 components show a different dependence on eccentricity. For PC1 all distributions are from radial dipoles. The source moves upward and outward with increasing eccentricity, while the

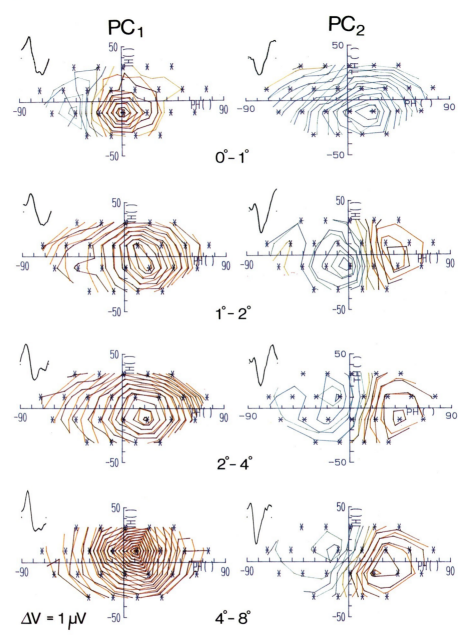

Fig. 4. Time functions and contour plots for the dipole source contributions that resulted from the procedure described in this paper for pattern appearance responses at different eccentricities in the visual field. Each row depicts the results for one eccentricity. The following stimulus parameters were employed: 0°–1°: 12' checksize, 30% contrast; 1°–2°: 24' checksize, 20% contrast; 2°–4°: 36' checksize, 20% contrast; 4°–8°: 55' checksize, 40% contrast. All stimuli were presented in the lower left quadrant of the visual field. The resulting time functions were either biphasic (PC1 with peak latencies of approximately 110 and 155 ms approx, *left*

strength of the contribution of PC1 to the variance changes hardly with eccentricity. For PC2 the source is radial for the most foveal stimulus, becomes tangential when eccentricity increases, and radial again but with different polarity for the largest eccentricity. The dipole moves only a little inward and upward. The strength of the contribution of PC2 to the total variance decreases with increasing eccentricity and the equivalent source lies deeper in the head.

The dependence of PC1 and PC2 on eccentricity is in complete agreement with the topologic representation of the visual field on the visual cortices. PC2 must originate in striate cortex, where the foveal projection lies on the occiput, while the periphery of the visual field projects to the medial wall. Assuming that the orientation of the equivalent dipole is at right angles with the surface of the activated cortex, this explains the rotation of the dipole orientation observed for PC2. The reoccurrence of radiality for the largest eccentricity indicates that part of the calcarine fissure is activated by that stimulus. It also explains the fixed position of the cortical source and why it moves deeper when eccentricity increases. PC1 must originate in extrastriate cortex, probably in area 18, which is rather unfolded and runs parallel to the cortical surface. In conclusion, the above analysis of the pattern-onset VEP as a function of eccentricity shows clearly that these responses cannot be described on the basis of their successive peaks and troughs. For example, our analysis reveals that the most marked negativity at about 100 ms after pattern onset (C_{II}) contains contributions from two cortical regions.

Reference

Maier J, Dagnelie G, Spekreijse H, Van Dijk B (1987) Principal components analysis for source localization of VEPs in man. Vision Res 27:165–177

---

column) or monophasic (PC2 with a peak latency of approximately 125 ms, *right column*). In the contour plots different colors were used for distribution values of different sign. The sign of the distribution value was chosen to be equal to the sign of the first peak of PC1 or the sign of the only peak of PC2. *Red lines* depict positive values, *yellow lines* zero values, and *blue lines* negative values. Also shown are the best fitting dipole distributions, represented by *orange, brown* and *sea-green* lines for positive, zero and negative potentials respectively

N100 Frontal Component and Influence of Reference Location in Pattern Visual Evoked Potential Studied with the Area Display Technique

M. GUIDI[1], O. SCARPINO[1], F. ANGELERI[1], and R.G. BICKFORD[2]

Introduction

The literature in the area of photic and pattern visual evoked potentials makes only scant reference to the distribution of potentials that appear beyond the primary visual area (Allison et al. 1977; Lehmann and Skrandies 1980; Skrandies 1986). A few recent reports (Hajdukovic et al. 1984; Spitz et al. 1986; Guidi and Bickford 1987) pointed out the existence of a negative frontal component that occurs about the same time as the occipital P100 in the majority of normal and pathological observations. This finding raises doubt about the relative inactivity of the midfrontal (MF) electrode as reference. In this study, the first aim was to evaluate the influence of different reference locations (cephalic and non-cephalic) in the recording of the 16 primary evoked responses and the possible change in interpretation that contour mapping could produce. The second aim was to define the spread of the N100 frontal component and to achieve some insight into the origin of this wave.

Methods

Forty normal volunteers (aged 28–51) with no history of neurological and ophthalmological diseases underwent a full field pattern visual evoked potential (PVEP). Twenty of them with a discernible N100 frontal component were divided into two groups of ten and studied with separate experimental procedures. The first group received three series of pattern shift stimuli, the reference electrode location being changed each time. Two cephalic (tip of the nose, N; linked ears, A1A2) and one non-cephalic (sternovertebral, SV) reference were employed. In the second group the only reference adopted was the linked ears. Each subject was submitted to a series of pattern stimuli. The pattern shift included a full-field stimulation with different checksize (1°7′, 34′2″) and a right and left hemifield. The time of the sweep analysis was 350 ms. The pattern shift stimulus was produced by a back-projected system (Biocomputronics) with a mirror moving at a repetition rate of 2/s. Full-field luminance and contrast respectively were 105 cd/m^2 and 0.75. Between 100 and 200 sweeps for full-field

---

[1] Clinica Neurologica, Università di Ancona, Ospedale di Torrette, 60020 Ancona, Italy
[2] Department of Neurosciences, School of Medicine, University of California, San Diego, La Jolla, CA 92093, USA

Topographic Brain Mapping of EEG and Evoked Potentials
Ed. by K. Maurer
© Springer-Verlag Berlin Heidelberg 1989

and hemifield pattern shift were recorded. The recording and processing system used in this study was a Minicears III (Bickford 1981). The evoked responses were recorded from 16 electrodes positioned according to the 10–20 international system. The bandwidth was 1–70 Hz. The electrode impedance was always below 4 kΩ. The signals were digitized at 256 samples/s/channel. The programs on Minicears III made it possible to produce 16-channel average traces and print out the voltage samples derived every 2 ms at chosen time windows after the stimulus. The voltage values were successively interpolated by a Zenith Z100 personal computer for the construction of color maps from different head perspectives (top of the head; frontal and occipital views; right and left side views) (Allen 1985).

Results

In all normal subjects, the main components (N75, P100, N145) could be identified from the occipital area. The N100 frontal component was present in 35

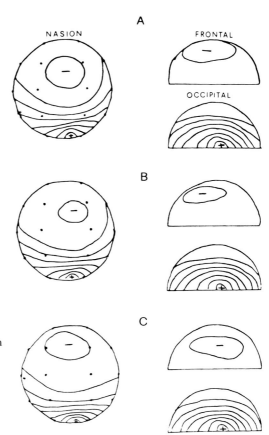

Fig. 1A–C. Contour maps obtained with the voltage values derived at 104 ms after the stimulus using different reference locations: **A** linked ears; **B** tip of the nose; **C** sternoclavicular junction connected with C7. The relative invariance to reference locations is evident

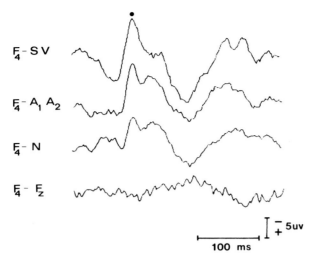

Fig. 2. Evoked responses to pattern stimulus recorded in the same subject from F4 using four reference locations: sternoclavicular junction connected with C7 (SV), linked ears (A1A2), tip of the nose (N), and Fz. The N100 has its maximal amplitude with the non-cephalic reference

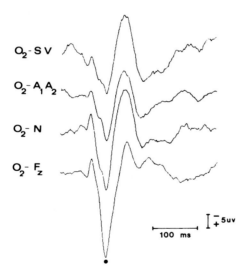

Fig. 3. Comparison of single PVEPs recorded in the same subject from O2 using four reference locations. The value of P100 increases in amplitude with the middle line references, especially with Fz

subjects (85%) with the maximal amplitude on F3 and F4. The evoked responses to full-field stimulation using three different reference locations (A1A2, N, SV) seem to be similar. However, a more thorough study of the individual components shows a variability in amplitude in the different situations. No changes were observed in polarity or latency of the major waves. Likewise, no differences were evident among the contour mapping of the same evoked potentials

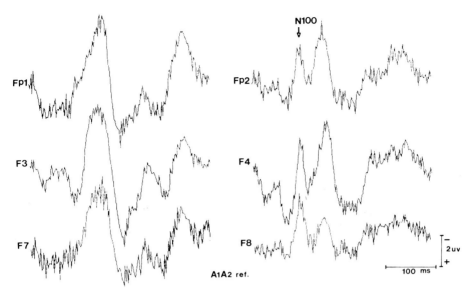

Fig. 4. Visual evoked responses to a left hemifield pattern recorded from frontal electrodes. The N100 is present in the hemisphere opposite to the visually stimulated hemifield

recorded with different references (Fig. 1). The N100 frontal component was always present in the three different recording situations. The value of the main components and of the N100, as recorded by using linked ears when compared with the nose reference, showed results closer to the non-cephalic reference. A recording using Fz as reference was also done in a few subjects. In this condition the N100 frontal component disappears in F3 and F4 as shown in Fig. 2. This is because the reference location has the same polarity and was close to the recording electrodes. On the other hand the P100 showed the highest voltage using Fz as reference, since in this condition the value of N100 was added (Fig. 3). We did not find any significant correlation between the amplitude of the N100 and that of the P100. In its latency relationship to P100, it may be a few milliseconds earlier or later. The negative frontal wave was always identified in full-field PVEP, both with small and with large checksize. These two different stimuli did not change the latency of the N100, and the amplitude was almost the same. On the other hand the P100 showed a slight shift in latency but a better definition of the wave using the small check. The N100 was always detected by using the right and the left hemifield in the hemisphere opposite to the hemifield presented, whereas the other hemisphere showed a significant reduction in amplitude or even disappearance of this wave in four cases (Fig. 4). The color map constructed with the voltage values derived 102 ms after the stimulus is shown in Fig. 5. The highest positive value found in the occipital area corresponds to the distribution of the P100, while the negative field centered on F3 and F4 is representative of the N100. In Fig. 6 is represented the electrical field distribution of the evoked response elicited by a right hemifield

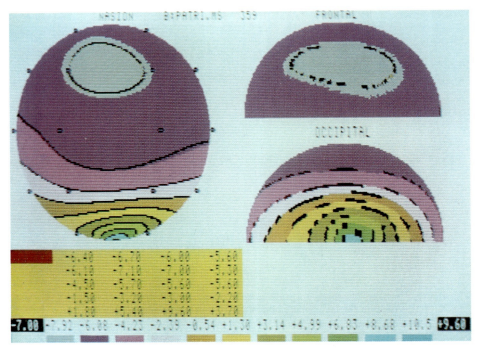

Fig. 5. Color map of PVEP representative of the electrical field distribution at 102 ms after the stimulus (full field; non-cephalic reference). The numbers at the bottom represent voltage values in microvolts

pattern at 96 ms after the stimulus. It is evident that the asymmetric response in the frontal area is more negative on the side opposite to the visual hemifield stimulus. In the same figure posteriorly, the paradoxical response is present.

Conclusions

The linked ears are relatively inactive and closer to the non-cephalic reference when compared with other cephalic references. The component arising from the references has its influence equally distributed over all the electrodes. No changes are observed on topographic display. A negative frontal component occurring at about the same time as the occipital P100 was encountered in the majority of normal observations. The hemifield stimulation elicited selectively the N100 in the hemisphere opposite the visual hemifield in 40% of cases, while in the rest an asymmetry in amplitude was constantly present. The comparison of components recorded by using cephalic and non-cephalic references ruled out the possibility that the N100 component originates from the reference. The invariability of this component with small and large stimulus check-size and its latency tend to exclude its possible correlation with the hypothetical

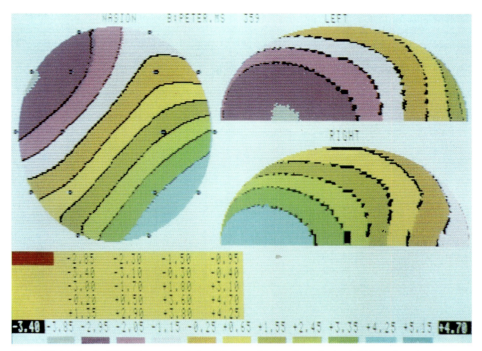

Fig. 6. Color map of PVEP constructed with the voltage values derived 96 ms after the stimulus (right visual hemifield; A1A2 reference)

fronto-occipital dipole (P100-N100). Thus, the origin of this frontal negative wave seems to be an event dissociated from the arrival in the striate cortex of the visual inputs. It could represent a far field potential from subcortical structures that are involved in the visual pathway (thalamus, superior colliculus) or a diffuse activation of the anterior head regions due to cortico-cortical or non-specific thalamocortical volleys. Experimental depth recordings or application of this method in pathological conditions might help to clarify the possible usefulness of the N100 component in clinical studies.

References

Allen BA (1985) Scope, accuracy, and limitations of computer toposcopic display of linearly interpolated electrophysiologic data. Thesis, University of California, San Diego

Allison T, Matsumiya Y, Goff GD, Goff WR (1977) The scalp topography of human visual evoked potentials. Electroencephalogr Clin Neurophysiol 42:185–197

Bickford RG (1981) A combined EEG and evoked potential procedure in clinical EEG (automated cerebral electrogram – Ace test). In: Jamaguchi N, Fujisawa K (eds) Recent advances in EEG and EMG data processing. Elsevier/North Holland Biomedical, Amsterdam, pp 217–235

Guidi M, Bickford RG (1987) Processing EEG and EP by area display techniques (case illustrations). Electroencephalogr Clin Neurophysiol 66:3

Hajdukovic R, Allen BA, Bickford RG (1984) Frontal processing of PVERs as indicated by contour studies. Electroencephalogr Clin Neurophysiol 58:13

Lehmann D, Skrandies W (1980) Reference free identification of components of checkerboard-evoked multichannel potential fields. Electroencephalogr Clin Neurophysiol 48:609–621

Skrandies W (1986) Visual evoked potential topography: methods and results. In: Duffy FH (ed) Topographic mapping of brain electrical activity. Butterworths, Boston, pp 7–28

Spitz MC, Emerson RG, Pedley TA (1986) Dissociation of frontal N100 from occipital P100 in pattern reversal visual evoked potentials. Electroencephalogr Clin Neurophysiol 65:161–168

Scalp Topography of Red LED Flash-Evoked Potentials: Normal and Clinical Data

E.J. Hammond[1], C.P. Barber[1], and B.J. Wilder[1,2]

Introduction

Clinical application of visual evoked potential (VEP) mapping will require extensive clinical correlation studies. Since the visual system has projections to many extrastriate regions (Van Essen 1979), there is reason to believe that VEP abnormalities might be detected in brain regions for from the "classical" visual system. Duffy and colleagues (1979, 1982, 1986) have shown that such VEP abnormalities can indeed be detected in certain patients.

Red light emitting diode (LED) goggles (Fig. 1) are available from several manufacturers, but there is very little in the literature concerning normative or clinical data obtained with these goggles. Such a stimulus device is useful in certain patients who cannot or will not fixate on the traditional stimuli used for VEP recording. Accordingly, we performed a prospective VEP mapping study (comparing pattern reversal, red LED, and xenon flash stimulation) in neurologic patients with confirmed structural lesions in order to determine how efficacious these procedures are in detecting brain lesions. Results of the red LED mapping study are reported here.

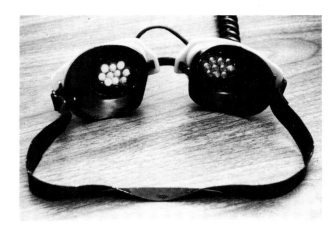

Fig. 1. Red LED goggles

---

[1] Neurology and [2] Medical Research Services, Veterans Administration Medical Center, Gainesville, FL 32602, USA

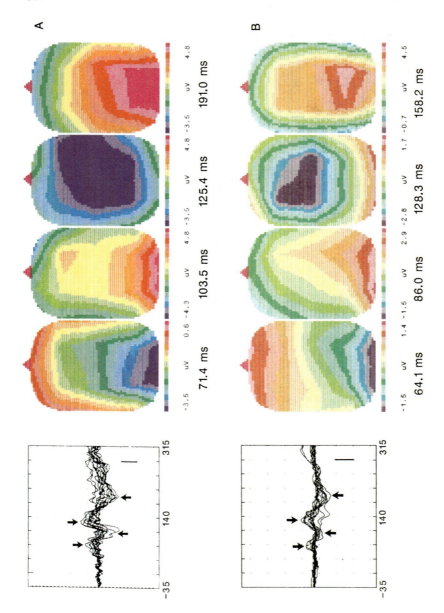

Methods

Subjects

Normative data recordings were made from 40 neurologically normal subjects (ages 20–45 years, mean 30.1 years), mostly hospital staff. Patients ($n=40$) with cerebral lesions (verified by computed tomography) were selected in a prospec-

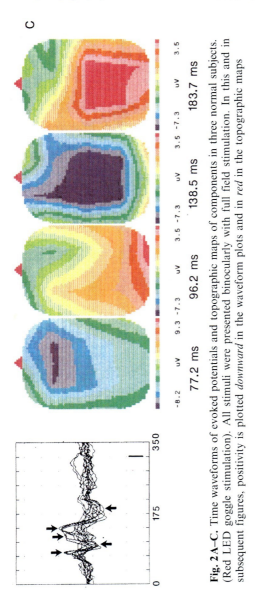

Fig. 2A–C. Time waveforms of evoked potentials and topographic maps of components in three normal subjects. (Red LED goggle stimulation). All stimuli were presented binocularly with full field stimulation. In this and in subsequent figures, positivity is plotted *downward* in the waveform plots and in *red* in the topographic maps

tive manner. Lesions included infarction, tumor, arteriovenous malformation, encephalomalacia, and lobectomy. Patients gave informed consent.

Stimulus

All stimuli were presented binocularly using LED goggles (Cadwell) with the subjects' eyes open. Stimuli were presented with a variable repetition rate; interstimulus intervals ranged from 600 ms to 5 s. The luminance of the stimulus was approximately 1.5 foot candles (16.5 lux).

Recording

All recordings were made on a 16-channel averager (Cadwell 8400). Amplifier band-pass was 1–100 Hz. Evoked potential waveforms were printed out on line and stored on a floppy disk. At least two trials were run of each stimulus condition, and each averaged response was comprised of 200 epochs. The averaging epoch was 350 ms, including a 35-ms prestimulus baseline. An average value (across 16 channels) of the voltage, calculated for averaged activity occurring in a 35-ms prestimulus segment, was used as the baseline for calculating the scalp potential fields. The computation performed for each of the 16 waveforms is

$$V = \frac{\sum_{i=t_1}^{t_2} d_i}{n}$$

where V = integrated voltage, d = data value at the i point in time, i = individual data points between t_1 and t_2, and n is the number of data points between t_1 and t_2. Electrodes were applied according to the international 10–20 system, and electrode impedances were maintained at less than 5 kΩ. Linked earlobes served as reference.

Results

Normal Subjects

A clear N70–80, P85–100, N140 complex was usually recorded at frontal and lateral frontal regions, an N70–80, P80–140, N140, N175 complex was recorded occipitally, and an N70–100, P80–110, N140 complex was recorded centrally. There are two main variants to this general picture and these are illustrated in Fig. 2. In one variant (Fig. 2B) there is a clear occipital positivity at the same time as the central N140. In another variant (Fig. 2C), there is a separate early negativity in frontal regions, and the central N140 starts more frontally then progressses over 35 ms to more central scalp locations. The latter component, N140, was the most consistent, and was recorded in almost all subjects. Often quite distinct, high-amplitude LED-evoked potentials were recorded in subjects who displayed only low-amplitude evoked potentials on pattern reversal. In seven subjects most components were larger in frontal regions. In four subjects occipital and frontal components appeared to be phase reversals of the same neural event, but in most subjects components generated in frontal, central, and occipital regions seemed quite distinct from each other on the basis of latency and amplitude.

Patients

The patients generally showed the same number of components and scalp topography as the normals controls. Two types of abnormalities were seen: In one type, one or more components were depressed over the site of a cerebral lesion. The second abnormality appeared as an apparent enhancement in amplitude over the site of a lesion.

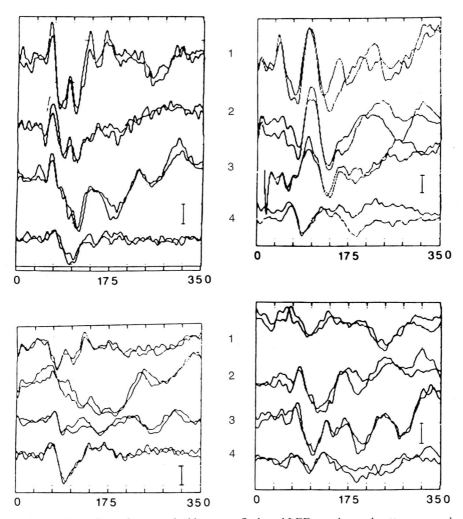

Fig. 3. Comparison of waveforms evoked by xenon flash, red LED goggles, and pattern reversal stimulation. Data from four normal subjects is shown. Amplitude calibration: 5 µV. *1*, White flash (eyes open); *2*, white flash eyes closed; *3*, red L.E.D.; *4* pattern reversal

Discussion

It is clear that pattern reversal, red LED goggles, and white xenon flash evoke potentials with differing waveforms and scalp distributions. Differences in waveform between the red LED goggle stimulus and the xenon flash stimulus are readily apparent (Fig. 3). Aside from stimulus intensity and color, other aspects of the red stimulus probably play a role: for example, the light is emitted from an array of diodes, so there is probably some aspect of pattern onset stimulation. The complex distribution of flash evoked potentials suggests that many cortical regions will be susceptible to physiological analysis using VEP topographic mapping.

Examination of typical waveforms of flash-evoked potentials (Fig. 4) shows considerable intersubject variability in time waveform, which would seem to indicate poor clinical applicability in comparison, say, to pattern reversal stimulation. This would be the case for single-channel recording, but multiple-channel recording provides for assessment of hemispheric asymmetries within a given patient.

The present results indicate that topographic mapping of VEPs can provide data on the location of lesions remote from the occipital area. Two types of abnormalities were seen: one in which a component was depressed over the site of a cerebral lesion and one in which the component appeared to be enhanced (see Fig. 5). A similar enhancement was also noted in the extensive studies by Kooi and Marshall (1979). Although this might be due to some hyperexcitability of neurons, and alternative explanation might be that this is a paradoxical lateralization phenomenon (Blumhardt and Halliday 1979) whereby potentials are best recorded over the hemisphere contralateral to the actual generator site due to the orientation of a dipole source. Thus, a lesion

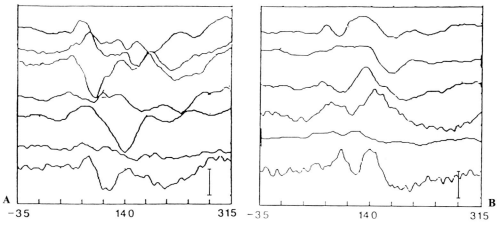

Fig. 4A, B. Variability of red flash-evoked potentials in six normal subjects. **A** Red stimulus, occipital electrode; **B** red stimulus, central electrode. Note variability in amplitude and latency across subjects for most components. Amplitude calibration: 5 µV

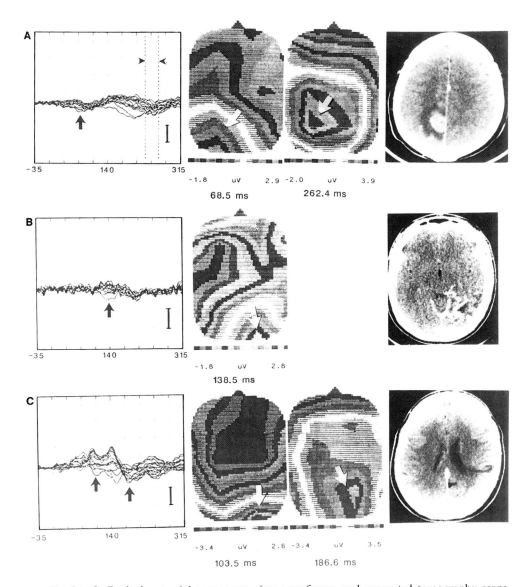

Fig. 5A–C. Evoked potential topograms, time waveforms, and computed tomography scans in patients with occipital lesions. *Black arrows* on topograms signify negative components and *white arrows* signify positivie components. Data presented here include cases showing an enhancement of the evoked potential over the affected side. Mechanisms for this enhancement are discussed in the text. Amplitude calibration: 5 μV. **A** Forty-year-old male with left falcine meningioma. No visual field defects noted. Patient presented with new onset of generalized tonic-clonic seizures. Note enhancement of red-evoked components of 68.5 ms and a late wave (figure shows integrated voltage from 230 to 262 ms) over the affected left occipital region. In this patient pattern reversal stimulation topograms were normal. **B** Forty-year-old male with a right occipital arteriovenous malformation presenting with seizures. The patient was unaware of a left heminopsia. Shown is an enhancement of red-evoked occipital component at 138 ms. **C** Forty-ear-old male with right parietal encephalomalacia of undetermined origin; shown are enhancements of red-evoked occipital components at 103 and 186 ms. Pattern reversal stimulation was normal

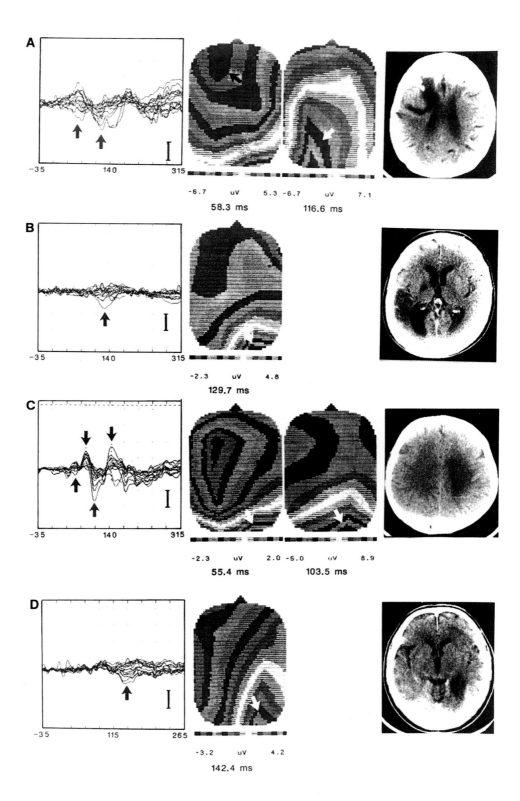

Fig. 6A–D. Evoked potential topograms, time waveforms, and computed tomography scans in patients with non-occipital lesions. *Black arrows* on topograms signify negative components and *white arrows* signify positive components. Amplitude calibration: 5 µV. **A** Thirty-two-year-old female with a left frontal glioblastoma. Red stimulation shows paradoxical lateralization of a frontal N58 and an occipital P116. Xenon flash also revealed focal left enhancement of several components (not shown). **B** Fifty-nine-year-old male with a left temporal lobe tumor. Patient presented with lethargy. Electroencephalogram was normal. **C** Fifty-eight-year-old male with a right temporoparietal tumor. **D** Sixty-year-old man with a parietal tumor

◁————————————————————————————————

affecting cells on the right would affect a potential recorded on the left. Normally functioning cells on the left would generate a normal potential on the right, thus giving the appearance of a paradoxical enhancement over the affected hemisphere.

Although the anatomy and physiology of human striate and peristriate cortex has been well studied, there is a paucity of information about visual projections to areas outside the occipital lobe. Anatomical (Kuypers et al. 1965; Pandya and Kuypers 1969) and physiological (Bignall and Imbert 1969; Boyd et al. 1971) studies have indicated cortico-cortical connections from visual association areas to the parietal lobe, premotor cortex, prefrontal cortex, and to the middle and inferior temporal gyri. Depth recordings in humans (Walter and Walter 1949; Brazier 1964) have shown VEPs in frontal and temporal regions. Our data and the extensive mapping studies of Kooi and Marshall (1979) have shown surface-recorded VEPs with amplitude maxima over central, temporal, and frontal regions, and certain components of the VEP can be affected by lesions in these regions.

It is our impression, from our clinical material, that it is necessary for one or more of the occipital-temporal or occipital-frontal projection pathways to be affected in order to alter a non-occipital VEP. Further studies in patients with discrete cortical lesions will help elucidate both the neural sources of the flash VEP and the functional relationships of the various visual areas.

Acknowledgement. The authors thank Janet Wootten and Anne Crawford for manuscript preparation.

References

Bignall KE, Imbert M (1969) Polysensory and cortico-cortical projections to frontal lobe of squirrel and rhesus monkeys. Electroencephalogr Clin Neurophysiol 26:206–215

Boyd EH, Pandya DN, Bignall KE (1971) Homotopic and nonhomotopic interhemispheric cortical projections in the squirrel monkey. Exp Neurol 32:256–274

Blumhardt LD, Halliday AM (1979) Hemisphere contributions to the composition of the pattern evoked potential waveform. Exp Brain Res 36:59–69

Brazier MAB (1964) Evoked responses recorded from the depth of the human brain. Ann NY Acad Sci USA 112:33–59

Duffy FH (1982) Topographic displays of evoked potentials – clinical applications of brain electrical activity mapping (BEAM). Ann NY Acad Sci USA 388:183–196

Duffy FH (ed) (1986) Topographic mapping of brain electrical activity. Butterworth, Boston

Duffy FH, Burchfiel JL, Lombroso CT (1979) Brain electrical activity mapping (BEAM): a new method of extending the clinical utility of EEG and evoked potential data. Ann Neurol 5:309–321

Kooi KA, Marshall RE (1979) Visual evoked potentials in central disorders of the visual system. Harper and Row, Cambridge

Kuypers HGJM, Szwarcbart MK, Mishkin M, Rosvold HE (1965) Occipitotemporal corticocortical connections in the rhesus monkey. Exp Neurol 11:245–262

Pandya DN, Kuypers HGJM (1969) Cortico-cortical connections in the rhesus monkey. Brain Res 13:13–36

Van Essen DC (1979) Visual areas of the mammalian cerebral cortex. Ann Rev Neurosci 2:227–263

Walter VJ, Walter WG (1949) The central effects of rhythmic sensory stimulation. Electroencephalogr Clin Neurophysiol 1:57–86

Topographic Mapping of Somatosensory Representation Areas

H. EMMERT and K.A. FLÜGEL[1]

Introduction

The primary somatosensory cortex is known to be somatotopically organized (Penfield and Rasmussen 1950). Afferent electrical activity evoked by stimulation of face, hand, foot etc. can be recorded from the postcentral cortex according to a homunculus-like distribution. An analogous placement of skull electrodes is suited to record the maxima of the early cortical complexes of somatosensory evoked potentials (SEP). The use of a multielectrode array and an electrical activity mapping system enables us to visualize the area of for example, the negativity at 20 ms following median nerve stimulation. The size of such an area could be used as a measure of the primary somatosensory representation field. Hence topographic brain mapping might give us a tool to record possible changes of cortical representation.

So far, brain mapping of short-latency SEP has mostly been used in conjunction with the stimulation of the median or the tibial nerve to demonstrate the activity of rather large and well-separated cortical areas. We attempted to see whether the resolution of the method was sufficient to distinguish smaller representation areas like those of the individual fingers or like the trigeminus versus the adjacent thumb area.

Material and Methods

We studied early cortical SEP maps in 13 normal subjects, seven females and six males, aged 20 to 42 years (mean age 34 years), who were free from neurological deficits and were not addicted to drugs. Square constant current pulses of 200 μs duration, an intensity of 3 times the sensory threshold and a repetition rate of 4.3/s were used for the stimulation of the median nerve trunk at the wrist, the tibial nerve trunk at the internal malleolus, the first and second finger (with the help of metal ring electrodes) and the trigeminus. In the latter case the second and third branch were stimulated together as proposed by Stöhr et al. (1982). Sixteen conventional EEG recording electrodes or silver cup electrodes were placed on the skull according to the 10/20 system or according to a unihemispheric montage which will be described below. Electrode imped-

---

[1] Abteilung Neurologie und Klinische Neurophysiologie, Krankenhaus Bogenhausen, Englschalkingerstr. 77, 8000 München 81, Federal Republic of Germany

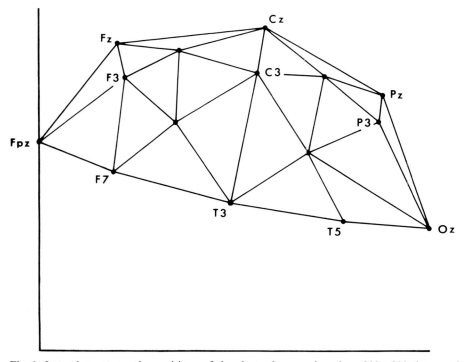

Fig. 1. Lateral montage: the positions of the electrodes are given in a 200 × 200 dot matrix. Four additional electrodes are grouped around C3. The *triangles* indicate the mode of interpolation

ances had to be below 3 kΩ throughout the entire measurement. The scalp potentials were recorded and averaged with a 5–1500-Hz bandpass, a sampling period of 50 ms plus a 10- to 20-ms prestimulus baseline, a bin width of 195 μs, a sweep number of 500 and two runs to assure reproducibility. In the case of trigeminus stimulation 1000 sweeps were taken per run with a change of stimulation polarity at the halfway stage in order to reduce the stimulation artifact. In all recordings the reference electrode was the earlobe contralateral to the side of stimulation because of the cancelling out of the N18 component (Desmedt and Bourguet 1985). In most cases a standard four-channel SEP with recording electrodes at Erb's point, C7, C2 and cortex was recorded to correct for arm length. All peaks were named according to the polarity-latency nomenclature. (Donchin et al. 1977).

The color imaging of the raw SEP data was achieved using the Nicolet Pathfinder mapping upgrade which calculated maps of up to 400 × 400 pixels and 45 colors by linear interpolation between the four nearest electrodes. The prestimulus period was used as zero baseline for the maps. Before mapping, the raw SEP data were visually inspected and the two runs were combined to a grand average which then was digitally filtered to 10–1200 Hz.

In addition to the usual top view, we chose a lateral montage in which 15 electrodes were located over one hemisphere and triangular linear interpolation was used. The mapping algorithm allowed a free choice of electrode placement, and electrode positions were given on a 200 × 200 dot matrix based on a spheric head model. Figure 1 shows the lateral montage electrode positions which we used for this study. There were four additional electrodes grouped around C3 or C4.

Results

The first series of SEP maps consisted of top-view montages which showed the scalp distribution of the early cortical components resulting from median nerve stimulation. Following the widespread positivity at about 14 ms (P14), the first focal peak is the N20, which is localized parietally, with maximal values at P4 and/or C4 in the 10/20 electrode arrangement (in the case of left side stimulation; Fig. 2A, left head). As shown previously (Desmedt and Bourguet 1985; Wood et al. 1985), the isopotential lines or colors for the N20 displayed a tangential orientation with a corresponding frontal positivity (which has to be discriminated from the precentral P22), suggesting a tangential dipolar source perpendicular to the fissure of Rolando. The spatial distribution and the field orientation of the consecutive peak, the P27, were found to be very similar (Fig. 2A, right head). Again, the maximum was limited to the C4/P4 region, and we could assume a dipolar source pointing from ipsilateral frontal to contralateral parietal (ipsilateral refers to the side of stimulation). In the color bar display shown in Fig. 2B, in which a whole recording period can be viewed, the P27 was somewhat better spatially confined than the N20.

In a second series the P27 peak was then used for the somatotopic postcentral cortex mapping. Figure 2C shows the mapping of the P27 following median nerve stimulation and of the P40 following tibial nerve stimulation. Both could easily be distinguished by the spatial distribution as well as by the field orientation. The maximum of the P40 was found at the parietal midline and its orientation was much less oblique than the N20, almost coinciding with the midline with a slight deviation to contralateral frontal. However, for further somatotopic discrimination, especially within the postcentral hand area, the 10/20 montage proved to be insufficient. Additionally, it was not possible to record from the 10/20 positions while stimulating the trigeminus; due to its very short distance from the site of stimulation the ipsilateral frontopolar electrode recorded a large stimulation artifact which constantly triggered the sweep rejection mode of the averaging system.

In the third series we mapped the P27, the P40 or the P19 in conjunction with the lateral montage shown in Fig. 1 and described above. Figure 2D gives, from top to bottom, a series of frozen maps taken at the maxima of the first cortical positivity, i.e., at the P40 in the case of tibial nerve, at the P27 in the case of finger or median nerve and at the P19 in the case of trigeminus stimulation. The P40 in the lateral montage was located at the very boundary

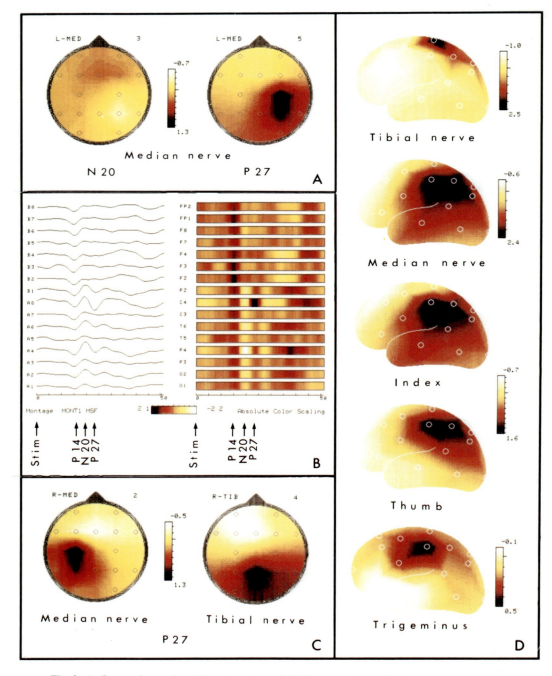

Fig. 2. A Comparison of culmination site and field orientation of N20 and P27 following median nerve stimulation. **B** Original SEP data resulting from median nerve stimulation (recorded with the 10/20 montage) and color bar display. Note N20 maximum at P4 and C4, P27 maximum at C4. **C** Comparison of culmination site and field orientation of median nerve and tibial nerve stimulation evoked P27 (10/20 montage). **D** Lateral montages as shown in Fig. 1: somatotopic distribution of P40, P27 or P19

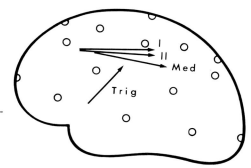

Fig. 3. Estimation of the positions of the assumed dipolar sources of the P27, resulting from stimulation of median nerve (*Med*), index (*I*), thumb (*II*) and trigeminus (*Trig*) (see text)

of the brain silhouette and was not free from artifacts. These originated from the interpolation between the electrodes with very high positive values (Cz, Pz), the electrodes with negative values (Oz) and the boundary points of the matrix which have plus/minus zero values by definition. This problem did not arise with P27 and P19. The P27 maps resulting from stimulation of the median nerve trunk or of digits could be discriminated by their spatial distribution, the median nerve P27 being roughly the size of the index and thumb P27 together (Fig. 2D). Discrimination by field orientation was only vaguely possible (Fig. 3). The lateral montage did not show most of the P27's corresponding negativity located frontally on the other hemisphere, but it did allow the estimation of the tangential dipoles, as shown in Fig. 3. The estimation was done by drawing an arrow that crossed the center of the positivity perpendicular to and bisected by the line of polarity reversal (Deiber et al. 1986). In contrast to the findings with digit SEP, the trigeminus P19 could be discriminated by field orientation better than by spatial distribution (Figs. 2D, 3). Its assumed dipole was found to run from the temporal pole to the caudal postcentral region.

Discussion

The first set of our data suggests that in addition to the N20, the P27 is suited for somatotopic postcentral cortex mapping. It is as spatially confined as the N20, and it can also be represented by a tangential dipole perpendicular to the fissure of Rolando. The use of the P27 has clear advantages when mapping the responses to digit or tibial nerve stimulation. Responses to digit stimulation (Fig. 4), like other segmental SEP, often have a rather low N20 which results in vague contours when mapped against the baseline. Responses to tibial nerve stimulation usually have no N33 at all. But in both cases, the first positivity of the early cortical complex is prominent.

A further necessary improvement was the use of more electrodes in the area of interest (Duff 1980). A lateral montage which concentrated 15 electrodes over one hemisphere was preferred, since the placement of more than 16 electrodes over the entire skull was found to be too time-consuming. The lateral

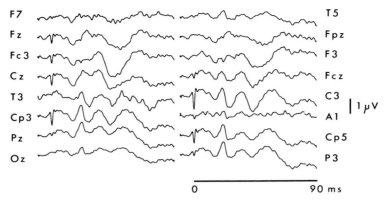

Fig. 4. Original data resulting from index stimulation as recorded with the lateral montage

montage used so far is subject to further change, with the aim of having an array of electrodes over the postcentral cortex. Alternatively, top-view montages which do not follow the 10/20 scheme have shown to be useful in SEP mapping (Desmedt et al. 1987).

The potential fields evoked by tibial nerve, median nerve and trigeminus stimulation can easily be discriminated. It is much more difficult to reveal the somatotopic arrangement of the fields within the upper limb representation. Both the sites of the P27 culmination and the field orientations show only small shifts. More pronounced are the differences of the spatial extension of the P27. Deiber et al. (1986) concluded that with respect to digit SEP, a homunculus-like distribution could not be found. However, they did depict the shift of the spatial orientation of the assumed dipole according to the stimulated finger. They also stated that the tangential orientation of the dipolar source which causes a wide spread of activity on the skull would partly mask small localization changes. Finally, the somatotopic arrangement of finger evoked responses has meanwhile been recorded using a different non-invasive technique, namely magnetic recording (Okada et al. 1984).

References

Deiber MP, Giard MH, Mauguierre F (1986) Separate generators with distinct orientations for N20 and P22 somatosensory evoked potentials to finger stimulation. Electroencephalogr Clin Neurophysiol 65:321–334

Desmedt JE, Bourguet M (1985) Color imaging of parietal and frontal somatosensory potential fields evoked by stimulation of median or posterior tibial nerve in man. Electroencephalogr Clin Neurophysiol 62:1–17

Desmedt JE, Nguyen TH, Bourguet M (1987) Bit-mapped color imaging of human evoked potentials with reference to the N20, P22, P27 and N30 somatosensory responses. Electroencephalogr Clin Neurophysiol 68:1–19

Donchin E, Callaway E, Cooper R, Desmedt JE, Goff WR, Hillyard SA, Sutton S (1977)

Publication criteria for studies of evoked potentials in man. In: Desmedt JE (ed) Attention, voluntary contraction and event-related cerebral potentials. Karger, Basel, pp 1–11 (Progress in clinical neurophysiology, vol 1)

Duff TA (1980) Topography of scalp recorded potentials evoked by stimulation of the digits. Electroencephalogr Clin Neurophysiol 49:452–460

Okada YC, Tanenbaum R, Williamson SJ, Kaufmann L (1984) Somatotopic organization of the human somatosensory cortex revealed by neuromagnetic measurements. Exp Brain Res 56:197–205

Penfield W, Rasmussen T (1950) The cerebral cortex of man. Macmillan, New York

Stöhr M, Dichgans J, Diener HC, Buettner UW (1982) Evozierte Potentiale. Springer, Berlin Heidelberg New York

Wood CC, Cohen D, Cuffin BN, Yarita M, Allison T (1985) Electrical sources in human somatosensory cortex: identification by combined magnetic and potential recordings. Science 227:1051–1053

Early Cortical Somatosensory and N1 Auditory Evoked Responses: Analysis with Potential Maps, Scalp Current Density Maps and Three-Concentric-Shell Head Models

F. Perrin, O. Bertrand, and J. Pernier[1]

Scalp Current Density Mapping

Scalp current density (SCD) mapping shows scalp areas where current either emerges (sources) from the brain into the scalp or enters (sinks) from the scalp into the brain (Nunez 1981). By definition the SCD of a point of the scalp is equal to the amount of current which flows (radially to the scalp surface) from the brain into a scalp unit volume surrounding the scalp point. SCD is reference-independent, the peaks and troughs of its distribution are sharper than those of the scalp potential (SP) and SCD, in contrast to SP, reflects mainly the activity of cortical generators. SCD maps may be estimated (Perrin et al. 1987b) by taking the spatial derivatives of SP maps. To obtain differentiable SP maps a bidimensional spline interpolation method was used (Perrin et al. 1987a).

Analysis of the Early Cortical Somatosensory Evoked Response

The somatosensory response evoked by constant current stimuli applied to the right middle finger was recorded on 16 electrodes concentrated in the left centro-parietal region with a left earlobe reference. In Fig. 1a are displayed three SP maps at 21.5, 24 and 32 ms after the stimulation showing the N20/P20, P22 and P30/N30 complexes respectively. Figure 1d shows the estimated SCD maps derived from the preceding SP maps. The numerous colored spots of these maps are difficult to interpret in terms of current sources or sinks associated with different brain generators. To better understand the underlying phenomena, the classical three-concentric-shell head model (Ary et al. 1981) was used. The methodology for model identification was similar to that described by Scherg and von Cramon (1985) for auditory responses. To fit the whole spatiotemporal distribution of the potential data between 20 and 32 ms, only three overlapping equivalent current dipoles were necessary, each having fixed position, fixed orientation and time-varying amplitude (Fig. 2). The rather tangential dipole peaking at 20.7 ms was responsible for the N20/P20 complex, the dipole peaking at 24 ms contributed mainly to the P22 peak and the third dipole, also rather

---

[1] U280 Inserm, 151 Crs A. Thomas, F-69003 Lyon, France

tangentially oriented, explained the P30/N30 complex. All these dipoles were located in the vicinity of the rolandic fissure. The results on the tangential dipoles are consistent with those obtained, although at only two fixed latencies, by magnetoencephalography (Wood et al. 1985; for a review see Desmedt and Bourguet 1987). The adequacy of the model (goodness of fit above 90% for all maps between 20 and 32 ms) is illustrated in Fig. 1b showing SP maps, interpolated from the 16 electrode values calculated from the model, which are very similar to those of Fig. 1a. Logically enough this similarity extends to the SCD maps (compare Fig. 1d and Fig. 1e). Having a model at our disposal, it is possible to compute pixel by pixel, without any interpolation, the "true" model maps of the potentials and of the SCDs. These are shown in Fig. 1c and Fig. 1f respectively. Although on one hand only slight differences, attributable to the interpolation method, can be noted between Fig. 1c and Fig. 1d (see map at 21.5 ms), on the other hand Fig. 1f is quite different from Fig. 1c. One may note the sharpness of the peaks and troughs, which are concentrated in a very restricted area whose diameter is of the order of the interelectrode distance. This indicates that the electrode spatial sampling used in this experiment was too large to estimate properly the SCDs produced by the extremely peripheral cortical somatosensory generators.

Analysis of the N1 Auditory Evoked Response

The same methodology was applied to the N1 auditory evoked response to 1000-Hz tone bursts delivered to the right ear and recorded on 16 electrodes with a nose reference. In Fig. 1g is shown a top view of the usual N1 SP map 100 ms after the stimulation with its broad frontocentral negativity. In Fig. 1j the corresponding experimental SCD map shows clearly distinct activities in each hemisphere, a predominance of the hemisphere contralateral to the stimulation and, moreover, since the SCD representation is reference-free, these observed sink-source patterns point without ambiguity to brain generators in the sylvian regions. This confirms previously obtained results (Wood and Wolpaw 1982; Elberling et al. 1982; Scherg and von Cramon 1985). To help determine the accuracy of the SCD maps, the three-concentric-shell head model was used but with two equivalent current dipoles of fixed locations, fixed orientation and time-varying amplitude (Fig. 3). These dipoles were found located in the vicinity of the sylvian regions and oriented tangentially. The adequacy of the model (goodness of fit above 98% for all maps between 90 and 120 ms) is illustrated in Fig. 1g, h. One may note that the maps in Fig. 1g, h, i on one hand and in Fig. 1j, k, l on the other are similar; this indicates that the electrode spatial sampling of this experiment was probably sufficient to obtain estimates of the SCDs due to the rather deeply located auditory brain generators.

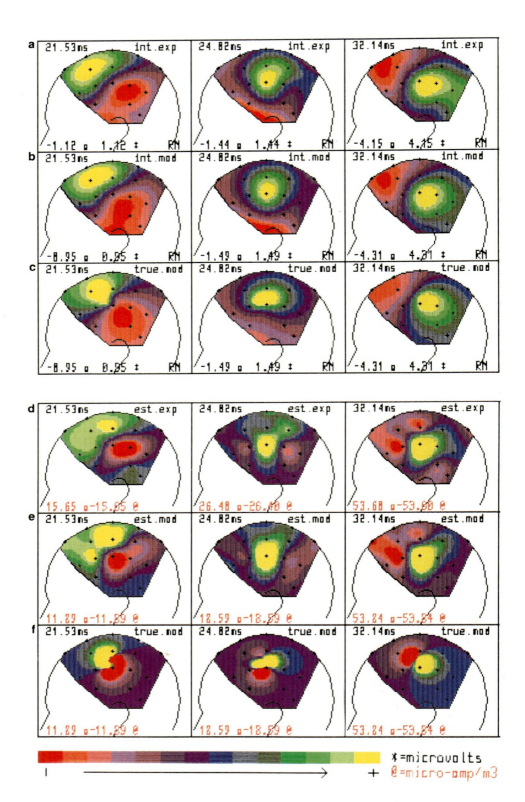

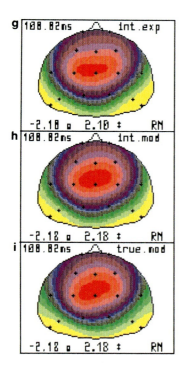

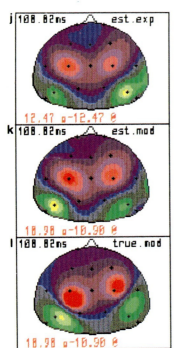

Fig. 1a–l. *Left:* somatosensory responses 21.5, 24 and 32 ms after the stimulation. *Right:* auditory responses 100 ms after the stimulation. *Top,* potential maps: **a, g** interpolated from experimental data; **b, h** interpolated from electrode model values; **c, i** non-interpolated "true" model SP maps. *Bottom,* scalp current density maps: **d, j** derived from **a, g**; **e, k** derived from **b, h**; **f, l** non-estimated "true" SCD model maps

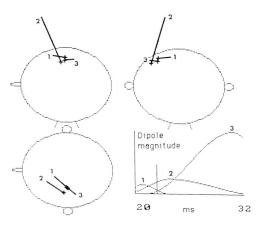

Fig. 2. Left, posterior and top plane projections of the head model showing the positions and orientations of the three equivalent current dipoles. The lengths displayed correspond to the 22.4-ms latency. The time varying dipole magnitudes are shown *lower right*

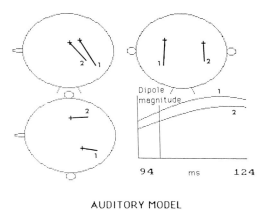

Fig. 3. Left, posterior and top plane projections of the head model showing the positions and orientations of the two equivalent current dipoles. The lengths displayed correspond to the 100 ms latency. The time varying dipole magnitudes are shown *lower right*

Conclusions

Analysis by means of SP maps and dipolar models of the early somatosensory cortical response to finger stimulation has confirmed the presence, between 20 and 32 ms, of at least three main brain generators in the central region. Because of the inadequacy of the spatial sampling, SCD mapping was not able to confirm these results.

Analysis of the N1 auditory response has shown concordance between SP maps, SCD maps and dipolar models, the results of which indicate at least one major brain generator in each sylvian region.

References

Ary JP, Klein SA, Fender DH (1981) Localization of sources of evoked scalp potentials: corrections for skull and scalp thicknesses. IEEE Trans Biomed Eng 28:447–452

Desmedt JE, Bourguet M (1987) Color imaging of parietal and frontal somatosensory potential fields evoked by stimulation of median and posterior tibial nerve in man. Electroencephalogr Clin Neurophysiol 62:1–17

Elberling C, Bak C, Kofoed B, Lebech J, Saermark K (1982) Auditory magnetic fields from the human cerebral cortex: location and strength of an equivalent current dipole. Acta Neurol Scand 65:553–569

Nunez PL (1981) Electric fields of the brain. Oxford University Press, New York

Perrin F, Pernier J, Bertrand O, Giard MH, Echallier JF (1987a) Mapping of scalp potentials by surface spline interpolation. Electroencephalogr Clin Neurophysiol 66:75–81

Perrin F, Bertrand O, Pernier J (1987b) Scalp current density mapping: value and estimation from potential data. IEEE Trans Biomed Eng (in press)

Scherg M, von Cramon D (1985) Two bilateral sources of the late AEP as identified by a spatio-temporal dipole model. Electroencephalogr Clin Neurophysiol 62:32–44

Wood CC, Wolpaw JR (1982) Scalp distribution of human auditory evoked potentials. II. Evidence for overlapping sources and involvement of auditory cortex. Electroencephalogr Clin Neurophysiol 54:25–38

Wood CC, Cohen D, Cuffin BN, Yarita M, Allison T (1985) Electrical sources in human somatosensory cortex: identification by combined magnetic and potential recordings. Science 227:1051–1053

The Topography of the N70 Component of the Visual Evoked Potential in Humans*

I. BÓDIS-WOLLNER, L. MYLIN, and S. FRKOVIĆ[1]

Introduction

The latency of the so-called P100 or major positive wave of the pattern visual evoked potential (VEP) is deservedly used as a most reliable indicator of retinal and optic nerve neuropathy. The fact that it occurs with such a long latency has given rise to considerable interest in the possibility of utilizing earlier VEP components for clinical diagnosis, in the hope of establishing at which anatomical level of visual processing an abnormality may have occurred. The earliest reported components, which occur as a short "burst" of oscillations, have been studied using very bright, brief flash stimulation. In the single study using pattern stimulation evidence was reported that components near 30 ms show spatial tuning and do not arise from the retina. Unfortunately, the amplitude of these oscillatory potentials is small and therefore at this stage of technology their clinical utility is rather doubtful. On the other hand, pattern elicited VEPs, which have nearly 10 times the amplitude of oscillatory scalp potentials, are reported to contain "unreliable" components preceding the P100. Nevertheless, there are components of the VEP which precede the P100. In particular, a negative wave, which we shall label N70 for convenience, has some physiologically and clinically intriguing properties. In this paper we shall summarize the evidence for the propostion that one of the reasons why N70 is considered unreliable is the use of inappropriate stimulation. We shall show that some of the properties of N70 express spatial tuning: it appears with reliability when one uses stimulation appropriate for foveal receptive fields in the human visual system. We shall also summarize the evidence that N70 is a cortical post-synaptic potential. Based on this evidence, it will appear that, using appropriate stimulation, the N70 component of the pattern VEP is clinically useable in the detection of paracentral visual field defects which may escape detection by routine visual field measurements. In fact we shall demonstrate the clinical use of N70, with topographic studies of patients. In some subjects the lesion involved the chiasmatic, in others the retrochiasmatic pathways. All lesions were diagnosed by means of CT scan or the magnetic resonance imaging (MRI) technique.

---

* The author and publisher gratefully acknowledge that the cost of colour prints was kindly subsidized by Dantec Elektronik

[1] VEP Laboratory, Departments of Neurology and Ophthalmology, The Mount Sinai School of Medicine of the City University of New York, 1200 Fifth Avenue, New York, NY 10029, USA

Method

Stimuli

Screen. Vertical gratings with sinusoidal luminance profile (Campbell and Green 1965) were generated on a Joyce Electronics display unit with a mean luminance of 100 cd/m^2 at a frame rate of 100 Hz. A square-shaped surround, illuminated from behind, had the same hue (whitish) and 0.2 log unit lower luminance than the display screen. The surround truncated the screen to a 9-degree circular field. Sinusoidal gratings were generated with the desired spatial and temporal frequencies of modulation. Contrast was calibrated for a range of spatial and temporal frequencies used in these studies, with the methods described by Bodis-Wollner and Hendley (1979). In hemifield studies a central 1-degree strip was left blank around the fixation point.

Patterns. The use of sinusoidal gratings with different spatial frequencies allowed us to investigate the relationship of the VEP N70 to foveal processing. Using sinusoidal gratings, human contrast sensitivity, established with psychophysical methods, is plotted as a function of spatial frequency (Schade 1956). Spatial frequency is defined as the number of alternating bands subtended in 1 degree of arc at the observer's eye; hence, spatial frequency is an equivalent description of pattern size. The contrast sensitivity curve is non-monotonic: its peak represents the optimal target size for foveal vision. It also corresponds to the size of the center of the most sensitive ganglion cells of the primate retina (Perry and Cowey 1985). These neurons, forming the optic nerve, have center-surround organization; hence, their receptive field center represents roughly the size of the pattern which is optimal for foveal stimulation. In humans and monkeys the contrast sensitivity curve has a peak near 5 cycles/degree (cpd). This measure corresponds to a square (check) element having a diagonal of 20' of arc, or roughly 13 min of arc checkwidth. We studied the VEP using spatial frequencies ranging from 1.1 cpd to 13.8 cpd. In this range was included 4.6 cpd, which falls closest to the human contrast sensitivity peak.

Subjects

Twenty-two normal observers with normal visual acuity and normal neurological status served as controls. Six of these observers had one or several recordings using topographical mapping of the VEP, obtained at least with three different spatial frequencies. Five patients with well-diagnosed and stable intracranial lesions were studied. Their initial diagnosis was based on CT scan and/or MRI data and neurological examination. In one other patient the diagnosis was first suggested by our recordings.

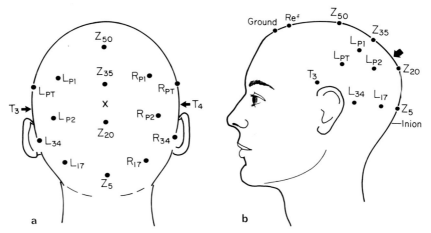

Fig. 1a, b. Placement of electrodes. **a** Vertical projection, 45 degrees inclined toward nasion; **b** left profile. Z Refers to the midline and the numbers represent the percentage of the inion-nasion distance. In the lower transverse electrode chain, *numbers* indicate the percentage of the distance between Z5 and the nasion. L, left; R, right; P, parietal; T, temporal. LP1 and RP1 are measured as one-third of the Z35 − T3 and the Z35-T4 distance respectively, and LPT, RPT as two-thirds of the same distance. LP2 and RP2 electrodes are placed at half of the LP1-L17 and the RP1-R17 distance. Reference electrode position was at Z63 and a ground electrode was placed at the forehead

Recordings

Electrode montage was as illustrated in Fig. 1. There were 16 active electrodes and two possible reference electrodes in addition to a theoretically calculated common average reference (Duffy 1982; Perrin et al. 1987; Maguire et al. 1985; Bertrand et al. 1985; Thickbroom et al. 1985). The locations of the 16 active electrodes were in essence as follows: a horizontal row of five electrodes centered on Z5, on the midline at the 5% inion-nasion distance. The others were placed evenly up to the vertex, in the midline and laterally. The reference electrode was either linked ears or Z63. The forehead was grounded. Signals were filtered between 0.3 and 100 Hz, amplified and averaged on line with a four-channel (Nicolet 1170) or eight-channel (Dantec Evomatic) averager and/or recorded with a Siegen "Sieg" for topographic analysis.

Results

N70 is the Earliest Cortical Component of the VEP

We have studied the VEP elicited with so-called dynamic random-dot correlogram (DRDC) patterns (Bodis-Wollner et al. 1981). This stimulus consists of two patterns projected in superimposition on the same screen. One pattern consists of red and white squares ("checks") in random sequence, the other of green and white squares, also in random sequence. An observer wearing a red filter can see only one of these patterns, wearing a green filter, only the other. An observer wearing a red filter over one eye and a green filter over the other will see both patterns, but each eye only sees one. Every time the two random patterns are changed in a such a way that they are in phase and then out of phase in respect to each other, the observer detects the change and also an EP can be recorded. Using this method of correlation-anticorrelation of the DRDC stimulus we found that the earliest statistically reliable component of the EP is a negative voltage recorded at Z5 around 70 ms. This voltage must represent signals which occur in the visual cortex at the level of, or beyond, binocular convergence. The implication of this finding is therefore that at around 70 ms the VEP contains a definitely postsynaptic potential. The results also suggest, though they do not prove, that by 70 ms following pattern stimulation, one records a surface negative cortical postsynaptic potential. However, as we shall see, the inferred generators of the foveal N70 do indeed suggest a cortical location.

N70 Is Determined by Foveal Neurons

We compared VEPs resulting from the following spatial frequencies of stimulation, using pattern onset-offset mode: 1.1, 2.3, 4.6, 6.9, 9.8 and 13.8 cpd. We studied both monocular and binocular responses. The results show, using either full-field or hemifield stimulation, that N70 amplitude grows with spatial frequency up to 4.6–6.9 cpd and then drops again. These results are broadly consistent with VEP studies by Jones and Keck (1978), Parker et al. (1982), Plant et al. (1983) and Paulus et al. (1984). Given that N70 is largest at spatial frequencies near the peak of human foveal contrast sensitivity, one is tempted to conclude that N70 is generated by the response of foveal neurons, from the retina onwards.

N70 Is Ipsilaterally Generated, One Generator in Each Hemisphere

The results we obtained in normals and in patients with well-known pathology and visual field defects, using full-field and hemifield stimulation, are in agreement with each other. As we have summarized above, the amplitude of N70 grows, with spatial frequency, from 1 to about 5 cpd. It is particularly evident using hemifield stimulation. We see an almost perfect polarity inversion of N70 across the midline in normal subjects: while the ipsilateral component is negative, contralateral recordings reveal a positive deflection in its place. We interpret these findings to show the presence of an N70 generator in each hemisphere. Their orientation is nearly opposite, thus in full-field recordings nothing or little of N70 is evident, due to electrical cancellation. Naturally, there is a fair amount of variability of cortical anatomy in normals (Stensaas et al. 1974), and perfect cancellation is not the rule. This interpretation is reinforced by our studies in patients with homonymous field defects, in whom the presence of the field defect is associated with an absence of the ipsilateral N70, and the N70 of the normal hemisphere is unmasked by pathology. Hence we should expect, and indeed we observe, an N70 which is more prominent in patients than in normals, using fullfield stimulation (Fig. 4B). It should be noted that while the patients we studied for the presence of a pathological N70 had large hemifield defects, what is relevant for the VEP is that their defect involved the paracentral 4–9 degrees of visual field.

Topographic Studies

We obtained monocular maps to 2.3, 4.6 and 6.9 cpd of stimulation in six normals and six patients. One of the latter had a craniopharyngioma involving the chiasmal region. In the other five the lesion was vascular: following infarct (3) or surgery for arteriovenous malformation (2). In each case there was CT scan confirmation and in each case the lesion was stable several months following the acute incident. The results on the whole confirm those obtained with only four- or eight-channel recordings (see Figs. 2, 3, 4). Topographic display can, however, reveal significant asymmetries that would have been missed) if we had only examined eight channels by visual inspection alone. Often the asymmetries were subtle, and only following the topographic display could be identify them in the "raw" recordings (Fig. 4). In fact, in one patient the presence of the arteriovenous malformation was revealed with appropriate radiological studies, after we obtained the VEP map which suggested the presence of a significant asymmetry. The referring diagnosis of the patient was suspected multiple sclerosis. In three of the patients the visual defect was evident only using red match or static perimetry (Humphrey), not using the Goldmann perimeter. In one patient a visual field defect could be demonstrated in only one eye, yet the VEP map revealed it to be present in both eyes.

Fig. 2a, b. Two sets of 16 VEP traces (*left*) and four maps obtained in normal subject A.G. (male, 45 years) with full-field stimulation of the right eye. Spatial frequency: **a** 2.3 cpd; **b** 4.6 cpd. The *upper maps* show N70 at latencies of 77.4 ms **a** and 81 ms **b**; the *lower maps* show P100 at 101.6 and 106.4 ms latency respectively. Electrode location is described in Fig. 1. The amplitudes of N70 and P100 for three selected electrode positions (Z5, L5, R5) are described above each set of the traces. In this figure, as in Fig. 3 and 4, the amplitudes were measured in microvolts. Downward deflection indicates positivity. Analysis time was 300 ms. Notice that N70 and P100 latency and amplitude increase with an increase in spatial frequency at the midline electrode, while there is a decrease of N70 amplitude over lateral electrodes. This differential effect of spatial frequency suggests that N70 following full-field stimulation is distributed more narrowly in respect to the inion as spatial frequencies of stimulation closer to foveal receptive field center size are selected

a A. G. normal, m 45, OD fullfield, 2.3cpd
top: N70map(77.4ms) low: P100map(101.6ms)
ampl. Z5: -0.5uV   +3.5uV
      R5: -0.8   +2.2
      L5: -0.7   +2.9
negative up;   maps: red+   blue-

b A. G. normal, 45 m, OD fullfield, 4.6cpd
top: N70map(81.0ms) low: P100map(106.4ms)
ampl.: Z5 -0.7   +4.0
       R5 -0.3   +3.0
       L5 -0.4   +3.2
negative up;   maps: red+; blue-

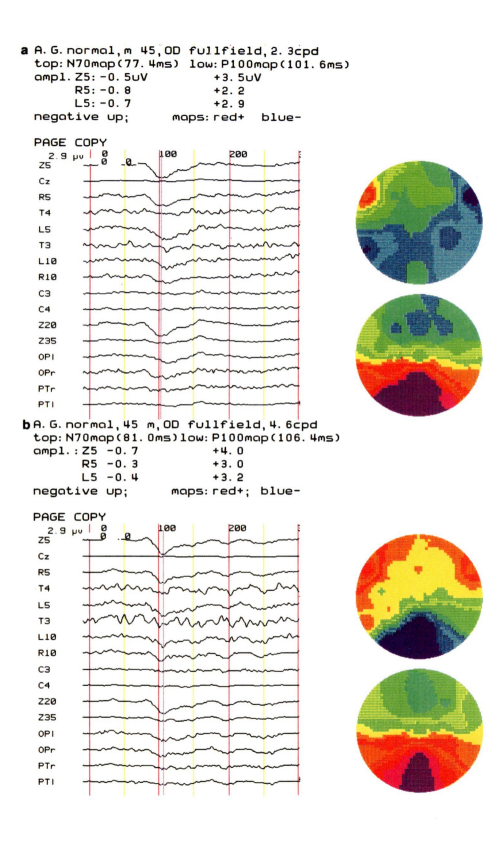

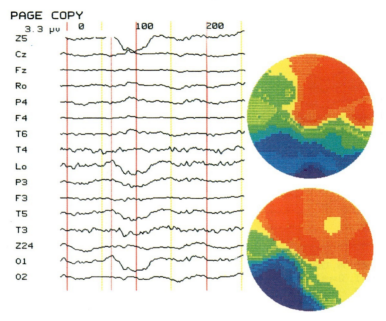

```
R.C., normal 18m, OS, 2.3cpd
maps of N70 (64.1ms, both) blue-; red+
top: FULLFIELD,    bottom: LEFT HEMIFIELD
ampl. Z5  -1.6uV   -1.4uV
      Ro  -0.7     +0.1
      Lo  -0.9     -2.0       negative up
```

Fig. 3. 16 VEP traces and two maps obtained in normal subject R.C. male, 18 years) with full-field (*top*) and left-field (*bottom*) stimulation of his left eye at spatial frequency of 2.3 cpd. The traces on the left of the figures correspond to the lower of the two maps. The amplitudes of N70 (in respect to the baseline) listed here are those following full-field (*F*) and left-field (*L*) stimulation for electrodes Z5, Ro and Lo. Ipsilateral negativity obtained with hemifield stimulation is clearly visible in the lower map, suggesting an ipsilateral origin of N70

Fig. 4a, b. Two sets of 16 VEP traces and four maps obtained in a female patient with right homonymous hemianopia. The amplitudes of three selected electrodes. (Z5, L5, R5) can be read above each set of traces. **a** Traces obtained and maps calculated with full-field stimulation of the patient's left eye at spatial frequency of 2.3 cpd. The *upper* map shows the distribution of N70 at 77.4 ms latency, and the *lower* map shows the distribution of P100 at 101.6 ms latency. **b** Traces obtained with full-field stimulation of the right eye at 4.6 cpd. The map of N70 displays the amplitudes at 82.2 ms latency and the P100 map shows the distribution of the amplitudes at 114.9 ms latency. P100 positivity with prolonged latency in R5, and polarity inversion in R10 derivation with the spatial frequency of 4.6 cpd suggest a right paracentral visual defect. In fact that this is not clearly evident with 2.3 cpd stimulation demonstrates the importance of foveal stimulation.

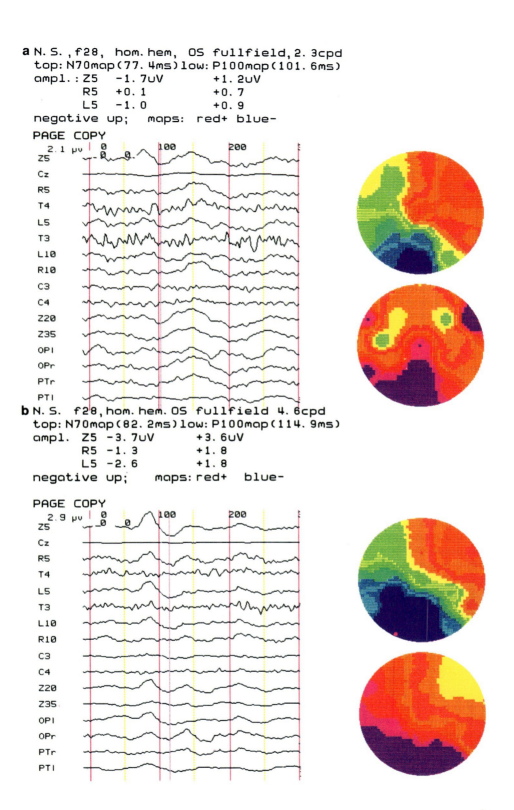

Discussion

While the N70 has been studied and occasionally described in some detail (Jones and Keck 1978; Parker et al. 1982; Plant et al. 1983), it has not on the whole received much attention, as it is thought to be an unreliable clinical indicator of visual pathway pathology. As we have shown, this reputation for unreliability stems from utilizing inappropriate stimulation for obtaining the VEP. Generally, clinical studies utilize check-sizes of 50 min of arc or larger (Halliday 1982; Chiappa 1983), while the human VEP is mostly dominated by foveal cortical neurons which respond best fo finer stimuli (Bodis-Wollner et al. 1986) (Fig. 2). This is particularly true for the N70 component, as has already been suggested in previous studies and as we have demonstrated. In addition, we have shown how the originization of the cortical generators of N70 can result in cancellation effects when using full-field stimuli, thus spuriously indicating a lack of a significant N70 component. We have also summarized the evidence concerning the cortical origin of VEP components around 70 ms, the evidence concerning the spatial tuning of N70 and, finally, using multichannel recordings and topographic display of VEP data of normals and patients, we have demonstrated the presence of two N70 generators, one in each hemisphere, responding to hemifield stimuli. For these reasons the N70 component cannot be identical to the components described by Jeffreys and Axford (1972) as CI. Their stimuli differed significantly from the ones we used, being more complex in both space and time. The closest analogy we find is with a component described as N60 by Lesevre and her collegues (1976, 1979, 1982). Our conclusion is that N70 has two generators; one was inferred in each hemisphere from studies of normals using hemifield stimuli and was evident in multichannel recordings. In patients N70 can best be verified by multichannel recording and topographic display. The effect of a paracentral scotoma is to attenuate the contribution of one of these generators and hence "unmask" a single N70 maximum, lateralized to one hemisphere. The effect of paracentral scotoma on the N70 suggests that the latter is a clinically relevant component of the VEP: using appropriate stimulation techniques and topographic recording, it can reveal hidden visual losses in the paracentral field. We (Onofrj et al. 1982) and others (e.g., Hoeppner et al. 1984) found that polarity inversion of P100, as originally described by Barrett et al. (1976), has fair diagnostic value for visual field defects caused by gross pathology. Our present data suggest that N70 is of greater significance in detecting paracentral visual field defects. The importance of the paracentral region of the visual field is that it is commonly affected not only in optic nerve lesions but also in incipient chiasmatic, optic tract (Bender and Bodis-Wollner 1978) and occipital lesions. Occipital lesions may cause perimetrically detected paracentral scotomas and, commonly, contrast sensitivity defects (Bodis-Wollner and Diamond 1976). In "bedside" neurology paracentral defects are best revealed by confrontation and using colored, primarily red, targets (Glaser 1978). Static perimetry is a superb but time-consuming technique where exact fixation is of prime importance. For obtaining the foveal-parafoveal VEP we used spatial frequencies which directly address foveal and parafoveal neurons. The pattern is presented as a "large" (9 degrees in diameter) stimulus. The patient's fixation may wander, yet his/her electrophysiological responses will by definition arise only from the central visual field, as the sensitivity of peripheral receptive fields rapidly becomes attenuated to the spatial frequencies (4.6 and 6.9 cpd) used for the foveal VEP (Robson and Graham 1981). Therefore, by using a foveal pattern and a full-field stimulus one does not need to rely on exact fixation. Exact fixation is difficult at the edge of a hemianopic field for most patients. Based on our initial experience, presented in this chapter, we believe that the VEP map provides a sensitive diagnostic tool in evaluating incipient chiasmatic lesions and optic tract lesions. Our experience with strict occipital lesions is limited, but classical data (Bender and Furlow 1945) concerning visual defects in occipital lobe lesions, using colour, flicker and completion as indices of normal visual functioning, suggest that novel visual stimuli may well have a role to play in diagnostic VEP mapping.

References

Barrett G, Blumhardt L, Halliday AM, Halliday E, Kriss A (1976) A paradox in the lateralisation of the visual evoked response. Nature 261:253–255

Bender MB, Furlow LT (1945) Visual disturbances produced by bilateral lesions of the occipital lobes with central scotomas. Arch Neurol Psychiatr 53:165–170

Bender MB, Bodis-Wollner I (1978) Visual dysfunctions in optic tract lesions. Ann Neurol 3:187–193

Bertrand O, Perrin F, Pernier J (1985) A theoretical justification of the average reference in topographic evoked potential studies. Electroencephalogr Clin Neurophysiol 62:462–464

Bodis-Wollner I, Hendley CD (1979) On the separability of two mechanisms involved in the detection of grating patterns in humans. J Physiol (Lond) 201:251–263

Bodis-Wollner I, Diamond S (1976) The measurement of spatial contrast sensitivity in cases of blurred vision associated with cerebral lesions. Brain 99:695–710

Bodis-Wollner I, Barris M, Mylin LH, Julesz B, Kropfl W (1981) Binocular stimulation reveals cortical components of the human VEP. Electroencephalogr Clin Neurophysiol 52:298–385

Bodis-Wollner I, Ghilardi MF, Mylin LH (1986) The importance of stimulus selection in the VEP practice: the clinical relevance of visual physiology. In: Bodis-Wollner I, Cracco RQ (eds) Evoked potentials. Liss, New York, pp 15–27

Campbell FW, Green DC (1965) Optical and retinal factors affecting visual resolution. J Physiol (Lond) 181:576–593

Chiappa KH (1983) Evoked potentials in clinical medicine. Raven, New York, p 28

Duffy FH (1982) Topographic display of evoked potentials: clinical applications of brain electrical activity mapping (BEAM). Ann NY Acad Sci 388:183–196

Glaser JS (1978) Neuro-ophthalmology. Harper and Row, Hagerstown, pp 18–19

Halliday AM (1982) The visual evoked response in healthy subjects. In: Halliday AM (ed) Evoked potentials in clinical testing. Churchill-Livingstone, Edinburgh, pp 71–120

Hoeppner TJ, Bergen D, Morell F (1984) Hemispheric asymmetry of VEPs in patients with well defined occipital lesions. Electroencephalogr Clin Neurophysiol 57:310–319

Jeffreys PA, Axford JG (1972) Source locations of pattern specific components of human VEPs I and II. Exp Brain Res 16:1–40

Jones R, Keck MJ (1978) Visual evoked response as a function of grating spatial frequency. Invest Ophathalmol Vis Sci 17:652–659

Lesevre N (1976) Topographical analysis of the pattern evoked response (PER): its application to the study of macular and peripheral vision in normal people and in some pathological cases. Doc Ophthalmol Proc Series 10:87–102

Lesevre N, Joseph JP (1979) Modifications of the pattern evoked potential in relation to the stimulated part of the visual field (clues for the most probable origins of each component). Electroencephalogr Clin Neurophysiol 47:183–190

Lesevre N (1982) Chronotopographical analysis of the human evoked potential in relation to the visual field (data from normal individuals and hemianopic patients). Ann NY Acad Sci 388:156–183

Mauguiere F, Giard MH, Ibanez V, Pernier J (1985) Sequential spatial maps of visual potentials evoked by checkerboard-pattern response topography Rev Electroencephalogr Neurophysiol Clin 15(2):129–137

Onofrj M, Bodis-Wollner I, Mylin LH (1982) VEP diagnosis of field defects in patients with chiasmatic and retrochiasmatic lesions. J Neurol Neurosurg Psychiatry 45:294–302

Parker DM, Salzen EA, Lishman JR (1982) Visual evoked responses elicited by the onset and offset of sinusoidal gratings: latency, waveform and topographic characteristics. Invest Ophthalmol Vis Sci 22:675–680

Paulus W, Homberg V, Cunningham K, Halliday AM, Rohde N (1984) Colour and luminance components of foveal visual responses in man. Electroencephalogr Clin Neurophysiol 58:107–119

Perrin F, Pernier J, Bertrand O, Giard MH, Echallier JF (1987) Mapping of scalp potentials by surface spline interpolation. Electroencephalogr Clin Neurophysiol 66:75–81

Perry VH, Cowey A (1985) The ganglion cell and cone distributions in the monkey's retina: implications for central magnification factors. Vision Res 25:1795–1810

Plant GT, Zimmern RL, Durden K (1983) Transient VEPs to the pattern reversal and onset of sinusoidal gratings. Electroencephalogr Clin Neurophysiol 56:147–158

Robson JG, Graham N (1981) Probability summation and regional variation in contrast sensitivity across the visual field. Vision Res 21:409–418

Schade DH (1956) Optical and photoelectric analog of the eye. J Opt Soc Am [A] 46:721–739

Stensaas SS, Eddington DK, Dobelle WH (1974) The topography and variability of the primary visual cortex in man. J Neurosurg 40:747–755

Thickbroom GW, Carroll WM, Mastaglia FL (1985) Dipole source derivation. Application to the half-field PEV. Biomed Comp 16:17

Surface Maps and Generators of Brainstem Auditory Evoked Potential Waves I, III, and V*

Introduction

Several reports on the distribution of brainstem auditory evoked potentials (BAEPs) on the scalp, although not in the form of topographical maps, are found in the literature (see, e.g., Picton et al. 1974; Terkildsen et al. 1974; Martin and Moore 1977; Streletz et al. 1977). More recently, Ihl et al. presented some examples of BAEP maps that agree reasonably well with the surface distributions reported by Grandori (1986), despite some differences in data analysis.

Surface BAEP electric fields have been analyzed in some recent papers aimed at extracting information about the sources of the fields with dipole localization methods (DLMs) at instants corresponding to the waves of major interest (Grandori 1984, 1986; Scherg 1984; Scherg and von Cramon 1985). DLMs have also been used to study BAEP fields in cats (Gaumond et al. 1983; Gaumond and Fried 1986). A simplified procedure describing the surface activity, similar to the technique known as vector ECG, has been proposed by some authors (see e.g., Pratt et al. 1985).

All these studies, despite the differences in data recording and processing, clearly pointed out that the electrical activity on the scalp can be summarized, at least during several time periods, by a simple model of the sources, the "equivalent" dipole; a fairly close agreement can be found for the estimated dipoles, in particular for orientation (Scherg 1984; Grandori 1986).

This paper presents examples of BAEP maps. The results of a DLM technique, in terms of equivalent dipoles for waves I, III and V, are then used in some simulations of a forward problem, to predict, at least as a first approximation, the magnetic fields (radial component) produced on the surface of a homogeneous sphere. It is thought that such predictions would be of some help in defining the experimental paradigm for the measurement of brainstem evoked magnetic fields.

Electric Fields: Maps and "Equivalent" Dipoles

Techniques for data recording and map computation are described elsewhere (Grandori 1984, 1986) and are summarized here. Data were collected from

---

* This paper was partially supported by grants from the Italian Ministry of Public Education, Project on Spatio Temporal Analysis of Evoked Potentials.

[1] Centro Teoria dei Sistemi, C.N.R., Dipartimento di Elettronica, Politecnico di Milano, Milano, Italy

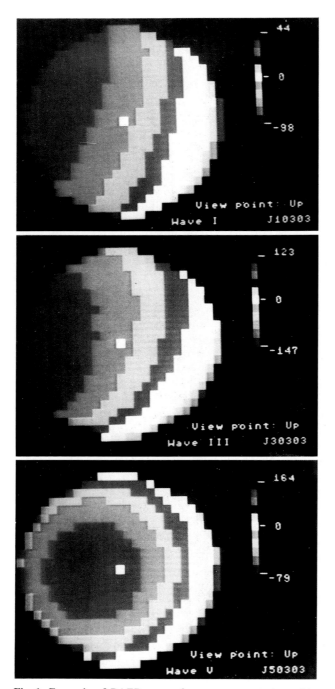

Fig. 1. Example of BAEPs maps from a representative subject at time points corresponding to the latency of waves I, III and V. Data shown are the orthogonal projections of the recorded fields from the top of the head. The *white squares* represent the vertex. Values in nV

subjects whose hearing was normal with monoaural clicks of alternated polarity (3000–4000 sweeps), at 110 dB peak equivalent sound pressure level from 31 electrodes located on the scalp (10/20 system and some additional locations), with common frontal reference, and re-referenced (average reference, with equal weight). Sampled data points were digitally filtered 250–2000 Hz. Maps were computed with a four nearest neighboring points interpolation algorithm, on a spherical surface, and then projected onto planes (orthogonal projections). An Amplaid MK 7 was used for data collection; signals were processed on a host computer for off-line map computation.

Field distributions obtained from a representative subject at time points corresponding to wave I, III and V are illustrated in Fig. 1. The "far field" character of the potential distributions is clear: field extremes are wide apart and gradients are low, as expected from sources located several centimeters below the skull. For wave I, the map shows the presence of a rather broad region of positive potentials on the hemisphere contralateral to the stimulated (right) ear; negative potentials are found mainly around the ipsilateral ear. It is clear that a vertex-ipsilateral mastoid – or earlobe – derivation will pick up a nearly maximal potential difference. For wave III, the situation is very similar, apart from a greater spread of positive potential values around the contralateral temporal region. At the latency of wave V, the field maximum is located around the vertex and this wave can be recorded with almost the same magnitude from any point located on horizontal planes, against the vertex.

As discussed in some previous papers (Grandori 1984, 1986; Scherg 1984; Scherg and von Cramon 1985), BAEP fields can be analyzed with DLMs. The results obtained using these techniques, in terms of equivalent dipoles, have been shown to summarize the activity of intracranial regions whose location and extent can be quantified with a reasonable degree of approximation (Grandori 1988).

Theoretical Predictions of Auditory Evoked Brainstem Magnetic Fields

Measurements of magnetic fields evoked from the brainstem structures are technically very difficult since the signal-to-noise ratio is extremely unfavorable. This is due mainly to the fact that the strength of the magnetic fields produced at the head surface by deep sources is very low.

Dipoles estimated at time points corresponding to the latency of waves I, III and V (Grandori 1986) have been used as sources in a forward problem to predict the magnetic fields produced by the brainstem structures at corresponding time points.

Model equations are those proposed by Cuffin and Cohen (1977) for the radial component of the field with a 9.2-cm radius spherical homogeneous model. No attempt was made to account for the pickup coil, as is usually done in DLMs for magnetic measurements. Fields were computed on a spherical grid (4° for latitude and longitude) and then projected onto orthogonal planes. Figure 2 shows the projections of the fields from the top, the back and the right of the sphere.

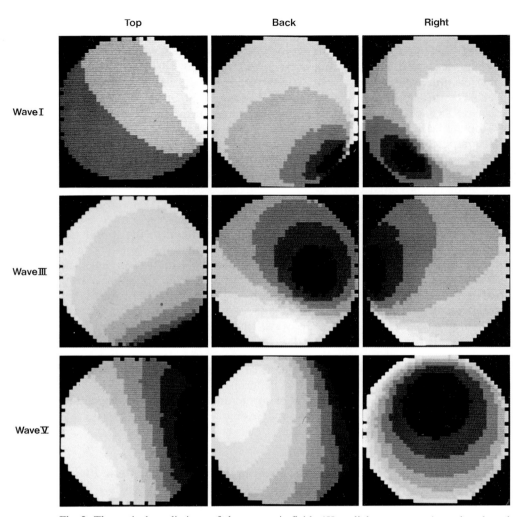

Fig. 2. Theoretical predictions of the magnetic fields (H, radial components) produced at the surface of a homogeneous spherical conductor. Sources of these magnetic fields are the equivalent dipoles estimated from the electric measurements at corresponding time instants. Maxima and minima for each map, from left to right, top to bottom (oersteds $\times 10^{-15}$): [(0.687, −0.186), (0.797, −0.996), (1.017, −1.021)] for wave I; [(0.225, −1.984), (2.058, −2.068), (1.974, −2.058)] for wave III; [(0.890, −0.890), (0.890, −0.890), (0.313, −0.089)] for wave V

Due to the rather deep location of the dipoles for brainstem waves I–V, positive and negative maxima are fairly well separated. It is interesting to observe that the magnetic fields computed for wave I and III are not as close as in the case of the electric potential fields; this is most likely due to the higher sensitivity of the magnetic fields to dipole location compared to that of the electric potentials, which are somewhat blurred by the resistivity of the skull.

Summary

Brainstem auditory evoked potential maps can be interpreted using a DLM procedure; dipoles corresponding to the waves of major interest are to be considered both as a means of summarizing the surface potentials and as a first approximate model of the sources, although the identification of the precise anatomical sites contributing to the surface potentials is affected by a considerable degree of uncertainty (Grandori 1987). Data are presented on the magnetic fields (radial component) at time points corresponding to the three potential waves I, III and V as predicted by a model. Although it is not clear at present whether the excitation processes underlying the generation of electric and magnetic fields are the same (Kaufman et al. 1981), it is thought that these predictions would be of some help in defining the experimental paradigm for the measurement of brainstem evoked magnetic fields.

Acknowledgement. Thanks are due to Gianluca Bambozzi for assistance in developing the computer programs for the computation of the magnetic fields.

References

Cuffin BN, Cohen D (1977) Magnetic fields of a dipole in special volume conductor shapes. IEEE Trans Biomed Eng 24:372–381

Gaumond RP, Fried SI (1986) Analysis of cat multichannel acoustic brainstem response data using dipole localization methods. Electroencephlogr Clin Neurophysiol 63:376–383

Gaumond RP, Lin JH, Geselowitz DB (1983) Accuracy of dipole localization with a spherical homogeneous model. IEEE Trans Biomed Eng 30:29–34

Grandori F (1984) Dipole localization methods and auditory evoked brainstem potentials. Rev Laryngol Otol Rhinol (Bord) 105:171–178

Grandori F (1986) Field analysis of auditory evoked brainstem potentials. Hearing Res 21:51–58

Grandori F (1988) Dipolar fields and generators of electric evoked potentials. Some limits in the use of DLMs for the description of the sources. In: Erne S, Romani GL (eds) Advances in biomagnetism. (in press)

Kaufman L, Okada Y, Brenner D, Williamson S (1981) On the relations between somatic evoked potentials and fields. Int J Neurosci 15:273–282

Martin ME, Moore EJ (1977) Scalp distribution of early (0 to 10 ms) auditory evoked responses. Arch Otolaryngol 103:326–328

Picton TW, Hillyard SA, Krausz HI, Galambos R (1974) Human auditory evoked potentials. I. Evaluation of components. Electroencephalogr Clin Neurophysiol 36:179–190

Pratt H, Bleich N, Martin WH (1985) Three-channel Lissajous' trajectory of human auditory brainstem evoked potentials. I. Normative measures. Electroencephalogr Clin Neurophysiol 61:530–538

Scherg M (1984) Spatio-temporal modelling of early auditory evoked potentials. Rev Laryngol Otol Rhinol (Bord) 105:163–170

Scherg M, von Cramon D (1985) A new interpretation of the generators of BAEPs waves I–V: Results of a spatio-temporal dipole model. Electroencephalogr Clin Neurophysiol 62:290–299

Streletz LJ, Katz L, Hohenberger M, Cracco R (1977) Scalp recorded auditory evoked potentials and sonomotor responses: an evaluation of components and recording techniques. Electroencephalogr Clin Neurophysiol 43:192–206

Terkildsen K, Osterhammel P, Huis in't Veld, F (1974) Far field electrocochleography, electrode position. Scand Audiol 3:123–129

Topographic Brain Mapping and Long Latency Somatosensory Evoked Potentials of Posterior Tibial Nerve and Dorsal Nerve of Penis

W.H. SCHERB[1], G. GALLWITZ[1], J. KNEIP-SCHERB[2], W. BÄHREN[3], and J. KRIEBEL[1]

Introduction

Medical and sexual histories, physical examination and laboratory testing have not been adequate in diagnosing the major causes of erectile dysfunction (ED). Knowledge of multiple invasive and noninvasive tests is important for the clinician involved in the evaluation of impotence (Jevtich 1984). Especially neurologic evaluation of ED is still a challenge. It should always be part of a multidisciplinary testing program to differentiate pathologic inflow, pathologic outflow, neurogenic and other causes of ED (Bähren et al. 1986). Neurophysiologic evaluation includes the direct method of evaluating penile somatic nerves utilizing the bulbocavernosus reflex arc introduced by Rushworth (1967). In this test, distal endings of the dorsal nerve of the penis (DNP) are stimulated by electrical impulses and the resultant response evoked in the bulbocavernosus muscle is recorded. Perineal electromyography is a recording of the motor unit potentials from the perineal striated muscles. It has been used to identify denervation states and to recognize occult subclinical disturbances in the motor pudendal pathway (Siroky et al. 1979). Cortical or spinal short latency somatosensory evoked responses of the posterior tibial nerve (PTN) or DNP measure the sensory component of nerve roots, spinal cord and cerebral lesions (Haldeman et al. 1982). To our knowledge, studies of long latency components and their spatial distribution after stimulation of DNP have not yet been performed.

The aim of this study was to get normative data of long latency somatosensory evoked potentials (LLSSEPs) of PTN and DNP with a commercial topographic brain mapping system.

Materials and Methods

Recordings were made from 30 unpaid male volunteers who gave their informed consent. Their age range was 18–45 years (mean 24.9 years), their height 168–

---

[1] Abteilung für Neurologie und Psychiatrie, Bundeswehrkrankenhaus Ulm, Oberer Eselsberg 40, 7900 Ulm, Federal Republic of Germany
[2] Abteilung für Neurologie der Universität Ulm, 7900 Ulm, Federal Republic of Germany
[3] Abteilung für Radiologie, Bundeswehrkrankenhaus Ulm, Oberer Eselsberg 40, 7900 Ulm, Federal Republic of Germany

196 cm (mean 177 cm). They were all left hemisphere dominant, in good health, free from neurological disease and non-addicted to drugs. They were comfortably seated in a reclining chair and remained awake but relaxed during the recording, which lasted about 45–60 min. Skin temperature of the foot was measured and stayed above 28° C.

Stimulation

Stimulation was applied through the skin close to the PTN at the popliteal fossa: both sides were stimulated sequentially. The DNP was stimulated just below the glans penis using ring electrodes with poles 25 mm apart and with the proximal pole the cathode. Single 0.2-ms pulses of 2–2.5 times sensory threshold were delivered at a rate of 1/s. The sensory threshold was 8–15 mA (mean 11.5 mA) and the motor threshold was 18–38 mA (mean 23.6 mA); stimulation level was 20–40 mA.

Recording

Recording was made with a 28-channel electro-cap according to the 10-20-system and ear-linked reference. Electrode impedance was under 2 kΩ. A Neu-

Table 1. Latencies and amplitudes in posterior tibial nerve and dorsal nerve of penis

	Range	Mean	SD
Posterior tibial nerve right			
Latencies (ms)			
Onset	134–172	153.7	8.6
Minimum	174–232	196.8	14.8
Maximum	238–322	270.5	20.1
Amplitude (µV)	4–16	10.0	4.0
Posterior Tibial nerve left			
Latencies (ms)			
Onset	136–184	154.2	12.8
Minimum	172–234	201.9	15.4
Maximum	234–318	272.1	18.4
Amplitude (µV)	3.5–16	9.1	17.0
Dorsal nerve of penis			
Latencies (ms)			
Onset	136–180	153.8	10.0
Minimum	178–214	194.9	8.7
Maximum	210–276	247.5	16.4
Amplitude (µV)	3.8–22	8.5	5.9

roscience Brain Imager System was used with an amplifier bandpass of 0.15–40 Hz. An analysis time of 600 ms began 16 ms after the stimulus and two sequential runs of 200 sweeps were averaged to check the constancy of the response. The dynamic range was 256 µV.

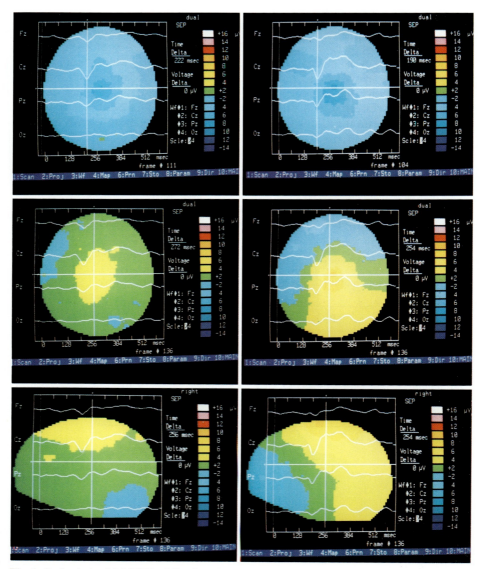

Fig. 1. Scalp-derived LLSSEPs following electrical stimulation of posterior tibial nerve (PTN; left): minimum 190 ms, maximum 240 ms; dorsal nerve of penis (DNP; right): minimum 176 ms, maximum 240 ms. Mapping shows spatial distribution with maximal response over centroparietal area of PTN and more widespread right posterior occipital distribution of DNP

Results

Ten totally artifact-free recordings were used for statistical calculation. In all recordings we found a P300-like response and measured the latency of the onset, of the first negativity (minimum) and of the first positivity (maximum) as shown in Fig. 1. Amplitude was measured between minimum and maximum (Table 1).

Discussion

In normals, LLSSEPs of PTN and DNP show a P300-like response. The major problems are to get artifact-free recordings without misleading mappings by using commercial brain mapping systems and to keep the proband at an equal state of consciousness. On topographic brain mapping spatial distribution shows a maximal response of PTN in the centroparietal area. In six of 10 cases the response after stimulating DNP was more widespread over the centroparietal and right parieto-occipital areas. This observation is in good agreement with Coslett and Heilman's findings of impairment of male sexual function after right hemisphere stroke (1986). According to the location of the stimulus, the maximum response is abnormal if tibial or pudendal pathways or subcortical or cortical sources are damaged.

The diagnostic implications of LLSSEPs are evident. They could prove to be a useful tool in the evaluation of conditions with central causes of neurogenic ED and perhaps even in some cases of functional (e.g., metabolic or drug-induced) or psychiatric and psychogenic ED, comparable to the P3b-like

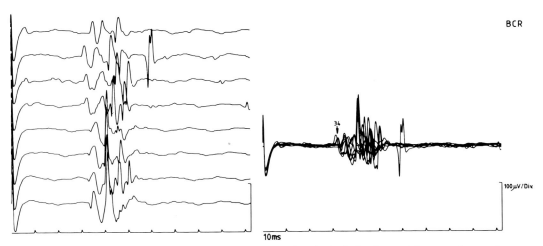

Fig. 2. Bulbocavernosus reflex. *Left:* eight consecutive single derivations; *right:* superimposed, minimum latency 34 ms

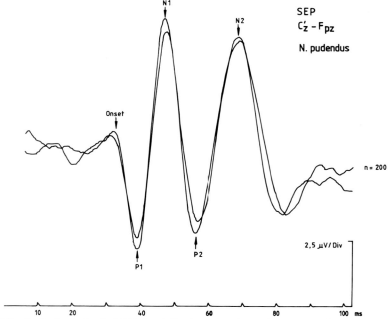

Fig. 3. Scalp-derived SLSSEPs following electrical stimulation of dorsal nerve of *penis*. P1 39 ms

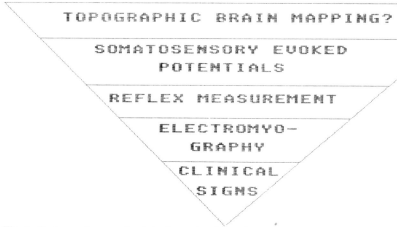

Fig. 4. System of neurophysiologic evaluation of erectile dysfunction: increasing complexity and amount of time

responses found in amygdala, hippocampus, and thalamus as well as over cortex (Courchesne et al. 1987).

A particular advantage might be, that LLSSEP could be carried out together with BCR measurements (Fig. 2), EMG-BC and SLSSEPs of DNP (Fig. 3) and so complete a neurophysiologic system of evaluation of neurogenic ED (Fig. 4).

References

Bähren W, Stief CH, Scherb W, Gall H, Gallwitz A, Altwein J (1986) Rationelle Diagnostik der erektilen Dysfunction unter Anwendung eines pharmakologischen Testes. Akt Urol 17:177–180

Coslett HB, Heilman KM (1986) Male sexual function: impairment after right hemisphere stroke. Arch Neurol 43:1036–1039

Courchesne E, Elmasian R, Yeung-Courchesne R (1987) Electrophysiological correlates of cognitive processing: P3b and Nc, basic, clinical, and developmental research. In: Halliday AM, Butler RS, Paul R (eds) A textbook of clinical neurophysiology. Wiley, London, pp 645–676

Haldeman S, Bradley WE, Bhatia NN, Johnson BK (1982) Pudendal evoked responses. Arch Neurol 39:280–283

Jevtich MJ (1984) Non-invasive vascular and neurologic tests in use for evaluation of angiogenic impotence. Inter Angiol 3:225–232

Rushworth G (1967) Diagnostic value of the electromyographic study of reflex activity in man. Electroencephalogr Clin Neurophysiol 25:65–73

Siroky MB, Sax DS, Krane RS (1979) Sacral signal tracing: the electrophysiology of the bulbocavernosus reflex. J Urol 122:661–664

Section VI Psychiatric Aspects

The Neuropsychology of Schizophrenia in the Context of Topographical Mapping of Electrocortical Activity

J. GRUZELIER and D. LIDDIARD[1]

Introduction

A preliminary study with EEG topographical mapping in carefully characterised schizophrenic patients will be reported in which patients were clearly differentiated from controls. The majority of test conditions involved functional activation with neuropsychological tests validated on neurological patients. Group differences were seldom found in the resting EEG. Before describing the results other reports using new EEG imaging procedures will be outlined and some contemporary approaches to the investigation of central nervous system dysfunction in schizophrenia will be briefly reviewed.

Topographical Mapping of EEG Power in Schizophrenia

In the resting EEG of schizophrenic patients Morihisa et al. (1983), using a 20-electrode array, found raised delta activity in virtually all areas but particularly in frontal regions. The effects were stronger in unmedicated patients. Fast frequency activity (28–31.5 Hz) was also elevated in patients in posterior regions, and medication was found to influence the lateral distribution of beta activity; a left parietal elevation occurred in unmedicated patients, whereas in the eyes closed condition in medicated patients there was a right central and temporal elevation. Though an increase in frontal delta in schizophrenia has also been reported by Morstyn et al. (1983) and Guenther et al. (1986), the significance of the frontal delta findings has been called into question by Karson et al. (1987) as possible artifacts of eye movement. After removal of traces contaminated by eye movements, unmedicated patients did not differ from controls in resting levels of delta, nor did they differ in any other bandwidth.

Functional activation of the EEG with psychological tasks has been explored by several investigators. In ten male, medicated, chronic schizophrenics, Morstyn et al. (1983) were unable to find task-specific effects over a range of activities including speech, music, learning and recognition of abstract figures, paired associates and reading. Effects were common to all psychological states but were reported to be somewhat more accentuated during activation. In general, more spectral energy in patients was found in delta, theta and fast beta (20–

---

[1] Department of Psychiatry, Charing Cross & Westminster Medical School, St. Dunstan's Road, London W6 8RP, United Kingdom

32 Hz). Increases in delta and theta were typically localised to the bilateral frontal regions, and hence may have been influenced by eye movements, whereas increases in fast beta were widespread posterior to the frontal lobe, and were maximal in the parieto-occipital and left anterior temporal regions.

Task-specific abnormalities in schizophrenia have been reported. Günther and Breitling (1985) and Guenther et al. (1986) compared EEG power, recorded from 16 electrodes, after a relaxation procedure with right hand motor tasks of variable complexity and dependence on sensorimotor integration. The patients, all of whom were medicated, failed to show increased activity in the primary sensory and motor areas of the left hemisphere, whereas often overactivation was seen in the right hemisphere.

Localisation of Dysfunction in Schizophrenia

The Temporolimbic System

In the 1960s there was a revival of interest in the likelihood of brain abnormalities in schizophrenia with growing awareness that organic conditions that mimicked schizophrenia could shed light on the brain mechanisms underlying the psychopathology, rather than simply being regarded as grounds for exclusion of a diagnosis of schizophrenia (Smythies 1969; Malamud 1967; Flor-Henry 1969; Davison and Bagley 1969). The temporal lobe, particularly of the left hemisphere (Flor-Henry 1974), was a possible locus of much florid, productive symptomatology, though the symptoms of the tumour cases of Malamud (1967) indicated that a full range of psychopathology in schizophrenia could arise from lesions in and around the hippocampal system. This was also the conclusion of Bragina's (1966) survey of temporal lobe lesions in neurological patients in whom a bipolarity in affect, motor activity and cognition was a particular hallmark.

The limbic hypothesis in schizophrenia also drew support from research with patients showing abnormalities of the autonomic orienting response and its habituation. This involves the matching of stimulus input to expectancies about the environment and the attenuation of response with stimulus repetition (Gruzelier and Venables 1972, 1973, 1974; Gruzelier 1973). Disruption of these processes occurred in primates after lesions to the amygdala and hippocampus and associated frontal regions (Pribram and McGuinness 1975). Strands of evidence from other sources have been reviewed in support of a temporolimbic locus of schizophrenic symptoms (Torrey and Peterson 1974), and recently dopamine concentrations have been reported to be abnormally elevated in the left-sided amygdala at post-mortem (Reynolds 1983; Reynolds and Czudek 1987).

Now topographical mapping of cortical evoked responses shows promise of clarifying the temporolimbic hypothesis. The P300 in some animal preparations has been shown to involve a hippocampal generator (Wood et al. 1980; Kaufman and Williamson 1982). Topographical investigation of the P300 in schizophrenia by Morstyn et al. (1983) has revealed a left posterior temporal deficiency, and P300 deficiencies in schizophrenia have been widely documented (Friedman 1987). Furthermore, investigation of the middle latency components which occur between 50 and 200 ms in response to flashes and tones of variable intensity from 16 electrodes sited over the left hemisphere has revealed reductions in amplitude in six unmedicated patients in the temporoparietal area (Buchsbaum et al. 1982).

The Frontal Lobe

Earlier this century there was interest in a possible frontal genesis of schizophrenia which led to surgical intervention through frontal leucotomy – interest which died down when the majority of patients operated on failed to recover. Interest was reawakened after claims of reductions in frontal blood flow from pioneering attempts at brain imaging following inhalation of xenon-133 (Ingvar and Franzen 1974). The phenomenon of "hypofrontality" is now thought to characterise a subgroup of patients with chronic negative symptoms such as blunted affect, emotional withdrawal and psychomotor poverty, while normal levels and sometimes elevations in frontal blood flow have been found during periods of acute exacerbation in remitting forms of schizophrenia (Sheppard et al. 1983).

Then followed computed tomography (CT) evidence such that in a proportion of schizophrenic patients there was ventricular enlargement and cortical atrophy which often encompassed the frontal lobe. Attempts to characterise the subgroup of patients with cortical atrophy have met with no clear-cut success despite initial promise (Johnstone et al. 1978), and though it is true that the clearer relationship is with negative symptoms, not all patients with the negative syndrome have CT signs, and not all patients with CT signs have negative symptoms. Furthermore, while negative symptoms in neurological patients are commonly associated with frontal pathology, they may also occur with both subcortical damage (Cummings and Benson 1984) and limbic lesions (Bragina 1966).

Neuropsychological testing has also revealed evidence of frontal losses of function in schizophrenia (e.g. Flor-Henry and Yeudall 1979; Kolb and Whishaw 1983), but as the frontal lobe is the final common pathway in response programming and execution it cannot be concluded that the genesis of the deficit is localised in the frontal lobe. A subcortical disturbance, say one that disrupts thalamofrontal interactions, may also lead to a disruption of the frontal lobe.

Posterior Parieto-Occipital Functions

Cortical evoked potentials in schizophrenia have revealed a variety of abnormalities in early and middle latency components which involve posterior sensory and polysensory brain functions (Shagass 1977; Connolly and Gruzelier 1982; Jutai et al. 1984; Gruzelier et al. 1985). Perceptual deficits are also well documented and these may involve non-verbal spatial perceptual functions (Venables

1964) or verbal abilities such as speech comprehension (Bull and Venables 1973). Attentional disturbance in schizophrenia has also been extensively documented (Kraepelin 1896; Bleuler 1950) and researched (Matthysee et al. 1978). Evidence of important attentional control mechanisms in the right parietal region has led to the speculation that this may be a region of dysfunction in schizophrenia (Mesulam and Geschwind 1978).

Hypofrontality is also relevant to posterior functions. The original finding was obtained with an anterior to posterior ratio measure. From the outset it was noticed that posterior blood flow was sometimes elevated, and in contrast to the frontal levels, which correlated with negative symptoms, posterior flow was found to correlate with symptoms having a perceptual-cognitive component (Franzen and Ingvar 1975).

Corpus Callosum

Enlargements in the corpus callosum in schizophrenia (Rosenthal and Bigelow 1972), have led to investigations with a range of techniques which had revealed interhemispheric transmission deficits in patients with callosectomy. The evidence to date is inconclusive (Gruzelier 1987b). Methodological and theoretical refinements are required, in order to be able to explore regional differences within the callosum, to differentiate subgroups of patients and to detect disordered callosal transfer as distinct from a failure of transfer akin to that of the split brain model. Abundant evidence of lateralised deficits, along with recurring evidence of left-right imbalances in function, also reinforces the need to elucidate interhemispheric functioning in schizophrenia via callosal and subcortical influences.

Lateralised Dysfunction in Schizophrenia

As there have been numerous reviews of lateralised dysfunction in schizophrenia (e.g., Walker McGuire 1982; Wexler 1980; Newlin et al. 1981; Gruzelier 1983), only recent developments in the author's laboratory will be summarised here. These developments cast a new light on the issue and are germane to the EEG topographical study that follows.

Re-examination of lateral asymmetries in electrodermal orienting responses in schizophrenia (Gruzelier 1973; Gruzelier and Venables 1974) with new diagnostic criteria (Wing et al. 1974) led to the discovery of two asymmetric patterns in undrugged schizophrenic patients (Gruzelier and Manchanda 1982). The two patterns delineated two syndromes in schizophrenia which had some affinities with the syndromes that Kety (1980) described as differentiating the malignant form of schizophrenia, originally defined by Kraepelin (1896) and Bleuler (1950), from remitting, drug-responsive schizophrenia. All of our patients had Schneiderian symptoms as this was required to fulfil the diagnostic criteria of schizophrenia (Wing et al. 1974). Accordingly all had positive symptoms (Crow 1980), but otherwise the syndromes could be differentiated by the positive-negative syndrome concept. The group with greater left than right hemispheric activity was characterised by hallucinations and delusions (non-Schneiderian), accelerated cognition and warm, positive affect, whereas the opposite syndrome was characterised by negative features such as poverty of speech, blunted affect and social withdrawal. It has been argued (Gruzelier 1984) that the electrodermal asymmetry is best thought of as reflecting a dynamic imbalance in hemispheric activation with the positive or *Active* syndrome revealing greater left hemispheric activation and the *Withdrawn* syndrome greater right hemispheric activation. This is consistent with a neuropsychological interpretation of the symptoms and with evidence of hemispheric asymmetries in affect, cognition and approach/avoidance behaviour (Sackheim et al. 1982; Kinsbourne 1982; Tucker and Williamson 1984), hence our labels Active and Withdrawn.

Many measures of cerebral laterality have revealed results compatible with the hemisphere imbalance syndromes (Gruzelier 1983) provided they tap dynamic processes as distinct from fixed, structural processes (Cohen 1982). Subsequent research in schizophrenia has shown that the syndrome classification has delineated a group with abnormal somatosensory evoked potentials coupled with impairments in interhemispheric transfer (Andrews et al. 1986, 1987) and has predicted patients' visual search performance, such that the serial type of processing of the Active group led to poorer performance than both that of the controls and the Withdrawn group, whose deployment of gestalt type holistic processing led to a more efficient performance (Gaebel et al. 1986). A range of Japanese studies (Gruzelier 1987a) also support the concept of two syndromes in schizophrenia associated with positive versus negative symptom pictures and underpinned by opposite states of hemispheric imbalance – here termed the Hemisphere Imbalance Syndrome model.

The concept of imbalance, however, does not specify the nature of hemispheric dysfunction. A study undertaken to clarify this issue used tests validated on neuropsychological patients to distinguish left from right-sided hippocampal and frontohippocampal impairments (Milner 1971; Petrides 1985). Tests of verbal fluency were also included. The pattern of deficits which distinguished the Active and Withdrawn syndromes (Gruzelier et al. 1987) was as follows: The Active syndrome had a predominance of deficits in the right hemisphere, with a relative integrity of function in the left hemisphere. The Withdrawn syndrome showed two patterns – either bilateral impairments, as may accompany the cognitive reduction associated with CT signs by Johnstone et al. (1978), or left hemispheric losses of function coupled with relative right hemispheric integrity of function, i.e. the opposite profile to the Active syndrome.

An Experimental Investigation in Schizophrenia

A Preliminary Study of Topographical Mapping with Neuropsychological Testing

Our investigation of schizophrenia with topographical mapping of EEG power was conceptualised within the framework of the Hemisphere Imbalance Syn-

Table 1. Conditions during recording of topographical EEG

Condition		Hemisphere involvement
I	Eyes open	
II	Eyes closed, focussed attention	
III	Index finger movement, bilateral	
IV	Nonverbal, unfamiliar faces: acquisition	Right
V	Nonverbal, unfamiliar faces: recognition	Right
VI	Words: acquisition	Left
VII	Words: recognition	Left
VIII	Index finger movement, bilateral	
IX	Left hand sequenced finger movements	Right/Left
X	Right hand sequenced finger movements	Left

drome model. Patients were first categorised with the Hemisphere Imbalance Syndrome scale: EEG was monitored while patients participated in neuropsychological tests which both lent themselves to EEG measurement and distinguished left from right hemisphere losses of function.

Five female hospitalised schizophrenic patients were compared with five age-matched female controls. During their current illness four patients displayed the Active syndrome while a fifth had a predominance of Active over Withdrawn symptoms as assessed by the Hemisphere Imbalance Scale. Symptomatology was also evaluated with the Present State Examination (Wing et al. 1974). The average age of the patients was 34 years, range 20–44 years, and they were on neuroleptics. Dextrality was measured with the Annett (1970) questionnaire; one of each group was sinistral but without familial sinistrality.

Brain electrical activity was monitored with a Brain Imager (Neuroscience Ltd.) from 28 scalp electrodes referenced to linked ears. Electrode placements were initially derived from the international 10–20 system. Electrodes were attached to a cap which was secured with elastic straps fastened to an elastic band placed around the chest. On average each test condition required 2 min recording to obtain 1 min of artefact-free EEG. The test conditions are shown in Table 1. They included 2 min of eyes closed EEG followed by 2 min with eyes open. To give structure to this condition and to minimise movements, subjects were instructed to focus on a white square, 2 cm in diameter, positioned on a dark-grey background 3.5 feet (107 cm) in front of them at eye level. The third condition involved the gentle raising of the index fingers, one at a time or simultaneously, at irregular intervals of about 6 s. This provided a control for the manual response in the memory tasks that followed. The same task was repeated after the memory tasks in condition VIII. The memory tasks involved the recognition of words and unfamiliar faces, 50 items in each task, with task order counterbalanced (Warrington 1984). Each task was divided into an acquisition and a recognition phase. The acquisition phase involved showing one item at a time with the instruction to raise one index finger if the items were regarded as pleasant and the other index finger if unpleasant. In the recognition phase items were shown in pairs, only one of each pair had been in the previous list, and the subjects had to indicate which one by raising the index finger on the same side as the item. If the subject was unable to remember both fingers were raised. Few subjects chose this option and subsequent work without this option gave the same pattern of results. The final condition involved a programmed movement task of Luria which involved tapping one finger at a time in sequence with the thumb of the corresponding hand. Hand order was counterbalanced across subjects. This was one of the tasks used by Günther and colleagues (Günther and Breitling 1985) to examine the effect of right hand movements on EEG power.

The laterality predictions were as follows. Warrington (1984) validated the memory task with neurological patients showing that patients with left-sided posterior temporal-parieto-occipital lesions revealed deficits in recognition of words and not faces, whereas the opposite was true of patients with equivalent right-sided lesions. Impairments in the programmed movement task are found after damage to sensory-motor areas of the contralateral hemisphere and bilateral frontal areas. According to the Hemisphere Imbalance Syndrome model patients with the Active syndrome would exhibit losses of function in the right hemisphere as revealed by deficits in memory for faces. In the topographical EEG, differences between controls and patients should generally be maximal in the right hemisphere, and the nature of these should reflect low functional activation, particularly in the right posterior temporo-parieto-occipital region. During the programmed movement task patients should be differentiated from controls during the left hand condition only.

EEG Analysis

The 2-min sections of trace were first examined by eye for evidence of movement artefacts. After deletion of artefacts a fast Fourier power spectrum analysis was carried out for delta 0.5–2 Hz, theta 3–9 Hz, alpha 10–12 Hz, beta I 13–16 Hz and beta II 17–30 Hz. The 2.5-s epoch topographical maps of the square root of power were examined for evidence of raised beta II at T3 and T4 which might indicate muscle artefact. One control subject showed evidence of this which prevented analysis of group differences in beta II at T3 and T4. The maps were also examined for evidence of raised bilateral frontal delta as a check on the adequacy of the movement artefact rejection. Any further contaminated samples were removed. Averages were then obtained for all the conditions in Table 1 for the five bandwidths for both the square root of power and the standard deviations in power of each group. In all cases the standard deviations for patients and controls were comparable, with the exception of beta II at T3 and T4 in controls due to the aberrant control subject mentioned above. Next, t tests were carried out on the standard deviations, and with the one exception just mentioned none approached significance. With assumptions of homogeneity of variance satisfied, the groups were compared with t tests for differences in power using two-tailed levels of significance.

Results

Recognition Memory

Whereas both controls and patients showed a discrepancy between verbal and non-verbal memory due to inferior face recognition (controls: words 97%, faces 75%; patients: words 80%, faces 51%), there was a significant interaction between group and task ($F_{1,8} = 7.18$; $P < 0.03$). These results confirm the predicted right hemisphere loss of function in patients.

Functional Activation and Topographical EEG

Of the 50 group comparisons between individual conditions (ten conditions, five bandwidths) significant regional differences were found in 21 comparisons; these are shown in Table 2. It is noteworthy that no significant effects were found in the eyes closed condition. In other words, functional activation was necessary to reveal differences between patients and controls, a conclusion also reached in recent studies of cortical bloodflow (Gur et al. 1983; Weinberger et al. 1986).

In support of many reports of power spectrum analysis in schizophrenic patients (Flor-Henry 1983), the major differences were found in the high and low beta range, where patients exhibited higher levels of beta than controls. In the event of elevations in beta power being indicative of pathology, they signify low functional activity (Gibbs and Gibbs 1961). The following conditions are characterised by high beta: recovery from head injury, the postencephalitic state, the effect of barbiturates, 50% of children under the age of 3 years.

Considering the lower bandwidths, it is of interest that group effects in alpha, which were in the direction of raised alpha in patients, occurred in the three tasks which on neuropsychological grounds involved predominantly the right hemisphere, namely face acquisition and recognition, and left hand programmed movements. Conversely differences in delta, which were in the direc-

Table 2. Conditions showing significant group effects

Condition	Bandwidth				
	Delta	Theta	Alpha	Beta I	Beta II
I					
II					
III					
IV			R	R	R
V			R	R	R
VI	L			L	L
VII				L	L
VIII					
IX			R	R	R
X	L				

L, left hemisphere; R, right hemisphere

tion of reduced delta in patients, involved two of three left hemisphere tasks: word acquisition and right hand sequenced movements. The effects will be mentioned further with respect to topography.

Topographical Maps

Beta II. Probability maps for the t values in conditions II–X are shown in Fig. 1, 1–9. In conditions II–VIII the areas differentiating the groups were in the posterior region, most often in the right posterior temporo-parieto-occipital area, sometimes extending centrally but localised to the left only in the eyes open, resting condition. This right-sided region corresponds to the area in which the memory tests revealed losses of function. Inspection of the group means showed that the patients (Fig. 2, 1), aside from a generalised increase in beta, showed a posterior elevation bilaterally around the circumference but predominantly on the right, whereas in controls there was a focal reduction in beta which coincided with the region of maximum difference in the probability maps (Fig. 2). Thus aside from an elevation in beta activity the patients failed to show the focal reduction in beta amplitude that has been found to accompany information processing in the normal brain – the expected dynamics of non-pathological beta according to Gibbs and Gibbs (1961).

In support of predictions for the programmed movement task only left hand movements showed group differences; these were in the right prefrontal area. In the eyes open focussed attention condition, the region of difference was in the left occipital area. This may be associated with a left hemispheric advantage for focussed as distinct from broadened attention (Dimond and Beaumont 1973; Gruzelier 1987c).

Averaging over the activation conditions, the major region of difference was in the posterior temporo-parieto-occipital region of the right hemisphere, which extended to the central posterior region (Fig. 2, 3).

Beta I. Patients showed higher levels of beta I activity than controls. Probability maps are shown in Fig. 3, 1–9 for conditions II–X. Two general conclusions are immediately apparent. Firstly, the group differences were all in the right hemisphere, with only one exception, word acquisition, where right-sided effects, which include both anterior and posterior focal regions, were joined by a left parietal elevation. Secondly, only those conditions that differentiated the groups in beta II showed significant effects in beta I, yet there was not necessarily a topographical correspondence.

The group regional differences in beta I appeared to vary more with the localisation of the neuropsychological functions involved in the various tasks. Considering first conditions III and VIII, which involved raising the index finger, on the first occasion (condition III) the task was novel and required concentration, whereas on repetition, in condition VIII, it was overlearned, as the same response had been required in conditions IV–VII. When the task was novel (condition III), the groups differed in the right anterior region, whereas when it was overlearned the effects were in the right posterior region, perhaps reflecting a shift from motoric prefrontal involvement to the attentional aspects of the task, in line with the role of the right parieto-occipital region as an attention control centre

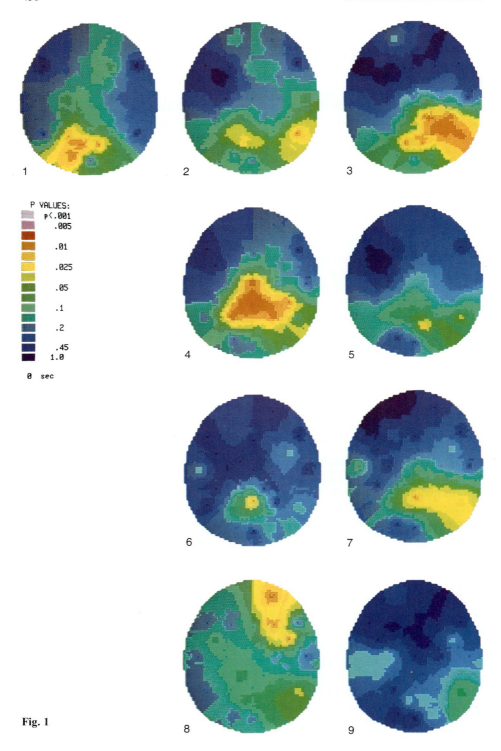

Fig. 1

The Neuropsychology of Schizophrenia in the Context of Topographical Mapping 431

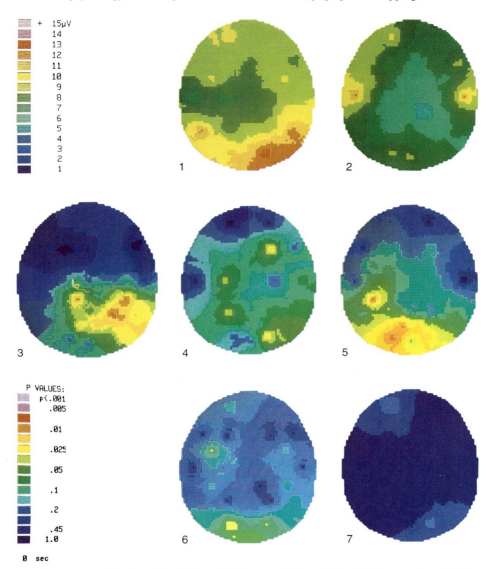

Fig. 2. Maps *1* and *2* show beta II power for face recognition. Maps *3–7* represent probability maps. Map *3* is the average of all activation conditions (II–X) for beta II. Maps *4–7* represent alpha for face acquisition (*4*) and recognition (*5*) and left (*6*) and right (*7*) programmed movement

◁─────────────────

Fig. 1. Topographical images as described in the text. Note that the probability scale is one-tailed; the values should be halved to obtain a two-tailed probability. Maps represent beta II probability maps for conditions II–X (Table 1) numbered left to right from top to bottom

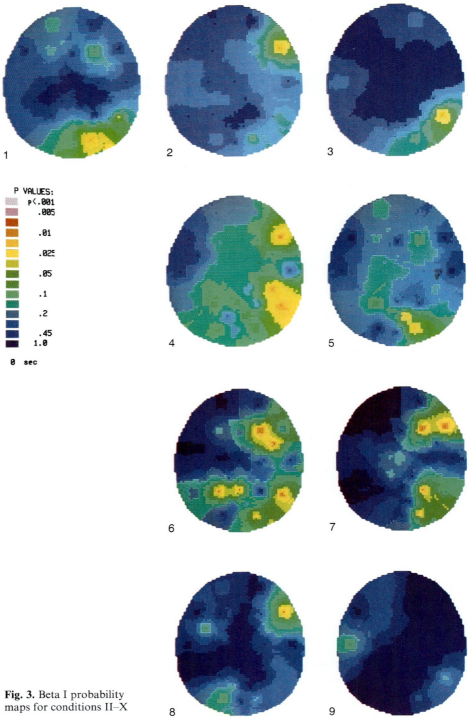

Fig. 3. Beta I probability maps for conditions II–X

(Mesulam 1981). The latter process may also be responsible for the right occipital regional difference in the focussed attention task in condition II.

Turning to the memory tasks, face acquisition and recognition involved the right posterior temporoparietal area, which has been implicated in non-verbal memory (Warrington 1984). The right frontal involvement may reflect the motor component of the task. In contrast, word acquisition and recognition revealed more widespread differences, with a right anterior temporofrontal effect, as well as a right posterior effect. Had these been in the left hemisphere they would have coincided with areas involved in verbal learning and memory. The fact that here the effects were in the right hemisphere may hint at inappropriate use of right hemispheric processes in the verbal task. Nevertheless the left hemisphere was implicated during the acquisition phase where the groups differed in the left central parietal area.

In the motor sequencing task again only use of the left hand revealed group differences, here in the right lateral frontal area. If these neuropsychological interpretations are correct, then quite apart from a circumscribed localised dysfunction, such as was apparent in the elevation of beta II in the right posterior region, the fact that the regional differences in beta I varied with processing demands suggests a generalised processing deficit in schizophrenia. This may be associated with allocation of processing resources for the specific task in hand, in which case it could implicate the focal activational functions of thalamocortical mechanisms.

Alpha. Levels of alpha activity were raised in patients compared with controls. In the majority of conditions there were no group differences: eyes open and closed, verbal acquisition and recognition memory, raising the index finger, and right hand programmed movements. The three conditions that showed group differences (Fig. 2, 4–6) were face acquisition and recognition and left hand programmed movements – all tasks involving right hemispheric functions. The regional group differences were not localised to the right hemisphere. In face acquisition they were widespread, involved both hemispheres, more so on the right than the left, and achieved probability levels mostly approaching significance. In contrast, face recognition showed highly significant differences in the left parietal region and a bilateral occipital effect reaching higher levels of significance on the left. Left hand programmed movements showed a slight difference in occipital regions, more so on the left side.

The significance of raised alpha power for information processing is not as clear as originally thought. Whether it signifies relative functional inactivity is called into question by recent topographic EEG studies comparing different psychological tasks. Petsche et al. (1985) engaged subjects in examining and memorising text and pictures, performing mental arithmetic and listening to music. Alpha power was found to increase in regions unambiguously involved in processing, such as the occipital lobe while reading.

Delta. In two left hemisphere tasks – word acquisition and right hand sequenced movements – there was a tendency towards a decrease in delta power in patients in a triangular region centering on P4 and extending to T6 and O2. This is the area most commonly implicated as dysfunctional in patients in this study.

However, as the significance of the effects at best reached $P<0.05$ to $P<0.10$, they will have to await replication before further discussion.

Conclusions

This preliminary study has shown the sensitivity of brain electrical activity mapping with a 28-electrode array in revealing regional differences in activity, particularly in beta power, between a small group of well characterised schizophrenic patients and controls. In accordance with previous reports mentioned in the section "Topographical Mapping of EEG Power in Schizophrenia" above, this was in the posterior regions. Our next step will be a replication study to compare different syndromes in schizophrenia stratified by gender, handedness and medication status. Until this is done only general conclusions will be drawn.

The validity of the major regional differences in topographical EEG discovered in the study is strenghtened by two factors. Their location was predicted on the basis of theory such that the Active syndrome characterising the patients has been shown to coincide with losses of right hemispheric function on neuropsychological tests (Gruzelier et al. 1987). Secondly, the study involved functional activation with validated neuropsychological tests which provided behavioural evidence of losses of function in the area most frequently implicated in the topographical EEG, namely the right posterior-temporo-parieto-occipital region.

However, we do not conclude that this region is necessarily the locus of pathology in patients with the Active syndrome. Most of the tasks in the experiment involved sustained concentration, and, as reviewed by Mesulam (1981), the right parietal region plays a critical role in the control of attentional processes. EEG recording procedures that require sampling over a 2-min task will commonly involve this mechanism. Subcortical systems such as those which encompass thalamus and limbic system and which have widely distributed cortical influences (Pribram and McGuiness 1975) may also be important. Systems such as these may underpin the task-dependent focal effects in beta I that appeared to vary with the neuropsychological localisation of processing components.

Finally, in the absence of group differences in the eyes closed condition, our results support the view that functional activation of the brain is necessary to reveal EEG abnormalities in schizophrenic patients. This is consistent with the failure by others to obtain evidence of dysfunction in the resting EEG in a topographical study (Karson et al. 1987), and the evidence of group differences in frontal blood flow occurring only when engaged in functionally specific neuropsychological tests (Weinberger et al. 1986). The strong effects in this study are remarkable given the small sample size, and raise the hope that comprehensive mapping techniques such as this may one day lead to the characterisation of a single clinical case and differentiation from a control sample. This is an essential aim of clinical science and has rarely been hinted at in schizophrenia research.

References

Andrews HB, Honse AO, Cooper JE, Barber C (1986) The prediction of abnormal evoked potentials in schizophrenic patients by means of symptom pattern. Br J Psychol 149:46–50

Andrews HB, Barber C, Cooper JE, Raine A (1987) Early somatosensory evoked potentials in schizophrenia: symptom pattern, clinical outcomes and interhemispheric functioning. In: Takahashi R, Flor-Henry P, Gruzelier J, Niwa SI (eds) Cerebral dynamics, laterality and psychopathology. Elsevier, Amsterdam, pp 175–186

Annett M (1970) Classification of hand preference by association analysis. Br J Psychol 61:303–321

Bleuler E (1950) Dementia praecox or the group of schizophrenias. New York International University Press, New York (translated from 1911 original)

Bragina NN (1966) Clinical syndromes of disorders of the hippocampus and adjacent areas of the brain. Klin Med (Mosk) 44:23–27

Buchsbaum MS, King AC, Cappelletti J, Coppola R, van Kammen DP (1982) Visual evoked potential topography in patients with schizophrenia and normal controls. Adv Biol Psychiatry 9:50–56

Bull HC, Venables PH (1974) Speech perception in schizophrenia. Br J Psychiatry 125:350–354

Cohen G (1982) Theoretical interpretations of lateral asymmetries. In: Beaumont JG (ed) Divided visual field studies of cerebral organisation. Academic, New York, pp 87–115

Connolly JF, Gruzelier JH (1982) A critical examination of augmenting/reducing methodology in schizophrenic patients and controls. In: Langnau ED (ed) Advances in biological psychiatry, vol 9. Karger, Basel

Crow TJ (1980) Molecular pathology of schizophrenia: more than one disease process? Br Med J 280:66–68

Cummings JL, Benson DF (1984) Subcortical dementia: review of an emerging concept. Arch Neurol 41:874–879

Davison K, Bagley CR (1969) Schizophrenia-like psychoses associated with organic disorders of the central nervous system: a review of the literature. In: Herrington RN (ed) Current problems in neuropsychiatry. Royal Medico-Psychological Association, London

Dimond SJ, Beaumont JG (1973) Difference in vigilance performance of the right and left hemisphere. Cortex 9:259–265

Flor-Henry P (1969) Psychosis and temporal lobe epilepsy: a controlled investigation. Epilepsia 10:363–395

Flor-Henry P (1974) Psychosis, neurosis and epilepsy. Br J Psychiatry 124:144–150

Flor-Henry P (1983) Cerebral basis of psychopathology. Wright, New York

Flor-Henry P, Yeudal LG (1979) Neuropsychological investigation of schizophrenia and manic-depressive psychoses. In: Gruzelier J, Flor-Henry P (eds) Hemisphere asymmetry of function and psychopathology. Elsevier/North Holland Biomedical, Amsterdam, pp 341–362

Franzen G, Ingvar DH (1975) Abnormal distribution of cerebral activity in chronic schizophrenia. J Psychiatr Res 12:199–214

Friedman D (1987) The endogenous scalp-recorded brain potentials in schizophrenia. In: Steinhauer S, Gruzelier JH, Zubin J (eds) Experimental psychopathology, neuropsychology & psychophysiology. Elsevier Science, Amsterdam (Handbook of schizophrenia, vol 4)

Gaebel W, Ulrich G, Frick K (1986) Eye-movement research with schizophrenic patients and normal controls using corneal reflection-pupil centre measurement. Eur Arch Psychiatry Neurol Sci 235:243–254

Gibbs FA, Gibbs EL (1961) Clinical and pharmacological correlates of fast activity in electroencephalography. J Neuropsychiatry 3:73–78

Gruzelier JH (1973) Bilateral asymmetry of skin conductance orienting activity and levels with schizophrenics. Biol Psychol 1:21–41

Gruzelier JH (1983) A critical assessment and integration of lateral asymmetries in schizophrenia. In: Myslobodsky MS (ed) Hemisyndromes, psychobiology, neurology and psychiatry. Academic, New York, pp 265–326

Gruzelier JH (1984) Hemispheric imbalances in schizophrenia. Int J Psychophysiol 1:227–240

Gruzelier JH (1987a) Commentary on neuropsychological information processing deficits in psychosis and neuropsychophysiological syndrome relationships in schizophrenia. In: Takahashi R, Flor-Henry P, Gruzelier J, Niwa S (eds) Cerebral dynamics, laterality and psychopathology. Elsevier Science, Amsterdam, pp 23–54

Gruzelier JH (1987b) Cerebral laterality in schizophrenia: a review of the interhemispheric disconnection hypothesis. In: Glass A (ed) Individual differences in hemispheric specialisation. Plenum, London, pp 357–376

Gruzelier JH (1987c) Individual differences in dynamic process asymmetries in the normal and pathological brain. In: Glass A (ed) Individual differences in hemispheric specialisation. Plenum, London, 301–330

Gruzelier JH, Manchanda R (1982) The syndrome of schizophrenia: relations between electrodermal response, lateral asymmetries and clinical subtypes. Br J Psychiatry 141:488–495

Gruzelier JH, Venables PH (1972) Skin conductance orienting activity in a heterogeneous sample of schizophrenics: possible evidence of limbic dysfunction. J Nervous Ment Dis 155:277–287

Gruzelier JH, Venables PH (1973) Skin conductance responses to tones with and without attentional significance in schizophrenic and non-schizophrenic patients. Neuropsychologia 11:221–230

Gruzelier JH, Venables PH (1974) Bimodality and lateral asymmetry of skin conductance orienting activity in schizophrenics: replication and evidence of lateral asymmetry in patients with depression and disorders of personality. Biol Psychiatry 8:55–73

Gruzelier J, Wilson L (1987) The hemisphere imbalance syndrome rating scale (in preparation)

Gruzelier JH, Jutai J, Connolly JF, Hirsch SR (1985) Cerebral asymmetries in unmedicated schizophrenic patients in EEG spectra and their relation to clinical and autonomic parameters. Adv Biol Psychiatry 15:12–19

Gruzelier J, Seymour K, Wilson L, Jolley A, Hirsch S (1987) Neuropsychological evidence for hippocampal and frontal impairments in schizophrenia, mania and depression. In: Takahashi R, Flor-Henry P, Gruzelier J, Niwa S (eds) Cerebral dynamics, laterality and psychopathology. Elsevier Science, Amsterdam, pp 273–286

Günther W, Breitling D (1985) Predominant sensorimotor area left hemisphere dysfunction in schizophrenia measured by brain electrical activity mapping. Biol Psychiatry 20:515–532

Günther W, Breitling D, Banquet JP, Marcie P, Rondot P (1986) EEG mapping of left hemisphere dysfunction during motor performance in schizophrenia. Biol Psychiatry 21:249–262

Gur RE, Skolnik BE, Gur RC et al (1983) Brain function in psychiatric disorders. Arch Gen Psychiatry 40:1250–1254

Ingvar DH, Franzen G (1974) Abnormalities of cerebral bloodflow distribution in patients with chronic schizophrenia. Acta Psychiatr Scand 50:425–462

Johnstone EC, Crow TJ, Frith CD, Husband J, Kreell (1978) The dementia of dementia praecox. Acta Psychiatr Scand 57:305–324

Jutai J, Gruzelier JH, Connolly J, Manchanda R, Hirsch SR (1984) Schizophrenia ad spectral analysis of the visual evoked potential. Br J Psychiatry 145:496–501

Karson CN, Coppola R, Morihisa JM, Weinberger DR (1987) Computed electroencephalographic activity mapping in schizophrenia. Arch Gen Psychiatry 44:514–517

Kaufman L, Williamson SJ (1982) Magnetic location of cortical activity. Ann Ny Acad Sci 388:197–213

Kety SS (1980) The syndrome of schizophrenia: unresolved questions and opportunities for research. Br J Psychiatry 136:421–436

Kinsbourne M (1982) Hemispheric specialisation and the growth of human understanding. Am Psychol 37:411–420

Kolb B, Whishaw I (1983) Performance of schizophrenic patients on tests sensitive to left or right frontal, temporal or parietal function in neurological patients. J Nerv Ment Dis 171:435–443

Kraepelin EE (1896) Lehrbuch der Psychiatrie. Barth, Leipzig

Malamud N (1967) Psychiatric disorders with intracranial tumours of the limbic system. Arch Neurol 17:113–123

Matthyssee S, Spring BG, Sugarman J (eds) (1978) Attention and information processing in schizophrenia. J Psychiatr Res 14:1–33

Mesulam M (1981) A cortical network for directed attention and unilateral neglect. Ann Neurol 10:309–325

Mesulam MM, Geschwind N (1978) On the possible role of neocortex and its limbic connections in the process of attention and schizophrenia. J Psychiatr Res 14:249–260

Milner B (1971) Interhemispheric differences in the localisation of psychological processes in man. Br Med Bull 27:272–277

Morihisa JM, Duffy FH, Wyatt RJ (1983) Brain electrical activity mapping (BEAM) in schizophrenic patients. Arch Gen Psychiatry 40:719–728

Morstyn R, Duffy FH, McCarley RW (1983) Computed P300 topography in schizophrenia. Electroencephalogr Clin Neurophysiol 40:729–734

Newlin DB, Carpenter B, Golden J (1981) Hemispheric asymmetries in schizophrenia. Biol Psychiatry 16:561–582

Petsche H, Pockberger H, Rappelsberger P (1985) EEG topography and mental performance. In: Duffy FH (ed) Topographic mapping of brain electrical activity. Butterworth, London

Petrides M (1985) Deficits on conditional associative-learning tasks after frontal lobe and temporal lobe lesions in man. Neuropsychologia 23:601–614

Pribram KH, McGuinness D (1975) Arousal, activation and effort in the control of attention. Psychol Rev 82:116–147

Reynolds GP (1983) Increased concentrations and lateral asymmetry of amygdala dopamine in schizophrenics. Nature 305:527–529

Reynolds GP, Czudek C (1987) Neurochemical laterality of the limbic system in schizophrenia. In: Takahashi R, Flor-Henry P, Gruzelier J, Niwa S (eds) Cerebral dynamics, laterality and psychopathology. Elsevier Science, Amsterdam, pp 451–456

Rosenthal R, Bigelow LB (1972) Quantitative brain measurements in chronic schizophrenia. Br J Psychiatry 121:259–264

Sackheim HA, Greenberg MS, Wynman AL et al (1982) Hemispheric asymmetry in the expression of positive and negative emotions: neurological evidence. Arch Neurol 39:210–218

Shagass C (1977) Early evoked potentials. Schizophr Bull 3:80–92

Sheppard G, Gruzelier JH, Manchanda R, Hirsch SR, Wise R, Frackowiak R, Jones T (1983) 15-O positron emission tomographic scanning in predominantly never-treated acute schizophrenic patients. The Lancet 2:1448–1452

Smythies JR (1969) The behavioural physiology of the temporal lobe. In: Herrington RN (ed) Current problems in neuropsychiatry. Royal Medico-Psychological Association, London

Torrey EF, Peterson MR (1974) Schizophrenia and the limbic system. Lancet 2:942–946

Tucker DM, Williamson PA (1984) Asymmetric neural control systems in human self-regulation. Psychol Rev 91:185–215

Venables PH (1964) Input dysfunction in schizophrenia. In: Mahar B (ed) Advances in experimental personality research, vol 1. Academic, New York

Walker E, McGuire S (1982) Intra- and inter-hemispheric information processing in schizophrenia. Psychol Bull 92:701–725

Warrington EK (1984) Recognition memory test manual. NFER-Nelson, Windsor

Weinberger DR, Burman KF, Zec RF (1986) Physiologic dysfunction of dorso-lateral prefrontal cortex in schizophrenia. I. Regional cerebral bloodflow evidence. Arch Gen Psychiatry 43:114–124

Wexler BE (1980) Cerebral laterality and psychiatry: a review of the literature. Am J Psychiatry 137:279–291

Wing JK, Cooper JE, Sartorius N (1974) The measurement and classification of psychiatric symptoms. Cambridge University Press, London

Wood CC, Allison T, Goff WR (1980) On the neural origin of P300 in man. Prog Brain Res 54:51–56

EEG Mapping in Psychiatry: Studies on Type I/II Schizophrenia Using Motor Activation

W. Günther, R. Steinberg, R. Petsch, P. Streck, and J. Kugler[1]

Introduction

Both in early (Ellingson 1954) and more recent (Itil 1977) reviews, the attempts to establish visually evaluated EEG features specifically related to schizophrenia have not had very promising results. However, the development of small digital computers and of the fast Fourier transform (FFT) algorithm have advanced the possibilities of quantitative EEG analysis, and led to interesting findings.

In the alpha frequency band, for instance, Itil proposed in 1964 that a "hypernormal rhythmical alpha EEG" may be related to "chronic therapy resistant schizophrenia," and suggested that increased alpha power may be used as a predictor for poor response to neuroleptic treatment. Igert and Lairy (1962) found a "hypernormal alpha-synchronisation EEG" in "chronic-process", but not in "acute-reactive" schizophrenics. Similarly, Etevenon et al. (1981) related a "high-alpha cluster" to the hebephrenic and a "low-alpha cluster" to the paranoid subtype of the disorder. Thus, in this frequency band, there is some evidence of EEG findings related to schizophrenia, and additionally for a possible role of biological heterogeneity in schizophrenia influencing such findings.

In beta frequency bands, there have been many reports of increased power values in schizophrenics (review Itil 1980). However, it has been suggested that this difference may result primarily from the influence of "treatment-responsive" schizophrenics; i.e., it is assumed that these patients have (when untreated!) larger amounts of EEG activity in beta bands (Itil et al. 1975). Since the "typical" EEG response to neuroleptic treatment is claimed to be attenuation of activity in the 13–30 cycles per second (cps) frequency range (Itil et al. 1980), this treatment should predominantly decrease beta power values in treatment-responsive patients. In direct support of this hypothesis, Itil (1972) reported a significant correlation (0.62) between the amount of drug-induced beta EEG attenuation and clinical improvement.

The results in slow frequency bands are plentiful, but controversial, and will be discussed later.

Using "mapping" facilities (topographical display of measured variables; for mapping of EEG parameters see. e.g., Petsche and Marko 1959; Lehmann 1971; Duffy et al. 1979) additional results were obtained.

Morihisa et al. (1983) reported (predominantly bifrontal) delta increases in schizophrenics. Morstyn et al. (1983) introduced musical, verbal and spatial "activation" into the EEG mapping studies in an attempt to increase the group

---

[1] Psychiatrische Universitätsklinik, Nussbaumstr. 7, 8000 München 2, Federal Republic of Germany

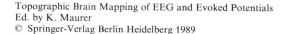

differences between schizophrenics and normals. The utility of such activation procedures for quantitative EEG (overview see Maurer and Dierks 1987) had been suggested by other neuroimaging techniques such as regional cerebral blood flow (rCBF; Gur et al. 1983, 1985), or positron emission tomography (PET; e.g., Brodie et al. 1984).

Based on the above findings and suggestions in the literature, we designed our series of EEG mapping studies in schizophrenia around the following considerations:

– There should be efforts to monitor for biological heterogeneity in the disorder. We decided to use Crow's clinically applicable "type I/II" concept (e.g. Crow 1985). Type I schizophrenia is characterized by "positive symptoms" such as delusions, hallucinations, good response to neuroleptic treatment, rather good prognosis, absence of intellectual impairment, and postulated dopaminergic transmission abnormality with an increased number of D2 receptors. The type II syndrome consists more of "negative symptoms" such as flattening of affect, poverty of speech, poor response to neuroleptic treatment, signs of intellectual impairment and possible structural brain alterations (e.g., cell loss in temporal areas or diffuse cortical atrophy).

– There should be "resting" conditions, defined as well as possible. We decided to apply a relaxation procedure as an attempt to reduce the variability of resting conditions.

– There should be "functional activation," compared to such a resting state, in order to obtain some information on "activation patterns" in different populations.

We decided to use motor activation for the following reasons:

– There are reports in the literature that, for instance, simple motor activation gives a "clear signal" in imaging methods examining the brain function of normal persons (e.g., the rCBF studies by Olesen 1971; Lauritzen et al. 1981).

– There is evidence that schizophrenic patients display deficiencies in motor tasks, especially more complex ones (Asarnow and McCrimmon 1978; Günther et al. 1986a; review, e.g., Manschreck 1986).

– In order to activate successively more complex brain areas, both simple and increasingly complex motor tasks should be used. Both simple and complex motor activation can be assumed to be *dysfunctional* in schizophrenic patients. This might be of value in the attempt to establish possibly correlated "pathological cerebral activation patterns" in patients, as compared to "normal activation patterns" (investigation of a "*functio laesa*").

EEG Mapping Study on Neuroleptic-Treated Type I Schizophrenic Patients During Simple Motor Tasks

Material and Methods

Subjects. The subjects were 10 schizophrenic inpatients of the Clinique des Maladies Mentales et de l'Encéphale, Hôpital Sainte Anne, Paris. The selection procedure, diagnostic process, the assessment of psychopathology and handedness, experimental situation and design are detailed elsewhere (Günther et al. 1986b). We restrict ourselves here to more general information:

10 right-handed schizophrenic patients (five hebephrenic and five paranoid) participated in the study. Their average age was 32.4 years and the male/female ratio was 6/4. Their average neuroleptic treatment was 540 units chlorpromazine daily. They were type I patients, with only little negative symptomatology as assessed by the Munich Version of the Scale of Assessment of Negative Symptoms (MV-SANS) (Dieterle et al. 1986; average score 12.3 in this scale). The right-handed control persons consisted of members of staff of the Service de Neurologie of the above hospital. Their average age was 31.6 years, the sex ratio was 5/5 and they were on no medication. The schedule of motor activation of the right hand was as follows:

- Relaxation program (6 min) using our version of autogenous training
- Simple movement: repetitive flexion of the index finger (1 min)
- Repetitive movement: (making a first repetitively in a self-paced rhythm (1 min)
- Programmed movement: (making a complex finger sequence opposing the thumb (1 min)
- Imaginary movement: (performing the programmed movement mentally (1 min)

Only the repetitive task can be described further here for space reasons. The other simple motor tasks are detailed by Günther et al. (1986b), and the multisensorimotor tasks are reported by Günther and Breitling (1985).

EEG. All subjects were studied with a 16-electrode EEG (plus one ground electrode). The system has its own nomenclature, which is demonstrated in Fig. 1 together with the placements of the electrodes. The data were recorded in a 16-channel polygraph, using mean reference leads. A 16-channel analog tape recorder (Alvar Reega XVI Duplex) was used to allow subsequent data treatment with an FFT algorithm and map representation.

Fig. 1. Statistical maps of repetitive movement of the right hand. *Top*, control persons; *middle*, type I schizophrenics; *bottom*, type II schizophrenics. *Left column*, significant *increases* (as compared to resting condition within the same group) in delta (1–4 cps in type I, 0.5–4.49 cps in type II patients); *right column*, significant *decreases* in beta 2 (18–24 cps in type I, 13.5–20.49 cps in type II). Only electrodes with significant ($p < 0.05$) changes in the t testing, based on multifactorial ANOVA, are in color (scale on the right); all non-significant ones remain blue. The change relative to resting condition (only in significant electrodes) is used as basis for attributing the colors to the electrodes. Note the contralateral (delta) or bilateral (beta 2) changes in control persons, the predominantly ipsilateral changes with left hemisphere hypofunction in neuroleptic-treated type I schizophrenic patients and the bilateral hypofunction in neuroleptic-treated type II patients (delta and beta). Electrode placement: *A*, Fp_2; *B*, C_4; *C*, P_4; *D*, O_2; *E*, Fp_1; *F*, C_3; *G*, P_3; *H*, O_1; *I*, F_z; *J*, T_4; *K*, T_6; *L*, F_2; *M*, F_7; *N*, T_3; *O*, T_5; *P*, P_z. For better visual comparison, all maps use the same scale (the scale of the map which shows the maximal changes in relative percent). This is not obligatory for *statistical* maps, and in fact only advisable if the relative power changes do not differ greatly between maps. However, it has to be kept in mind that there are *increases* in delta, but *decreases* in beta!

EEG Mapping in Psychiatry

DELTA	REPETITIVE MOVEMENT RIGHT HAND	BETA
SIGN. INCR. IN REL. %	(VERSUS RESTING CONDITION)	SIGN. DECR. IN REL. %

CONTROL PERSONS

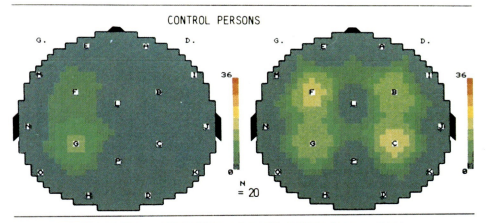

SCHIZOPHRENICS TYPE I. NEUROLEPTIC-TREATED LONGER THAN 4 WEEKS

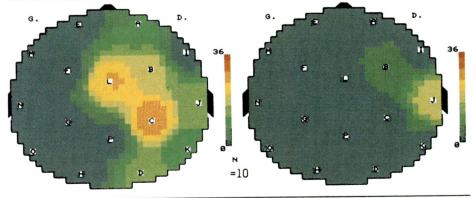

SCHIZOPHRENICS TYPE II. NEUROLEPTIC-TREATED LONGER THAN 4 WEEKS

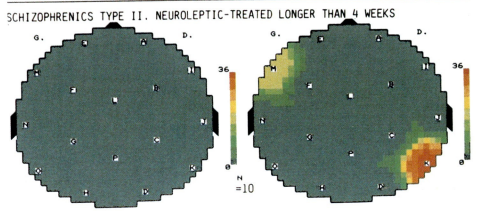

Two minutes of the relaxation condition and 45 s of each task were recorded. The paper traces were visually inspected for artifacts and 30 s of (as nearly as possible) artifact-free EEG was chosen for off-line FFT treatment. Data were filtered from 1 to 30 cps to avoid interferences from higher frequencies (especially muscle artifacts). Each task was analyzed in consecutive periods of 6 s; 30 s FFT was averaged to a mean FFT, which was used as a basis for histograms of power values in each frequency band within the range of 1–30 cps.

The EEG mapping system is detailed further by Günther and Breiling (1985) and Günther et al. (1986b)

Statistical Analysis. The numerical values of the FFT were grouped into power-subject-electrode-state-frequency tables. We examined the frequency bands delta (1–4 cps), theta (4–8 cps), alpha (8–12 cps), beta 1 (12–18 cps) beta 2 (18–24 cps) and beta 3 (24–30 cps). In a first statistical approach, we used a principal component analysis in order to create a more manageable reference system, based on intercorrelation matrices. We than ran Friedman tests over the factor loadings of each subject on the first factor of the principal component analysis. This first factor was extracted from the intercorrelation matrices of all 20 subjects in all task/resting conditions in the six frequency bands examined. We than ran analyses of variance (ANOVA) of power values within each group, involving 16 (electrodes) × 5 (task conditions) × 10 (subjects), to provide the basis for further t test group comparison statistics (i.e., for independent measurements: comparison of *resting conditions between the groups*). In an analogous manner, the results of the Friedman tests of the factor loadings on the first principal component provided the basis for subsequent Wilcoxon test analysis of the *motor activation conditions within the groups*.

Results

Resting Conditions

Delta. Higher power values in patients in *all* electrodes, with a predominance in the frontal regions (t values between 4.67 and 10.35, $p < 0.01$).

Theta. Higher power values in patients in bifrontal and centroparietal regions (t between 2.48, $p < 0.05$, and 4.03, $p < 0.01$).

Alpha. Lower power values in patients in posterior regions, the differences being more marked over the left hemisphere (t 1.74 to 2.63, $p < 0.05$).

Beta 1–3. Lower power values in patients in nearly all electrodes (t between 2.10, $p < 0.05$, and 7.87, $p < 0.01$). For further details see Günther et al. (1986b, p. 253).

Motor Activation State, Repetitive Movement Right Hand

Delta. The average power values *increased* in both type I schizophrenics and controls. However, as Fig. 1 (left half) demonstrates, the distribution of electrodes which showed significant power changes in comparison to resting conditions differed between two groups. Whereas in normal persons (Fig. 1, top line) there were increases predominantly in centroparietal areas *contralaterally*, in schizophrenics (Fig. 1, middle), these changes seemed to be more *ipsilaterally* (i.e., over the right hemisphere).

Theta. The average power values *decreased* in both groups. However, whereas schizophrenics showed *no* significant decreases in C3 or P3, the electrode P3 is "active" in this (and all other) "simple" tasks.

Alpha. There was no separation of the two groups in the principal component analysis, indicating similar activation patterns. Thus, there was no basis for further repetitive testing and probability mapping.

Beta 1–3. The three beta bands (12–18, 18–24 and 24–30 cps) showed a similar activation pattern in both groups. Therefore, only one (beta 2, 18–24 cps) is demonstrated in Fig. 1 (right half). The average power *decreased* in both groups during motor activation. However, the motor activation pattern seemed to display differences in normal and schizophrenic groups similar to those shown previously for delta and theta: in healthy control persons, there were rather *bilateral* decreases of power (Fig. 1, top); in type I schizophrenics, there was a hyporeactivity over the left hemisphere during repetitive movement of the right hand (Fig. 2, middle), as well as in other simple motor tasks (further details 1986b, pp. 253ff).

EEG Mapping Study on Neuroleptic-Treated Type II Schizophrenic Patients During Simple Motor Tasks

Material and Methods

Subjects. The subjects were 10 schizophrenic inpatients of the Clinique des Maladies Mentales et de l'Encéphale, Hôpital Sainte Anne, Paris. The selection procedure, diagnostic process, assessment of psychopathology and handedness and experimental situation were analogous to those for the EEG mapping studies on type I patients and are detailed by Günther et al. (1988). Some general information: Ten right-handed schizophrenic patients (six chronic, two paranoid, two disordered) participated in the study. Their average age was 34.7 years, the male/female ratio 4/6, the mean duration of illness 6.2 years and the mean educational level 13.3 years. The average score on the Munich version of the SANS was 31.4 (SD 5.1; this indicates rather distinct "negative symptomatology"). The average neuroleptic treatment was 500 chlorpromazine units daily.

In a statistical screening, there was no significant difference in age, distribution of gender, educational level or neuroleptic treatment level in comparison to type I patients; however, there was a significant ($p<0.001$) difference between type I and type II patients in regard to the score on the SANS.

A separate control group was matched to the type II patients for the following reasons: modifications of the EEG mapping system, the motor activation procedures, and the frequency bands examined (see below). Their average age was 33.2 years (SD 5.2), the mean educational level 13.6 years, sex ratio 5/5; no person was receiving any medication at the time of the study.

The schedule for motor activation was as follows:
- Reference state (obtained after a 6-min relaxation procedure)
- Repetitive movement right (1 min)/repetitive movement left (1 min)/visuomotor movement right (1 min)/visuomotor movement left (1 min).

Only the repetitive movement right will be described for space reasons see Günther et al. 1988).

EEG. There was a slight modification of the frequency bands, partially due to changes of the system (using 1/2 cps units instead of 1 cps units). The delta band was 0.5–4.49 cps, theta 4.50–7.49 cps, alpha 7.50–13.49 cps, beta $1+2$ 13.50–30 cps.

Statistical Analysis. The procedure was similar to that described for type I patients. However, there was no principal component analysis available for a first-step descriptive analysis. The combination of ANOVA and repetitive univariate testing (using t tests both for independent *resting conditions* and dependent *motor activation conditions*) was applied in an analogous manner as detailed above.

Results

Resting Conditions

Delta. Higher power values in type II schizophrenics (only) in four central and posterior electrodes (only!) ($0.02<p<0.04$).

Theta. No differences between type II patients and controls.

Alpha. Tendency toward higher (!) values in patients.

Beta $1+2$. Higher values in T4 and P_z ($0.02<p<0.04$).

The inspection of these results in comparison to those obtained for type I patients indicates that there seems to be less power in type II patients in slow frequencies delta and theta, but higher power values in alpha and beta bands. However, both groups were treated with neuroleptics, and so great caution should be exercised in the interpretation of the findings.

Motor Activation State, Repetitive Movement Right Hand

Delta. The average power during motor activity *increased* in normal persons. The activation pattern was very similar to that of the control group in the type I study (Fig. 1, top). However, in type II patients the average power *decreased* (!), although in the comparison with resting states no decrease attained significance (Fig. 1, bottom).

Theta. Minimal overall changes with no significance in either group.

Alpha. The average power *decreased* in both groups. However, there was a more widespread "alpha blockage" in type II patients than in controls (for further discussion of this discrepancy of "alpha activation" and "non-reactivity" in all other frequency bands, see Günther et al. 1987).

Beta 1 + 2. The major results were found in beta 1 (13.50–20.49), where the average power *decreased* in both groups. However, whereas the controls showed rather bilateral decreases in the probability maps, analogously to the control persons in our type I study (Fig. 1, top), there were almost no significant changes in type II schizophrenics (Fig. 1, bottom).

EEG Mapping Study on Untreated Schizophrenics During Motor Activation: First Results of the Possible Influence of Neuroleptic Medication

For this ongoing study, using methodology analogous to that in the above EEG mapping investigations, we demonstrate some preliminary results in Fig. 2. The top line of Fig. 2 demonstrates the results of "probability mapping" (using the same ANOVA/t test statistics as described above) in 16 male control persons (average age 29.1 years, range 20–46 years) during repetitive movement with the right and left hand in the delta (0.5–4.45 cps) frequency band. (In theta there were only very slight changes both in these patients and the control persons; in alpha there were similar activation patterns; the statistical analysis of the beta bands has not yet been finished.)

In control persons, there seems to be a predominantly contralateral increase of delta during repetitive movement of the right hand and a bifrontal increase during movement of the left hand. Although we made efforts to exclude eye and/or blinking artifact-contaminated EEG periods from the FFT analysis, this possibility cannot entirely be ruled out, especially in view of these results.

However, in type I schizophrenic patients (Fig. 2 middle; $n=16$, average age 25.5 years, range 21–32 years, not currently being (and predominantly never having been) treated with neuroleptics; SANS score 18.3, i.e., rather extreme type I patients) the bilateral diffuse increases of delta during movement of the right and left hands spread onto central areas (which is not explained by artifacts).

DELTA REPETITIVE MOVEMENT
RIGHT HAND SIGN. INCR. IN REL. % (VS. RESTING CONDITION) LEFT HAND

MALE (M.) CONTROL PERSONS

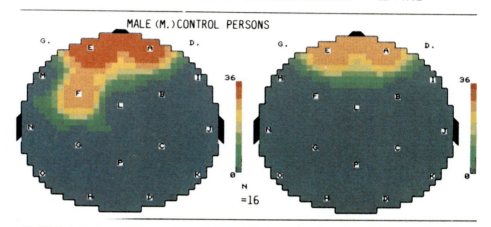

N=16

SCHIZOPHRENICS "TYPE I". NOT/NEVER TREATED WITH DRUGS BEFORE

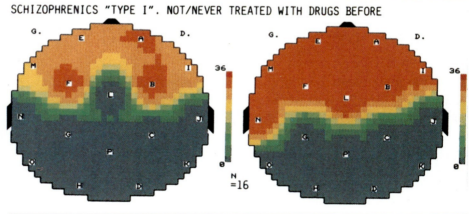

N=16

SCHIZOPHRENICS "TYPE I". NEUROLEPTIC-TREATED LESS THAN 10 DAYS

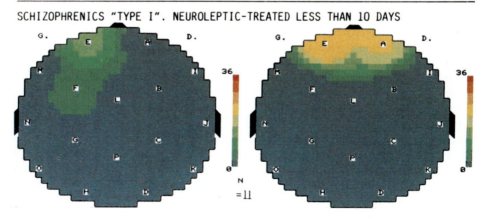

N=11

Additionally, if one reexamines these patients (possible only for a subgroup; $n=11$, average age 21.8 years, range 21–35 years) (Fig. 2 bottom) after short-term administration of neuroleptic treatment (on average less than 10 days; average dosage 480 units chlorpromazine daily), there seems to be a reduction of the "bilateral diffuse activation" (in this frequency band) approaching "normal patterns". This preliminary result could be of clinical value, if it holds true in the further evolution of the study (to be reported).

Discussion

Resting Conditions

The results of our studies on (neuroleptic-treated) type I and II schizophrenics seem to indicate the following:
– In type I schizophrenics there is (relative to normals) more power in slow frequency bands and less power in alpha and beta frequencies.
– In Type II patients, however, there is (relative to normals) some minor evidence of increases in delta and no such evidence for theta. In contrast, there seems to be more power in alpha and a tendency toward more power in the beta bands. Since there were no significant differences in age, duration of illness, mean educational level and average level of neuroleptic medication, none of these factors should be considered as a likely explanation for the "power shift" from slower to faster EEG frequencies along the type I/II dimension. However, the cross-validation in *untreated* patients must be completed in order to check the reliability of this difference. There is more support in the literature for the importance of biological heterogeneity along a positive-negative dimension of schizophrenia for EEG investigations.

As we stated in the Introduction, there are discrepancies for EEG power findings (resting conditions) in slow frequencies: Some authors have found increased values in delta and sometimes in theta (Fink et al. 1965; Itil et al. 1972; Lifshitz and Gradijan 1972, 1974; Etevenon et al. 1979; Stevens and Livermore 1982; Morstyn et al. 1983; Morihisa et al. 1983). Other authors have not reported such increases (d'Elia et al. 1977; Coger et al. 1979; Flor-Henry et al. 1979; Merrin et al. 1986). If one reevaluates the patient groups involved in

---

Fig. 2. Statistical maps of repetitive movement of the right and left hands: delta (0.5–4.49 cps). *Top*, control persons; *middle*, type I schizophrenics never or not currently on neuroleptics; *bottom*, subgroup of these patients after short-term administration of neuroleptics (and considerable amelioration of positive symptoms such as hallucinations, delusions). Construction of the maps as in Fig. 1. Note the predominantly contralateral *increase* in movement of the right hand and a bifrontal increase (artifact contamination?) in movement of the left hand in controls. Note also the widespread, bilateral increases in drug-free, predominantly drug-naive type I patients (not likely to be explained by artifacts) and the reduction of such "hyperactivation" toward normal patterns after short-term neuroleptic treatment (not likely to be explained by artifacts). Electrode placement and map scale as in Fig. 1

these studies, there is indeed some evidence that biological heterogeneity may influence the controversial results:

Stevens and Livermore (1982; p 392) studied schizophrenics who "displayed acute catatonic and/or hallucinatory symptoms." Morstyn et al. (1983; p 264) investigated patients who "all had current symptomatology of thought disorder and/or delusional cognition and auditory hallucinations." Other author groups described increased deltas in "paranoid", but not "residual" patients (Fink et al. 1965; Itil et al. 1972; Lifshitz and Gradijan 1972, 1974; Etevenon et al. 1979). This seems to be consistent with our findings of increased power values in slow frequencies in type I schizophrenia.

In contrast, Merrin et al. (1986), for example, did not find increased deltas in the following patients: "schizophrenia, paranoid, chronic ($n=6$); disorganised, chronic (1), undifferentiated, chronic (1)" (p 456), with only one "subchronic" patient and no "acute" patients. This again seems to be in line with our findings of only minor increases in delta and no such increases in theta for type II schizophrenia.

Further evidence supporting for the possible role of the type I/type II dimension on findings in other frequency bands has been stated in the introduction and is discussed in more detail elsewhere (Günther et al. 1988). However, the relations of acute-chronic, paranoid-nonparanoid/residual and other dimensions to our operationally defined type I/type II dimension remain unclear. Much more work will be needed to reveal intercorrelations of different dimensions through the "group of schizophrenias" (Bleuler 1911).

Motor Activation Conditions

Although there are signs of brain dysfunction in schizophrenia during verbal and spatial activation, for example using rCBF (Gur et al. 1983, 1985), there is not much such evidence for the "motor window." Our rCBF results (Günther et al. 1986c) yielded signs of a "bilateral diffuse hyperactivation" in (never treated) type I patients and a "non-reactivity" in (not currently medicated) type II schizophrenics (during repetitive movement of the right hand. There might be some congruence between these rCBF findings and our EEG mapping findings of a "diffuse hyperactivation" (in delta) in untreated type I patients during simple motor activity (see Fig. 2). Unfortunately, the delta band (in which many EEG findings for schizophrenia are reported) is most susceptible to artifact contamination. Since this issue seems insoluble efforts toward external validation of functional EEG data are urgently needed (including PET facilities). However, for several purposes – especially the evaluation of the course of a particular brain dysfunction parameter – the innocuous and low-cost quantitative EEG will retain its great advantages over other neuroimaging methods.

Thus, EEG mapping may be the future method of choice for long-term brain function monitoring in clinical psychiatry, providing further advances in theory and clinical application of the method can be achieved.

Acknowledgement. We thank Promonta GmbH, Hamburg for financial support.

References

Asarnow RF, McCrimmon DJ (1978) Residual performance deficit in clinically remitted schizophrenics. A marker of schizophrenia? J Abnorm Psychol 87:597–608

Bleuler E (1911) Dementia praecox oder die Gruppe des Schizophrenien. In: Aschaffenburg G (ed) Handbuch der Psychiatrie. Deuticke, Leipzig

Brodie JD, Christman DR, Corona JF et al. (1984) Patterns of metabolic activity in the treatment of schizophrenia. Ann Neurol 15 (Suppl):166–169

Coger RW, Dymond AM, Serafetinides EA (1979) Electroencephalographic similarities between chronic alcoholics and chronic, nonparanoid schizophrenics. Arch Gen Psychiatry 36:91–94

Crow TJ (1985) The two-syndrome concept. Origins and current status. Schizophr Bull 11:471–486

d'Elia GD, Jacobsson L, von Knorring L, Mattison B, Mjörndal T, Oreland L, Perris C, Rapp W (1977) Changes in psychopathology in relation to EEG variables and visual averaged evoked responses (V.AER) in schizophrenic patients treated with penfluridol or thiotixene. Acta Psychiatr Scand 55:309–318

Dieterle DM, Albus MI, Eben E, Ackenheil M, Rockstroh W (1986) First results with the Andreasen scale (Munich version). Assessment of productive and negative symptoms in chronic schizophrenic patients. Psychopharmacology 19:96–100

Duffy FH, Burchfield JL, Lambroso CT (1979) Brain electrical activity mapping (BEAM): a method for extending the clinical utility of EEG and evoked potential data. Ann Neurol 5:309–321

Ellingson RJ (1954) The incidence of EEG abnormality among patients with mental disorders of apparently nonorganic origin. Am J Psychiatry 111:263–275

Etevenon P, Ridoux P, Rioux P, Peron-Magnan P, Verdeaux G, Deniker P (1979) Intra- and interhemispheric EEG differences quantified by spectral analysis. Acta Psychiatr Scand 60:57–68

Etevenon P, Peron-Magnan P, Rioux P, Pidoux P, Bisserbe JC, Verdeaux G, Deniker P (1981) Schizophrenia assessed by computerized EEG. In: Perris C, Kemali D, Vacca L (eds) Electroneurophysiology and psychopathology. Adv Biol Psychiatry, vol 6. Karger, Basel, pp 29–34

Fink M, Itil TM, Clyde D (1965) A contribution to the classification of psychoses by quantitative EEG measures. Proc Soc Biol Psychiatry 2:5–17

Flor-Henry P, Koles ZJ, Howarth BG, Burton L (1979) Neurophysiology studies of schizophrenia, mania, and depression. In: Gruzelier J, Flor-Henry P (eds) Hemisphere asymmetries of function in psychopathology. Elsevier, Amsterdam, pp 481–521

Günther W, Breitling D (1985) Predominant sensorimotor area left hemisphere dysfunction in schizophrenia measured by brain electrical activity mapping. Biol Psychiatry 20:515–532

Günther W, Günther R, Eich FX, Eben E (1986a) Psychomotor disturbances as a possible basis for new attempts at differential diagnosis and therapy. II. Eur Arch Psychiatry Neurol Sci 235:301–308

Günther W, Breitling D, Banquet JP, Marcie P, Rondot P (1986b) EEG mapping of left hemisphere dysfunction during motor performance in schizophrenia. Biol Psychiatry 21:249–262

Günther W, Moser E, Müller-Spahn F, Öfele Kv, Büll U, Hippius H (1986c) Pathological cerebral blood flow during motor function in schizophrenic and endogenous depressed patients. Biol Psychiatry 21:889–899

Günther W, Davous P, Godet JL, Guillibert F, Breitling D, Rondot P (1988) Bilateral brain dysfunction during motor activation in type II schizophrenia measured by EEG mapping. Biol Psychiatry 23:295–311

Gur RE, Skolnick BE, Gur RC, Caroff S, Obrist WD, Younkin D, Reivich M (1983) Brain function in psychiatric disorders. I. Regional cerebral blood flow in medicated schizophrenics. Arch Gen Psychiatry 40:1250–1254

Gur RE, Gur RC, Skolnick BE, Caroff S, Obrist WD, Resnick S, Reivich M (1985) Brain function in psychiatric disorders. III. Regional cerebral blood flow in unmedicated schizophrenics. Arch Gen Psychiatry 42:329–334

Igert C, Lairy GC (1962) Interêt prognostique de l'EEG au cours de l'evolution des schizophrènes. Clin Neurophysiol 14:183–190
Itil TM (1964) Elektroencephalographische Studien bei Psychosen und psychotropen Medikamenten. Ahmet Sait Matbaasi, Istanbul
Itil TM (1977) Qualitative and quantitative EEG findings in schizophrenia. Schizophr Bull 3:61–79
Itil TM (1980) Computer analysed electroencephalogram to predict the therapeutic outcome in schizophrenia. In: Baxter CF, Melnechuk T (eds) Perspectives in schizophrenia research. Raven, New York
Itil TM, Saletu B, Davis S (1972) EEG findings in chronic schizophrenics based on digital period analysis and analog power spectra. Biol Psychiatry 5:1–13
Itil TM, Marasa J, Saletu B, Davis S, Mucciardi AN (1975) Computerized EEG: predictor of outcome in schizophrenia. J Nerv Ment Dis 160:188–203
Lauritzen M, Henriksen L, Lassen NA (1981) RCBF during rest and skilled hand movements by Xenon-133 and emission computerized tomography. J Cereb Blood Flow Metab 1:385–389
Lehmann D (1971) Multichannel topography of human alpha EEG fields. Electroencephalogr Clin Neurophysiol 31:433–449
Lifshitz K, Gradijan J (1972) Relationships between measures of the coefficient of variation of the mean absolute EEG voltage and spectral intensities in schizophrenics and control subjects. Biol Psychiatry 5:149–163
Lifshitz K, Gradijan J (1974) Spectral evaluation of the electroencephalogram: power and variability in chronic schizophrenic and control subjects. Psychophysiology 11:479–490
Manschreck TC (1986) Motor abnormalities in schizophrenia. In: Nasrallah HA, Weinberger DR (eds) Handbook of schizophrenia, vol 1. Elsevier, New York, pp 65–96
Maurer K, Dierks T (1987) Brain Mapping-topographische Darstellung des EEG und der evozierten Potentiale in Psychiatrie und Neurologie. Z EEG-EMG 18:4–12
Merrin EL, Fein G, Floyd TC, Yingling CD (1986) EEG asymmetry in schizophrenic patients before and during neuroleptic treatment. Biol Psychiatry 21:455–465
Morihisa JM, Duffy FH, McCarley RW (1983) BEAM in schizophrenic patients. Arch Gen Psychiatry 4:719–728
Morstyn R, Duffy FH, McCarley RW (1983) Altered topography of EEG spectral content in schizophrenia. Electroencephalogr Clin Neurophysiol 56:263–271
Olesen J (1971) Contralateral focal increase of cerebral blood flow in man during hand work. Brain 94:635–645
Petsche HA, Marko A (1955) Toposcopische Untersuchungen zur Ausbreitung des Alpha-Rhythmus. Wien Z Nervenheilkd 12:87–100
Stevens JR, Livermore A (1982) Telemetered EEG in schizophrenia: spectral analysis during abnormal behavior episodes. J Neurol Neurosurg Psychiatry 45:385–395

Coherence Mapping Reveals Differences in the EEG Between Psychiatric Patients and Healthy Persons

H. Pockberger[1], K. Thau[2], A. Lovrek[1], H. Petsche[1], and P. Rappelsberger[1]

Introduction

The purpose of this pilot study was to test both the usefulness and reliability of a mapping method that was described in its most recent version by Rappelsberger et al. (1986). Unlike other mapping methods, this one takes into account coherence estimates. Up to the present time, it has been applied for extracting features characteristic of changes of the ongoing EEG due to cognitive tasks (Petsche et al. 1985, 1986; Pockberger et al. 1985). It turned out that the parameter "coherence" yields additional and valuable hints to how information is processed by the cortex.

Material and Methods

Ten depressive and 11 schizophrenic patients were compared with 10 healthy male persons who had no neurological or psychiatric history and no previous drug or alcohol abuse. The 10 depressive patients met the diagnostic criteria 296.1 and 296.3 in DSM-III and ICD-9 respectively, the 11 schizophrenic patients the criteria 295.1 and 295.3 in DSM-III and ICD-9 respectively. The mean age was 27.2 years in the schizophrenics, 36.8 years in the depressives, and 26.8 years in the normal controls. All patients attended the clinic in an acute period of their disease and had taken no medication for at least 3 days before EEG recordings. These were performed between the 1st and the 4th day after attending the clinic.

The EEG was recorded at rest with eyes closed and during different mental conditions (monaural listening, right and left ear, two different kinds of music and text). Each recording lasted 1.5 min. The periods of acoustic stimulation were interrupted by periods of rest. Total continuous recording time was 15.5 min (a total of 6 min during the acoustic tasks and 7.5 min at rest before, between and after the tasks; the recording started with an initial resting period of 2 min for adaptation).

In this paper, only the resting periods are considered, with respect to two questions: (1) Are there reliable differences between depressives, schizophrenics

---

[1] Institut für Hirnforschung, Österreichische Akademie der Wissenschaften, Institut für Neurophysiologie der Universität Wien, Währingerstr. 17
[2] Psychiatrische Universitätsklinik, 1090 Wien, Austria

and healthy persons with respect to the parameters examined? (2) Since the level of vigilance certainly did not remain the same within the 13.5 min during which the five subsequent recordings of EEG at rest were obtained, are the differences constant within the groups of patients with time? A positive answer to these questions would be a confirmation of the usefulness and validity of this method for studying psychopathological conditions.

Since a detailed description of the method is given by Rappelsberger et al. (1986), only a brief account of its essential features is given here: During the EEG examination, the persons were resting in a comfortable armchair. The electrodes were placed according to the 10/20 system; EEG was recorded with respect to linked earlobe electrodes from 19 electrodes and the data stored on analogue tape for off-line processing.

After digitization at 256/s, eye and muscle artifacts were eliminated by visual inspection. For spectral analysis, 15 sections of 2 s each were chosen for computation. After Fourier transformation of the 2-s epochs, averaged power and cross-power spectra were computed, the latter between adjacent electrodes and between electrodes at homologous locations on both hemispheres. The amount of data was reduced by extracting broad band parameters for five frequency bands: theta (4–7.5 Hz), alpha (8–12.5 Hz), beta 1 (13–18 Hz), beta 2 (18.5–24 Hz) and beta 3 (24.5–31.5 Hz). The broad band parameters are absolute power and coherence.

The statistical procedure in this study aims at the evaluation of significant differences of the resting EEG between groups of depressives, schizophrenics and healthy persons. Randomization tests according to Fisher (Edgington 1980; Lebart et al. 1982) were applied. The results are presented in color-coded topographic maps indicating the probability of differences.

Fig. 1. Significant probability mapping of absolute power, local coherence, and interhemispheric coherence (vertically arranged). Five frequency bands, theta to beta 3 (3.5–31.5 Hz, horizontally arranged). The colors indicate error probabilities for the rejection of the null hypothesis, i.e., no differences between patients and normal persons: *red*, low error probability, or the respective parameter is significantly larger at the respective location in patients; *blue,* low error probability, but the corresponding parameter is significantly lower in patients; *green,* no difference between the two groups compared. The figure comprises the data of resting periods II and III together (time delay between the two recordings 1.5 min). *Top:* comparison of 10 depressive patients and 10 normal persons. Depressives show more beta power than normals. Local coherence in the beta range is lower in depressives, particularly in the left temporal region; interhemispheric coherence is larger in frontal regions in the alpha and beta 1 band. *Bottom:* comparison of 11 schizophrenic patients and 10 normal persons. Schizophrenics show lower local coherence in all frequency ranges, particularly in the central and the right temporal and parietal regions. On the other hand, in schizophrenics, temporo-occipital interhemispheric coherence is larger in all bands except the alpha band

Differences in the EEG Between Psychiatric Patients and Healthy Persons 453

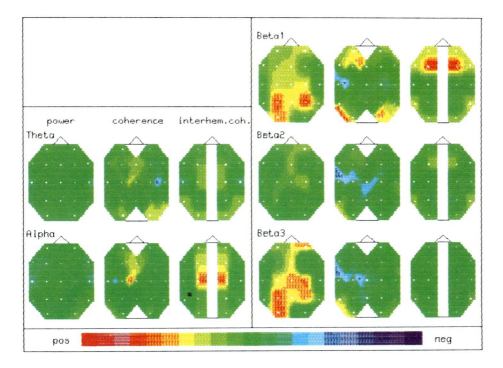

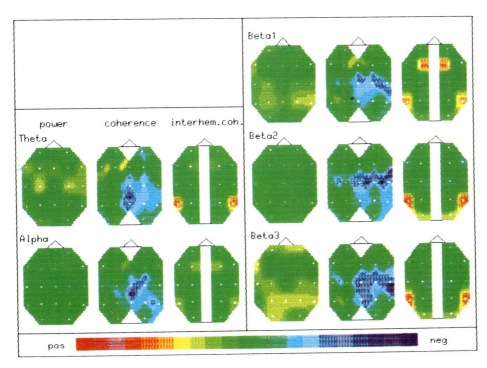

Results

Question 1 above, whether differences exist between each of the two groups of patients and healthy persons, can be answered positively, as illustrated in Fig. 1. The following conclusions can be drawn:

Depressive patients have somewhat more beta power than the normal group. Coherence differences are also most pronounced in the beta range: in beta 1, depressives have a larger degree of local coherence than normal persons in the temporo-occipital regions on both sides, and in the left frontal region; in the total beta range, local coherence in the left temporal area is lower in depressives than in the normal group. In interhemispheric coherence, the depressive groups shows larger values in the precentral region in the alpha band and in the frontal region in beta 1.

The power of the resting EEG of *schizophrenic* patients, on the other hand, is hardly different from power in the normal group. For local coherence, however, there are most impressive differences in all frequency bands. In schizophrenic patients, this parameter is in all bands lower than in the healthy group: the most distinct differences are found in the central area, with a further extension to the right hemisphere, particularly to temporal and parietal areas. The most impressive difference between schizophrenics and healthy persons with respect to interhemispheric coherence concerns the temporo-occipital region, with its larger coherence in schizophrenics in all bands except the alpha; in the beta 1 band, in addition, the frontal region displays larger interhemispheric coherence values than in normal persons.

Figure 1 also shows that the topographic distribution of differences is not the same in the two groups of patients, particularly with respect to coherence. The most impressive finding in this regard is the asymmetry of local coherence: in schizophrenics, lower local coherence is found in the central area and more to the right hemisphere in all frequency bands, in depressive patients more to the left side and restricted to the beta bands.

Question 2, whether such differences are stable, certainly cannot be answered affirmatively by this study. Nevertheless, a comparison of the four resting periods of 1.5 min recorded within a total period of 10.5 min is illustrated in Fig. 2, where the changes in local coherence are shown for the four periods of EEG at rest that were separated by 1.5-min EEG periods with acoustic stimulation. (Coherence was selected as the parameter displaying the majority of changes.) It turns out that, in spite of certain differences between the four periods of rest and regardless of the oscillations of degree of attention, the trend toward a predominance of lower coherence in the right hemisphere is recognizable in all four recordings of schizophrenic patients.

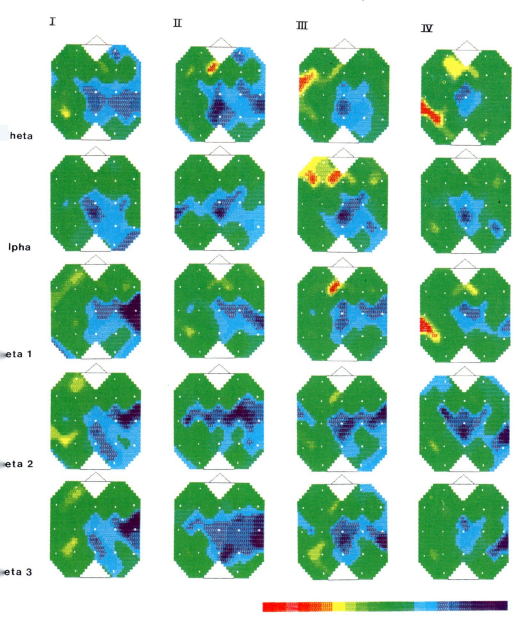

Fig. 2. Four subsequent control periods (EEG at rest) of 1.5 min each (I–IV), separated by three periods of equal length with different acoustic stimuli (total period 10.5 min). Only local coherence differences between the schizophrenic patients and the normal group are shown. Note the largely stable patterns of the differences of local coherence within this relatively long period of time. 11 Schizophrenic patients, 10 healthy persons; EEG at rest, periods (90 s) I–IV

Discussion

These results demonstrate that the efficiency of brain mapping in psychoses seems to depend largely on the choice of parameters. When comparing groups of psychoses with normal persons, a mapping of significant differences of absolute power of the EEG at rest turned out to be less informative than a mapping of differences of coherence: both local and interhemispheric coherence differences tend to be stabler over time. This supports anew the view that the main aim of mapping methods should be to register interareal cortical connections rather than to detect strictly localized disorders, a point emphasized as early as 1978 by Shaw et al.

The above findings of characteristic differences in resting EEG, not only between psychotic and normal persons but also between schizophrenics and depressives (the former displaying lower values of local coherence essentially in the right hemisphere and in central regions, the latter in the left temporal area, both with respect to healthy persons), again raise the question of lateralization of psychotic dysfunctions. This problem has recently been examined by different groups, mainly by Flor-Henry and Koles (1984), Etevenon et al. (1983) and Gruzelier (this volume). Unfortunately, their data, though hinting at a certain lateralization of functions, cannot be discussed in the light of the above findings because of the great differences of methodology in collection and processing of the data in different laboratories. The same holds true for the question of hypofrontality that was raised by blood flow studies in schizophrenia (Ingvar and Franzen 1974).

How difficult it will probably turn out to be to subsume the dysfunctions underlying psychoses under a unified concept may also be guessed from our data: in spite of the significantly lower coherence estimates in schizophrenic resting EEG than in normals, the interhemispheric coherence between the occipitotemporal regions is larger in schizophrenics than in healthy persons in all bands except the alpha band (in depressives, it is larger only in the beta 1 band). Even though we are still far from understanding the meaning of these findings, one is inclined to hypothesize that this pronounced interplay between the temporo-occipital regions of the two hemispheres could be an expression of tendencies on the part of the brain to compensate for the lower degree of information exchange in the central and the right temporo-occipital regions.

References

Edgington ES (1980) Randomization tests. Dekker, New York

Etevenon P, Person-Magnan P, Campistron D, Verdeaux G, Deniker P (1983) Differences in EEG symmetry between patients with schizophrenia and normals assessed by Fourier analysis. In: Flor-Henry P, Gruzelier J (eds) Laterality and psychopathology. Elsevier, Amsterdam, pp 269–290

Flor-Henry P, Koles ZJ (1984) Statistical quantitative EEG studies of depression, mania, schizophrenia and normals. Biol Psychiatry 19:257–279

Ingvar DH, Franzen G (1974) Abnormalities of cerebral blood flow distribution in patients with chronic schizophrenia. Acta Psychiatry Scand 50:425–462

Lebart L, Morineau A, Fenelon JP (1982) Traitement des donnees statistiques: methodes et programmes. Dunod, Paris

Petsche H, Pockberger H, Rappelsberger P (1985) EEG studies in musical perception and performance. In: Spintge R, Droh R (eds) Music and medicine. Roche, Basel, pp 31–60

Petsche H, Pockberger H, Rappelsberger P (1986) EEG topography and mental performance. In: Duffy FH (ed) Topographic mapping of the brain. Butterworth, Stoneham, pp 63–98

Pockberger H, Petsche H, Rappelsberger P, Zidek B, Zapotoczky HG (1985) On-going EEG in depression: a topographic spectral analytic study. Electroencephalogr Clin Neurophysiol 61:349–358

Rappelsberger P, Pockberger H, Petsche H (1986) Computer aided EEG analysis: evaluation of changes during cognitive processes and topographic mapping. EDV Med Biol 17:45–53

Shaw JC, O'Connor K, Ongley C (1978) EEG coherence as a measure of cerebral functional organization. In: Brazier MAB, Petsche H (eds) Architectonics of the cortex. Raven, New York, pp 245–256

Mapping of Evoked Potentials in Normals and Patients with Psychiatric Diseases

K. Maurer, T. Dierks, R. Ihl, and G. Laux[1]

Introduction

Studies on the clinical use of evoked potentials (EP) in psychiatry date back to the mid-1960s, when Callaway et al. (1965) and Rodin et al. (1964) described EP alterations in schizophrenia. The first book about the use of EP in psychiatry appeared in 1972 (Shagass 1972). The most consistent finding in the following studies by Roth et al. (1981) and Pfefferbaum et al. 1984b) was a reduction of P300 amplitudes in schizophrenia and dementia. For schizophrenia, this reduction seemed to be the most robust and replicable waveform alteration indicating biological deficits in this disease. Despite all these valuable results, the EP method did not gain the degree of clinical significance that would have been necessary for routine use of EP for differential diagnosis and drug monitoring. One reason might be the nonspecificity of EP alterations, which are often similar in different diseases.

Duffy et al. (1979) were the first to describe the method and the clinical utility of brain electrical activity mapping (BEAM) of EEG and EP. Later, Morihisa et al. (1983) applied mapping of visual and auditory evoked potentials (VEP, AEP) to untreated and treated schizophrenic patients. The P300 maps gained by Morstyn et al. (1983) and McCarley et al. (1985) in schizophrenia showed lateralization of P300 activity in this disease.

Whereas the "exogenous" waves – VEP, AEP and somatosensory EP(SEP) – are generated in corresponding nuclei, pathways and representation areas, one assumes that the "endogenous" wave P300 originates not only in the cortex but also in brain structures such as the hippocampus and amygdala (Halgren et al. 1982; Okada et al. 1983). These areas are thought to be involved in the pathogenesis of psychoses and of dementia.

The aim of the present study is to show the topography of EP in normals (VEP, AEP and SEP) and the topography of the auditory elicited P300 in control subjects and patients with various psychiatric disorders such as dementia, schizophrenia and major depression. With topographic pharmaco-AEP300, a new method in the field of psychopharmacology will be introduced.

Methods

EP were elicited according to methods described thoroughly by Maurer et al. (1982, 1987) and Lowitzsch et al. (1983). A reversing checkerboard was used

[1] Department of Psychiatry, University of Würzburg, Füchsleinstr. 15, 8700 Würzburg, Federal Republic of Germany

to evoke VEP, a click or tone for AEP and AEP300 and an electric shock for SEP. For eliciting the auditory P300 we recorded AEP after frequent low-pitched (1000 Hz, 80 dBHL) and infrequent high-pitched tones of 50 ms duration (10 ms rise and fall time). The tones were presented in a random sequence with a 20% probability of hearing the infrequent high-pitched tone. The subjects were asked to pay attention and to count the rare tones ("target" stimuli). After separate averaging of the responses after target and nontarget stimulation a positive wave of high amplitude could be recorded with a latency of about 300 ms due to target stimuli. The electrical activity of the brain was recorded from 20 electrodes applied to the scalp according to the 10–20 system. Two mastoid electrodes served as reference. The analogue data from the 20 EEG electrodes then underwent analogue-to-digital conversion and were processed into topographic maps of electrical field distribution. The areas around the original 20 electrodes were filled in by linear interpolation based upon the values of the four nearest electrodes. For baseline definition a predelay interval of 100 ms duration was used. Further analysis involved construction of group averages and t-statistical maps to delineate the differences in peak values of P300 between the control and patient groups.

Subjects

Control subjects were ten right-handed students (mean age 28.8 years) and ten elderly people (mean age 74.2 years) with no history of psychiatric illnesses. They were medication-free. Thirty schizophrenic patients were investigated. Selection criteria were right-handedness, no history of organic brain damage, normal computed tomography (CT) and diagnosis meeting the DSM-III and ICD-9 criteria. Ten patients had been classified as being of the hebephrenic subtype (DSM-III and ICD-9: 295.1) 10 as the paranoid subtype (DSM-III and ICD-9: 295.3) and 10 as the residual subtype (DSM III and ICD-9: 295.6). The average age of the patients was 25.5 years for the hebephrenic, 28.7 years for the paranoid and 41.2 years for the residual group. The average current treatment lay between 440 and 560 chlorpromazine equivalent units. In addition we investigated 10 patients suffering from major depression (DSM-III: 296.1, 296.3, 296.4, 300.4) with a mean age of 45.9 years and eight patients diagnosed as having senile dementia of the Alzheimer type (SDAT). One patient had dementia due to Wilson's disease. The P300 was also recorded in six volunteers after administration of phosphatidylserine to introduce the "topographic pharmaco-AEP 300". Since P300 topography is also changed by organic brain lesions, the case of one patient with an arachnoidal cyst will be presented. All patients underwent audiological examination and an early AEP (EAEP) test to exclude a hearing disorder which would have interfered with AEP generation.

Results

EP and AEP300 Maps in Normals

Figures 1–3 show the typical topographic pattern of the main components of EP. After pattern reversal a symmetrical positive field representing the P2 component could be obtained with an occipital distribution (Fig. 1). The major positive and negative SEP peaks after electrical stimulation are shown in Fig. 2a–d with topography of the N20, P40 and N120 components. The binaural auditory stimulation modality showed a more centralized pattern for components N100 and P180, with a shift toward frontal for the negative and toward parietal for the positive components (Fig. 3a, b).

The P300 can be elicited in any modality (visual, somatosensory, auditory) as long as the target stimulus is meaningful. Only the auditory paradigm will be considered in this report. Figure 4 shows a group average waveform for a single electrode (Cz) and the topographic distribution of P300 activity. The topographic pattern showed a positive maximum at P3, Pz and P4, with amplitude values in the range of 15 µV, and at Pz and slightly greater activity over the right hemisphere. The P300 amplitude became diminished toward temporal and frontal structures.

Age-dependent Alteration of AEP300 Maps

With increasing age, latencies of the P300 become longer and amplitudes lower (Hegerl et al. 1985). The same result was obtained in our control groups, where the old population (mean age 74.2 years) showed amplitudes of 12.5 µV and

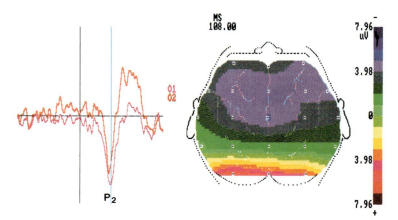

Fig. 1. Visual evoked potential (*VEP*). P2 component after pattern-reversal stimulation with a maximum of positivity of points O1, Oz and O2. *Left:* Single curve of points O1 and O2. *Right:* Topographic display of the P2 component at 108 ms. (All figures in this contribution were prepared using equipment from Bio-logic Systems Corporation, Mundelein, IL, USA)

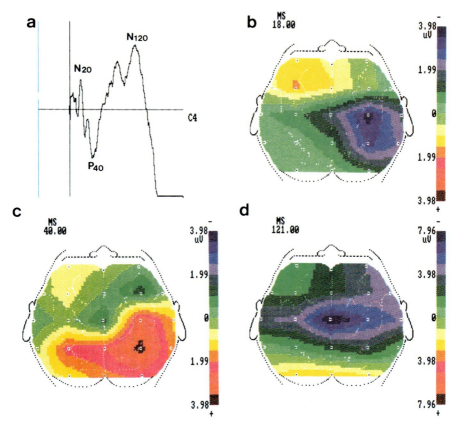

Fig. 2a–d. Somatosensory evoked potential (SEP) after stimulation of the left median nerve. **a** Single curve recorded at point C4. **b** N20 component with a maximum of negativity at point C4. **c** P40 component with a maximum of positivity at point P4. **d** N120 component with a maximum of positivity at point Cz and C4

latencies of 380 ms at Pz; the corresponding values were 17.5 µV and 332 ms for the young collective (mean age 28.8 years). The topographic distribution of P300 activity was identical in the old and young populations (Figs. 4, 5a).

P300 Topographic Mapping in Psychiatric Patients

Dementia. P300 data obtained from eight patients with SDAT were compared with P300 fields of eight age-equivalent controls. The age of the patients ranged from 65 to 80 years. All patients underwent several tests to differentiate between vascular and degenerative manifestation and to determine the degree of dementia, which was defined according to the Brief Cognitive Rating Scale (BCRS; Reisberg 1983) as mild (<23), moderate (24–32) and severe (>33). Only patients with a score of 24–32 (intermediate) were chosen for further testing. To delineate

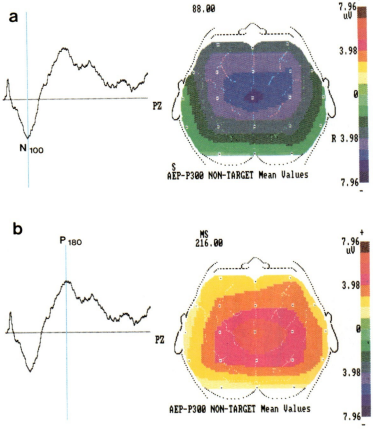

Fig. 3a, b. Late auditory evoked potential (AEP). **a** N100 component with a centrally located negative field after binaural stimulation. (group mean of 10 control subjects). **b** P180 component with a centrally located positive field (group mean)

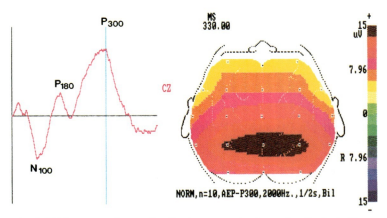

Fig. 4. P300 topography. *Right:* Single curve gained at point Cz. *Left:* Topographic distribution of P300 with a maximum of positivity at points P3, Pz and P4 (group mean of 10 control subjects)

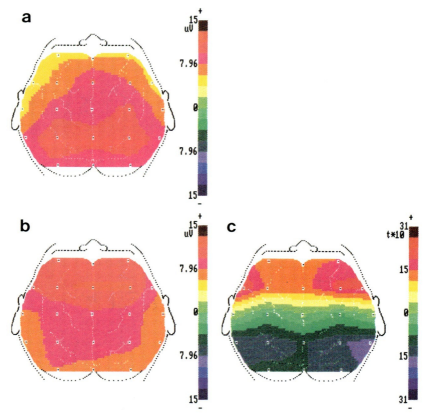

Fig. 5. a P300 topography in a geriatric control group. **b** P300 topography in SDAT patients with an amplitude loss compared to the geriatric control group in temporal, central, parietal and occipital areas. Bifrontally augmented amplitudes were observed. **c** A t value map showing differences between SDAT patients and geriatric controls. Positive values indicate an increase and negative values a decrease of amplitude compared to normals

regions in which SDAT patients differ from age-matched controls, the two groups were compared using t statistic techniques. As shown in Fig. 5b the demented patients exhibited higher amplitudes frontally, no difference centrally and an amplitude decrement in the parietal region in which the group differences reached t values of 1.8 and even more (Fig. 5c). Only the bifrontal P300 amplitude increase achieved statistical significance ($p < 0.05$).

In one patient with dementia due to Wilson's disease we were able to perform a follow-up study over a period of 3 months during therapy with penicillamine. The corresponding maps are shown in Fig. 6a–d. Most obvious was the displacement of the positive field from frontal to more central and parietal areas. The change of P300 field was accompanied by improvement in the neuropsychological test scores and normalization of reaction time.

a

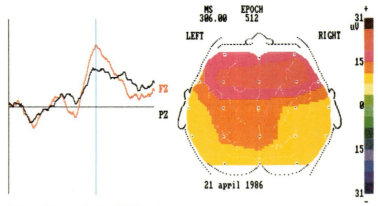

F channel intensity is: 22.05 uV

b

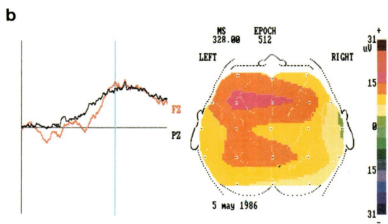

F channel intensity is: 16.42 uV

c

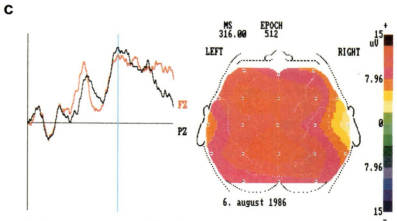

F channel intensity is: 11.76 uV

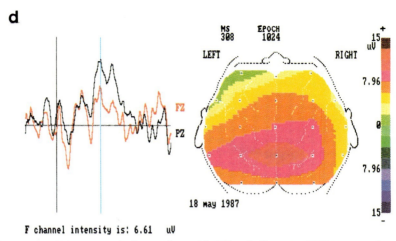

Fig. 6 a–d. Follow-up of P300 topography in a patient with Wilson's disease. **a** P300 topography in the untreated state (21.4.1986), with a frontal accentuated pattern. **b** P300 topography after initiation of therapy with penicillamine (5.5.1986), with a slight expansion towards central structures. **c** P300 topography with a widespread positive field (6.8.1986). **d** P300 topography with stabilization in the parietal area (18.5.1987)

Schizoaffective Disorder. We were able to record the P300 in a 24-year-old female student with no history of previous mental illness suffering from schizoaffective disorder (ICD-9: schizoaffective psychosis, 295.7; DSM-III: schizophreniform disorder). Family history, drug screening, laboratory tests (including virology) and CT were all negative. Her psychopathology showed catatonic (excitement/mutismus), paranoid (delusions of reference, verbal hallucinations) and hebephrenic (incoherence, inappropriate silly affect) symptoms. On first brain mapping (21.1.87) she was drug-free, at the time of the second examination (4.2.87) she was on 10 mg haloperidol and 150 mg perazine daily. The subject was able to perform the P300 task correctly. In the psychotic state she failed to exhibit a discernible P300 at all, whereas after treatment with neuroleptics and a concomitant amelioration of the psychopathological condition a normalization of the former altered P300 took place, with a topography similar to that of normals. Only in the frontal area was an amplitude decrement maintained which resembled that of the hebephrenic subtype (Fig. 7a, b).

Schizophrenia. After the single case study just described, P300 topography was determined in 30 medicated schizophrenic patients. According to their symptomatology they were classified into the three subtypes of hebephrenic, paranoid and residual. Figure 8b–g shows P300 field distributions. The t statistic maps confirmed areas where the differences between normals and schizophrenics attained significance. The maximal difference in the hebephrenic subgroup occurred in frontal areas (Fp1, F3 and Fz), where t values of 1.7 were obtained. Areas exhibiting maximal differences for the paranoids were C4, P4 and T6 (t value 2.7), and for the residuals, C4 and P4 (t value 2.5; $p<0.05$).

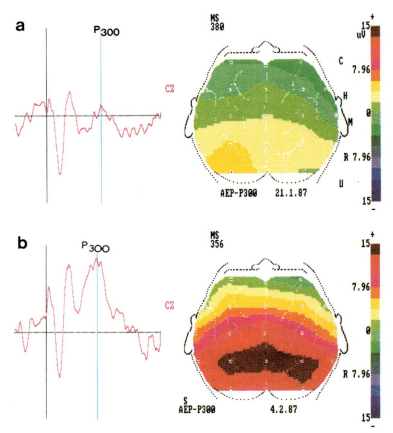

Fig. 7. a, b Topography of P300 in a patient with a schizoaffective disorder. **a** P300 field in the untreated condition with only a spurious P300 component at 380 ms. **b** P300 field after treatment with a clearly definable P300 wave at the points P3, Pz and P4 at 356 ms

Major Depression. Ten patients with a major depressive syndrome were investigated in this study, all free of medication. In comparison to an age-matched control population, an amplitude reduction was observed at P3, Pz and P4 with t values in the range of 1.4–1.5; this reduction was not significant (Fig. 9a–c).

Fig. 8 a–g. P300 fields in schizophrenic patients. **a** P300 map in the control group. **b** P300 topography in the hebephrenic subgroup, with a frontal decrement. **c** A t value map with negative values bifrontally. **d** P300 topography in the paranoid subgroup, with an imbalance between left and right hemisphere. **e** A t value map with sign of right-sided underactivation. **f** P300 topography in the residual subgroup, with more generalized amplitude reduction. **g** A t value map with signs of parietal amplitude reduction with an accentuation at points P4 and T6

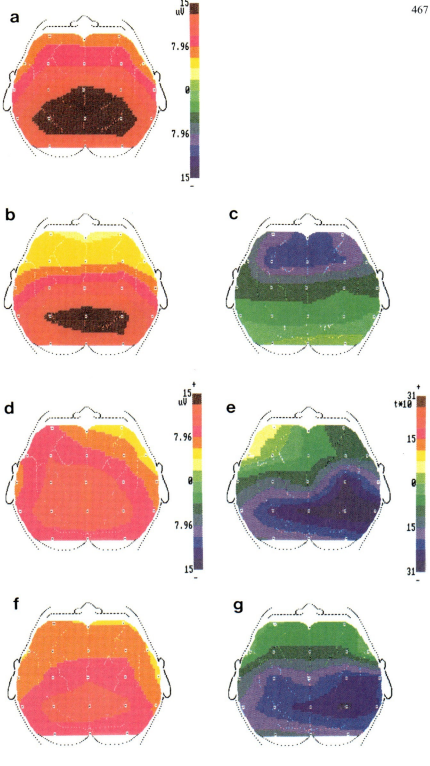

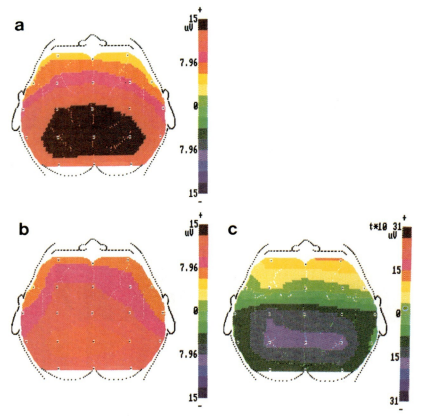

Fig. 9a–c. P300 topography in patients with major depressive syndrome. **a** P300 topography in an age-matched control group. **b** P300 topography in depressive patients with signs of parietal amplitude reduction. **c** A t value map with negative t values at points P3, Pz and P4

Topographic Pharmaco-AEP300

Few reports have yet appeared describing the use of endogenous event-related potentials such as P300 in psychopharmacology. This report is to our knowledge the first describing the topography of P300 after administration of a nootropic substance (phosphatidylserine, PS). A dose of 60 mg PS was given intravenously. Measurements of the P300 fields were carried out before drug ingestion and 60 and 120 min afterwards. The baseline P300 field and corresponding maps after medication are shown in Fig. 10a–c. There was an increase of amplitude within the first hour from 12 to 15 µV at Pz and a decay to the original measured values after 2 h.

Mapping of Evoked Potentials in Normals and Patients with Psychiatric Diseases

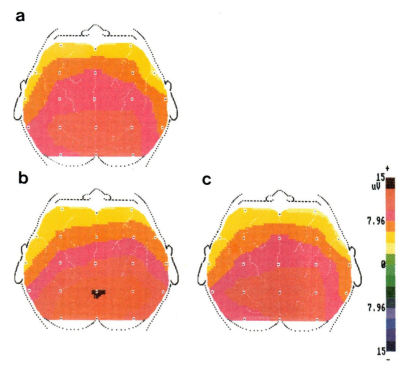

Fig. 10a–c. P300 topography in a control subject before and after administration of phosphatidylserine (PS). **a** P300 field before PS ingestion. **b** P300 field 60 min after administration of 50 mg PS with an amplitude increase at Pz. **c** P300 field 120 min after drug ingestion (P300 topography similar to **a**)

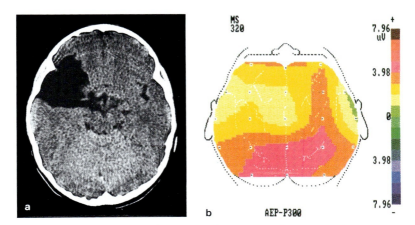

Fig. 11a, b. P300 topography in a patient with a left-sided arachnoid cyst. **a** Lesion detected by CT. **b** P300 field with amplitude loss on the left side frontally and centrally

P300 Topography in a Patient with an Organic Brain Lesion

The mapping of the P300 in organic brain lesions opens a new field in electrodiagnosis. Of special interest is the P300 field distribution in cases with a normal EEG and evidence of a brain lesion due to CT findings. Figure 11a shows the CT of a patient with a left-sided arachnoidal cyst in the temporal area. Whereas the EEG maps were not able to reveal an abnormality, the P300 field (Fig. 11b) exhibited an area of reduced amplitudes at points F3, C3, F2 and Cz which corresponds to the lesion found in CT.

Discussion

After testing exogenous potentials such as VEP, AEP and SEP and the endogenous potential P300 in normals and in various psychiatric conditions, we came to the conclusion that the auditory elicited P300 is a reliable measurement for evaluation of the electrical function of cortical and hippocampal structures. The P300 enables the examination of, and yields more insight into, the function not only of cortical but also of limbic and paralimbic structures, and we assume from our results that these are affected in psychoses and dementia. We therefore concentrated upon the AEP300, studying its electrical fields in young and old control groups, in dementia, schizophrenia and depression, and in one patient with an organic brain lesion. In this report we have shown for the first time the surface topography of P300 after administration of a psychotropic substance (PS).

The topographic distribution of the P300 field, with its maximum at Pz and concentric decrement toward temporal and frontal structures, is in accordance with the findings described by Pfefferbaum et al. (1984a) for a limited number of scalp electrodes and coincides with P300 maps published by Morstyn et al. (1983) and McCarley et al. (1986). Remarkable was the symmetry of P300 fields in the young and old control groups, with a persistence of the maximum at P3, Pz and P4. The wave proved to be reliable enough for the evaluation of psychiatric clinical conditions. The amplitude values in the elderly group were reduced at Pz to just over half of the values found in the young population and the latencies were slightly prolonged, although neither alteration was significantly correlated with age.

In dementia our findings with P300 topography were similar to those already known from neuroanatomic, rCBF and PET studies. Brun and Gustafson (1976) studied seven cases from a neuropathological point of view. Maximal cortical degeneration occurred in the medial temporal (limbic) area and in a field expanding from the posterior inferior temporal areas to the adjoining portions of the parieto-occipital lobes. The frontal lobes were less severely involved. Stigsby et al. (1981) described a "hyperfrontal flow distribution," i.e., high relative flow precentrally and a low relative flow postcentrally in spite of a reduced mean hemisphere blood flow. Foster et al. (1984) found a low glucose utilization in the SDAT group (10%–40% below that of control individuals) affecting almost all of the posterior parietal cortex and adjacent portions of the posterior temporal and anterior occipital lobes; the frontal cortex was found to be relatively intact. Similar findings were reported by Friedland et al. (1983), who described relatively lower [^{18}F] fluorodeoxyglucose (FDG) uptake in the temporoparietal cortex bilaterally which was related to the severity of dementia. Mapping of P300 together with the results of neuropathology rCBF and regional cerebral glucose metabolism showed a similar pattern of temporoparietal involvement, with the frontal lobes less severely affected, in dementia. The findings of a similar pattern of cortical and subcortical structural and functional damage raises the hope that the noninvasive AEP300 mapping may be used as an index of neuronal activity and for follow-up studies, and may serve as an indicator for the more invasive PET method.

Our single case study delineating P300 alterations in a case of an untreated schizoaffective disorder showed clearly that the P300 amplitude reduction was not due to medication with neuroleptics. Rather, the neuroleptic therapy had a normalizing effect upon the waveform. This is in line with the findings of Spohn et al. (1977), who showed that attention dysfunction and impaired information processing, both indispensable for proper P300 generation, are normalized by neuroleptic treatment. Two other studies that have examined this question found little or no alteration of the P300 by neuroleptics.

We investigated the three subtypes of schizophrenia and our results in hebephrenics, paranoids and residuals are not similar in every respect to with the findings described by Morstyn et al. (1983) and McCarley et al. (1985). The results in hebephrenics with a frontal lobe decrement might be consistent with EEG, rCBF and PET studies indicating reduced neuronal activity in frontal regions. All parameters measured by means of functional imaging procedures (rCBF, PET, P300 mapping) support the hypothesis of "hypofrontality" and are a further indication that frontal lobe dysfunction may be one of various pathological processes relevant to our understanding of the hebephrenic subgroup of schizophrenia. It is worth mentioning, however, that in our EEG research no frontal slowing could be found in the three subgroups of schizophrenia (Dierks et al., this volume).

Findings of decreased amplitudes in the right temporoparietal area and relatively increased amplitudes in the left temporal lobe were found in the paranoid and residual subgroups. The reduction in P300 in the right posterior temporoparietal area of paranoid schizophrenics is consistent with the findings of Gruzelier et al. (this volume), who found in paranoid schizophrenics firstly evidence of reduced right temporal functioning in terms of neuropsychological tests of learning and long-term memory, and secondly evidence from EEG topographic mapping of an abnormal elevation in fast beta in the right posterior temporoparietal area during a test of recognition memory of unfamiliar faces, a function which involves the same area and on which the patients were also deficient.

The results in the residual subtype of schizophrenia, which were similar to those described in the paranoid subtype cannot at present be explained in terms of over- and underactivation. It may be of interest that Gruzelier et al. (this volume) found either left-sided or bilateral impairments in patients with negative symptoms in the learning and memory tests.

Several investigations have stated the hippocampus and nucleus amygdalae to be the major sources of P300. Precisely in this area, Reynolds (1983) found an increase of dopamine concentrations in schizophrenics, with an accentuation in the left hemisphere amygdala. It one assumes that dopamine uptake correlates with P300 amplitude (augmentation of P300 after ingestion of PS) the relatively increased P300 amplitudes in the left temporoparietal region in the paranoid subgroup may be of interest.

For depressive patients, the P300 findings were found not to be lateralized and the t values did not indicate significance of the alterations compared to those in an an age-matched control group. These results may be consistent with those of Pfefferbaum et al. 1984, who also found decreased P300 amplitudes after auditory stimuli. It might be of interest that the pattern was quite similar to that described for the elderly control group.

It is known from the work of Bruni and Toffano (1982) that PS interferes with the dopamine uptake, which increases in limbic and paralimbic structures. The findings of an augmentation of P300 amplitudes after ingestion of PS may be explained in terms of an increased dopamine turnover in subcortical structures which contributes to the generation of the P300 complex. Evidently the cognitive function can be increased by a nootropic substance not only in demented but also in control persons. The question arises of whether the P300 topography may be used to test whether or not so-called nootropic substances develop a cognitive enhancing test.

In summary, P300 topography can be utilized in a wide range of psychiatric illnesses. The clinical results confirm the hypothesis that the P300 originates in considerable part in limbic and paralimbic structures. In dementia, the cell degeneration and the bilaterally reduced FDG uptake in the temporoparietal cortex may explain the symmetrically reduced P300 amplitudes in the same area with a "hyperfrontal" electrical behavior, whereas in schizophrenia, especially the paranoid subtype, the dopamine concentration in the amygdala may play an important role and may explain in part the lateralized P300 findings in this subtype. The experiment with PS also points to a short-lasting functional alteration mainly caused by an altered uptake of transmitters. The P300 test and its topography may be used for evaluation of electrical behavior of limbic and paralimbic structures and may illuminate our understanding of dementia and psychosis. If the correlation between transmitter activity and P300 wave alterations is better understood, this test may be used to improve the regional in vivo diagnostis of neurotransmitter function and topology. The advantages over other methods such as PET and rCBF are noninvasiveness and extremely short analysis times which allow the study of very short-lasting cognitive and emotional states.

References

Brun A, Gustafson L (1976) Distribution of cerebral degeneration in Alzheimer's desease. Arch Psychiatry Neurol 223:15–33

Bruni A, Toffano G (1982) The principles of phospholipid pharmacology. In: Antolini E

et al. (eds) Transport in biomembrana: model systems and reconstruction. Raven, New York, pp 235–242
Callaway E, Jones RT, Lyne RS (1965) Evoked responses and segmental set of schizophrenia. Arch Gen Psychiatry 12:83–89
Duffy HF, Buchfield JL, Lombroso CT (1979) Brain electrical activity mapping (BEAM): a method for extending the clinical utility of EEG and evoked potentials data. Ann Neurol 5:309–321
Foster NL, Chase TN, Mansi L, Brooks R, Fedio P, Patronas NJ, Chiro G (1984) Cortical abnormalities in Alzheimer's disease. Ann Neurol 16:649–654
Friedland RP, Budinger TF, Ganz E, Yano Y, Mathis CA, Koss B, Ober BA, Huesman RH, Derenzo SE (1983) Regional cerebral metabolic alteration in dementia of the Alzheimer type: positron emission tomography with Fluorodeoxyglucose. J Comput Assist Tomogr 7:590–598
Halgren E, Squires NK, Wilson CL, Crandall PH (1982) Brain generators of evoked potential: the late (endogenous) components. Bull Los Angeles Neurol Soc 47:108–123
Hegerl K, Klotz S, Ullrich G (1985) Späte akustisch evozierte Potentiale – Einfluß von Alter, Geschlecht und verschiedenen Untersuchungsbedingungen. Z EEG-EMG 16:171
Lowitzsch K, Maurer K, Hopf HC (1983) Evozierte Potentiale in der klinischen Diagnostik. Thieme, Stuttgart
Maurer K, Leitner H, Schafer E (1982) Akustisch evozierte Potentiale. Enke, Stuttgart
Maurer K, Lowitsch K, Stöhr M (1987) Evozierte Potentiale, Einführung und Atlas. Enke, Stuttgart
McCarley RW, Torello M, Shenton M, Duffy FH (1985) The topography of P300 and spectral energy in schizophrenics and normals. In: Chagass RC, Bridger WH, Weiss KJ, Stoff D, Simpson GM (eds) Biological psychiatry. Elsevier, Amsterdam, 389–391
Morihisa JM, Duffy FH, Wyatt RJ (1983) Brain electrical activity mapping (BEAM) in schizophrenic patients. Arch Gen Psychiatry 40:719–726
Morstyn R, Duffy FH, McCarley RW (1983) Altered P300 topography in schizophrenia. Arch Gen Psychiatry 40:729–734
Okada YC, Kaufman L, Williamson SJ (1983) The hippocampal formation as a source of the slow endogenous potentials. Electroencephalogr Clin Neurophysiol 55:417–426
Pfefferbaum A, Ford JM, Wenegrat BG, Roth WT, Kopell BS (1984a) Clinical application of the P3 component of event-related potentials in normal aging. Electroencephalogr Clin Neurophysiol 59:85–103
Pfefferbaum A, Wenegrat BG, Ford JM, Roth WT, Kopell BS (1984b) Clinical application of the P3 component of event-related potentials: II. Dementia, depression and schizophrenia. Electroencephalogr Clin Neurophysiol 59:104–124
Reisberg B, London E, Ferris SH, Borenstein J, Scheier L, de Leon MJ (1983) The brief cognitive rating scale: language motoric and mood, concomitants in primary degenerative dementia (PDD). Psychopharmacol Bull 19:702–708
Reynolds GP (1983) Increased concentration and lateral asymmetry of amygdala dopamine in schizophrenia. Nature 305:527–528
Rodin E, Zacharopoulos G, Beckett P, Frohman C (1964) Characteristics of visually evoked responses in normal subjects and schizophrenic patients. Electroencephalogr Clin Neurophysiol 17:451
Roth WT, Pfefferbaum A, Kelly AF, Berger PA, Kopell BS (1981) Auditory event-related potentials in schizophrenia and depression. Psychiatry Res 4:199–212
Shagass C (1972) Evoked potentials in psychiatry. Plenum, New York
Spohn HE, Lacoursiere RB, Tompson K (1977) Phenothioazine effects on psychological and psychophysiological dysfunction in chronic schizophrenics. Arch Gen Psychiatry 34:633–644
Stigsby B, Johanneson G, Ingvar D (1981) Regional EEG analysis and regional cerebral blood flow in Alzheimer's and Pick's disease. Electroencephalogr Clin Neurophysiol 51:537–547

Event-Related Potential (N100) Studies in Depressed Patients Treated with Electroconvulsive Therapy

J.A. COFFMAN and M.W. TORELLO[1]

Introduction

Impairment of attention and concentration is a hallmark of clinically significant depression. The impairment in intentional processes induced by depressive disorders has been verified with electrophysiological measures of attention. The N100 component of the long latency auditory evoked response, a negative wave which occurs in the range of 90–150 ms post-stimulus, has been generally regarded as reflecting changes in selective attention (Hillyard and Kutas 1983), and diminutions in N100 amplitude appear to be a feature associated with significant depression (Giedke et al. 1981; Shagass 1983; Knott and Lapierre 1987). However, findings have not been consistent in all studies, as elevations in sensory evoked potential amplitudes have been reported in severe (Friedman and Meares 1979), psychotic (Borge 1973) and bipolar (Borge et al. 1971) depressives. Little or nothing has been reported regarding the natural history of evoked potential changes in depression or the response of such changes to effective treatment for depression. A particular difficulty in the evaluation of changes in evoked potential measures subsequent to treatment for depression is that drug treatments commonly used to relieve depression themselves have large effects on brain event-related potential (ERP) features. One study reflecting this is the recent report by Blackwood et al. (1987), who determined in a group of individuals with depression treated by pharmacotherapy that N100 amplitude actually decreased from baseline levels. In addition, many of the previous studies of ERP have not utilized a full electrode montage for recording.

In order to address the issue of ERP changes in depression, particularly of the N100 component, this study was initiated, taking advantage of a full 28-lead montage and avoiding drug-induced changes in evoked potential components by focusing study on depressed patients receiving electroconvulsive therapy (ECT). We hypothesized that depressed patients would show diminished N100 amplitude and increased latency prior to treatment and that subsequent to effective treatment with ECT these evoked potential differences from control values would disappear. In addition, we hoped to take advantage of topographic display of the N100 response in order to discern any relevant spatial component of the ERP changes observed.

---

[1] The Ohio State University, Department of Psychiatry, 473 West 12th Avenue, Columbus, OH 43210, USA

Method

Subjects

The group of depressed subjects (major depressive disorder, DSM-III) was recruited from patients referred for ECT who gave informed consent for their participation in the study outlined below. A total of 11 subjects consented to and completed the study. Two of these subjects, both female, were excluded from analysis, one due to the development of a neurological disorder and the other due to insufficient evoked potential data collection. The remaining nine subjects, six men and three women, all except one right-handed, had a mean age of 50 ± 15 years. All subjects received ECT stimuli through bilateral electrodes with a brief pulse apparatus. Twelve normal subjects were recruited from the community at large by newspaper advertising and were selected from a larger pool of individuals in order to provide controls matched for age and handedness. The group consisted of two males and 10 females, with one male control being dropped due to the development of a depressive episode. The remaining 11 controls had a mean age of 50 ± 13 years and were free of any history of psychiatric disorder.

Controls were medication-free when studied. Five of the depressed subjects had been receiving tricyclic antidepressants before the first study. These drugs were stopped at least 4 days (on average 7 days) before the first study. Three were on neuroleptics prior to the first study and these were stopped a minimum of 3 days before study. Four received short-acting sedative hypnotics (three temazepam, one chloral hydrate) for sleep prior to the first study. Prior to the second study, one depressed subject received a single dose of lithium carbonate, one received temazepam and one chloral hydrate for sleep the night prior to study. All subjects in both groups were free of neurological illness and alcohol or drug abuse and were in good physical health when tested.

Extent and severity of depressive symptomatology were established using the Carroll Scale (Carroll et al. 1981), a self-rated version of the 17-item Hamilton Depression Rating Scale (HDRS; Hamilton 1960).

Evoked Potential Recording Procedures

In this study we examined brain electrical activity in a group of drug-free depressed individuals before and after ECT and in control subjects, employing the power of ERP topographic mapping methods in order to define clearly any ERP abnormalities. These new methods are powerful enough to (1) reduce the mass of ERP data to interpretable electrophysiological features, and (2) display the ERP data in a simpler format (color-coded maps). We used a data acquisition and analysis system for the ERP imaging in the Department of Psychiatry at the Ohio State University. We applied this new non-invasive imaging technology to the study of ECT in depression in the confident expectation that reliablel ERP features specific to depression and effective treatment would be discovered. Topographic mapping of ERPs (TME) has been used successfully in psychiatric research, where specific ERP features have been found in groups of schizophrenic patients (Torello and Duffy 1985; Torello and McCarley 1986; McCarley et al. 1985; Morstyn et al. 1983; Faux et al. 1986).

In this study, the international 10/20 system was used for the placement of 28 electrodes in standardized scalp locations. Monopolar recordings were made with linked ears as a reference. EEG testing of the depressed subjects was performed 1 day before the first bilateral ECT treatment and 1 day after the sixth bilateral ECT treatment (14-day interval). The normal control subjects were tested similarly. There were 2-min rest periods between the test conditions. The entire EEG test session took about 2 h for each subject to complete. A registered EEG technician accurately and symmetrically placed the 28 electrodes within a 5 mm tolerance. This was felt essential if we were to collect reliable data and eliminate EEG asymmetries associated with nothing more than inaccurate electrode placements.

Subjects were seated in a comfortable chair while EEG data were collected in 2.5-s epochs. In order to determine whether each subject had a normal resting EEG, brain electrical activity was collected with the eyes open and fixated forward and with the eyes closed.

Event-related brain potentials are brain waves which are time-locked to a specific stimulus event. The N100 waveform is seen approximately 100 ms following an event to which a subject attends. Multiple presentations of a stimulus are necessary to average out background EEG and extract the N100. The N100 paradigm provides a greater degree of experimental control over and comparability of subjects' mental activity than other paradigms which look at spontaneous EEG. Moreover, the absence of strict time-locking of any artifacts with stimulus onset simplifies artifact control.

During the N100 task, brain activity was collected immediately following the presentation of a randomly occurring, infrequent (15%) high-pitched tone (1000 Hz) which the subject counted. Periodic breaks were given to each subject as needed to maintain attention to the task and subjects were reinforced verbally for correct discriminations. Thirty-two EEG epochs, following the infrequent tone, were summed, averaged and displayed as a series of topographic maps from 16 ms prior to stimulus onset to 600 ms post-stimulus. Similarly, 32 epochs of EEG were collected after the presentation of the frequent tone (500 Hz) for comparison purposes with the infrequent epochs.

During ERP averaging, the computer automatically rejected segments containing any high-voltage artifact (usually blinks). A single ERP average was constructed for each electrode was 256 sampled data points spaced over a 600-ms interval, with the stimulus occurring during this interval so that the points occurring during the first 16 ms formed a baseline.

Artifacts represent a potentially serious confounding factor interfering with the assessment of brain activity. Thus, our general strategy was to attend to the wide variety of artifacts at each step in data acquisition and processing, using strict control procedures. To this end, we employed the following protocol:

1. Use of three sets of electrodes, which allowed artifact recognition to help minimize artifact from eye movements, blinks and muscle activity
2. Minimization of muscle and eye artifact at the source (the subject) during the experiment
3. Monitoring of the effectiveness of 1 and 2 by watching a printout of the EEG
4. Use of the artifact-detection electrodes at the time of analysis to detect any possible effects of artifacts on the analysis

Specifically, the control electrode channels showing blink, eye movements, and muscle activity were monitored during the recordings and a number of techniques were used in the experimental session to reduce the frequency and amplitude of all artifact activity. For example, subjects were requested to suppress eye blinks and minimize eye movements and were asked to relax in order to diminish muscle artifact during the experimental conditions. Further, during the test session, each subject sat in a comfortable, reclining chair to minimize muscle tension. Finally, frequent rest periods were provided.

Data Analysis

For each subject the topographic display of averaged evoked potential data was examined to determine the maximal negative peak in the 90–150 ms poststimulus interval. From this, peak latency and peak-to-peak amplitude were determined. Spatial localization of the N100 component was determined by lined sorting of evoked potential maps and rating of each map as to leftward, central, or rightward distribution of the N100 peak. Group comparisons were made by two-tailed t test for continuous data between control and depressed groups. Intragroup comparison of the depressed subjects' continuous data was performed using the two-tailed paired t test. Comparisons of categorical data specifically spatial orientation of the N100 component, were made using Fisher's exact test.

Results

N100 Findings

Amplitude and latency data for the N100 component of the auditory ERP for 11 controls and nine depressed patients before and after six ECT treatments are shown in Table 1. Pretreatment N100 amplitude in depressed patients was significantly lower, while their pretreatment N100 latency was greater than that seen in controls. Post-treatment N100 amplitude and latency did not differ from control values.

Spatial distribution of the N100 component tended to distinguish controls from the depressed group prior to treatment (Fisher's exact test, $p < 0.09$), with one of 11 controls and four of nine depressed patients showing a rightward

Table 1. N100 component of the auditory event-related potential in depressed patients and controls

Group	N100 feature	
	Amplitude (μV, mean ± SD)	Latency (ms, mean ± SD)
Depressed subjects before ECT ($n=9$)	-11.2 ± 4.4[a]	125.8 ± 12.7[a]
Depressed subjects after ECT ($n=9$)	-15.9 ± 3.4[b]	122 ± 17.2
Control subjects ($n=11$)	-15.3 ± 3.8	115.2 ± 6.7

[a] Depressed and control subjects differ significantly ($p<0.05$, two-tailed, t test)
[b] Depressed subjects differ before and after treatment ($p<0.02$, two-tailed paired t test)

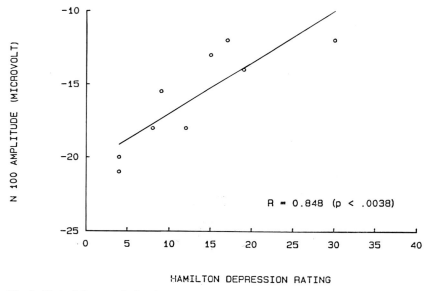

Fig. 1. Plot of the correlation between post-treatment N100 amplitude (μV peak-to-peak) and Hamilton Depression Rating Scale scores in nine patients who received electroconvulsive therapy

orientation of the N100 peak. Following treatment this right ward orientation of the N100 peak was seen in two of nine depressed patients.

The correlation of the severity of depression with N100 was explored in two ways. Correlations between self-rated HDRS and N100 pretreatment amplitude and latency were not significant. Post-treatment latency also did not correlate significantly with post-treatment HDRS. However, as shown in Fig. 1, post-treatment N100 amplitude correlated robustly with post-treatment HDRS ($r = 0.85$; $p < 0.0038$). Overall, there was a significant drop in mean HDRS from 27.1 ± 8.2 to 13.1 ± 8.3 ($p < 0.001$, two-tailed paired t test). No relation was found between evoked potential (EP) measures or depressive ratings and incidental drug treatment.

P300 Findings

No significant differences were noted between controls and depressed patients before or after treatment in amplitude, latency, or spatial distribution of auditory P300.

Conclusions

A number of important results emerged from this study. For the first time, to our knowledge, full-montage ERP recordings were obtained from depressed patients undergoin ECT and from a group of matched controls. The advantages of such an approach are several. First, N100 and P300 peak determinations were derived from the electrode showing the highest activity rather than from one of a randomly chosen limited sample of electrodes. Second, computer processing of the data allows for enhanced discrimination of spatial distribution in the ERP. Overall, these methodological advances seem likely to augment the reliability of the results obtained.

In summary, the findings of this study confirm the hypothesis that depression of a severity necessitating inpatient treatment is associated with differences from control values in N100 but not P300 components of the auditory ERP. Specifically, N100 latency was increased, amplitude was diminished, and peak location tended to show a righward displacement. These group differences disappeared with treatment. Interestingly, two measures appeared to be strongly related to the severity of the depressive symptoms. Among the three patients who failed to improve with treatment (those whose depression rating dropped by less than 50%), rightward spatial orientation of the N100 peak tended to persist. More significantly, N100 amplitude following treatment correlated highly with severity of depression.

Enthusiasm concerning the value of such a finding must be tempered by consideration of a few cautionary comments. Results such as those noted above could have arisen from changes over the 2-week interval between studies in depressed patients, especially as there were no interval studies of the controls. At least two factors weaken such an argument. Random changes in ERP measurements over time in controls ought to have emerged sufficiently in the control group to create variance in the data, which did not in fact appear. Further, the strong relationship of the severity of depressive symptoms to amplitude supports rather than refutes a systematic relationship between the variables. We believe that the observed lack of correlation between pretreatment amplitude and depression ratings resulted from a "floor" effect in the data and was related to inadequate spread in the data (i.e., all subjects had very large HDRS scores and very small N100 amplitudes before treatment).

Another aspect calling for caution might be generalization of the findings to the broad group of individuals suffering from clinically significant depression. The group of depressed patients constituted a highly selected, severely affected group, and associated factors may account for the changes seen in ERP as well as the variability of ERP findings in previous reports of depression (Giedke et al. 1981; Shagass 1983; Knott and Lapierre 1986).

The importance of the findings reported here lies in the demonstration of a potentially valied and reproducible electrophysiological parameter linked to the severity of clinically important psychiatric symptomatology. Such a parameter, if it can be reproducibly demonstrated, would lend itself to diagnostic and treatment studies which might aid in rationalizing the clinical approach to depression. One readily apparent use would be in judging the need for continuation of ECT. At present, such decisions are made empirically by the treating physician, who must assess the extent of response based only on observation and on the patient's reports of symptoms. These findings may also shed light on some pathophysiological aspects of depression.

The validity of alterations of N100 amplitude, latency, and distribution as markers for depression is supported by the understanding of N100 as it relates to selective attention processes (Hillyard and Kutas 1983) and the clinical impression of depressed patients showing impaired concentration and attention. The cognitive difficulties of depressed patients stand in contrast to those of schizophrenics, who show greater difficulty in discriminating the relevance of stimuli than in attending to them, as reflected in their P300 performance (Pfefferbaum et al. 1984). As noted above, our depressed subjects showed no P300 differences from controls.

Further studies will be needed to verify the lack of significant changes in ERP parameters in controls over time, as well as to demonstrate the populations of depressed patients in whom the present results can be corroborated. One factor confounding the wide application of such studies will be the difficulty of separating drug effect directly on EP parameters from drug therapeutic effect on depression and resultant EP changes.

Acknowledgements. The authors would like to thank Daniel J. Martin, M.D. for his clinical assistance in this study. The availability of high-quality data for this study was assured by the careful attention of Linda D. Fortin, R. EEG T. and Catherine E. Lewis, M.S.B.E. Kathryn Tilson provided able secretarial support.

References

Blackwood DHR, Whelley LJ, Christie JE, Blackburn IM, St Clair DM, McInnes A (1987) Changes in auditory P3 event-related potential in schizophrenia and depression. Br J Psychiatry 150:154–160

Borge G (1973) Perceptual modulation and variability in psychiatric patients. Arch Gen Psychiatry 29:760

Borge G, Buchsbaum M, Goodwin F, Murphy D, Silverman J (1971) Neuropsychological correlates of affective disorders. Arch Gen Psychiatry 24:501

Carroll BJ, Feinberg M, Simouse PE, Rawson SG, Greden JF (1981) The carroll rating scale for depression I. Development, reliability and validation. Br J Psychiatry 138:194–200

Faux SF, Torello M, McCarley RW, Shenton ME, Duffy FH (1986) Altered P300 topography in schizophrenia: a replication study. In: Proceedings of the Eighth International Conference on Event-Related Potentials of the Brain, Stanford, June 1986

Friedman J, Meares J (1979) Cortical evoked potentials and severity of depression. Am J Psychiatry 138:1441–1448

Giedke H, Thier P, Bolz J (1981) The relationship between P3-latency and reaction time in depression. Biol Psychol 13:31

Hillyard SA, Kutas M (1983) Electrophysiology of cognitive processing. Annu Rev Psychol 34:33–61

Knott VJ, Lapierre YD (1987) Psychomotor responsivity in depression. Biol Psychiatry 22:313–324

McCarley RW, Torello MW, Shenton ME, Duffy FH (1985) The P300 and spectral topography in schizophrenics and normals. In: Proceedings of the IV World Congress of Societies of Biological Psychiatry, Philadelphia, September 1985

Morstyn R, Duffy FH, McCarley RW (1983) Altered P300 topography in schizophrenia. Arch Gen Psychiatry 40:729–734

Pfefferbaum AF, Wenegrat BG, Ford JM, Roth WT, Kopell BS (1984) Clinical application of the P3 component of event-related potentials. II. Dementia, depression and schizophrenia. Electroencephalogr Clin Neurophysiol 59:104–124

Shagass C (1983) Evoked potentials in adult psychiatry. In: Hughes JR, Wilson WP (eds) EEG and evoked potentials in psychiatry and behavioral neurology. Butterworth, Boston, pp 149–168

Torello MW, Duffy FH (1985) Using brain electrical activity mapping to diagnosis learning disabilities. Learn Brain 24:95–99

Torello MW, McCarley RW (1986) The use of BEAM topographic mapping techniques in clinical studies in psychiatry. In: Duffy F (ed) Topographic mapping of brain electrical activity. Butterworth, Boston

EEG Imaging of Brain Activity in Clinical Psychopharmacology

B. SALETU[1]

Introduction

Although Berger described electroencephalographic (EEG) changes for barbiturates, morphine, cocaine and scopolamine as early as 1933, systematic pharmacological EEG (pharmaco-EEG-)studies were not initiated until the mid-1950s (Bente and Itil 1954; Fink 1959). However, only with the introduction of modern computer facilities did pharmaco-EEG gain momentum. It soon became obvious that every drug with psychotropic properties induces statistically significant EEG changes. Moreover, drugs with similar therapeutic effects induce similar CNA changes, resulting in similar pharmaco-EEG profiles (Itil 1974; Goldstein et al. 1974; Fink 1975; Saletu 1976, 1987; Matejcek and Devos 1976; Herrmann 1982). The pharmaco-EEG proved to be a reliable classification instrument as well as a technique with which one could evalute quantitatively and objectively a drug's bioavailability in the target organ – the human brain. Furthermore, it is easy to apply, without pain or discomfort for the subjects and the only non-invasive technique for investigation of brain function continuously, repetitively and at relatively low cost.

Some difficulties with the classification have been thought to derive from the fact that most investigators analyzed only one or at most only a few leads. Inconsistency of results from different research centers may be due to local brain differences, which suggests the importance of a comprehensive regional topographic approach, already postulated by Künkel (1982), Buchsbaum et al. (1985) and Itil et al. (1985). Walter and Shipton (1951) demonstrated a new toposcopic system as early as 1951, followed by the photocell toposcopic system of Petsche and Marco (1954). Further early articles on spatiotemporal EEG mapping were published by Lehmann (1971), Petsche (1973, 1976), Ueno et al. (1975) and Ragot and Remond (1978). In 1979 Duffy et al. published the first article on the brain electrical activity mapping (BEAM) technique, followed by Dubinsky and Barlow (1980), Buchsbaum et al. (1982). Coppola et al. (1982), Etevenon et al. (1983), Persson and Hjorth (1983), Pidoux et al. (1983) and Pfurtscheller et al. (1984). Up to this time, minicomputers were utilized for mapping EEG rather than microcomputers, although Persson and Hjorth (1983) had already described EEG topograms obtained using microcomputers. Gaches and Etevenon (1984) and Sebban et al. (1984) published the first results obtained also using microcomputers.

---

[1] Bereich für Pharmakopsychiatrie, Psychiatrische Universitätsklinik, Währinger Gürtel 18–20, 1090 Wien, Austria

The aim of the present paper is to describe the utilization of topographic brain mapping of EEG in psychopharmacology and pharmacopsychiatry based on data obtained by means of our own quantitative EEG (Q-EEG) imaging system (Anderer et al. 1987; Saletu et al. 1987b). This system consists of a server Hewlett-Packard Vectra microcomputer functioning as an acquisition unit, a workstation Hewlett-Packard Vectra microcomputer for statistical analysis and a printer and a colour plotter for subsequent documentation of data.

Classification of Psychotropic Drugs Based on Topography Pharmaco-EEG Imaging

Representative drugs of the five psychopharmacological classes demonstrated significant and systematic changes in EEG brain maps as compared with placebo. Data were obtained exclusively from double-blind, placebo-controlled trials carried out in normal, healthy volunteers (Saletu et al. 1986a, b, 1988, this volume). Findings described below were obtained mostly in the 2nd h post drug except those for pyritinol, obtained in the 1st h after oral drug administration. Statistical probability maps are computed based on t values as described by Duffy et al. (1981).

Neuroleptics

A dose of 30 mg chlorprothixene (a representative sedative neuroleptic) produced no changes in the vigilance-controlled EEG (V-EEG) in regard to total power 2 h after oral administration compared with placebo (Fig. 1). The centroid of the total activity (1.3–35 Hz) showed significant ($P<0.01$) slowing over the whole scalp except the left F_p (frontopolar) regions (Fig. 1). The deviation of the centroid, of the total activity, also declined over the F_p, F (frontal) and FT (frontotemporal) regions. The dominant frequency of the alpha activity declined significantly over the left F, C (central), T (temporal) and TO (temporooccipital) regions and over the right T, C, vertex and F_p area (Fig. 1). The absolute (Fig. 2) and relative (Fig. 3) power of the dominant frequency remained unchanged.

Absolute power of the combined delta/theta activities increased over F, right T and TO areas (Fig. 2). There were no significant changes in absolute power of the combined alpha and beta activities. Alterations in each single frequency band are described in detail elsewhere (Saletu et al. 1987b).

Relative power of the combined delta/theta activities was augmented all over the scalp, while the combined alpha activities showed an attenuation, specifically over the right O and OT (occipitotemporal) regions (Fig. 3). The combined beta activities also showed a significant decrease over the F, FT, C, and OT regions.

The centroid of the combined delta/theta activities remained unchanged (Fig. 4) as did its deviation (Fig. 5). The alpha centroid decreased specifically over the posterior regions (up to the interauricular line). The deviation of the

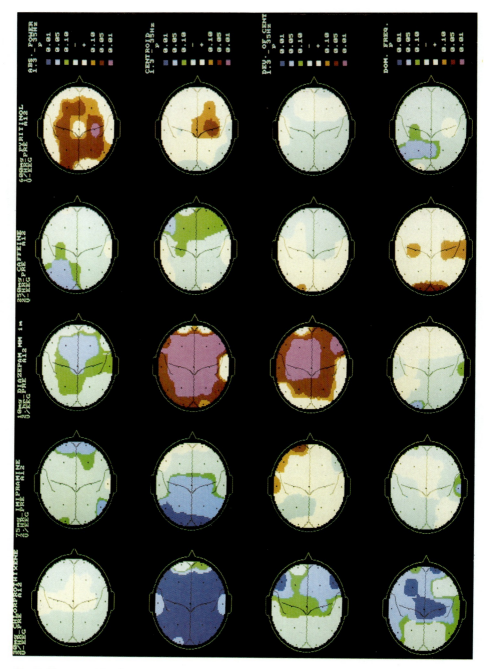

Fig. 1. Topographic pharmaco-EEG changes of total power (absolute power, 1.3–35 Hz), the centroid and centroid deviation of total activity (Hz) and of the dominant frequency (Hz) after representative drugs of five psychopharmacological classes. Each pharmaco-EEG significance probability image represents the results of a statistical comparison by t test of drug-

alpha centroid remained unchanged. The centroid of the combined beta activities slowed down over all regions (except the T regions) (Fig. 4). There were no changes in the deviation of the beta centroid (Fig. 5).

Antidepressants

A dose of 75 mg imipramine (representative for antidepressants of its type) produced in the V-EEG a significant attenuation of the total power over both F_p and right OT regions 2 h after oral drug administration as compared with placebo (Fig. 1).

In regard to the centroid of the total activity, we noticed a slowing over the left and right O, OT, P (parietal) and C regions (Fig. 1), while its deviation remained unchanged (except for an increase over the left F_{pl}). For more information concerning other time periods after oral drug administration see Saletu et al. (1988).

There were no changes in regard to the dominant alpha frequency (Fig. 1), while the absolute power of the dominant frequency decreased – mostly over both F_p, FT and F but also over the vertex, C, left T and left O regions (Fig. 2). Relative power of the dominant frequency decreased over all regions except F_p, P, and right T, with a significant decrease over both O regions (Fig. 3).

Absolute power of the combined delta/theta activities did not change significantly after 75 mg imipramine (except for a decrease over both F_p regions), while the combined alpha activity demonstrated a significant attenuation over all anterior regions up to the interauricular line (Fig. 2). In addition, there was an attenuation over the left O and right OT regions. Absolute power of the total beta activity remained unchanged.

Relative power of the delta/theta activities showed a significant increase in both O and OT, left P, both C, vertex, both F and right T regions (Fig. 3), while the relative power of the combined alpha activity was attenuated almost over all the scalp except for both F_p and the right P regions. Combined beta activity decreased only to a minor extent over the right O region.

◁───

induced to placebo-induced changes. The eight-color scale shows differences between drug-induced and placebo-induced changes (based on t values expressed in p values): *dark blue*, decrease at $p<0.01$ level; *light blue*, decrease at $p<0.05$; *dark green*, decrease at $p<0.10$; *light green*, trend toward decrease; *light yellow*, trend toward increase; *dark yellow*, increase at $p<0.10$; *red*, increase at $p<0.05$; *lilac*, increase at $p<0.01$. A dose of 30 mg chlorprothixene slows the centroid all over the brain and decreases the centroid deviation and dominant frequency over the anterior regions ($n=8$). A dose of 75 mg imipramine attenuates total power over the Fp region and slows the centroid mostly over the O, P and C regions ($n=15$). A dose of 10 mg diazepam MM i.m. attenuates total power frontally and at the vertex but increases centroid and centroid deviation all over the brain and maximally over the C and F regions ($n=15$). A dose of 250 mg caffeine decreases total power over the left O and P regions and accelerates the dominant frequency occipitally ($n=8$). A dose of 600 mg pyritinol, in contrast, increases total power and accelerates the centroid but slows the dominant frequency ($n=12$)

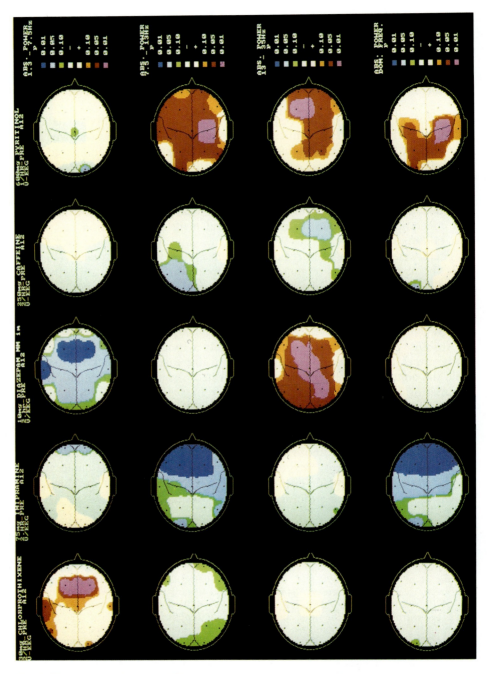

Fig. 2. Topographic pharmaco-EEG changes in absolute power of delta/theta, alpha, and beta activities as well as in the dominant frequency after representative drugs of five psychopharmacological classes. For description of the color key see Fig. 1. A dose of 30 mg chlorprothixene increases delta/theta power; 75 mg imipramine attenuates power in the alpha activity and

The centroid of the combined delta/theta activities was accelerated over the F_p regions (Fig. 4) as was the corresponding centroid deviation (Fig. 5). The deviation of the centroids of these slow activities decreased significantly over the right OT region. There were no changes in regard to the alpha centroid, although the deviation of the alpha centroid increased significantly over both F_p and F regions as well as in the right P and OT areas. There were no changes in the beta centroid except for a slight increase in the deviation of the beta centroid in the left T area.

Tranquilizers

A dose of 10 mg diazepam MM (mixed micelles solution) produced an attenuation of total power over both F and the vertex regions 2 h after intramuscular injection as compared with placebo (Fig. 1).

The centroid of the total activity was accelerated in all areas (except the right T and both F regions) (Fig. 1). The deviation of the centroid of the total activity increased as well, again mostly over the vertex and anterior areas (Fig. 1).

The dominant frequency of the alpha activity was slowed over the left O region. The absolute and relative power of the dominant frequency did not show significant changes (Fig. 2 and 3).

Absolute power of the combined delta/theta frequencies showed a decrease mostly over both F regions but also over both C, P and T regions (Fig. 2). Absolute power in the combined alpha activity declined in the 1st h after 10 mg diazepam MM i.m. over both P, C, and T regions, but not in the 2nd h (described in this paper). Combined beta activity increased in the 2nd h over all regions but F_p, FT and T, with a maximum over the vertex.

Relative power of combined delta/theta activity was attenuated after 10 mg diazepam MM i.m., mostly over the anterior regions (up to the interauricular line) (Fig. 3). In addition, there was a decrease over the left O and right OT regions. Combined alpha activity did not change. Combined beta activities were augmented all over the scalp except in the right T region.

The centroids and centroid deviations of the combined delta/theta, alpha and beta activities remained unchanged at 2 h (Fig. 4). There was an increase in the centroid deviation of the slow activities in the left F region (Fig. 5).

Psychostimulants

A dose of 250 mg caffeine produced a significant attenuation of total power in the V-EEG 2 h after oral administration as compared with placebo, specifically over the left O, OT and P regions (Fig. 1).

◁―――

dominant frequency; 10 mg diazepam MM decreases delta/theta power and increases beta power; 250 mg caffeine decreases alpha activity over the left posterior region and beta power over the right F region; 600 mg pyritinol markedly augments power in alpha and beta activity as well as in the dominant frequency

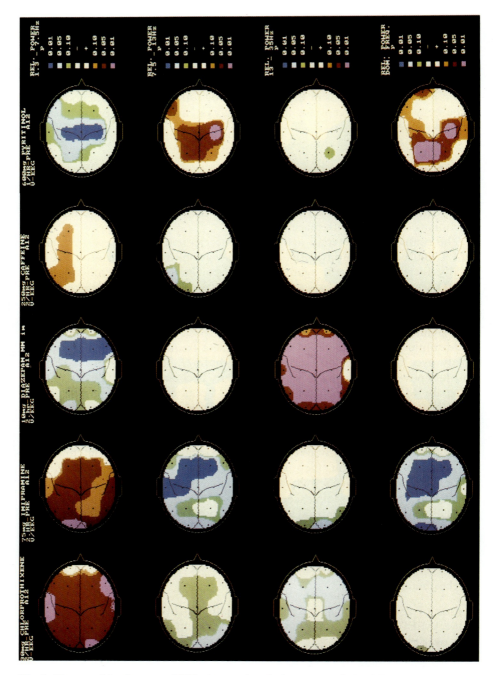

Fig. 3. Topographic pharmaco-EEG changes in relative power of the delta/theta, alpha and beta bands and of the dominant frequency after representative drugs of five psychopharmacological classes. For technical description and color key see Fig. 1. A dose of 30 mg chlorprothixene increases relative power in the delta/theta activity and decreases alpha and beta activity;

The centroid of the total activity declined slightly and specifically over the right F_p. The centroid deviation remained the same (Fig. 1). Absolute and relative power of the dominant frequency was unchanged, but an acceleration was observed over both O regions (Fig. 1).

Absolute power of the combined delta/theta activities remained unchanged (Fig. 2). That of the combined alpha bands was attenuated over the left O, OT and P regions, while that of the combined beta activities decreased significantly only over the right F region.

Relative power remained generally unchanged in the three combined frequency bands (delta/theta, alpha and beta activities) (Fig. 3).

The centroid of the combined delta/theta activity remained unchanged (Fig. 4). No changes were seen in regard to the deviation of the delta/theta centroid (Fig. 5). The alpha centroid was significantly accelerated over the left and right O, P and OT regions (Fig. 4). Its deviation remained unchanged except for an increase over the left C region. The centroid of the total beta activity remained unchanged (Fig. 4), while its deviation increased minimally over the left FT region (Fig. 5).

Nootropics/Antihypoxidotics

A dose of 600 mg pyritinol produced in the V-EEG a significant increase in total power over the left and right P and C regions and the left O and F regions 1 h after oral administration as compared with placebo (Fig. 1). The centroid of the total activity became faster over the right C region, while the centroid deviation remained unchanged.

The dominant frequency of the alpha activity slowed over the left P and OT regions (Fig. 1), while the absolute power of the dominant frequency increased markedly over both C and regions and the left O region (Fig. 2). Relative power of the dominant frequency showed an increase as well, predominantly in both C and P regions (Fig. 3).

Absolute power of the combined delta/theta activities remained unchanged (Fig. 2). There was a significant increase of total alpha power all over the brain except in the right O, T, and FT regions and the left O and F_p regions. A maximal increase was observed over the right C area. Total beta power was significantly augmented in the left and right F_p and F regions, the right C and P regions and the vertex.

Relative power of the combined delta/theta band decreased significantly over the vertex and in both C and left P, and FT regions, while there was an increase in regard to total alpha activity over the vertex and over left and

◁—————————————————————————————

75 mg imipramine also augments slow activities while attenuating slow alpha activity and relative power of the dominant frequency; 10 mg diazepam MM i.m. produces, as compared with placebo, a decrease of delta/theta activity and increase of beta activity; 250 mg caffeine shows only minimal changes; 600 mg pyritinol attenuates delta/theta and augments alpha activity and relative power of the dominant frequency

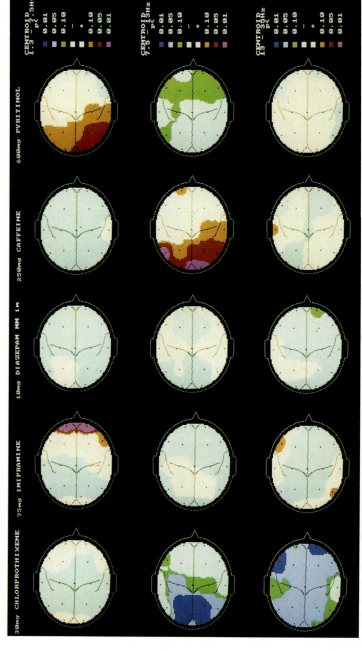

Fig. 4. Topographic pharmaco-EEG changes in the centroids of the combined delta/theta, alpha and beta activities after oral administration of representative drugs of five psychopharmacological classes. For color key see Fig. 1. A dose of 30 mg chlorprothixene slows the centroid of the alpha and beta activity; 75 mg imipramine slightly accelerates the delta/theta centroid over the F_p regions; 250 mg caffeine accelerates the alpha centroid; 600 mg pyritinol accelerates the delta/theta centroid mostly over the right O, OT and P regions

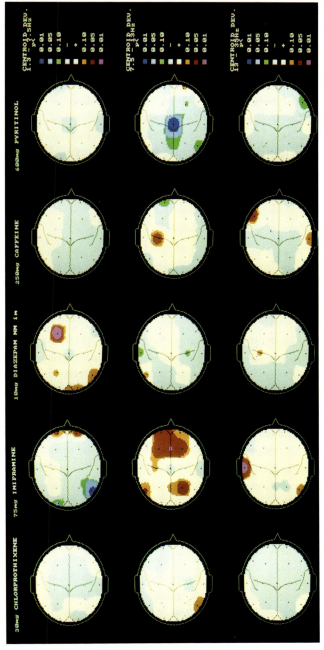

Fig. 5. Topographic pharmaco-EEG changes in the centroid deviations of the delta/theta, alpha and beta activity after oral administration of representative drugs of five psychopharmacological classes. For color key see Fig. 1. A dose of 75 mg imipramine attenuates the centroid deviation over the right OT region, while, in contrast, it augments it in the alpha band over both F_p and F regions and the right P region. An augmentation of the centroid deviation of beta activity can be seen over the left T region. A dose of 250 mg caffeine increases the centroid deviation of the alpha activity over the left C region. A dose of 600 mg pyritinol attenuates the centroid deviation in the alpha band over the vertex

right C and left P and FT regions (Fig. 3). Relative power of the total beta activity remained unchanged.

The centroid of the combined delta/theta activity was accelerated over the right O, P and OT regions (Fig. 4), while the centroid deviation was unchanged in this band (Fig. 5). The alpha centroid remained unchanged but its deviation declined over the vertex. Centroid and centroid deviation of the beta activity did not change significantly as compared with placebo.

Cerebral Bioavailability Determined by Topographic Pharmaco-EEG

Dose-Efficacy Relations

Topographic pharmaco-EEG images may demonstrate dose-efficacy relations, as can be seen in Fig. 6. Fengabine – a novel GABA agonist – produced in regard to total power a significant increase, specifically over the left C and P regions in the 4th h after oral administration in doses between 200 and 800 mg (the results of this study are described in detail by Saletu et al. 1987c). Interestingly, the higher the dosage, the less augmentation was observed. However, dose-efficacy relations may differ over various regions. Therefore, an overall dose-efficacy relation is calculated utilizing Friedman's test and the multiple Wilcoxon test of sign-free changes in 28 V-EEG and R-EEG (resting EEG variables) (combined variables were excluded for redundancy) in all 17 derivations. Generally, 200 and 800 mg fengabine and the reference compound, 75 mg imipramine, could be significantly differentiated from placebo (Table 1). However, as can be seen based on the high χ^2 values, there were topographical differences in regard to the significance levels. It seems of interest that the differentiation was easier over the right Fp, F, C, T and P regions and over the left O and OT regions. There were no linear dose-efficacy relations after fengabine.

Bioequipotency

Bioequipotency may be evaluated in a way similar to dose-efficacy relations. Figure 7 demonstrates topographic differences in changes of relative power in the typical 16–20 Hz beta activity band between two different formulations of a drug in this case the standard solution of diazepam and a novel MM solution. While there were no significant differences between the two formulations after intravenous application, the MM solution was superior to the standard solution from the 2nd to the 6th when the drug was given intramuscularly. This pharmacodynamic superiority was obviously due to a better absorption in the muscle, which in turn is due to better water solubility of the new formulation (Saletu et al. 1986a). If one ranks the cerebral effectiveness of 10 mg diazepam i.v., 10 mg diazepam MM i.v., 10 mg diazepam i.m., 10 mg diazepam MM i.m. and placebo, based on sign-free changes in all 28 V-EEG + R-EEG variables

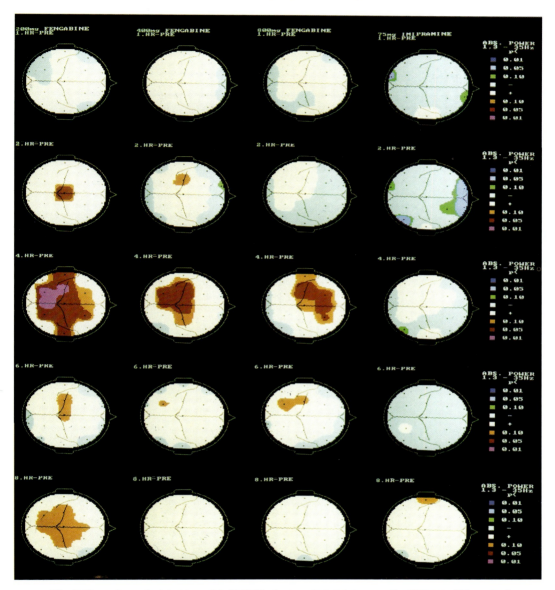

Fig. 6. Dose-dependent topographic V-EEG changes in total power after 200 mg, 400 mg and 800 mg fengabine as well as 75 mg imipramine as compared with placebo at 1, 2, 4, 6 and 8 h ($n=15$). For color key see Fig. 1. A dose of 75 mg imipramine induces a decrease in total power over the left and right F_p and right OT regions in the 2nd h post drug. In contrast, fengabine produces an increase in power, specifically in the 4th h over the left C region, which decreases with increasing doses

Table 1. Regional dose-efficacy relations (based on changes in all EEG variables obtained at all times)

	χ^2	Rank sums				
		A	B	C	D	E
FP1	21.4***	754.0	863.5	829.0	922.0	831.5
FP2	27.3***	757.5	868.5	776.0	887.0	911.0
F7	6.0***	798.5	824.5	833.5	879.5	864.0
F3	32.4***	730.5	914.5	888.0	869.0	798.0
F4	58.7***	707.0	948.5	779.0	927.0	838.5
F8	15.9***	759.5	852.5	840.0	841.5	906.5
T3	40.2***	719.5	826.5	846.5	853.5	954.0
C3	29.3***	760.5	927.5	798.5	902.0	811.5
C4	90.6***	695.0	974.5	773.5	969.0	788.0
T4	78.8***	694.0	886.5	758.0	994.0	867.5
T5	35.3***	827.5	852.5	730.0	950.0	840.0
P3	42.2***	743.5	913.0	762.0	932.0	849.5
P4	46.5***	746.5	925.5	761.0	939.0	828.0
T6	32.3***	820.0	907.5	719.0	883.5	870.0
O1	42.2***	837.0	867.0	695.0	890.5	910.5
O2	24.2***	843.5	866.5	728.0	872.5	889.5
CZ	79.1***	726.0	965.0	788.5	967.0	753.5
M	25.6***	760.0	893.2	782.7	910.5	853.6
FP1	A : B *	A : D **	C : D +		
FP2	A : B *	A : D **	A : E **	B : C +	C : D *
	C : E **				
F7					
F3	A : B **	A : C **	A : D **	B : E *	
F4	A : B **	A : D **	A : E **	B : C **	B : E *
	C : D **				
F8	A : B +	A : E **			
T3	A : B *	A : C **	A : D **	A : E **	B : E **
	C : E *	D : E +			
C3	A : B **	A : D **	B : C **	B : E *	C : D *
C4	A : B **	A : D **	A : E +	B : C **	B : E **
	C : D **	D : E **			
T4	A : B **	A : D **	A : E **	B : C **	B : D *
	C : D **	C : E *	D : E **		
T5	A : C +	A : D **	B : C **	B : D +	C : D **
	C : E *	D : E *			
P3	A : B **	A : D **	A : E *	B : C **	C : D **
P4	A : B **	A : D **	B : C **	B : E +	C : D **
	D : E *				
T6	A : C +	B : C **	C : D **	C : E **	
O1	A : C **	B : C **	C : D **	C : E **	
O2	A : C *	B : C **	C : D **	C : E **	
CZ	A : B **	A : D **	B : C **	B : E **	C : D **
	E : E **				
M	A : B **	A : D **	A : E +	B : C *	C : D **

A, placebo; B, 200 mg fengabine; C, 400 mg fengabine; D, 800 mg fengabine; E, 75 mg imipramine

*** $p < 0.01$ (Friedman); + $p < 0.10$; * $p < 0.05$; ** $p < 0.01$ (Multiple Wilcoxon)

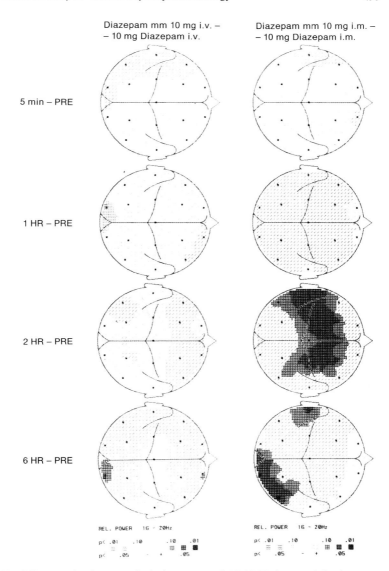

Fig. 7. Topographic differences in changes of relative power of 16–20 Hz beta activity between two different formulations of a drug (mixed micelles (MM) solution versus standard solution of diazepam 10 mg) given intravenously and intramuscularly ($n=15$; V-EEG; A12). While no significant differences can be observed between the two formulations after intravenous injection, the new MM solution is superior to the standard solution of diazepam in the 2nd and even in the 6th h when given intramuscularly. The greater increase in beta activity over the C and T regions indicates better absorption of the drug in the muscle

obtained in all 17 leads at all times, one obtains the following rank sums: 1113.3, 990.7, 1042.6, 1152.4 and 741.1 respectively (χ_r^2 126.3, $p<0.01$). Thus, the lowest values were seen after placebo and the highest after 10 mg diazepam i.v. and diazepam MM i.m. The two formulations differed from each other at the $p<0.05$ level (multiple Wilcoxon test) and from placebo at the $p<0.01$ level.

Time-Efficacy Relations

Time-efficacy relations may be demonstrated by imaging drug-induced changes in a specific EEG variable. As can be seen in Fig. 8, diazepam i.v. induces the maximum beta augmentation right after the injection (5th min), while the central effect of diazepam i.m. takes some time to develop. An overall time-efficacy relationship can also be calculated utilizing Friedman's test and the multiple Wilcoxon test of sign-free and placebo-corrected changes in 28 V-EEG and R-EEG variables obtained in 17 derivations. An example is shown in Table 2, which depicts time-efficacy relations after standard and MM solutions of diazepam i.v. and i.m. based on sign-free placebo-corrected changes in all 28 V-EEG and R-EEG variables. While diazepam i.v. showed the most CNS effects immediately after the injection, the pharmacodynamic peak effect after the intramuscular injection falls into the 1st h post drug, which was also consistent with our blood level data.

Topographic Pharmaco-EEG in Pharmacopsychiatry

Topographic pharmaco-EEG changes may mediate valuable information about the central effects of a drug and – in the case of nootropics/antihypoxidotics – about the therapeutic efficacy of a drug in a specific patient or in a specific group of patients. Figure 9 demonstrates topographic brain maps of two multi-infarct dementia patients before and after 8 weeks therapy with 900 mg propentofylline – a new xanthine derivative – daily. One patient was a 74-year-old woman with a large left F-T-P and left periventricular cystic degenerated infarct. Her pretreatment Sandoz Clinical Assessment-Geratric (SCAG) score was 48. A markedly augmented delta activity could be seen over the left F, C, T, and P regions which diminished significantly after 8 weeks of treatment (Fig. 9), although the focus could still be observed. This decrease in delta activity is obviously due to the functional improvement of the surrounding brain tissue and can be demonstrated in terms of change values or p values using statistical probability mapping (Fig. 9). There was a highly significant decrease, specifically over the left hemisphere but also to some extent over the right hemisphere. This neurophysiological improvement in vigilance was reflected clinically by a decrease of the SCAG score to 36.

The other patient was an 87-year-old woman with a bilateral frontal hygroma, an interhemispheric frontal hygroma, more pronounced on the right than

EEG Imaging of Brain Activity in Clinical Psychopharmacology 497

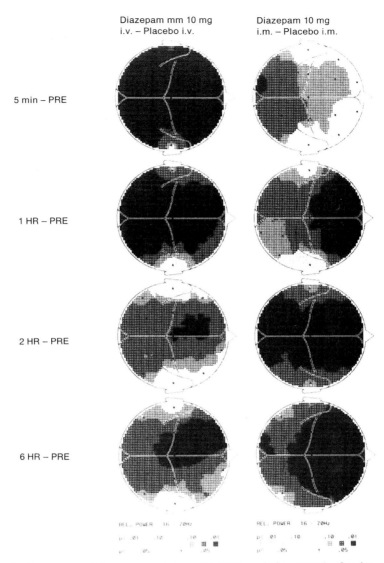

Fig. 8. Differences in time-course of beta augmentation (16–20 Hz, relative power) after i.v. and i.m. administration of 10 mg diazepam (based on significance probability maps; differences to placebo; ($n=15$). While after intravenous injection beta augmentation is highest right after the injection and declines thereafter, the peak effect after the intramuscular injection may be observed in the 2nd h

Table 2. Relationship between time-courses in CNS effect (shown in rank sums based on sign-free placebo corrected changes in 28 V-EEG + R-EEG variables, means of 17 leads) and blood levels after standard and a mixed micelles (MM) solutions of diazepam i.v. and i.m. ($n=15$)

Treatment	Time-course EEG (rank sums)						χ_r^2	Multiple Wilcoxon test ($*p<0.05$; $**p<0.01$)
	5 to 20 min	1 H	2 H	4 H	6 H	8 H		
A Diazepam 10 mg i.v.	**283.9**	201.9	182.1	174.1	168.9	165.2	52.2**	5 min:1 H; 5 min:2 H; 5 min:4 H; 5 min:6 H; 5 min:8 H**
B Diazepam MM 10 mg i.v.	**282.8**	221.7	164.5	160.4	175.4	171.2	59.1**	5 min:1 H*; 5 min:2 H**; 5 min:6 H**; 5 min:8 H**; 1 H:2 H*; 1 H:4 H
C Diazepam 10 mg i.m.	180.3	**251.1**	187.9	182.6	202.6	171.4	21.3**	5 min:1 H**; 1 H:2 H*; 1 H:4 H**; 1 H:8 H**
D Diazepam MM 10 mg i.m.	181.8	**225.6**	217.4	173.9	207.5	169.8	14.6*	1 H:4 H; 1 H:8 H*

Treatment	Time-course blood levels (ng/ml)					
	30 min	1 H	2 H	4 H	6 H	8 H
A Diazepam 10 mg i.v.	**370.3**	313.9	250.6	198.9	175.2	170.5
B Diazepam MM 10 mg i.v.	**285.9**	257.0	193.9	168.7	162.8	161.4
C Diazepam 10 mg i.m.	174.1	**188.0**	167.0	159.3	155.6	150.3
D Diazepam MM 10 mg i.m.	197.1	**234.6**	220.1	185.8	153.8	155.7

on the left, and a left periventricular infarct (Fig. 9). The pretreatment SCAG score was 47. The delta activity was most pronounced over the F_p regions and decreased with treatment, significantly so over the right F_p and also left FT and T regions. This improvement in vigilance was also seen in the SCAG, the score decreasing to 36.

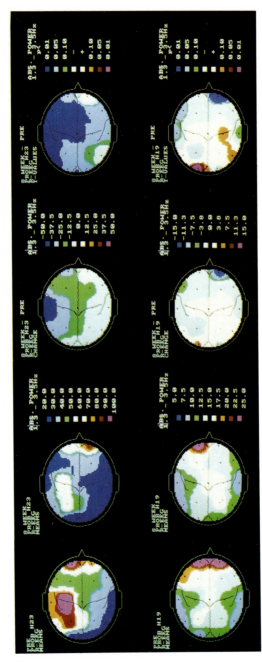

Fig. 9. Topographic brain maps of the absolute power in the delta activity in two MID dementia patients before and 8 weeks after therapy (900 mg propentofylline/day). *Left*, mean values before and 8 weeks after treatment; *right* changes (from pretreatment) and significance levels. *Upper row*, maps of a 74-year-old female patient with a large left F-T-P and periventricular cystic degenerated infarct; *lower row*, maps of an 87-year-old woman with a bilateral frontal hygroma, an interhemispheric frontal hygroma (right more than left) and a left periventricular infarct are demonstrated. Augmented delta activity is seen mostly over the pathological regions (*red*): in the the first patient over the left F_p, T, C and P regions and in the second patient over both F_p regions (pretreatment). Eight weeks after treatment (300 mg propentofylline t.i.d) a significant decrease of delta activity can be observed, although the infarcts can still be recognized

Discussion

Topographic pharmaco-EEG maps after single doses of representative substances of the five psychopharmacological classes are in relatively good agreement with our classical pharmaco-EEG profiles obtained from the O2-Cz lead as well as the limited body of data concerning pharmaco-EEG images in the literature.

Chlorprothixene, as a representative of the low-potency neuroleptics, increased absolute delta/theta power and tended to decrease alpha and beta power. In regard to relative power there was a marked increase in delta and theta and a decrease in alpha and beta activity. Moreover, chlorprothixene slowed the centroid of the total activity and the dominant frequency of the alpha activity. This is consistent with our pharmaco-EEG profiles based on single-lead recordings (O2–Cz) after sedative low-potency neuroleptics which were characterized mostly by an increase of delta/theta activity and a decrease of alpha activity (Grünberger et al. 1985; Herrmann 1982; Itil 1974; Langer et al. 1986; Saletu 1976, 1987; Saletu et al. 1983, 1987a). However, the less consistent beta changes were often characterized by an increase. By comparison, high-potency non-sedative neuroleptics like haloperidol showed (at least in low doses in normal volunteers) an increase in alpha or alpha-adjacent beta activity (Saletu et al. 1983, 1986b).

From the topographic point of view, we saw in the present study, as in a previous detailed analysis considering more narrowly defined frequency bands (Saletu et al. 1987b) the maximum delta augmentation over the posterior regions (such as the OT, T, P and C regions), eventually reaching the F regions, while the theta augmentation was best seen over the F_p and T regions. This is consistent with the data of Itil et al. (1985), who described after 50 mg chlorpromazine also an increase of slow activity in the T regions). Herrmann and Schaerer (1986) reported after 75 mg chlorpromazine an increase in delta but also in theta power. Alpha activity – in our own study – was attenuated significantly over the right O, OT and P regions. Concerning beta activity, we observed a significant attentuation in relative power of the medium-fast beta frequencies, which is in agreement with Itil's description of a decrease, while Herrmann's reported increase of slow and fast beta activity is in agreement with our trend toward an increase of absolute beta 1 and beta 3 power.

Imipramine produced a significant decrease of absolute power in alpha activity and dominant frequency. In relative power there was a marked augmentation of slow activity. In detail, we observed a significant increase of delta activity specifically over the posterior regions and of theta activity specifically over the anterior but also over the posterior regions, while the T regions were spared (Saletu et al. 1987b). In regard to alpha activity, a significant attenuation was observed (slightly more over the left than the right hemisphere), predominantly over the T, C and F regions, while total beta activity remained unchanged with the exception of a decrease in the right O region. However, subdividing the beta band, we saw that slow beta 1 activity was augmented over the anterior regions, while beta 2 and beta 3 activity were attenuated over the posterior regions. These topographic pharmaco-EEG data are in agreement with our O2-Cz pharmaco-EEG profiles after administration and antidepressants of the imipramine type (Saletu 1976, 1982, 1987; Saletu et al. 1983). This pharmaco-EEG profile of the imipramine type, described also by other investigators (Fink 1975; Herrmann 1982; Itil 1974; Matecjek and Devos 1976), was quite different from the profile of the desipramine type of antidepressant (Herrmann 1982; Saletu 1982; Saletu et al. 1983).

From the topographic point of view it was of interest that the delta augmentation was seen mostly over the posterior brain, while the theta augmentation was seen predominantly over the anterior region, as was also the case with the increase of slow beta activity. Alpha 1 attenuation was seen best over the F to left C and T regions. Itil et al. (1985) described after 50 mg amitriptyline an increase of slow waves in the F and T regions, a marked decrease of alpha activity in the O and P regions and an increase of fast beta activity in the C region. Herrmann and Schaerer (1986) described an increase of delta waves after 75 mg amitriptyline, reflecting a decline in vigilance. In the O region they found a reduction of alpha power but an increase of beta 1 and beta 3 power, while absolute beta 3 power declined.

A dose of 10 mg diazepam, the classical tranquilizer, produced a decrease of delta/theta activity and in increase of beta activity in both absolute and relative power. There was also attenuation of total power, acceleration of the centroid and centroid deviation, in agreement with our single-lead pharmaco-EEG profiles of tranquilizers (Saletu 1986; Saletu et al. 1981) and with the pharmaco-EEG profiles reported by other investigators (Fink 1975; Herrmann 1982; Itil 1974; Matecjek and Devos 1976). Topographically, the decrease of delta power occurred mostly over the posterior, that of theta power over the anterior regions, while the augmentation of beta activity was seen best over the C and F regions (Saletu et al. 1987b). This is consistent with the report by Itil et al. (1985) of a marked increase in fast activity, particularly in the F and C regions of the brain. Herrmann and Schaerer (1986) also described an increase of slow and medium-fast beta activity over the C regions. They noted as well a decrease of alpha 1 and alpha 2 power, reflecting the decline in vigilance after diazepam. The latter was only observed as a trend in our own study.

The psychostimulant caffeine showed, in the given dose of 250 mg, only subtle changes, characterized by an attenuation of total power and of alpha and beta power. Relative power showed similar alterations. The most obvious findings were the acceleration of the alpha centroid and of the dominant frequency. Etevenon et al. (1986) also described an EEG activation characterized by a simultaneous increase in alpha (and beta) mean frequency together with a decrease of mean amplitude (absolute and relative power). Topographically, we observed the alpha attenuation and alpha acceleration over the posterior regions while the attenuation of beta power was seen best over the right F region. As we described in a detailed analysis, the decrease of medium-fast beta power occurred mostly over the C region and the vertex. Beta 1 power was attenuated mostly over both P regions, while, in contrast, the relative power of the slow beta activity was attenuated mostly over the left FT regions (Saletu et al. 1987b). Etevenon et al. (1986) noted an increase in alpha frequency and decrease in alpha amplitude in centroposterior EEG leads together with the right P and right PF areas. They speculated about a possible somatosensory specific activation of the right hemisphere, which was, however, seen on our own study only in the 20–25 Hz beta band. Beta 1 amplitudes were also described as decreased by Etevenon et al. (1986). Itil et al. (1985) described after another psychostimulant, dextroamphetamine, a decrease in slow waves over the F and T regions and an increase in alpha activity, mostly over the P and O regions.

Pyritinol, as a representative of the nootropic/antihypoxidotic class of drugs, induced an increase of total power, an augmentation of absolute alpha and beta power, a decrease of relative power in the delta/theta band and an increase of relative power in the alpha band. It seems of interest to note that fast alpha actually decreased, while relative power of the slow alpha activity increased significantly (Saletu et al. 1987b). Dominant alpha frequency slowed down, while its absolute and relative power increased. The centroid of the total activity was accelerated, as was the centroid of the combined delta/theta activities. Similar changes have been described by us as typical for nootropics/antihypoxidotics based on single-lead recordings and are indicative of improvement in "vigilance" as defined by Head (1923) (Saletu 1981a, b; Saletu and Grünberger 1980, 1985). Topographically speaking, the main effect took place over the C and anterior regions, providing a typical example of the fact that the analysis of the right O lead alone may fail to show typical drug-induced changes. Our findings are in agreement with recent results of Herrmann et al. (1986) concerning vigilance improvement in elderly patients with symptoms of mental dysfunction treated with either 3×200 mg pyritinol daily or placebo under double-blind conditions. Absolute delta power was lower under the active medication than with placebo, while the alpha/slow wave index was, as expected, higher in the active treatment group. As early as 1970, Künkel and Westphal had reported that in young healthy subjects, oral administration of 200 mg pyritinol resulted in EEG alterations indicating activation and raised vigilance. Brain protective properties of pyritinol were also demonstrated recently by us utilizing the experimentally-induced hypoxic/hypoxidosis model (Saletu et al., this volume). Inhalation of a fixed gas combination of 9.8% oxygen and 90.2% nitrogen (equivalent to 6000 m altitude) induced an increase in delta/theta activities and a decrease of alpha activity; the decrease was attenuated significantly by pyritinol. Psychometric data added further evidence for the nootropic/antihypoxidotic nootropic properties of pyritinol; psychometric performance under hypoxia deteriorated by 68% after placebo but by only 21% and 12% after 600 mg and 1000 mg pyritinol respectively.

Although our above-described topographic pharmaco-EEG images are certainly an encouraging step toward more accurate neurophysiological classification of psychotropic drugs in man, further systematic investigations with different dosages of classical psychopharmacological substances, as well as time-course studies, seem necessary. The determination of dose-efficacy and time-efficacy relationships based on alterations of the brain electrical activity, on the other hand, was already a hallmark of the pharmaco-EEG method (Saletu

1987) and thus also of the topographic pharmaco-EEG. It seems of interest that there are topographic differences in the significance levels of such dose time efficacy relations. The exact meaning of the latter, as well as the significance of topographic changes in specific EEG variables in general, has to be explored in the future utilizing behavioral and psychopathological evaluation techniques. Correlation analyses involving clinical and topographic EEG data as performed, for instance, by Buchsbaum et al. (1985), may add more valuable information about the mode of action of psychotropic drugs. Last but not least, topographic brain mapping of the EEG during drug treatment of psychiatric patients may enable us to monitor the therapeutic efficacy of drugs and eventually to select the optimal psychopharmacotherapeutic agent for each individual patient. Moreover, one may hope that the new methodology will increase our knowledge concerning the pathophysiology of the brain in psychiatric and neurological disorders.

Summary

Since the early systematic pharmacoelectroencephalographic (pharmaco-EEG) studies in the mid-1950s and the increasing utilization of computer facilities in the mid-1960s, quantitative analysis of the human EEG in combination with certain statistical procedures ("quantitative pharmaco-EEG") has proved to be a valuable method in clinical psychopharmacology. It has served as a classification instrument and even more so as a reliable technique to determine a drug's cerebral bioavailability. However, some difficulties with the classification have been thought to derive from the fact that most investigators analyzed only one or at most only a few leads. With the advent of modern mini- and microcomputers, multilead analysis and subsequent imaging of topographic pharmaco-EEG maps have become possible and practicable. This paper has surveyed topographic analysis of pharmaco-EEG data obtained from systematic double-blind placebo-controlled studies in normal volunteers involving representative drugs of different psychopharmacological classes: neuroleptics (chlorprothixene), antidepressants (imipramine), tranquilizers (diazepam), psychostimulants (caffeine) and nootropics/antihypoxidotics (pyritinol). Further, examples have been given of the determination of cerebral bioavailability utilizing time-efficacy and dose-efficacy relations as well as evaluation of the bioequipotency of different formulations of a compound. Finally, it has been demonstrated how the topographic brain mapping of drug-induced EEG changes can be utilized to demonstrate therapeutic efficacy of drugs in pharmacopsychiatry.

References

Anderer P, Saletu B, Kinsperger K, Semlitsch H (1987) Topographic brain mapping of EEG in neuropsychopharmacology. Part I: Methodological aspects. Methods Find Exp Clin Pharmacol 9(6):371–384

Bente D, Itil TM (1954) Zur Wirkung des Phenothiazinkörpers Megaphen auf das menschliche Hirnstrombild. Arzneimittelforschung 4:418–423

Berger H (1933) Über das Elektroencephalogramm des Menschen. VIII. Mitteilung. Arch Psychiatr Nervenkr 101:452–469

Coppola T, Buchsbaum MS, Rigal F (1982) Computer generation of surface distribution maps of measures of brain activity. Comput Biol Med 12:191–199

Buchsbaum MS, Rigal F, Coppola R, Cappelletti J, King C, Johnson J (1982) A new system for gray-level surface distribution maps of electrical activity. Electroencephalogr Clin Neurophysiol 53:237–242

Buchsbaum MS, Hazlett E, Sicotte N, Stein M, Wu J, Zetin M (1985) Topographic EEG changes with benzodiazepine administration in generalized anxiety disorder. Biol Psychiatry 20:832–842

Dublinsky J, Barlow JS (1980) A simple dot-density topogram for EEG. Electroencephalogr Clin Neurophysiol 48:473–477

Duffy FH, Burchfield JL, Lombroso CT (1979) Brain electrical activity mapping (BEAM): a method for extending the clinical utility of EEG and evoked potential data. Ann Neurol 5:309–321

Duffy FH, Bartels PH, Burchfield JL (1981) Significance probability mapping: an aid in the topographic analysis of brain electrical activity. Electroencephalogr Clin Neurophysiol 51:455–462

Etevenon P, Peron-Magnan P, Verdeaux G, Gaches J, Deniker P (1983) Electroencéphalographie quantitative en neurologie et psychiatrie: images topographiques d'EEG, effects d'agents psychotropes, typologie de la schizophrénie (Poster 422, 473A). Colloque Natn "Génie Biologique et Médical". Toulouse 1982 Gebiomip/Faculté de Médecine, Toulouse; p 43

Etevenon P, Peron-Magnan P, Boulenger JP, Tortrat D, Guillou S, Troussaint M, Gueguen B, Deniker P, Zarifian E (1986) EEG cartography profile of caffeine in normals. Clin Neuropharmacol 9 (S4):538–540

Fink M (1959) EEG and behavioral effects of psychopharmacology agents. In: Bradley PB, Deniker P, Radouco-Thomas C (eds) Neuropsychopharmacology, vol 1. Elsevier, Amsterdam, pp 441–446

Fink M (1975) Cerebral electrometry-quantitative EEG applied to human psychopharmacology. In: Dolce G, Künkel H (eds) Computerizing EEG analysis. Fischer, Stuttgart, pp 271–288

Gaches H, Etevenon P (1984) Topographie loco-régionale du spectre EEG chez l'homme: cartographie de deux cas d'accident vasculaire cérébral (dont l'un suivi sous sommeil). In: Lassen NA, Cahn J (eds) Maladies et médicaments/drugs and diseases. Libbey, London; Eurotext, Paris, pp 182–191

Goldstein L (1974) Psychotropic dry-induced EEG changes as revealed by the amplitude integration method. In: Ihl TM (ed) Psychotropic drugs and the human EEG. Karger, Basel, pp 131–148

Grünberger J, Saletu B, Linzmayer L, Stöhr H (1985) Determination of pharmacokinetics and pharmacodynamics of amisulpride by pharmaco-EEG and psychometry. In: Pichot P, Berner P, Wolf R, Thau K (eds) Psychiatry: the state of the art. Plenum, New York, pp 681–686

Head H (1923) The conception of nervous and mental energy. II. Vigilance: a physiological state of the nervous system. Br J Psychol 14:125–147

Herrmann WM (1982) Development and evaluation of an objective procedure for the electroencephalographic classification of psychotropic drugs. In: Herrmann WM (ed) Electroencephalography in drug research. Fischer, Stuttgart, pp 249–351

Herrmann WM, Schärer E (1986) Das Pharmako-EEG und seine Bedeutung für die klinische Pharmakologie. In: Kuemmerle DS, Hinterhuber G, Spitzy KU (eds) Klinische Pharmakologie, 4th edn. Landberg, München, pp 1–71

Herrmann WM, Kern U, Röhmel J (1986) Contribution on the search for vigilance-indicative EEG variables. Results of a controlled, double-blind study with pyritinol in elderly patients with symptoms of mental dysfunction. Pharmacopsychiatry 19:75–83

Itil TM (1974) Quantitative pharmaco-electroencephalography. Use of computerized cerebral biopotentials in psychotropic drug research. In: Itil TM (ed) Psychotropic drugs and the human EEG: modern problems of pharmacopsychiatry. Karger, Basel, pp 43–75

Itil TM, Shapiro DM, Eralp E, Akman A, Itil KZ, Garbizu C (1985) A new brain function diagnostic unit, including the dynamic brain mapping of computer analyzed EEG, evoked potential and sleep (a new hardware/software system and its application in psychiatry and psychopharmacology). New Trends Exp Clin Psychiatry 1:107–177

Künkel H (1982) On some hypotheses underlying pharmaco-electroencephalography. In: Hermann WM (ed) EEG in drug research. Fischer, Stuttgart, pp 1–16

Künkel H, Westphal M (1970) Quantitative EEG analysis of pyrithioxine action. Pharmakopsychiatry 3:41–49

Langer G, Ackenheil M, Dixon AK, Kurtz-May G, Möller HJ, Müller-Spahn F, Pitzcker A, Saletu B, Schönbeck G (1986) The psychopharmacology and neuroendocrinology of neuroleptics: the state of the art from a clinical perspective. Pharmacopsychiatry 19:145–148

Lehmann D (1971) Multichannel topography of human alpha EEG fields. Electroencephalogr Clin Neurophysiol 31:439–449

Matejcek M, Devos JE (1976) Selected methods of quantitative EEG analysis and their applications in psychotropic drug research. In: Kellaway P, Petersen I (eds) Quantitative studies in epilepsy. Raven, New York, pp 183–205

Persson A, Hjorth B (1983) EEG topogram – an aid in describing EEG to the clinician. Electroencephalogr Clin Neurophysiol 56:399–405

Petsche H (1973) EEG topography. In: Remond (ed) Handbook of electroencephalography and clinical neurophysiology. Elsevier, Amsterdam

Petsche H (1976) Topography of the EEG: survey and prospects. Clin Neurol Neurosurg 79:15–28

Petsche H, Marko A (1954) Das Photozellentoposkop. Arch Psychiatr Z Neurol 192:447–462

Pfurtscheller G, Ladurner G, Maresch H, Vollmer R (1984) Brain electrical activity mapping in normal and ischemic brain. In: Pfurtscheller J, Jonkman EJ, Lopes da Silva FH (eds) Brain ischemia – quantitative EEG and imaging techniques. Elsevier, Amsterdam

Pidoux B, Etevenon P, Campistron D, Peron-Magnan P, Bisserve JC, Verdaux G, Deniker P (1983) Topo-électroencéphalographie quantitative par ordinateur (TEQO). Rev Electroencéphalogr Neurophysiol Clin 13:27–34

Ragot RA, Remond A (1978) EEG field mapping. Electroencephalogr Clin Neurophysiol 45:417–421

Saletu B (1976) Psychopharmaka, Gehirntätigkeit und Schlaf. Karger, Basel

Saletu B (1981a) Nootropic drugs and human brain function. In: Wheatley D (ed) Stress and the heart. Raven, New York, pp 327–359

Saletu B (1981b) Application of quantitative EEG in measuring encephalotropic and pharmacodynamic properties of antihypoxidotic/nootropic drugs. In: Scientific International Research (eds) Drugs and methods in CVD Int Cerebrovascular Diseases. Pergamon Press, Paris, pp 79–115

Saletu B (1982) Pharmaco-EEG profile of typical and atypical antidepressants. In: Costa E, Racagni G (eds) Typical and atypical antidepressants. Clinical practice. Raven, New York, pp 257–268

Saletu B (1986) Zur Bestimmung der Pharmakodynamik alter und neuer Benzodiazepine mittels des Pharmako-EEGs. In: Hippius H, Engel RR, Laakmann G (eds) Benzodiazepine: Rückblick und Ausblick. Springer, Berlin Heidelberg New York Tokio, pp 45–68

Saletu B (1987) The use of pharmaco-EEG in drug profiling. In: Hindmarch I, Stonier PD (eds) The human psychopharmacology series. Wiley, Chichester, pp 173–200

Saletu B, Grünberger J (1980) Antihypoxidotic and nootropic drugs: proof of their encephalotropic and pharmacodynamic properties by quantitative EEG investigations. Prog Neuropsychopharmacol Biol Psychiatry 4: 469–489

Saletu B, Grünberger J (1985) Memory dysfunction and vigilance: neurophysiological and psychopharmacological aspects. Ann NY Acad Sci 444: 406–427

Saletu B, Grünberger J, Linzmayer L, Flener R (1981) Anxiolytics and beta blockers: evaluation of pharmacodynamics by quantitative EEG, psychometric and physiological variables. Aggressologie 22: 5–16

Saletu B, Grünberger J, Linzmayer L, Dubini A (1983) Determination of pharmacodynamics of the new neuroleptic zetidoline by neuroendocrinologic, pharmaco-EEG, and psychometric studies – Part I. Int J Clin Pharmacol Ther Toxicol 21: 489–495

Saletu B, Grünberger J, Anderer P, Sieghart W (1986a) Comparative bioavailability studies with a new mixed-micelles solution of diazepam utilizing radioreceptor assay, psychometry and Q-EEG imaging. Clin Neuropharmacol 9 [Suppl]: 532

Saletu B, Küfferle B, Grünberger J, Anderer P (1986b) Quantitative EEG, SPEM, and psychometric studies in schizophrenics before and during differential neuroleptic therapy. Pharmacopsychiatry 19: 434–437

Saletu B, Grünberger J, Linzmayer L, Anderer P (1987a) Comparative placebo-controlled pharmacodynamic studies with zotepine and clozapine utilizing pharmaco-EEG and psychometry. Pharmacopsychiatry 20: 12–27

Saletu B, Anderer P, Kinsperger K, Grünberger J (1987b) Topographic brain mapping of EEG in neuropsychopharmacology. Part II: Clinical applications (pharmaco-EEG imaging). Methods Find Exp Clin Pharmacol 9(6): 385–408

Saletu B, Anderer P, Kinsperger K, Grünberger J, Musch B (1988) On the central effects of the GABA agonist fengabine: psychometric and pharmaco-EEG studies utilizing imaging methods. Drug Dev Res 11: 251–279

Sebban CL, Debouzy CL, Berthaux P (1984) EEG quantifié et cartographie numérisée. In: Lassen NA, Cahn J (eds) Maladies et médicaments/drugs and diseases. Libbey, London; Eurotext, Paris, pp 176–181

Ueno S, Matsuoka S, Mizuguchi T, Nagashima M, Cheng CL (1975) Topographic computer display of abnormal EEG activities in patients with CNS diseases. Mem Fac Eng Kyushu Univ 24: 196–209

Walter G, Shipton H (1951) A new toposcopic display system. Electroencephalogr Clin Neurophysiol 3: 281–292

Evaluation and Interpretation of Topographic EEG Data in Schizophrenic Patients

T. DIERKS, K. MAURER, R. IHL, and A. SCHMIDTKE[1]

Introduction

As early as 1936 Lemere published reports of EEG changes in schizophrenic patients which showed a reduction of alpha rhythm. This was 1 year before Berger himself described an EEG recording of a 17-year-old schizophrenic patient who exhibited prominent beta activity. Berger interpreted beta waves as "material concomitant of cognitive processes". The large number of reports about EEG alterations, which cannot be reviewed in detail here, described more or less similar peculiarities in schizophrenics, such as "disorganized EEG's dominated by choppy activity" (Ellingson 1954). Attempts to quantify EEG data go back to 1932, when Dietsch described a Fourier analysis of human EEG, and 1939, when Gibbs used an analogue frequency analyzer to investigate cortical frequency spectra of schizophrenic individuals. The quantitative procedure was able to verify the former descriptive and qualitative EEG findings. The development of small digital computers and the fast Fourier transform algorithm (Cooley and Tukey 1965) have made real quantitative frequency analysis of the EEG technically feasible. Worthy of mention in this context are the frequency profiles of schizophrenic patients made by Itil et al. (1972), who confirmed an appearance of excessive fast activity along with some slow waves and the lack of alpha activity. The more recent quantitative studies have been reviewed by Itil (1978).

Attempts to localize these abnormalities topographically have been limited by recording from a small number of electrodes. EEG cartography became possible, however, when Duffy et al. (1979) introduced the newly developed method of brain electrical activity mapping. Since then the topographic display of EEG data has been described by Morihisa et al. (1983), Morstyn et al. (1983) and Guenther and Breitling (1985) in resting conditions and in multisensory motor and mental activation states. The findings common to both drug-free and medicated patients were increased slow activity, mainly in frontal regions, and more fast activity in postcentral areas.

The aim of the present study was (a) to subdivide a schizophrenic population of 30 persons into the three subtypes according to DSM-III and ICD-9 criteria and (b) to delineate the corresponding EEG pattern in the delta, theta, alpha and beta range by means of topographic brain mapping of the EEG. Several test procedures, including the F test, Student's t test and the test of practical significance, were applied to compare controls with patients.

---

[1] Department of Psychiatry, University of Würzburg, Füchsleinstr. 15, 8700 Würzburg, Federal Republic of Germany

Subjects

Of the total number of 30 schizophrenic patients, 10 had been classified as being of the hebephrenic subtype (DSM-III and ICD-9: 295.1), 10 of the paranoid subtype (DSM-III and ICD-9: 295.3) and 10 of the residual subtype (DSM-III and ICD-9: 295.6). The average age of the patients was 24.5 years for the hebephrenic, 28.7 years for the paranoid and 41.2 years for the residual group. The male/female ratio was 1/1. The average current treatment lay between 440 and 560 chlorpromazine equivalent units. All patients were right-handed. The controls ($n = 10$) had a mean age of 28.8 years, a male/female ratio of 1/1 and were receiving no medication whatsoever.

Methods

Data were recorded from 19 electrodes applied to the scalp according to the 10–20 format. The following electrode sites were used: Fp1, Fp2, F7, F3, Fz, F4, F8, T3, C3, Cz, C4, T4, T5, P3, Pz, P4, T6, O1 and O2.

All data were referenced to linked mastoids. A brain-mapping system (Brain-Atlas III, Bio-logic Systems Corp.) was used including a biomedical software system and a statistical system which was developed by Maurer and Dierks (1987). Up to 5 min EEG was recorded for each subject in the eyes open alert (EO) and eyes closed alert (EC) states. Subjects were carefully instructed to minimize eye movement and blinks. In the EO condition subjects were asked to focus on a black point. Raw EEG data for controls and patients were stored on magnetic disk (10 M Byte Bernoulli Box) to enable subsequent off-line data processing. For further analysis 12 visually inspected artifact-free 2-s EEG epochs were taken. Analysis of EEG data comprised computerized spectral analysis of the data from each electrode by means of fast Fourier transform algorithm. For the purpose of analysis only the 0–31.5 Hz segment was examined. This was divided into the following eight frequency bands: delta (0–3.5 Hz), theta (4–7.5 Hz), alpha (8–11.5 Hz), $beta_1$ (12–15.5 Hz), $beta_2$ (16–19.5 Hz), $beta_3$ (20–23.5 Hz), $beta_4$ (24–27.5 Hz) and $beta_5$ (28–31.5 Hz).

Single measurements from each of the 19 electrodes which represented the amplitude (µV) for a particular frequency band were used for further analysis. The scalp areas around the original 19 electrodes were filled in by linear interpolation based upon the values at the four nearest electrodes. The original values were then mapped upon a 64 by 64 matrix of numerical values. These values were used for display on a computer monitor.

The first step in data analysis comprised the calculation of group means and variances for each point. Thus for each frequency band and in both the EO and the EC state two group-average spectral distribution images were calculated for the control group and the three subgroups of schizophrenic patients. The F test was used to determine if the variances were equal or nonequal. For comparison among the different groups calculations of Student's t statistic were performed. For display the t values of each channel were transformed into statistical t value maps where the areas around the original 19 electrodes were interpolated. It is common practice to construct t value maps using unsigned t values, but this procedure does not enable differentiation between positive and negative values. Our method, however resulted in positive t values if the mean activity was augmented in comparison to controls and in negative t values if the contrary happened (i.e., decrease of the mean activity compared to control values).

The method evinces weaknesses if in the mapping field only statistically significant differences are taken into account. This occurs especially when, owing to the size of the sample groups, small effects attain statistical significance.

Table 1. EEG results in the eyes closed state for eight frequency bands and for the three subtypes of schizophrenia. The results indicate differences between the control and schizophrenic groups

Eyes closed	Schizophrenia subtype		
	Hebephrenic	Paranoid	Residual
0–3.5 Hz	Augmented activity over C3, P3 and Pz (PS ≈ 10%) (Fig. 1)	No significant difference to controls	Slightly increased activity over C3, P3, P4 and Cz compared to controls
4–7.5 Hz	No significant difference to controls	Decreased activity over O1, Oz and O2 (PS ≈ 10%)	No significant difference to controls
8–11.5 Hz	Significant decrease of activity over all electrodes, especially over O2 (PS ≈ 45%) (Fig. 2)	Same findings as in the hebephrenic group (Fig. 3A)	Same findings as in the hebephrenic group (Fig. 3B)
12–15.5 Hz	Slight decrease of activity over left occipital electrodes	No significant difference to controls	No significant difference to controls
16–19.5 Hz	Decrease of activity over occipital electrodes (PS ≈ 15%)	Decrease of activity over occipital electrodes (PS ≈ 20%) compared to controls	Significant decrease of activity over T3, T5, O1 and O2 (PS ≈ 45%)
20–23.5 Hz	Findings as in the band 16.0–19.5 Hz		
24–27.5 Hz	Findings as in the band 16.0–19.5 Hz		
28–31.5 Hz	Findings as in the band 16.0–19.5 Hz		

PS, practical significance

Even though the difference of mean values may be significant, the area of overlap may be so large that such differences are really meaningless when looking at individual cases. In this case the danger is that of "overinterpreting" a significant result.

Taking this disadvantage into account, we decided to apply values indicating in which way the proportion of variance of dependent variables (EEG) can

Table 2. EEG results in the eyes open state for eight frequency bands and for the three subtypes of schizophrenia. The results indicate differences between the control and schizophrenic groups

Eyes open	Schizophrenia subtype		
	Hebephrenic	Paranoid	Residual
0–3.5 Hz	No significant difference compared to controls	A slight decrease ($t \approx 1.6$) over Fp1, F3 and T3 compared to controls	No significant difference compared to controls
4–7.5 Hz	Increase of activity over frontal electrodes (PS $\approx 10\%$) and especially over occipital electrodes (PS $\approx 25\%$)	Increase over parietal electrodes (PS $\approx 10\%$)	No significant difference compared to controls
8–11.5 Hz	Significant increase of activity, especially over the left hemisphere (PS left $\approx 15\%$, right $\approx 10\%$) (Fig. 4A)	As the hebephrenic group but a PS of the left side about 25% (Fig. 4B)	Increased activity over F8 (PS $\approx 25\%$) and F3, C3 and P3 (PS $\approx 10\%$) (Fig. 4C)
12–15.5 Hz	Increase of activity over Pz and P3 (PS $\approx 10\%$) (Fig. 5)	Increased activity over F8 (PS 25%) and T5, C3 and P3 (PS 10%)	Increased activity over F8 (PS $\approx 25\%$)
16–19.5 Hz	No significant difference compared to controls	Slight increase over all electrodes (PS ≈ 5–10%), and a significant increase over F8 (PS $\approx 25\%$)	Increase over frontal electrodes (PS $\approx 15\%$), especially F8 (PS $\approx 40\%$)
20–23.5 Hz	No significant difference compared to controls in any group		
24–27.5 Hz	No significant difference compared to controls	No significant difference compared to controls	A slight increase of activity over F4 and P4 (PS $\approx 15\%$)
28–31.5 Hz	Same findings as in the band 24.0–27.5 Hz		

PS, practical significance

be attributed to independent variables (clinical classification). We chose ω^2 as a conservative value for the estimation for the population (=lower limit; Wolf and Brandt 1982). These so-called practical significance maps (PSM) are shown in Figs. 2–4 for the three subgroups of schizophrenics. The PSM allow evaluation of whether an alteration (e.g. augmented beta activity) is marked enough to provide meaningful support for any particular scientific hypothesis. A value with a high "practical significance" which is defined in percent of variance is then able to delineate the real relevance of clinically obtained data in groups with different diagnoses.

In this study we were able to construct practical significance maps for different states (EO and EC state) and for the three subgroups of schizophrenia, the hebephrenic, the paranoid and the residual form. The aim was to find out whether defined psychopathological conditions are correlated to a special pattern in the PS maps.

Results

Tables 1 and 2 contain data of topographic amplitude spectra (µV), t value maps and PSM in the EC and EO states for the three subgroups of schizophrenic patients.

There were higher amplitude values in the delta range only in the hebephrenic subgroup in the EC state, with a predominance centrally and parietally and a slight accentuation on the left hemisphere (Fig. 1).

The theta band showed a decrease of amplitude values occipitally in the paranoid subgroup in the EC state, but an increase in the EO state in the hebephrenic and paranoid subgroups.

Most obvious and consistent were our findings of decreased alpha activity in the EC state, especially in the hebephrenic subgroup (Fig. 2a–d) but also in the paranoid and residual collectives (Fig. 3a–b), whereas the contrary occurred in the EO state, i.e., a significant increase with an accentuation in all three subgroups (Fig. 4a–c).

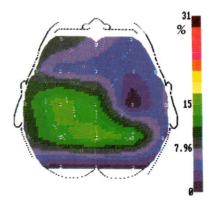

Fig. 1. Practical significance map for the delta band (0–3.5 Hz) gained by comparison of the control group with the hebephrenic subgroup. Maximal values are measured over the midline and left central and parietal electrodes, indicating an increase of delta activity in these regions. (All figures in this contributions were prepared using equipment from Bio-logic Systems Corporation, Mundelein, IL, USA)

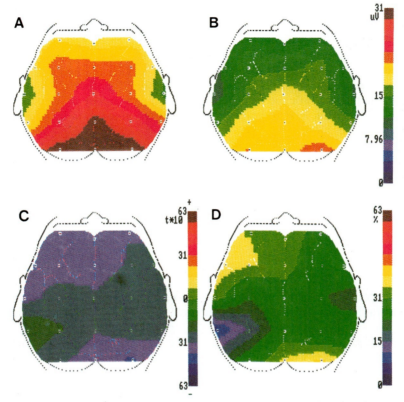

Fig. 2 A–D. Comparison between the controls and the hebephrenic subgroup for the alpha band (8–11.5 Hz) in the eyes closed state. **A** Mean value for 10 normals. **B** Mean value for 10 hebephrenics. **C** A *t* value map exhibiting the difference between controls and hebephrenics. The color scale indicates *t* values multiplied by the factor 10. Positive *t* values mean augmented and negative *t* values decreased activity in hebephrenics compared to controls. **D** Practical significance map indicating the clinical relevance of a finding. The map is constructed using *t* values

For the beta bands the same alterations occurred as in the alpha range, i.e., a decrease in the EC state and an increase in the EO state. Remarkable was an increase of activity in the slow beta band (12–15.5 Hz) in the EO state, with a maximum over Pz and P3 in the hebephrenic subgroup (Fig. 5).

Discussion

Not all findings in our study can be compared to others and discussed thoroughly because of the subdivision of our schizophrenic patients into the three subgroups according to DSM-III and ICD-9 criteria. Considering that our patients

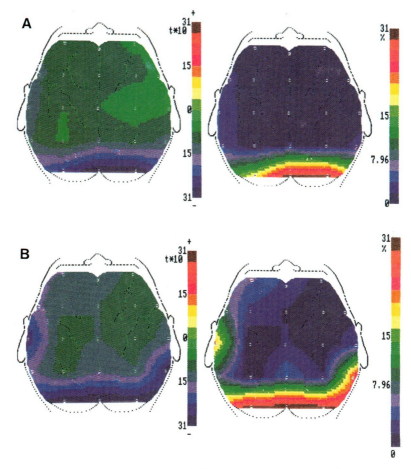

Fig. 3A, B. *Left:* *t*-value maps; *right:* practical significance maps. **A** Results of comparison between the controls and the paranoid subgroup for the alpha band (8–11.5 Hz) in the eyes closed state, indicating an occipital decrease. **B** Results of comparison between the controls and the residual subgroup for the alpha band (8–11.5 Hz) in the eyes closed state, indicating an occipital decrease

were not drug-free, some topographic features in defined frequency ranges may be due to the neuroleptic treatment.

The most obvious finding in the EC and EO states was the absence of frontal slowing (0–3.5 Hz). Instead, we saw a mild increase in delta activity in the hebephrenic and residual subgroups over centroparietal areas, with a modest accentuation at C3 in the hebephrenics. This lack of frontal slowing is not in accordance with findings described by others (Morihisa et al. 1983; Morstyn et al. 1983; Guenther and Breitling 1985). It is worth mentioning in this context that great care was taken to suppress eye movements and blinks: in addition, only artifact-free EEG segments were chosen for spectral analysis.

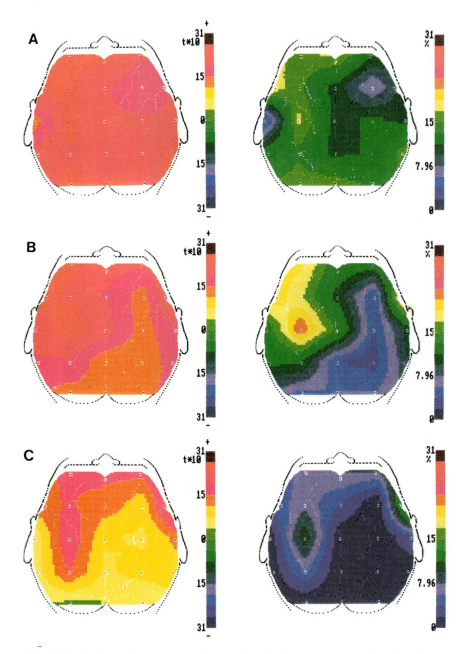

Fig. 4A–C. *Left:* *t* value maps; *right:* practical significance maps. **A** Results of comparison between the controls and the hebephrenic subgroup for the alpha band (8–11.5 Hz) in the eyes open state, indicating a generalized increase. **B** Results of comparison between the controls and the paranoid subgroup for the alpha band (8–11.5 Hz) in the eyes open state, indicating a left-sided increase. **C** Results of comparison between the controls and the residual subgroup for the alpha band, indicating a frontal and left centroparietal increase

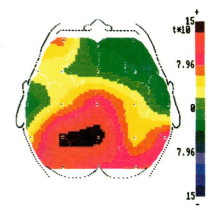

Fig. 5. A *t* value map indicating the difference between the controls and the hebephrenic subgroup for the beta$_1$ band (12–15.5 Hz) in the eyes open state

Our results, however, are in line with those recently described by Karson et al. (1987), who found a mild increase in delta activity only at midsagittal electrode locations, with no tendency for frontal localization of this slow activity. Although frontal slowing is a consistent EEG finding in schizophrenia, our results and those of Karson et al. support the notion that frontal delta may be due to eye movement and blinking. Even in the EO state, the increase of frontal slowing that could have been expected did not take place. Excessive frontal delta, if present, may be connected with the clinically well-known fact that schizophrenic patients exhibit more eye movement and blinking than normal control subjects.

Instead of frontal slowing, we saw augmented delta activity over central and parietal structures with a slight preference over the left hemisphere (Fig. 1). If we assume that the delta activity correlates with blood circulation and metabolism, our results on generalized slowing are more consistent with those rCBF and PET studies that suggest an overall reduction in brain metabolic activity (Berman and Weinberger 1986). Signs of selective frontal lobe hypofunction (hypofrontality) were not present in our population of schizophrenic patients in the resting state. A medication effect cannot be ruled out in our patients, since some neuroleptics decrease the very slow wave activity in the range 0–3.5 Hz (Itil 1972). A study with untreated schizophrenics is planned to clarify this problem.

The alterations in the theta band were somehow contradictory. Only in the EO state did an increase of activity occur in hebephrenic patients over frontal and occipital electrodes. Karson et al. (1987) described a significant difference in theta activity in the right parasagittal leads with eyes closed, the they described no significance differences between groups in any univariant comparison in this frequency band.

The most consistent finding in the EC state was a decrease in alpha activity over all electrodes, pronounced at the occiput. Reduced alpha activity is the most replicable finding in EEG research in schizophrenia and has been described by many authors (Itil et al. 1972; Itil 1978; Fenton et al. 1980). In the report by Fenton et al. (1980), the reduction in alpha power in the EC state was found mainly in temporal leads bilaterally. In contrast, we found an alpha decrease in all our three subgroups with a preference for the occipital area. One reason for the suppression of occipital alpha could be a "hyperarousal state" which leads to a desynchronization of alpha waves. Another explanation for the lower observed alpha activity is proposed by Itil (1978) from studies of the EEG frequency pattern induced by indole and anticholinergic dopamine-blocking drugs. This view would support Friedhoff's notion (1973) of a genetically determined imbalance between dopaminergic and cholinergic activity (increased dopaminergic activity and/or decreased cholinergic activity).

The meaning of an increase of alpha power especially over the left hemisphere in the EO state can cautiously be interpreted in terms of reduced alpha blocking, which occurs normally in the EO state on both sides. If this proves right, the lesser blocking of alpha in the left hemisphere in all three subgroups may be a further sign of a left-sided dysfunction in schizophrenia.

Findings similar to those described for the alpha band occurred in some of the beta frequency ranges, i.e., a decrease in the EC state and an increase in the EO state. The practical significance, however, was much less. Worth mentioning is the increase of slow beta over parietal and occipital sites, with a slight left-sided accentuation (Fig. 5).

Increased posterior fast beta activity, especially on the left side, is a feature often described in schizophrenic patients and has been interpreted in terms of irritable if not epileptogenic cortex (Lombroso and Duffy 1980). An increase in the 16–19.5 beta band was observed over frontal electrodes, with a practical significance of 40% only in the residual subgroup in the EO state. The meaning of this local beta pattern cannot be explained at present and a medication effect may be responsible.

In summary, our data showed a wide sprectrum of frequency changes in the EEG of schizophrenics compared to values in controls. Some of the features, such as alpha decrease and changes in the beta band, were consistent with findings in the literature. Inconsistencies may be due to the fact that medicated patients were investigated and to the division into three subgroups. Most remarkable was the fact that we did not observe frontal slowing, a most consistent finding in other studies.

The next step will be the analysis of EEG data in carefully characterized schizophrenic patients belonging to different psychopathological syndromes, either untreated or treated with standardized medication in order to exclude variables which may be responsible for some of the inconsistencies.

References

Berman FK, Weinberger R (1986) Cerebral blood flow studies in schizophrenia. In: Nasrolle HA, Weinsberger R (eds) Handbook of schizophrenia, vol 1. Elsevier, Amsterdam, p 300

Cooley JW, Tukey JW (1976) An algorithm for the machine calculation of complex Fourier series. Math Comput 19:297–301

Dietsch G (1932) Fourier-Analyse von Electroencephalogrammen des Menschen. Pflügers Arch Ges Physiol 230:106–112

Duffy HF, Buchfield JL, Lombroso CT (1979) Brain electrical activity mapping (BEAM): a method for extending the the clinical utility of EEG and evoked potentials data. Ann Neurol 5:309–321

Ellingson RJ (1954) The incidence of EEG abnormality among patients with mental disorders of apparently nonorganic origin: a critic review. Am J Psychiatry 111:263

Fenton GW, Fenwick PBC, Dollimore J, Dunn TL, Hirsch SR (1980) EEG spectral analysis in schizophrenia. Br J Psychiatry 136:445–455

Friedhoff AM (1973) Biogenic amines and schizophrenia. In: Mendels J (ed) Biological psychiatry. Wiley, New York

Gibbs FA (1939) Cortical frequency spectra of schizophrenic, epileptic and normal individuals. Trans Am Neurol Assoc 65:141–144

Guenther W, Breitling D (1985) Predominant sensomotor area left hemisphere dysfunction in schizophrenia measured by brain electrical activity mapping. Biol Psychiatry 20:515–532

Itil TM (1978) Qualitative and quantitative EEG-Befunde bei Schizophrenen. Z EEG-EMG 9:1–13

Itil TM, Saletu B, Davis S (1972) EEG findings in chronic schizophrenics based on digital computer period analysis and analog power spectra. Biol Psychiatry 5:1–13

Karson CN, Coppola R, Morihisa JM, Weinberger DR (1987) Computed electroencephalographic activity mapping in schizophrenia. Arch Gen Psychiatry 44:514–517

Lemere F (1936) The significance of individual differences in the Berger Rhythm. Brain 59:366–375

Lombroso CT, Duffy FH (1980) Brain electrical mapping as an adjunct to CT scanning. In: Canger R, Angeleri F, Perry JK (eds) Advances in epileptology. Raven, New York, pp 83–88

Maurer K, Dierks T (1987) Brain Mapping – topographiche Darstellung der EEG und der evozierten Potentiale in Psychiatrie und Neurologie. Z EEG EMG 18:4–12

Morihisa JM, Duffy FH, Wyatt RJ (1983) Brain electrical activity mapping (BEAM) in schizophrenic patients. Arch Gen Psychiatry 40:719–726

Morstyn R, Duffy FH, McCarley RW (1983) Altered P300 topography in schizophrenia. Arch Gen Psychiatry 40:729–734

Wolf B, Brandt W (1982) Über Maße der praktischen Signifikanz bei Varianzen und Regressionsanalysen. Z Empir Pädagog 6:57–73

EEG Mapping During Cholinergic Drug Challenge with RS-86

J. Fritze, T. Dierks, and K. Maurer[1]

Introduction

The cholinergic-adrenergic balance hypothesis of affective disorders postulates cholinergic overactivity in depression (Janowsky et al. 1972, 1985). Indeed, patients suffering from affective disorders have been found supersensitive to cholinergic drugs like physostigmine and arecoline in behavioral, neuroendocrine, and electrophysiological parameters. Cholinomimetics inducing an anergic-anhedonic syndrome in healthy volunteers elicited full-blown depressive symptoms even in the euthymic interval. Following cholinomimetics the rise of ACTH/β-endorphin/cortisol secretion has been found greater than in controls. The reduction of REM sleep latency was more pronounced. Thus, cholinergic supersensitivity was proposed to represent a trait marker. Findings in split-brain patients suggest REM sleep to be generated primarily in the right hemisphere, i.e., the one not dominant for speech (Gazzaniga and LeDoux 1978). Based on various lines of evidence, including electrophysiological findings, the lateralization hypothesis suggests the right hemisphere to be overactive and dysfunctioning in depression (Coffey 1987; Flor-Henry 1983; Nasrallah 1982). Attempting to establish a bridge between the cholinergic and lateralization hypotheses, the present study investigated whether topographic changes of electrical brain activity under cholinergic drug challenge might mimic some of the lateralized findings in depression.

Methods

One healthy volunteer ingested single doses of 2, 3, 4 and 5 mg RS-86 (2-ethyl-8-methyl-2,8-diazospiro-(4,5)-decan-1,3-dion hydrobromide), a centrally active muscarinic agonist (Palacios et al. 1986), and placebo in randomized order under double-blind conditions with wash-out intervals of 1 week. The psychotropic effects were estimated by the activation-inhibition scale of Janowsky et al. (1973) before and 1, 3, 6, and 7 h after administration. Topographic EEG was recorded using the Brain Atlas III (Bio-logic Systems Corp.) 1 h before and 30 min and 2 h after drug ingestion. It was evaluated off line, selecting by visual inspection artifact-free segments which were transformed to frequency spectra by Fourier analysis. Mean spectra for the following frequency bands were calculated for

---

[1] Department of Psychiatry, University of Würzburg, Füchsleinstr. 15, 8700 Würzburg, Federal Republic of Germany

each recording: theta (4.0–7.5 Hz), alpha (8.0–11.5 Hz), beta (12.0–31.5 Hz). Delta activity could not be reliably analyzed because of drug-induced sweating artifacts.

The psychotropic effects were analyzed by correlating the means of the postdrug changes from baseline to the dosages using Kendall's τ. Kendall's τ was also used as the criterion for dose-dependent effects on electrical brain activity, constructing correlation maps for each frequency band and comparing the postdrug correlations with those occurring by chance in the predrug recordings.

Results

The centrally active muscarinic agonist RS-86 induced an anergic-anhedonic syndrome the severity of which was done-dependent ($\tau = 0.9$; Fig. 1).

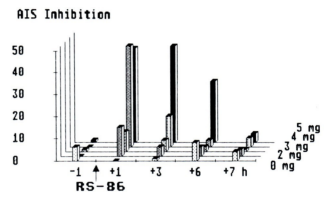

Fig. 1. Subscale inhibition of the activation-inhibition scale. Scores of the observer's ratings before and after administration of RS-86

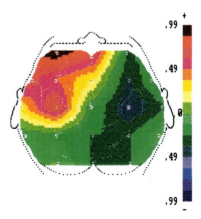

Fig. 2. Kendall's τ correlation map relating the regional 24–27.5 Hz postdrug EEG activity to the dosages of RS-86. Activation of the left frontotemporal region

The predrug electrical brain activity showed, by chance, correlations of $\tau \leq 0.3$ in the various frequency bands. In the postdrug recordings there were no dose-related changes of theta activity in any brain region. The alpha activity decreased in the left frontocentral and right occipitoparietal regions in a clearly dose-dependent manner ($\tau = -0.7--1.0$). The 12–15.5 Hz activity decreased in the right frontocentral region ($\tau = -0.8--1.0$) and, with less clear dose dependency, bifrontally ($\tau = -0.5$). The 24–27.5 Hz activity increased in the left frontotemporal region ($\tau = 0.5-1.0$; Fig. 2).

Discussion

The present dose-response study of the central cholinomimetic RS-86 confirmed that the so-called behavioral physostigmine syndrome is mediated by muscarinic receptors. Moreover, it revealed localized drug effects on brain electrical activity in distinct frequency bands. Although it is astonishing that a systemically applied drug induces localized effects, this corresponds to the ideas of Geschwind and Galaburda (1985). The results can, however, be interpreted only cautiously in view of the preliminary character of this single case study. They are suggestive of activation of the left frontal lobe relative to the right and of the right parietal lobe relative to the left, and thus do not indicate global differences between the hemispheres. Comparisons with findings in psychiatric disorders described in the literature are difficult because of differences in methodology. The results are not compatible with the findings of right greater than left EEG activation over the frontal lobes following experimental induction of dysphoric mood in normal volunteers (Tucker et al. 1981) and in spontaneous depression (Schaffer et al. 1983). Rather, they are reminiscent of the left hemispheric activation in schizophrenia (Newlin et al. 1981). Interestingly, the anergic-anhedonic behavioral syndrome resembles negative symptoms in schizophrenia, where an involvement of cholinergic systems is also discussed (Singh 1985).

References

Coffey EC (1987) Cerebral laterality and emotion: the neurology of depression. Compr Psychiatry 28:197–219
Flor-Henry P (1983) The cerebral basis of psychopathology. Wright, Boston
Gazzaniga MS, LeDoux JE (1978) The integrated mind. Plenum, New York
Geschwind N, Galaburda AM (1985) Cerebral lateralization. Biological mechanisms, associations, and pathology: III. Arch Neurol 42:634–654
Janowsky DS, El-Yousef MK, Davis JM, Sekerke HJ (1972) A cholinergic-adrenergic hypothesis of mania and depression. Lancet ii:632–635
Janowsky DS, El-Yousef MK, Davis JM, Sekerke HJ (1973) Parasympathetic suppression of manic symptoms by physostigmine. Arch Gen Psychiatry 28:542–547
Janowsky DS, Risch SC, Judd LL, Huey LY, Parker DC (1985) Brain cholinergic systems and the pathogenesis of affective disorders. In: Singh MM, Warburton DM, Lal H (eds) Central cholinergic mechanisms and adaptive dysfunctions. Plenum, New York, pp 309–352

Nasrallah HA (1982) Hemispheric asymmetry in affective disorders. Psychopharmacol Bull 18:62–67

Newlin DB, Carpenter B, Golden CJ (1981) Hemispheric asymmetries in schizophrenia. Biol Psychiatry 16:561–582

Palacios JM, Bolliger G, Closse A, Enz A, Gmelin G, Malanowski J (1986) The pharmacological assessment of RS-86 (2-ethyl-8-methyl-2,8-diazospiro-(4,5)-decan-1,3-dion hydrobromide). A potent, specific muscarinic acetylcholine receptor agonist. Eur J Pharmacol 125:45–62

Schaffer CE, Davidson RJ, Caron C (1983) Frontal and parietal electroencephalogram asymmetry in depressed and nondepressed subjects. Biol Psychiatry 18:753–762

Singh MM (1985) Cholinergic mechanisms, adaptive brain processes and adaptive psychopathology. In: Singh MM, Warburton DM, Lal H (eds) Central cholinergic mechanisms and adaptive dysfunctions. Plenum, New York, pp 353–397

Tucker DM, Stenslie CE, Roth RS (1981) Right frontal lobe activation and right hemisphere performance. Arch Gen Psychiatry 38:169–174

Topographic Mapping of Event-Related Potentials as a Diagnostic Tool for Identification of Dyslexic Persons

J. LYCKLAMA À NIJEHOLT[1], W. VAN DRONGELEN[2], and B.E.J. HILHORST[1]

Introduction

There is substantial evidence that event-related pontentials (ERPs) may provide a useful index of brain processes that underlie *grapheme-phoneme conversions*. These conversion abilities have been indicated as one of the skills lacking in dyslexics. The topography of visual ERPs during geometric and phonetic discrimination tasks has been studied by Lovrich et al. (1986) in normal adults. Topographic mapping as described by Duffy et al. (1980) is a method to study the topographic distribution of potential amplitudes or frequencies by means of colored maps. We used the same stimulation conditions as described by Lovrich et al. (1986) and compared the results of topographic mapping of the ERPs in normal adults and a small age-matched group of persons with a long history of dyslexia, with the aim of diagnosing dyslexia on neurophysiological criteria.

Material and Methods

Our method is essentially the same as that described by Lovrich et al. (1986). In brief, letters from the standard alphabet are presented on a computer-driven TV screen in a randomized way. Sixteen-channel EEG (10–20 system, reference linked ears) is recorded during 1 s post stimulus and the waveforms are averaged over 128 presentations. Three different trials are recorded:
1. No instruction to the test person: simple response (SR).
2. Form identification: the test person is instructed to identify closed letters by pushing a button. Closed letters are target (T), others are non-target (NT). Waveforms associated with T and with NT are stored in separate memory blocks. This results in two sets of waveforms: T and NT.
3. Rhyme identification: the next instruction is to identify the letters with an "e" sound (b, c etc.). The same data sampling is performed as in the second trial, resulting in two sets of waveforms, T (rhyming letters) and NT (non-rhyming letters).

---

[1] Ziekenhuis Ziekenzorg, Haaksbergerstraat 55, 7513 ER Enschede, The Netherlands
[2] Nicolet Instrument Benelux, Meidoornkade 19, 3992 AG Houten, The Netherlands

For data analysis the SR waveform is substracted from the other waveforms, resulting in three waveforms for the form condition and three for the rhyme condition.

Form
T-SR
NT-SR
(T-SR)−(NT-SR)

Rhyme
T-SR
NT-SR
(S-SR)−(NT-SR)

Eventually these waveforms are topographically mapped with intervals of 34 ms in the 300–800 ms post-stimulus period; resulting in three different sets of maps for the form and rhyme conditions. The grand mean average ERPs of normal adults were compared with the grand mean average ERPs of eight adults with a long history of dyslexia.

Results

Description of Maps in Normal Controls and Adult Dyslexics

In the *form condition* in normal adults the NT-SR and T-SR maps both show a well-defined centroparietal negativity at 300 ms which disappears at 368 ms. Next, a posterior-located positivity appears in the T-SR condition, starting at 436 ms, reaching a maximum at 538 ms and then slowly diminishing until it disappears at 674 ms post stimulus.

In the NT-SR condition the posterior positivity is located centroparietally and has a maximum at 572 ms. Thus the positivity appears later, reaches a maximum later and has a slightly different localization. Substracting (NT-SR) from (T-SR) yields an occipitally located maximal positivity at 504 ms. The increase and decrease of the positive field is between 436 and 572 ms, with a slight shift of the maximum to the left occipital region. When we compare this with the "dyslexic pattern," we see that the latter lacks the initial centroparietal negativity. In the T-SR maps from dyslexics the centroparietal negativity is absent and a frontal positivity develops at 334 ms, slowly increasing until 436 ms, when two positive maxima are defined at Pz and Fz. At 470 and 504 ms a positivity is located at Pz which has disappeared at 572 ms. In these maps the posterior positivity also has a maximum earlier in time with a centroparietal location.

In the NT-SR calculation in dyslexics there is a centroparietal positive maximum at 436 ms which has disappeared by 572 ms, shifting to the vertex area. So the maximal positivity has the same location, but reaches that maximum much earlier and is of shorter duration.

Subtraction of NT-SR from T-SR gives a pattern different from normals in the respect that the greatest positivity is frontal at 368–402 ms and that the posterior positivity is of low intensity with a maximum at 504 ms.

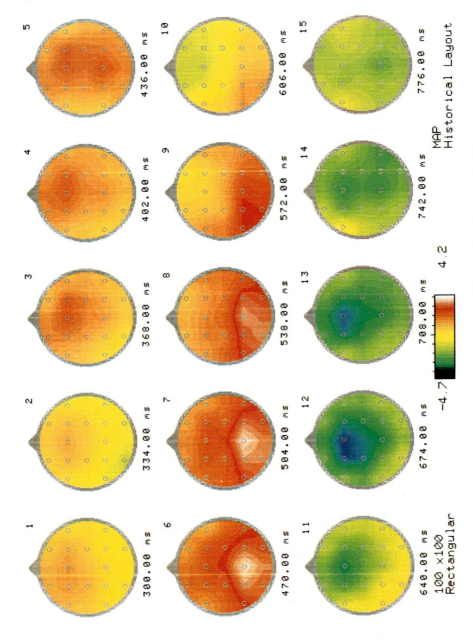

Fig. 1. Rhyme condition, grand mean average ERPs: (T-SR) − (NT-SR) maps in eight normal adults

Topographic Mapping of Event-Related Potentials as a Diagnostic Tool 525

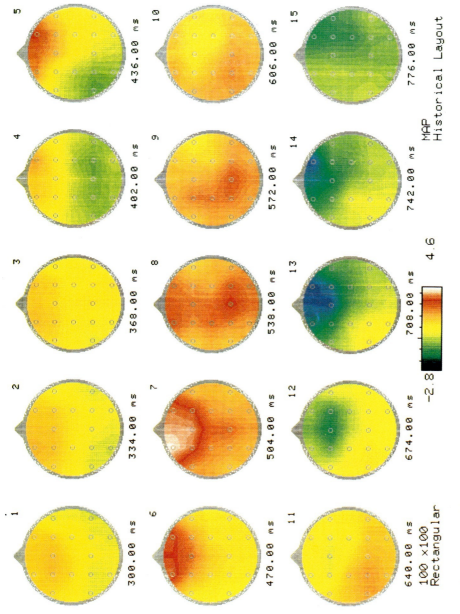

Fig. 2. Rhyme condition, grand mean average ERPS: (T-SR) – (NT-SR) maps in eight dyslexics

For the *rhyme condition* we followed the same procedure: T-SR, NT-SR and (T-SR)−(NT-SR). In normals there is again an initial negativity at 300 ms maximal in the Pz region. The T-SR maps show a well-defined posterior positivity between 436 and 606 ms, also predominantly left and more sharply delineated than in the NT-SR maps.

In the NT-SR maps posterior positivity is first seen at 436 ms, increases slowly in intensity until 572 ms and spreads over the scalp until a maximum is reached at 674 ms, predominantly over the left hemisphere. The (T-SR)−(NT-SR) maps show a well-defined posterior positivity between 470 and 538 ms.

Again, the dyslexics show different patterns. In the NT-SR maps, a frontal positive maximum is seen at 402 ms. There was no posterior positivity between 470 and 640 ms. In the (T-SR) maps we seen essentially the same: frontal positivity, but over a longer period, between 368 and 538 ms, maximal at 436 ms. The most evident difference in the (T-SR)−(NT-SR) maps is a maximal frontal positivity at 504 ms; the normals have positive maxima in the Pz region at this latency.

Conclusion

Although the numbers are small, this study suggests that mapping of visual ERPs can depict clear differences in potential field distributions between normal and dyslexic persons. We will continue this study in order to define neurophysiological criteria for diagnosing dyslexia.

References

Duffy FH, Wenckla MB, Bartels PH, Sandini G, Kiessling LS (1980) Dyslexia: automated diagnosis by computerized classification of brain electrical activity. Ann Neurol 7:421–428

Lovrich D, Simson R, Vaughan HS Jr, Ritter W (1986) Topography of visual event-related potentials during geometric and phonetic discriminations. Electroencephalogr Clin Neurophysiol 65:1–12

Topographic EEG Brain Maps and Mental Performance Under Hypoxia After Placebo and Pyritinol

B. SALETU, P. ANDERER, K. KINSPERGER, and J. GRÜNBERGER[1]

Introduction

In recent years we have demonstrated that the hypoxia model may be successfully utilized in human psychopharmacology to assess the brain-protecting properties of antihypoxidotic/nootropic drugs – specifically if quantitative EEG (Q-EEG) and psychometric analyses are carried out (Saletu and Grünberger 1983, 1984; Saletu et al. 1987a). In our past experiments, however, we were restricted to the right and left occipital and parietal regions. Recently, we have had the opportunity to employ our newly developed topographic Q-EEG mapping system for the above-mentioned problems (Saletu et al. 1986, 1987b; Anderer et al. 1987).

Method

Twelve healthy volunteers in the age range 24–34 (mean 27) years received the following treatments randomized at weekly intervals: placebo, 600 mg pyritinol and 1000 mg pyritinol under normobaric hypoxic conditions (9.8%, O_2, 90.2% N_2), and placebo under normoxia (21% O_2, 79% N_2). The reversible hypoxic hypoxidosis was induced repetitively for 23 min (before and 1, 3, 5 and 7 h after oral drug administration) by inhalation of a hypoxic gas mixture (equivalent to 6000 m altitude). Hypoxemia was checked by *blood gas analyses* of arterialized capillary blood samples from the hyperemized earlobe (PO_2, PCO_2, pH, base excess, standard bicarbonate).

EEG recordings, psychometric tests and evaluation of pulse, blood pressure and side effects were carried out at the 0, 1, 3, 5 and 7 h. Seventeen leads (Fp1, Fp2, F7, F3, F4, F8, T3, C3, Cz, C4, T4, T5, P3, P4, T6, O1 and O2 to averaged mastoids) were recorded on paper (Nihon Kohden 4317 F polygraph) and digitized off line by a Hewlett-Packard Vectra system with a sampling frequency of 102.4 Hz (Anderer et al. 1987; Saletu et al. 1987b). Spectral analysis from 0 to 35 Hz was performed using the fast Fourier transform technique resulting in 36 variables. The latter were processed into topographic maps utilizing a 64 × 64 numerical matrix. Each interpolated value was based on the cubic distance from the values at the three nearest electrodes. Differences in the distribution of particular EEG variables before and after drug administration were

---

[1] Bereich für Pharmakopsychiatrie, Psychiatrische Universitätsklinik, Währinger Gürtel 18–20, 1090 Wien, Austria

displayed by significance probability mapping (Duffy et al. 1981). Subsequently, the same method was utilized to demonstrate differences between drug-induced and placebo-induced alterations under hypoxia and normoxia (pharmaco-EEG images) (Saletu et al. 1987b).

Psychometric investigations included the measurement of noopsychic functions such as attention, concentration, attention variability, fine motor activity, numerical memory and reaction time performance, as well as of thymopsychic variables such as mood, drive, affect and sedation (Grünberger 1977).

Results

Blood Gas Analysis

Inhalation of the hypoxic gas mixture resulted in a drop of PO_2 from a pretreatment value of 95 mm Hg to 39 mm Hg after 14 min PO_2 remained stabile thereafter until the end of the recording session (39 mm Hg in the 23rd min) (Table 1). Changes in other blood gases are shown in Table 1. Moreover, blood gas alterations were identical in the recording sessions at 1, 3, 5 and 7 h.

Topographic EEG Changes

Absolute power of delta/theta activity increased under hypoxia/placebo as compared to normoxia/placebo all over the brain, but specifically over the left

Table 1. Stability of blood gases during a 23-min inhalation of a hypoxic gas mixture (9.8% O_2 90.2%, N_2)

Blood gases	Means (standard deviations)			Multiple Wilcoxon test
	A 0 min	B 14 min	C 23 min	
PO_2 (mm Hg)	96.0 (5.2)	39.3 (5.8)	39.2 (7.1)	A:B*; A:C**, B:C n.s.
PCO_2 (mm Hg)	37.7 (2.4)	32.4 (4.0)	32.4 (3.5)	A:B**; A:C**; B:C n.s.
pH	7.4 (0.0)	7.5 (0.0)	7.5 (0.1)	A:B**; A:C**; B:C n.s.
Base excess (nmol/l)	0.9 (1.1)	0.6 (0.8)	1.5 (2.5)	A:B*; A:C*; B:C n.s.
Standard bicarbonate (nmol/l)	24.1 (0.8)	24.8 (0.6)	25.5 (1.9)	A:B n.s.; A:C n.s.; B:C n.s.

* $p<0.05$; ** $p<0.01$ ($n=9$)

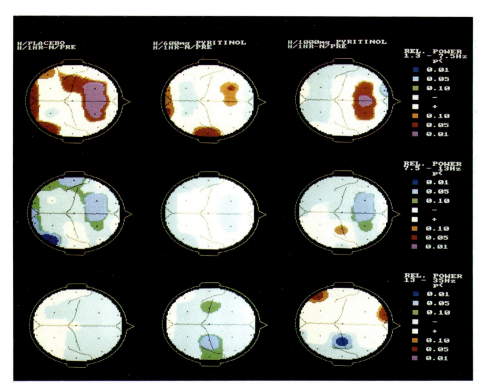

Fig. 1. Topographic EEG changes (relative power of delta/theta, alpha and beta activity) under hypoxia (*H*) (9.8% O_2) 1 h after placebo, 600 mg and 1000 mg pyritinol as compared with normoxia (*N*) (21% O_2) ($n = 12$). An eight-color scale shows differences between drug-induced and placebo-induced changes (based on *t* values expressed in *p* values): *dark blue*, decrease at $p < 0.01$; *light blue*, decrease at $p < 0.05$; *dark green*, decrease at $p < 0.1$; *light green*, trend toward decrease; *light yellow*, trend toward increase; *orange*, increase at $p < 0.1$; *red*, increase at $p < 0.05$; *lilac*, increased at $p < 0.01$. Under placebo/hypoxia conditions, delta/theta activity increases specifically over both F, the left C and O and the right O and OT regions, while alpha activity decreases. Doses of 600 and 1000 mg pyritinol attenuate these hypoxia-induced brain activity changes. There are no marked alterations in the beta band

occipital (O), parietal (P), temporal (T) and central (C) regions. The changes were most pronounced in the 1st and 7th h, while in the 3rd and 5th h differences between hypoxia and normoxia were smaller, obviously due to a spontaneously occurring decline in vigilance at noon and in the early afternoon. Doses of 600 mg and 1000 mg pyritinol attenuated the hypoxia-produced changes. One hour post 1000 mg pyritinol, slow activities tended even to decrease over the O and P regions. *Relative power of delta/theta activity* also demonstrated a significant increase under hypoxia/placebo as compared with normoxia/placebo, mostly over the frontal (F), the left C, both O and the right occipitotemporal (OT) regions (Fig. 1). In the 7th h i.e., at the end of the recording day, the hypoxia-induced augmentation of delta/theta activity was even more pro-

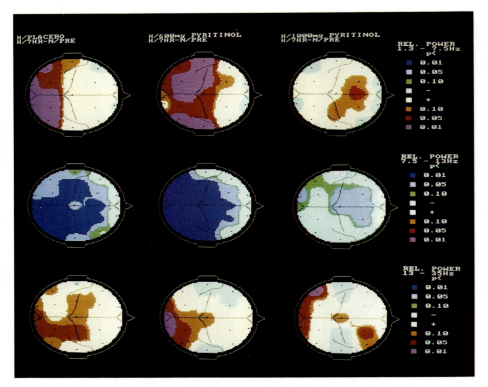

Fig. 2. Topographic EEG changes (relative power of the delta/theta, alpha and beta activity) under hypoxia (*H*) (9.8% O_2) 7h after placebo, 600 mg and 1000 mg pyritinol as compared with normoxia (*N*) (21% O_2) (*n* = 12). For color key see Fig. 1. Hypoxia induces 7 h after placebo a marked increase in delta/theta activity, decrease of alpha activity and increase of beta activity, which is attenuated at that late time only by the higher dosage of pyritinol (1000 mg)

nounced (Fig. 2). Doses of 600 mg and 1000 mg pyritinol attenuated the hypoxia-induced augmentation of slow activity.

Absolute alpha power showed only minor changes under hypoxia, such as an increase over both T and C regions and the vertex in the 1st h. However, in the 7th h there was a decrease over the right O and OT region. Under 600 mg pyritinol there were no significant differences from placebo, except for an alpha attenuation over the right O region. A dose of 1000 mg pyritinol significantly augmented alpha power over the left T region in the 1st, 3rd and 7th h. *Relative alpha power* demonstrated under hypoxia/placebo an attenuation over the left F and T regions as well as over the O and right OT regions (Fig. 1). At the end of the recording day this alpha attenuation was more pronounced and evident all over the brain, except the frontopolar (FP) and frontotemporal (FT) areas (Fig. 2). Pyritinol attenuated these hypoxia-induced changes markedly; in the 7th h this was best seen after the 1000 mg dosage.

Absolute beta power increased under hypoxia over the left T region and

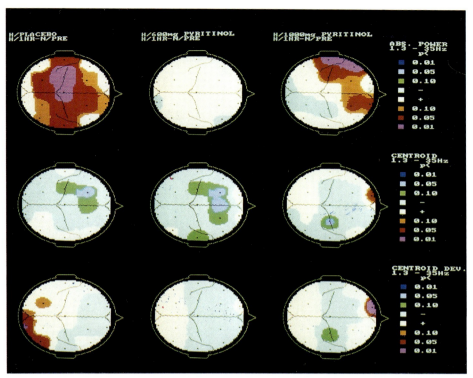

Fig. 3. Topographic EEE changes – total power, centroid and centroid deviation of total activity (1.3–35 Hz) – under hypoxia (H) (9.8% O_2) 1 h after placebo, 600 mg and 1000 mg pyritinol as compared with normoxia (N) (21% O_2) ($n=12$). For color key see Fig. 1. Hypoxia induces after placebo an increase in total power and the centroid deviation which is attenuated by pyritinol. The centroid itself shows only a slight decrease (slowing) over the F regions, which is blocked by 1000 mg pyritinol

the vertex in the 1st h and all over the brain in the 7th h. After 600 mg pyritinol there was an increase in the 1st and 7th h and an even greater increase in the 5th h. After 1000 mg pyritinol beta activity increased in the 1st h over both the FT and F regions, as well as over the left F, T, C, P and TO regions. In the 7th h beta activity was augmented all over the brain as compared with normoxia/placebo (except both T regions and the right C region). *Relative beta power* remained rather stabile in the initial hour of the recording day (Fig. 1), while in the 7th h there was an increase over the right O, P and C regions under hypoxia. After pyritinol there were only minor changes in the 1st h, characterized by a decrease over the right C region after 600 and 1000 mg pyritinol and an increase over the left FP and OT regions after the higher dosage. In the 7th h post 600 mg pyritinol, beta activity was increased over both O and the right P and OT regions (Fig. 2). After 1000 mg similar findings were observed with an additional increase of beta activity over the right F and left OT regions.

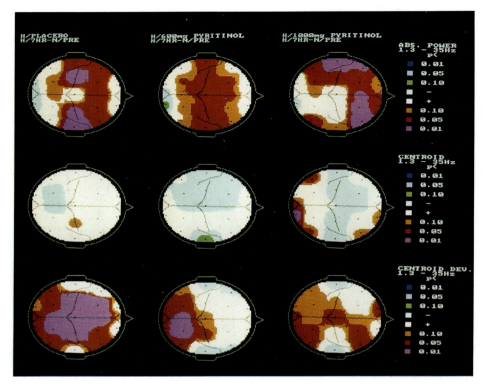

Fig. 4. Topographic EEG changes – total power, centroid and centroid deviation of total activity (1.3–35 Hz) – under hypoxia (H) (9.8% O_2) 7 h after placebo, 600 mg and 1000 mg pyritinol as compared with normoxia (N) (21% O_2) ($n=12$). For color key see Fig. 1. Hypoxia increases total power (absolute power in 1.3–35 Hz). This is attenuated slightly by 600 mg pyritinol, while 1000 mg even induces a slight increase due to its drug-specific effect. The centroid deviation is markedly increased under hypoxia after placebo, which is attenuated dose-dependently by pyritinol. The centroid itself is accelerated over the O and T areas after 1000 mg dose

Total power increased significantly under hypoxia as compared with normoxia over almost the whole brain. This increase was attenuated by 600 mg pyritinol in the 1st h (Fig. 3) as well as the 7th h (Fig. 4). After 1000 mg pyritinol an attenuation was seen in the 1st h, while in the 7th h there was a slight increase. Pyritinol under normoxic conditions augmented total power (Saletu et al. 1987b).

The *centroid of the total activity* slowed down under hypoxia/placebo. In contrast, there was an acceleration over the FP, O and OT regions after the administration of the higher dose of pyritinol (Figs. 3, 4). The latter may be regarded as a drug-specific effect, as we saw an acceleration of the centroid after pyritinol under normoxia (Saletu et al. 1987b).

The *centroid deviation of the total activity* increased markedly under hypoxia all over the brain in the 7th h. This increase was attenuated dose-dependently by pyritinol (Figs. 3, 4).

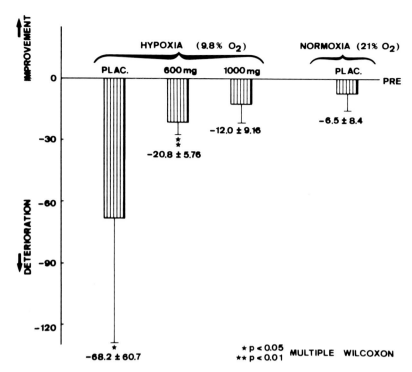

Fig. 5. Mental deterioration under hypoxia and normoxia after placebo and pyritinol based on changes (2–8 h post drug) in 13 psychometric variables (in % of baseline values, means ± SEM). After placebo, mental performance deteriorates under hypoxia by 68% of baseline values; after 600 mg and 1000 mg pyritinol, by only 2% and 12% respectively. The dose of 1000 mg pyritinol provides so much brain protection that there is no significant difference from normoxic pretreatment values

Psychometric Findings

Evaluation of the changes in all 13 psychometric variables obtained at all times demonstrated that mental performance deteriorated under hypoxia/placebo by 68% compared with baseline values. This deterioration was attenuated by 600 mg and 1000 mg to 21% and 12% respectively (Fig. 5). Under normoxia the performance decrement was 7%.

Conclusions

1. Utilizing topographic brain mapping of the EEG and psychometry, changes in human brain function and mental performance under hypoxic hypoxidosis were studied in a double-blind, placebo-controlled trial, as were antihypoxidotic properties of pyritinol.

2. Hypoxic hypoxidosis was induced by a fixed gas combination of 9.8% O_2 and 90.2% N_2 – equivalent to 6000 m altitude – which was inhaled for 23 min under normobaric conditions by 12 healthy volunteers. After an adaptation session they received, randomized at weekly intervals, placebo under hypoxia and nor moxia as well as 600 mg and 1000 mg pyritinol under hypoxia. Evaluation of blood gases, O-EEG recording and psychometry were carried out at 0, 1, 3, 5 and 7 h after oral drug administration.

3. Blood gas analysis demonstrated a drop in PO_2 from 95 to 39 and 39 mm Hg in the 14th and the 23rd min of inhalation respectively. PCO_2 also decreased (from 38 to 35 and 33 mm Hg), while pH increased (from 7.39 to 7.45 and 7.46). Base excess showed only minor changes in the 23rd min, while standard bicarbonate remained unchanged.

4. Topographic brain mapping of the EEG exhibited under hypoxia an increase of delta/theta activities, decrease of alpha activity and inconsistent changes in beta activity, as well as a slowing of the centroid, an increase in total power and centroid deviation as compared with normoxia. These changes indicate a deterioration in vigilance. Doses of 600 mg and 1000 mg pyritinol attenuated these hypoxia-induced brain dysfunctions. In the 7th h post drug, however, only the 1000 mg dosage provided protection.

5. Psychometric data added further evidence for antihypoxidotic/nootropic properties of pyritinol. Psychometric performance under hypoxia deteriorated by 68% after placebo, while after 600 mg and 1000 mg pyritinol the decrease was only 21% and 12% respectively. Under normoxia/placebo the performance decrement was 7%.

References

Anderer P, Saletu B, Kinsperger K, Semlitsch H (1987) Topographic brain mapping of EEG in neuropsychopharmacology. Part I: methodological aspects. Methods Find Exp Clin Pharmacol 9(6): 371–384

Duffy FH, Bartels PH, Burchfield JK (1981) Significance probability mapping: An aid in the topographic analysis of brain electrical activity. Electroencephalogr Clin Neurophysiol 51: 455–462

Grünberger J (1977) Psychodiagnostik des Alkoholkranken. Ein methodischer Beitrag zur Bestimmung der Organizität in der Psychiatrie. Maudrich, Vienna

Saletu B, Grünberger J (1983) Cerebral hypoxic hypoxidosis: neurophysiological, psychometric and pharmacotherapeutic aspects. Adv Biol Psychiatr 13: 146–164

Saletu B, Grünberger J (1984) The hypoxia model in human psychopharmacology: neurophysiological and psychometric studies with aniracetam iv Hum Neurobiol 3: 171–182

Saletu B, Grünberger J, Anderer P, Sieghart W (1986) Comparative bioavailability studies with a new mixed-micelles solution of diazepam utilizing radioreceptor assay, psychometry and Q-EEG imaging. Clin Neuropharmacol 9(4): 532

Saletu B, Grünberger J, Anderer P (1987a) Proof an antihypoxidotic properties of tenilsetam by quantitative EEG and psychometric studies in experimental hypoxic hypoxidosis. Drug Dev Res 10: 135–155

Saletu B, Anderer P, Kinsperger K, Semlitsch H (1987b) Topographic brain mapping of EEG in neuropsychopharmacology. Part II: clinical applications (pharmaco-EEG imaging). Methods Find Exp Clin Pharmacol 9(6): 385–408

Section VII   Magnetoencephalographic Aspects

Cortical Auditory Evoked Magnetic Fields: Mapping of Time and Frequency Domain Aspects*

M. Hoke, K. Lehnertz, B. Lütkenhöner, und C. Pantev[1]

Introduction

Less than a decade has passed since the auditory evoked magnetic field was first described by Reite et al. (1978). Since then, not only auditory evoked magnetic fields, but also magnetic fields evoked by stimuli of different sensory modalities as well as endogenous and motor fields have been studied, not to mention spontaneous brain magnetic activity as recorded in the magnetoencephalogram (MEG), the magnetic complement of the electroencephalogram (EEG). Before dealing with brain magnetic activity, one important question to be posed is whether, why and to what extent mapping of brain magnetic fields is superior to mapping of brain electric potentials. Basically, biomagnetic fields and bioelectric potentials have the same source, are generated by the same (populations of) current dipoles and thus reflect the same physiological processes. The decisive difference is that the electric potential distribution over the surface of the scalp is brought about by *volume* currents flowing in the conductive medium of the head from the source to the sink of the individual dipole generators, whereas the radial magnetic field component measurable outside the head is essentially generated by the *intracellular* ("impressed") current flowing within the dipole. At least for spherical bodies – and the head is a rough approximation of a sphere – volume currents do not contribute to the radial magnetic field component outside the skull, nor do secondary sources originating at boundaries between media of different conductivity. Furthermore, the propagation of volume currents is considerably distorted by the anisotropic tissues of brain, skull and scalp, whereas all tissues are "transparent" to a magnetic field provided its frequency is below the kilohertz range. Hence it follows that the spatial resolution of biomagnetic fields is superior to that of bioelectric potentials. A further advantage is that, unlike EEG measurements, there is no need for a reference electrode. However, the advantages of magnetic field measurements are counterweighted in part by one essential shortcoming: In a spherical body, only the tangential component of a current dipole gives rise to a (radial) magnetic field measurable outside (Grynszpan and Geselowitz 1973). There are two major implications of this: The more radial the dipole is oriented, or the closer the dipole is located to the center of the sphere, the smaller is the field which can be measured outside the body, i.e., deep sources are difficult or impossible to detect.

---

* This work has been supported by grants from the Deutsche Forschungsgemeinschaft and the Heinrich-Hertz-Stiftung.

[1] Institut für Experimentelle Audiologie der Westfälischen Wilhelms-Universität Münster, Kardinal-von-Galen-Ring 10, 4400 Münster, Federal Republic of Germany

Similar to evoked potentials, evoked magnetic fields can be distinguished from the background MEG only if a population of neural generators in the brain, lying closely together and, to a large extent, oriented in parallel fashion in space, are simultaneously brought to discharge. The single current dipoles representing the intracellular current flow in the dendrites of the individual neurons can then be regarded in terms of a so-called equivalent current dipole (ECD) which is the vectorial integral of all individual dipoles and is located in the "center of gravity" of the excited neuronal population. We know from histological studies as well as from evoked potential studies that this prerequisite is met for most of the nuclei and fiber tracts of the primary auditory pathway. With respect to cortical evoked responses, sources of neural activity seem to be ensembles of dipolar current sources oriented parallel to each other and perpendicular to the cortical surface (Okada 1983). If the activated cortical area happens to be located in a sulcus, then the main ECD component is lying tangential to the surface of the skull. That this is obviously true for the auditory cortex was recently demonstrated by Scherg and von Cramon (1986), who applied dipole localization methods (DLM) to the scalp distribution of auditory evoked potentials and described the slow cortical auditory evoked potential in terms of tangential and radial dipole source components. (DLM are mathematical procedures which, under certain limiting assumptions, allow localization of a dipole in a body by approximating a calculated surface distribution of electric potentials or magnetic fields to the observed one.) One major outcome of their study is that the main dipole component is the tangential one which is, as mentioned above, a prerequisite for neuromagnetic measurements. It can be concluded, therefore, that magnetic field measurements are a powerful instrument for studying neural activity, both spontaneous and evoked, of the human cortex.

Characteristic Features of the Auditory Evoked Magnetic Field

Auditory stimuli evoke a magnetic field which is maximal at both ends of the Sylvian fissure. The field distribution resembles that of a current dipole, located 20–40 mm below the scalp and oriented almost perpendicular to the Sylvian fissure (e.g., Hari et al. 1980; Elberling et al. 1980; Elberling et al. 1982; Aittoniemi et al. 1981). The waveform of the magnetic response is basically similar to that of the simultaneously recorded electric potential (Hari et al. 1980), apart from a polarity reversal to both sides of a line coinciding with the surface projection of the dipole. (Due to the polarity reversal, a different terminology is used to designate the response components: the magnetic equivalent of the electric wave N1, or N100, is referred to as M100, that of the electric wave P2, or P200, as M200.) The location of the ECD in the superior-inferior direction shows only little dependence on stimulus parameters or on the hemisphere measured. In contrast, the side of stimulation highly influences not only the ECD location in the anterior-posterior direction but also the strength of the magnetic field: the ECD is located approximately 14 mm more posteriorly over the *left* hemisphere if the contralateral ear is stimulated (the difference is less pronounced with ipsilateral stimulation), and the dipole moment is generally stronger over the *left* hemisphere rather than over the right one (e.g., Elberling et al. 1981; Arlinger et al. 1982; Pantev et al. 1986c). This, however, is true only for right-handed subjects. As was demonstrated by Hoke (1985, 1988), the reverse is true in left-handed subjects: The dipole is located approximately 14 mm more posteriorly over the *right* hemisphere, and the ECD moment is stronger over the *right* hemisphere. Independent of right- or left-handedness, contralateral stimulation produces stronger fields than ipsilateral or binaural stimulation does, and the 100-ms component occurs approximately 9 ms earlier with contralateral stimulation than with ipsilateral stimulation (e.g., Elberling et al. 1980, 1981; Pantev et al. 1986c; Reite et al. 1981). Needless to say, these hemispheric differences should be considered when neuromagnetic studies are planned.

Time Domain Aspects: Key to the Functional Organization of the Auditory Cortex

The application of DLM to the scalp distribution of the auditory evoked magnetic field allows inferences about the location of the underlying neural processes, if some limiting assumptions are made. The necessary assumptions which constitute a model used to solve the inverse problem can be divided into two categories: (a) assumptions concerning the geometry of the head and its physical properties ("head model"), and (b) assumptions concerning the primary current sources within the neural generators ("source model"). Basically, assumptions of the first category cause less severe difficulties. Simple models which allow an analytical solution can be satisfactorily used, e.g., a semi-infinite volume model for the (fairly plane) temporal region (as in this case) or a sphere model for the (more spherically shaped) frontal or occipital regions. (The real shape of the head could be accounted for by using more realistic head models, e.g., boundary element models). More difficulties are encountered in the second category. The most commonly used assumption is that of a single ECD, though there are strong indications that an ECD does not describe the real situation. Much emphasis should be put on this issue because the conclusions drawn in the following stand and fall with the validity of the model. Our results of dipole localization emphasize that the single ECD model is obviously not an adequate description for all components of the auditory evoked response ("waves"), but it seems to produce satisfactory results in the case of wave M100.

If ECD localizations can be made with sufficiently high accuracy, as it seems in the case of wave M100, then auditory evoked magnetic fields will play a key role in the study of the functional organization of the human auditory cortex. Functional organization implies that structural elements are arranged in space according to that stimulus parameter to which they respond best. This may be stimulus frequency ("best" or "characteristic" frequency, CF), stimulus intensity ("best" or "characteristic" intensity) or any other stimulus parameter.

Basics of Stimulation, Data Collection and Processing

Before dealing with special aspects of the functional organization, a brief outline shall be given of the technique of stimulation, data collection and data processing which has been published elsewhere in great detail (Pantev et al. 1986a–c). Subjects were four normal-hearing, paid volunteers, two of whom were right-handed and two left-handed. To obtain maximum possible field amplitudes, the left hemisphere was investigated in right-handed subjects and vice versa, using contralateral stimulation with tone bursts with a duration of 500 ms and rise/decay times of 15 ms. To study the frequency dependence, the carrier frequency of the tone burst was varied between 250 and 4000 Hz in octave steps with the intensity kept constant at 60 dB HL, while the intensity dependence was studied with 1000 Hz tone-bursts whose intensity was varied between 30 and 80 dB HL in 10-dB steps. Measurements were carried out in an electrically, but not magnetically shielded room. The radial field component of the evoked field was measured at 50–60 positions over the scalp using a single-channel SQUID (BTi) equipped with a second-order gradiometer. Partial averages or individual responses were stored in a Prime computer system. Off-line data processing consisted in compilation of data matrices for each sampling instant from corresponding samples recorded at each position. These matrices served to generate isocontour plots after interpolation and filtering as well as to calculate the ECD parameters, including the goodness of fit, from which time func-

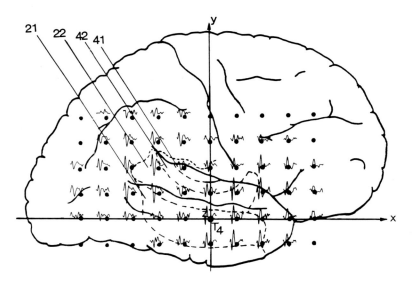

Fig. 1. Matrix of sampling positions (reference position T4), projected onto the contours of the supralateral surface of the right cerebral hemisphere. The auditory area AI (Brodmann areas 41 and 42) and the secondary auditory area AII (Brodmann areas 21 and 22) are indicated. Waveforms of an exemplary set of raw data are inserted on top of the respective sampling positions

tions were composed and plotted. Figure 1 shows a synopsis of raw data projected onto a lateral view of the head, from which the polarity reversal becomes evident.

Tonotopic Organization

Tonotopic organization is present as peripheral as at the cochlear level. Even before the mechanoelectric transduction takes place, the sound signal – conducted to the inner ear with equal group delay – undergoes a remarkable spatiotemporal dispersion: It gives rise to a travelling wave which assumes an amplitude maximum at a place whose distance from the stapes depends on frequency. High-frequency components of the sound signal are represented at the beginning, lower ones at the end of the cochlear partition, and the scale of this "tonotopic" representation is a logarithmic one. In this way, *frequency* information is encoded as *place* information at the cochlear level. Closely related to this spatial dispersion is a temporal dispersion caused by the different travel time which increases exponentially with increasing distance from the stapes. But not only frequency determines the representation of a sound signal along the cochlear partition, it is also influenced by the intensity of the sound signal in a highly nonlinear manner: the excitation spreads with higher intensity in basal direction, recruiting additional nerve fibers (with higher CF) into the active population (Green 1976), which again is an expression of a place mechanism.

Hence it has been intriguing to investigate to what extent such place mechanisms can be traced throughout the central auditory pathways. Place mechanisms in frequency coding have been considered for more than a century. The idea of a tonotopic organization was conceived long before physiological measurements could be done. It is as old as the renowned hearing theory of Helmholtz (from 1862) according to which radial fibers of the basilar membrane in the cochlea form a set of resonators, like the strings of a piano. Though this resonance theory was later superseded by more sophisticated hearing theories, one principle remained unchallenged – the place principle. This is, of course, not sufficient to explain all pitch sensations, e.g., that of complex tones, but physiological research – from G. von Békésy (1928) to S.M. Khanna (1982) – have safely established the basis for the tonotopy at the cochlear level: the mechanics of the cochlea. Microelectrode studies gave further evidence that the tonotopic organization is maintained in different nuclei and fiber tracts of the central auditory pathway (Harrison and Howe 1974), and this is even true for the primary auditory cortex as was established in several experimental animal species, e.g., for the monkey (Merzenich and Brugge 1973), the squirrel (Merzenich et al. 1976) and the cat (Merzenich et al. 1975).

But investigations in humans failed. Celesia (1976) who recorded auditory evoked responses from the exposed human cortex during neurosurgery could not find significant differences between responses to tone bursts of 600 and 1000 Hz. Neuromagnetic measurements done by Elberling et al. (1982, tone-

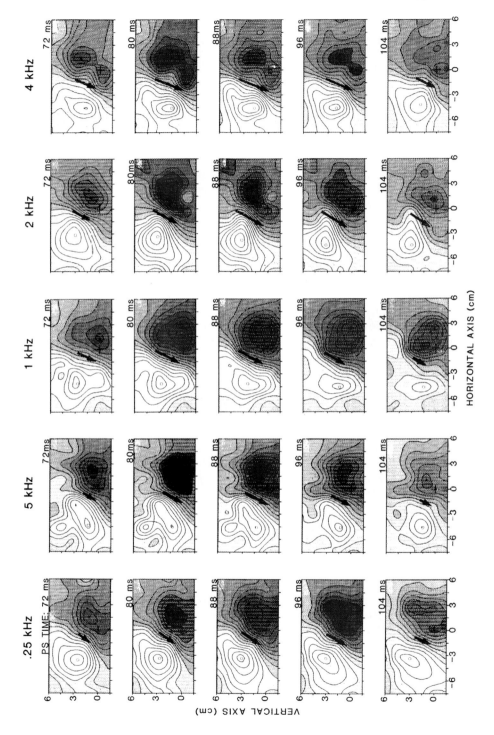

burst stimulation) and Romani et al. (1982, steady-state stimulation) gave first evidence of a tonotopic organization of the human auditory cortex.

The tone burst evoked field distribution depends on both time elapsing since stimulus onset and stimulus frequency (Pantev et al. 1987). However, time slices (Figs. 2 and 3) taken around the maxima of waves M100 and M200 for all frequencies investigated are more likely to visualize common features than to quantify the effect of both variables.

Temporal aspects of the ECD parameters become evident from their time functions (Fig. 4). Except for the angle, there is obviously different behavior of the ECD parameters of the two waves. In the case of wave M100, the position in the tangential plane remains fairly constant around the maximum of the dipole moment, for most frequencies also the depth. In the case of wave M200, however, we find a certain systematic change with time of the position in the tangential plane, while no systematic behavior can be detected with respect to depth. With the sole exception of the angle of the ECD, the functions do not coincide with each other, which indicates that the location of the ECD not only varies with time but also differs for different frequencies. As to be expected, the goodness of fit is highest around the maxima of the dipole moment.

The influence of stimulus frequency becomes more obvious when the ECD parameters of both waves are plotted as a function of frequency (Fig. 5). This was done for those times when the ECD moment assumes a maximum, because a maximal dipole moment implies a maximum of neural excitation and the most favorable signal-to-noise ratio. Furthermore, the high goodness of fit at those moments also indicates a high correspondence of the observed field distribution with that of a single current dipole. A general observation is that the data of wave M100 are more consistent than those of the later wave M200, which exhibit more pronounced interindividual variability. The dipole moment of wave M100 changes only gradually with frequency. The mean is virtually constant, independent of frequency, except at the lowest test frequency investigated, where it is slightly diminished. This suggests that, independent of test frequency, approximately the same number of neurons was excited. The data of the dipole moment computed for wave M200 are less consistent, but again the mean does not show a significant frequency dependence. The functions obtained for the dipole angle do not show a systematic frequency dependence, either for wave M100 or for wave M200. The interindividual variability would be basically similar for both waves if there were not one case with a distinct smaller angle for wave M200.

◁───

Fig. 2. Isofield contour maps computed for five test frequencies at five consecutive instants around wave M100 (time elapsed since stimulus onset is inserted on top of each map). Field strength encoded by a gray scale (spacing between isocontour lines 40fT; *darker areas:* outward-going flux; *brighter areas:* inward going flux). *Heavy line:* zero field strength; *cross:* reference position of the sampling matrix (corresponding to T3/T4); *arrow:* location and direction of the equivalent current dipole in the tangential plane, with length proportional to the dipole moment (length of arrowhead: 10 nAm)

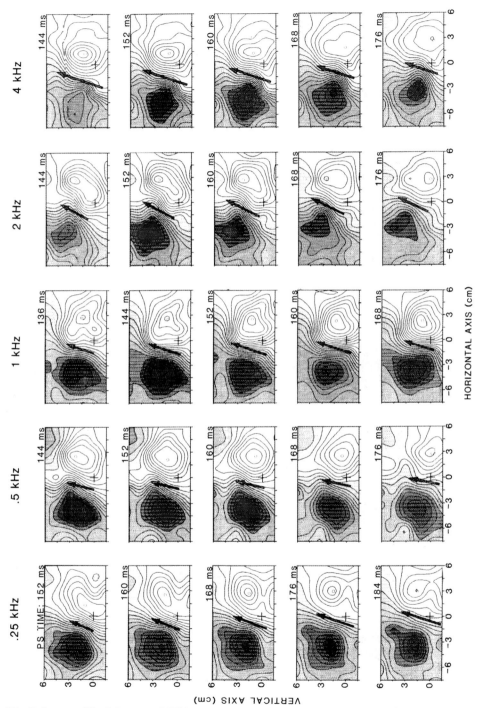

Fig. 3. Same as Fig. 2 for wave M200

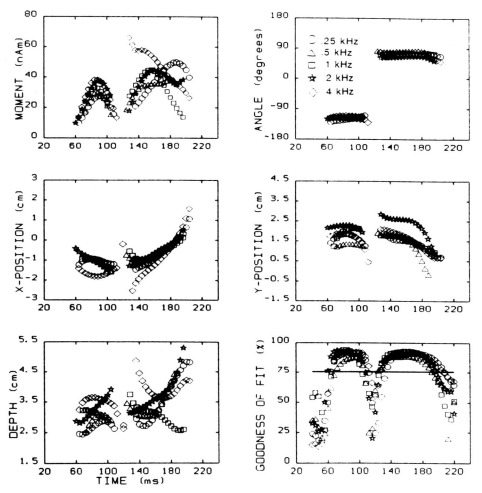

Fig. 4. Time dependence of ECD parameters and of the goodness of fit. The functions were obtained from data of one representative subject. Nonsignificant parts of the functions where the goodness of fit was less than 75% were omitted. Different symbols were used to distinguish between different subjects

With respect to the projection of the dipole locations onto the tangential plane, the x–y coordinates of both waves (M100 and M200) form circumscribed clusters in each subject, though they scatter a little more for wave M200. If the frequency is increased from 250 to 4000 Hz the mean x position of wave M100 is shifted in posterior direction by approximately 6 mm while no significant shift was observed in superior-inferior direction. The values of depth calculated for wave M100 are very consistent with negligible interindividual variability, and show an almost pure logarithmic dependence on frequency, but this is not the case with wave M200, which exhibits pronounced deviation from a logarithmic function as well as distinct interindividual variability.

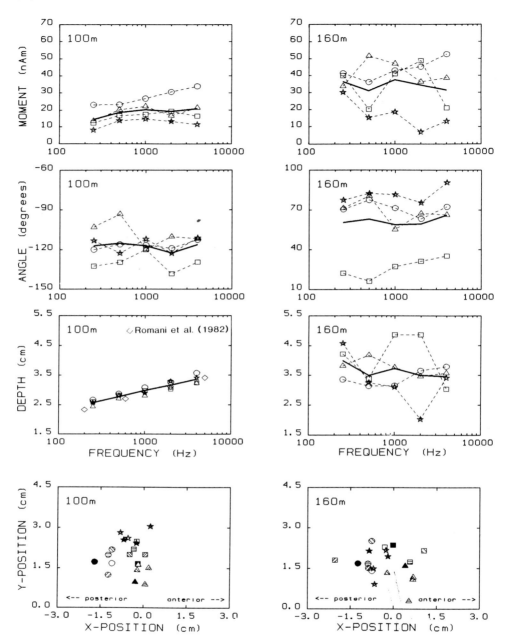

Fig. 5. Dependence on frequency of dipole moment (*top row*), angle (*second row*), depth (*third row*) and location in the tangential plane (*bottom row*) of the equivalent current dipole, computed for waves M100 (*left column*) and M200 (*right column*). Different symbols and different patterns are used to distinguish between different frequencies and subjects

If we compare the location in space of waves M100 and M200, we find no significant difference of the x coordinates, but wave M200 is found to be located 3 mm inferior to (t-test for paired data: $p<0.03$) and 6 mm deeper than ($p<0.01$) wave M100.

The data obtained in our tonotopy study obviously support the existence of a tonotopic organization of the human auditory cortex, at least as far as wave M100 is concerned. They are also in excellent agreement with data previously reported by Romani et al. (1982a, 1982b) and Elberling (1982). As Fig. 5 shows (third row, left panel), the values obtained by Romani et al. (1982) for the depth of the ECD location of the steady-state response practically coincide with those obtained in our study for wave M100 of the transient response. We also observed a similar mean horizontal shift of the ECD location of wave M100, as did Elberling et al. (1982) in their study. The similarity of results derived from steady-state and transient responses allows the hypothesis that the major contribution to the steady-state response originates from the same source as wave M100, but the significant differences between the y and z coordinates of waves M100 and M200 components point to a different source for the later component. The estimated location in space of wave M100 corresponds fairly well with that of the temporal transverse gyri (Heschl) as revealed by concomitant anatomical preparations. The estimated location in space of wave M200 may point to a slightly more medial aspect of the Heschl gyri, but in view of their greater variability this conclusion should be considered with care.

Amplitopic Organization

Less attention has been paid so far to place mechanisms for intensity coding. Phillips et al. (1985) recently detected cells in the AI cerebral cortex of the cat and the monkey displaying nonmonotonic rate-vs-intensity functions. The most effective stimulus intensity differed from one cell to the next, i.e., similar to the best frequency there is an intensity to which the cells respond best. Changing the sound pressure level results in a shift in the active neuronal population such that many neurons once maximally active become less so, while others marginally active or unresponsive are brought to maximal response (Brugge and Merzenich 1973). This finding inevitably leads to the hypothesis of a place mechanism of intensity coding which has not been tested yet in either cat or monkey. However, evidence for an "amplitopic organization" has been obtained for the primary auditory cortex of the mustache bat (Suga 1977).

Unlike the influence of stimulus frequency, the effect of changing stimulus intensity becomes obvious from the isocontour maps computed for both waves M100 and M200 (Fig. 6). Especially clear are the increase of the ECD moment and the shift of the ECD location in the tangential plane with increasing stimulus intensity (Pantev et al. 1988a–c).

Temporal changes of the ECD parameter and of the goodness of fit are shown in the time functions of Fig. 7, exemplary for a stimulus intensity of 40 dB HL. Noteworthy is that the values of all dipole parameters remain fairly

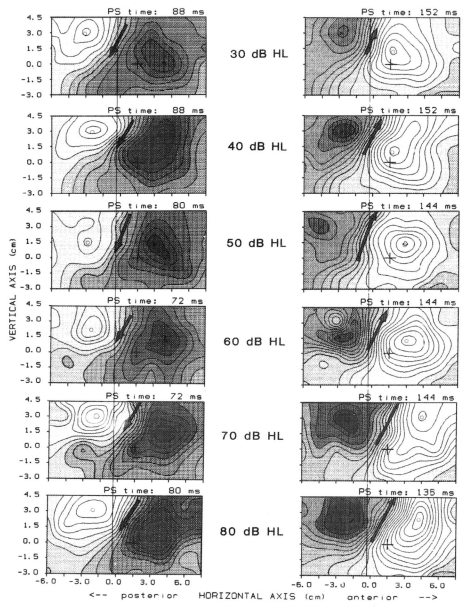

Fig. 6. Dependence of the magnetic field distribution on intensity. Isofield contour maps for all stimulus intensities are reproduced for those instants (inserted on top of each map) when the moment of the equivalent current dipole assumes a maximum. The *vertical line* was inserted for better visualization of the shift of the ECD location

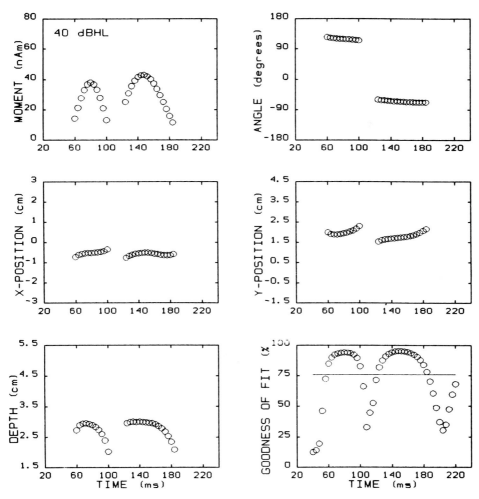

Fig. 7. Time dependence of the ECD parameters and of the goodness of fit, computed for a stimulus intensity of 40 dB HL. Nonsignificant parts of the functions where the goodness of fit was less than 75% were omitted

constant around the maxima of both components, and that even at such a low stimulus intensity the goodness of fit exceeds 90% around the maxima.

The influence of stimulus intensity is shown in Fig. 8. Unlike the influence of stimulus frequency, we generally find a systematic behavior of all dipole parameters of wave M100 but not of all parameters of wave M200. The dipole moment of both waves increases with increasing stimulus intensity assuming a maximum at 50–60 dB HL, and then diminishes. The function of the dipole angle of wave M100 also deviates from a monotonic course: it is maximal at 50 dB HL and diminishes with increasing and decreasing stimulus intensities except for a slight increase at 30 dB HL. The dipole angle of wave M200 does

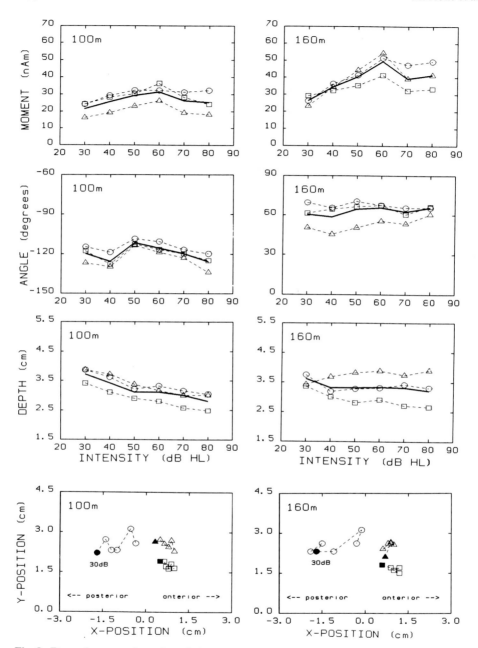

Fig. 8. Dependence on intensity of the ECD moment (*top row*), angle (*second row*), depth (*third row*) and location in the tangential plane (*bottom row*), computed for waves M100 (*left column*) and M200 (*right column*). Different symbols are used to distinguish between different subjects. *Filled symbols:* lowest intensity of 30 dB HL

not show a significant dependence on intensity. The depth of wave M100 decreases almost linearly with increasing stimulus intensity, whereas the depth of wave M200 does not show any systematic change. The ECD location of both waves is shifted with increasing stimulus intensity in anterior direction (on average 8 mm for wave M100 and 7 mm for wave M200), but this again is more obvious for wave M100. No significant intensity-related shift in superior-inferior direction could be observed for either wave.

The most intriguing finding of this study, which has never been described before and which was consistently observed in all subjects investigated, is the influence of stimulus intensity on the depth of the ECD location of wave M100. The higher the stimulus intensity, the more superficial is the cortical excitation. This goes along with an anterior shift of the ECD location with increasing intensity. This result can be interpreted in terms of an amplitopic organization of the auditory cortex, as was hypothesized by Brugge and Reale (1985): the place of maximal excitation moves along an isofrequency line whose existence has been well established in animal studies.

The amplitopic organization is obviously different from the tonotopic organization, and this is best demonstrated by the dependence of the depth of the ECD on stimulus frequency. While the depth *increases* with increasing stimulus *frequency*, it *decreases* with increasing stimulus *intensity*. This implies that the cortical mechanism of intensity coding is quite different to the peripheral one. The cochlear excitation pattern spreads with increasing intensity in basal direction, i.e., increasingly more neurons with higher CF are recruited into the active population. If the cortical representation of intensity was also cochleotypical, the ECD location would move towards the place of higher frequency, i.e., the depth would increase with higher stimulus intensity. This is definitely not the case: the depth increases with increasing stimulus intensity. Our data do not suggest that the place of maximal excitation is shifted towards lower frequencies, since the displacement in horizontal direction is also opposite to that induced by an increase in stimulus frequency. Rather, they suggest that the cortical representation of frequency and intensity is bidimensional, i.e., an isointensity line exists for each frequency just as an isofrequency line exists for each intensity. Isofrequency lines and isointensity lines form two sets of parallel trajectories crossing each other.

Another most interesting finding is the behavior of the ECD moment of both waves, which agrees with the data of Reite et al. (1981) as well as with our previous data (Pantev et al. 1986b). Though it is speculative, the nonmonotonic intensity function of the dipole moment can be explained with an ECD location approaching the edge of a sulcus so that the ECD orientation changes from tangential to radial. This implies that the only dipole component measurable outside the skull, the tangential dipole component, becomes increasingly smaller due to the dipole rotation, though the overall vector of the dipole continues to increase.

Single Equivalent Current Dipole Assumption Revisited

Our results emphasize that it is dangerous to regard the goodness of fit between observed and theoretical field distribution as sole indication of tenability of a single dipole assumption. The dipole parameters obtained in the tonotopy study behave fairly consistently around the first peak, but not around the second peak at 160 ms. Some parameters, especially the dipole coordinates, change dramatically with time, but the high goodness of fit still mediates the impression that the calculated location would not be subject to large errors.

Examination of the frequency or intensity dependence of specified ECD parameters gives a different view of the validity of data. If we look at the influence of frequency on the depth of wave M100, we observe a result which is physiologically and anatomically meaningful: the monotonic, almost logarithmic dependence of the depth on frequency reveals the established tonotopic organization of the auditory cortex. On the other hand, the exceptionally high interindividual differences obtained for wave M200 raise doubts about the applicability of a single ECD model.

Similar findings were obtained in the amplitopy study. Again we find a sufficiently high goodness of fit for both waves, and the dipole parameter change only gradually around the maxima of both peaks. But only the depth of the first wave shows clear dependence on intensity and systematic behavior in all subjects which is the first clear-cut neuromagnetic evidence of an amplitopic organization of the human auditory cortex. This also indicates that the results are physiologically and anatomically meaningful.

Hence, one common aspect of the results of both the tonotopy study and the amplitopy study is that the single ECD model seems to give satisfactory results for wave M100 but obviously fails to do so in the case of wave M200. Various explanations are possible for the unsatisfactory results: not one, but multiple dipoles may be active simultaneously, the excitation in the population forming the ECD may propagate slowly (Særmark 1988), or several dipoles may be activated subsequently (spatiotemporal dipole model, Scherg and von Cramon 1986). Especially the spatiotemporal dipole model of Scherg and von Cramon is very intriguing and seems to be supported by our data. Figure 9 shows in a kind of slow-motion picture the transition in field distribution between waves M100 and M200. The area of outward-going flux (darker area) is continuously present during the transition between the maxima of both waves, but it is monotonically shifted to that place where previously the area of inward-going flux was located. While the area of outward-going flux is shifted, the area of inward-going flux vanishes and a new one occurs at the place previously occupied by that of outward-going flux. The same phenomenon can be observed during the transition between waves M200 and M250 (Fig. 10). Again we find a monotonic shift of the area of outward-going flux, while that of inward-going flux ceases to exist and a new one emerges. This slow-motion picture reveals that a single ECD model be a permissible assumption for times around the maximum of the first peak, but possibly not for the second one, and definitely not for the time of transition, and the finding suggests the need to reanalyze the data with a spatiotemporal model, which still remains to be done.

Cortical Auditory Evoked Magnetic Fields

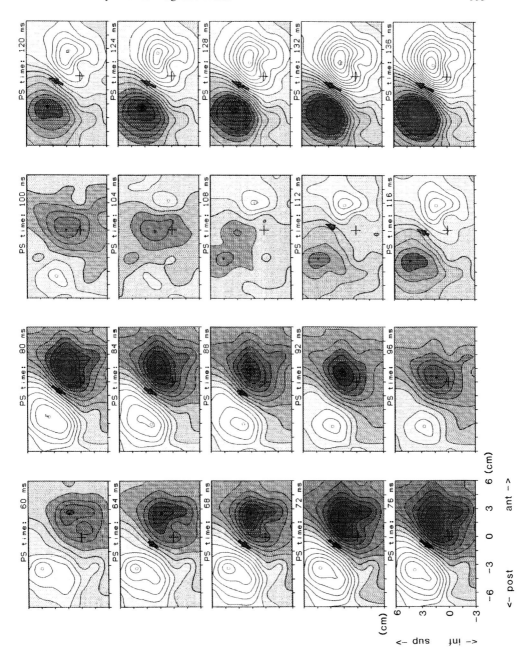

Fig. 9. Transition of the field distribution between the maxima of wave M100 and M200. The area of outward-going flux, though becoming smaller, does not cease to exist at the time of polarity reversal but is continuously shifted from its old position (maximum of wave M100) to its new one (maximum of wave M200). For full explanation, refer to the legend of Fig. 2

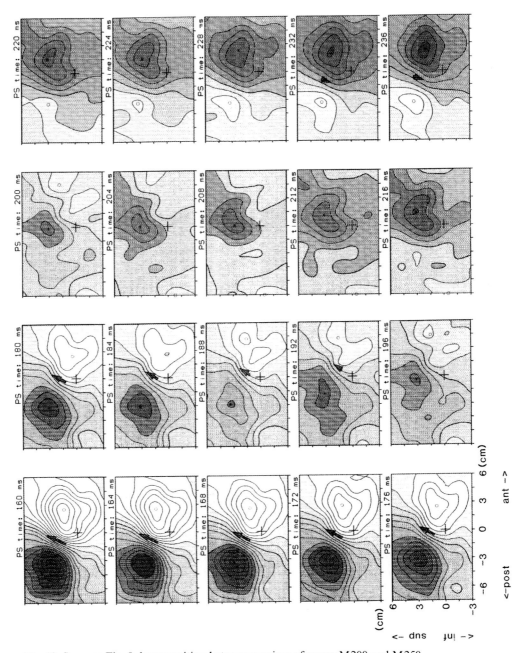

Fig. 10. Same as Fig. 9, but transition between maxima of waves M200 and M250

Frequency Domain Aspects: Phase Coherence

The relations between ongoing EEG and evoked potentials (EP) have been studied in numerous investigations. Sayers et al. (1974a, b, 1979) found that phase constraints, derived from a response to a high-level stimulus, imposed on the Fourier harmonics of the background EEG can produce a typical auditory EP (AEP). They concluded that AEP are due to a recordering of the phases in each realization of the background EEG due to the stimulus rather than to the evoking of a response which is *additive* to the background EEG. Phase recordering was found to increase with stimulus intensity. The effect of the evoking stimulus can be imagined in terms of triggering or synchronizing a set of harmonic oscillators tuned to the same frequency. The conclusion of Sayers et al. was supported by the finding that the energy content of the prestimulus EEG is the same as that of the EP. Beagley et al. (1979) later found indications that, at high stimulus levels, additive energy can be observed. Jervis et al. (1983) applied several different statistics to ensembles of pre- and poststimulus EEG epochs and found that all the EP studied contained additive energy in at least one harmonic component. Başar (1980, 1983a, b) and Başar et al. (1976a, b) most vividly compared the phasor representation of neuronal population activity with that of elementary magnets in para- and ferromagnetic substances. The higher the entropy, the higher is the effect of magnetization, or, in terms of neurophysiology, the degree of synchronization of neural elements which may be regarded as relaxation oscillators. The external stimulus was claimed to push the spontaneous, fluctuating, incoherent electric activity of the brain into the coherent state of a single harmonic oscillator for a coherence time after which fluctuations set in again.

Since MEG measurements permit much higher spatial resolution than do EEG recordings, it seemed natural also to study the spatial distribution over the scalp of coherent neural activity evoked by auditory stimuli and to compare it with the distribution of the auditory evoked magnetic field at the same times. Since the procedures of data processing are being published in detail elsewhere (Hoke et al. 1988), they will be reported only in outline here. An overlapping short-time spectral analysis was applied to the ensembles of stimulus-related epochs by moving a Hanning window (160 ms, padded with zeros yielding a 256-ms time window) over the individual epochs (duration 1024 ms, sampling interval 4 ms). A limitation of this procedure results from the uncertainty principle, which implies that better spectral resolution (longer Hanning window) decreases the temporal resolution. Methods of directional statistics (Mardia 1972) were then applied to the phase angles of the Fourier components in order to obtain the circular variance for each Fourier component in the frequency range below 20 Hz. For each Fourier component we then compiled time functions of the mean spectral amplitude and of the complement of the circular variance to 1, which is a direct measure of interepochal *phase coherence*. The time functions of phase coherence and mean amplitude were used to compile, for all instants every 4 ms (corresponding to the sampling interval), data matrices containing the respective values from all sampling positions, from which isocontour plots were generated.

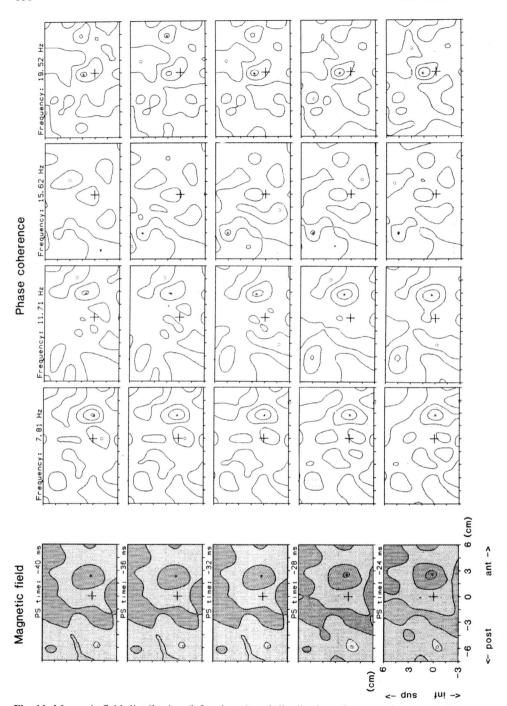

Fig. 11. Magnetic field distribution (left column) and distribution of phase coherence (column 2 to 5) of the 2nd to 5th Fourier component for time slices taken approx. 40 ms before stimulus onset (inserted on top of each map). Dark (columns 2 to 5): higher coherence

Cortical Auditory Evoked Magnetic Fields

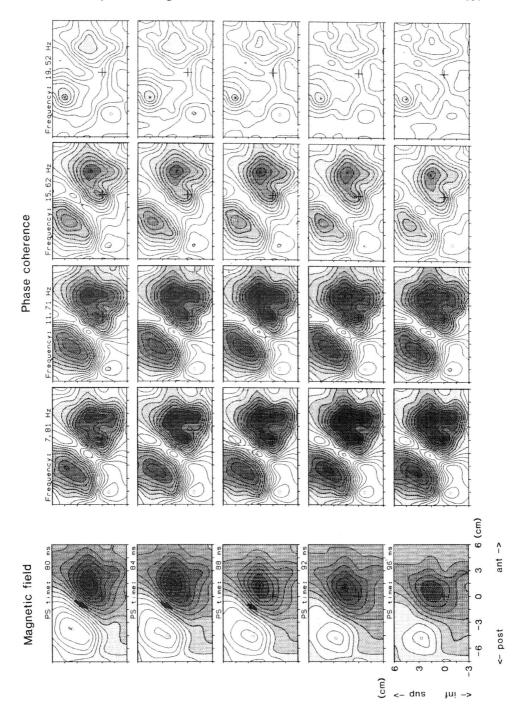

Fig. 12. Same as Fig. 11, but time slices around the maximum of wave M100

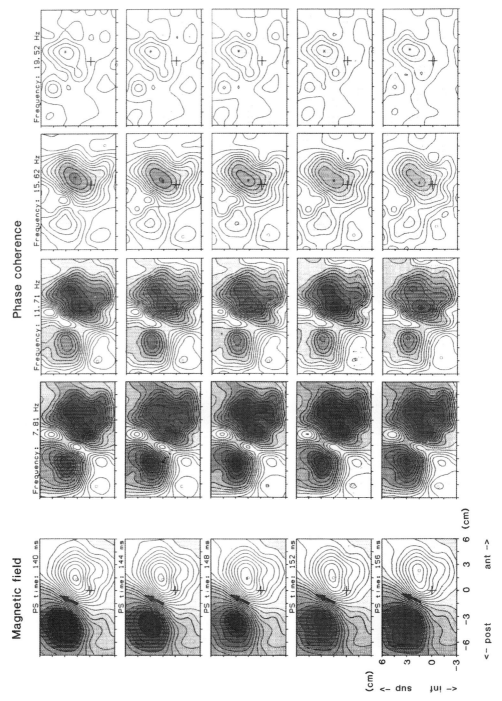

Fig. 13. Same as Fig. 11, but time slices around the maximum of wave M200

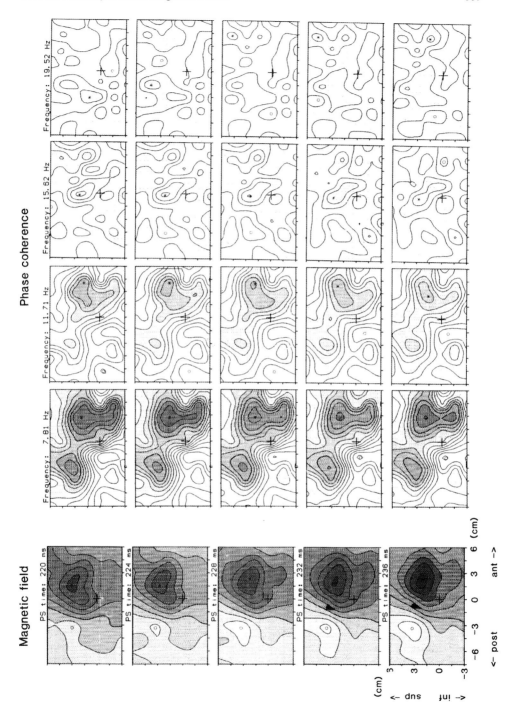

Fig. 14. Same as Fig. 11, but time slices around the maximum of wave M250

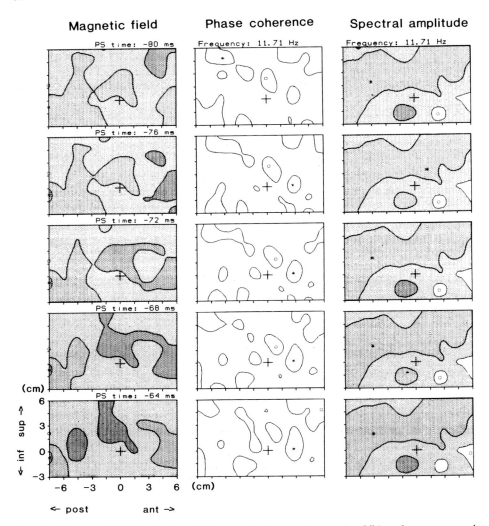

Fig. 15. Magnetic field distribution (*left column*), phase coherence (*middle*) and mean spectral amplitude (*right column*) calculated for the third Fourier component. Five time slices taken approximately 80 ms before stimulus onset are reproduced. Nothing than noise can be detected in all distributions

The instantaneous distribution of phase coherence of the second to fifth Fourier components is compared with the distribution of the evoked magnetic field in Figs. 11–14. (It should be emphasized that the change in the distribution of phase coherence is smoother than the respective change in the field distribution, since the Hanning window exerts a smoothing influence on the results.) Time slices calculated for five successive prestimulus times are reproduced in Fig. 11. The only regularity both in the field distribution and in that of the second Fourier component may be due to the periodic stimulation employed

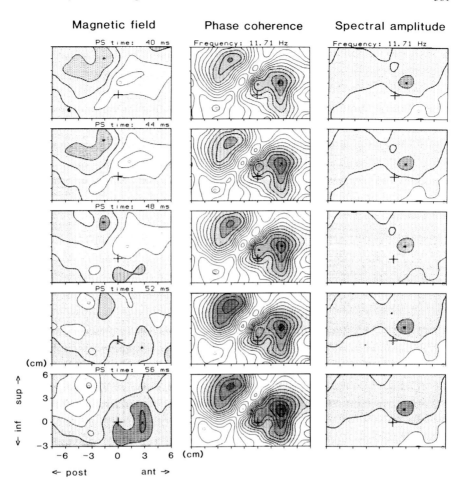

Fig. 16. Magnetic field distribution (*left column*), phase coherence (*middle*) and mean spectral amplitude (*right column*) calculated for the third Fourier component. Five time slices taken approximately 40 ms after stimulus onset are reproduced. While the amplitude distribution does not significantly differ from that reproduced in Fig. 15 (prestimulus times), the phase coherence maps show a clear-cut pattern of high coherence

(expectancy wave). Around the maximum of wave M100 (Fig. 12), the distribution of phase coherence is basically similar to that of the magnetic field. The second Fourier component exhibits the strongest phase coherence. It is noteworthy that the shape of the areas of higher coherence is not as circular as would be expected from a dipolar source; rather, they show an indentation. A deformation of these areas is also evident around the peak of wave M200 (Fig. 13). It is also plain that the contribution of the two higher Fourier components becomes smaller as time elapses. Around wave M250 (Fig. 14), there are no more contributions from the two higher Fourier components, and the shape of the areas of higher coherence (corresponding to those of outward-going flux) again deviates from a circular one.

As mentioned before, the evoking stimulus is thought to cause two effects: generating additive energy (= triggering additional discharges) and reordering the phases (= synchronizing spontaneous discharges). The second effect is generally present while the first one may be missing, e.g., in specified Fourier components and at lower stimulus intensities. This phenomenon is illustrated in Figs. 15 and 16, in which the magnetic field distribution, the distribution of the mean spectral amplitude of the third Fourier component and that of the phase coherence of the same Fourier component are compared. Before stimulus onset (Fig. 15), every representation contains background noise only. However, 40 ms after stimulus onset (Fig. 16) some areas exhibit clear-cut phase recordering, though the spectral amplitude does not deviate from the noise level.

Conclusions: Power and Pitfalls of Neuromagnetic Measurements

The results presented here demonstrate both the power and the pitfalls of neuromagnetic measurements. It has been shown that neuromagnetic measurements are a powerful research instrument: they gave the first evidence of an amplitopic organization of the human auditory cortex, and were the first technique to allow study of the spatiotemporal aspects of synergetic processes of the human brain. The nonmonotonic intensity function of the magnitude of the ECD moment, however, revealed a strong limitation of neuromagnetic measurements: only tangential dipole components can be detected outside the head. We are convinced that, if used to answer the right questions, neuromagnetic studies will continue to be an indispensable tool for basic research and will become equally indispensable also for clinical applications (Hoke 1988b). One potential clinical application, not only for audiology but also for neurology, is the use of evoked magnetic field measurements to calculate the magnitude of the ECD moment, which allows estimation of the number of excitable neurons, which is difficult to assess from evoked potential measurements.

Acknowledgements. Part of this material was first published by the Advisory Group for Aerospace Research and Development, North Atlantic Treaty Organization (AGARD/NATO) in the Proceedings No. 432 of the AGARD Workshop "Electric and Magnetic Activity of the Central Nervous System: Research and Clinical Applications in Aerospace Medicine." (1988), AGARD, pp. 11-1–11-12

References

Aittoniemi K, Hari R, Järvinen ML, Katila T, Varpula T (1981) Localization of neural generators underlying auditory evoked magnetic fields of the human brain. In: Erné SN, Hahlbohm HD, Lübbig H (eds) Biomagnetism. de Gruyter, Berlin, pp 463–472

Arlinger S, Elberling C, Bak C, Kofoed B, Lebech J, Særmark K (1982) Cortical magnetic fields evoked by frequency glides of a continuous tone. Electroencephalogr Clin Neurophysiol 54:642–653

Başar E (1980) EEG-Brain dynamics: relation between EEG and brain evoked potentials. Elsevier/North-Holland, Amsterdam

Başar E (1983a) Synergetics of neuronal populations. A survey on experiments. In: Başar E, Flohr H, Haken H, Mandell AJ (eds) Synergetics of the brain. Springer, Berlin Heidelberg New York, pp 183–200

Başar E (1983b) Toward a physical approach to integrative physiology. I. Brain dynamics and physical causality. Am J Physiol 244:510–533

Başar E, Gönder A, Ungan P (1976a) Important relation between EEG and brain evoked potentials. I. Resonance phenomena in subdural structures of the cat brain. Biol Cybern 25:27–40

Başar E, Gönder A, Ungan P (1976b) Important relation between EEG and brain evoked potentials. II. A systems analysis of electrical signals from the human brain. Biol Cybern 25:41–48

Beagley HA, Sayers BM, Ross JA (1979) Fully objective ERA by phase spectral analysis. Acta Otolaryngol (Stockh) 87:270–278

Békésy G von (1928) Zur Theorie des Hörens. Die Schwingungsform der Basilarmembran. Phys Z 29:793–810

Brugge JF, Merzenich MM (1973) Patterns of activity of single neurons of the auditory cortex in monkey. In: Møller AR (ed) Basic mechanisms of hearing. Academic, New York, pp 745–772

Brugge JF, Reale RA (1985) Auditory cortex. In: Peters A, Jones EG (eds) Cerebral cortex, vol 4. Plenum, New York, pp 229–271

Celesia GG (1976) Organization of auditory cortical areas in man. Brain 99:403–414

Elberling C, Bak C, Kofoed B, Lebech J, Særmark K (1980) Auditory magnetic fields from the human brain. Scand Audiol 9:185–190

Elberling C, Bak C, Kofoed B, Lebech J, Særmark K (1981) Auditory magnetic fields from the human cortex: influence of stimulus intensity. Scand Audiol 10:203–207

Elberling C, Bak C, Kofoed B, Lebech J, Særmark K (1982) Auditory magnetic fields. Source location and "tonotopical organization" in the right hemisphere of the human brain. Scand Audiol 11:61–65

Green DM (1976) An introduction to hearing. Erlbaum, Hillsdale

Grynszpan F, Geselowitz DB (1973) Model studies of the magnetocardiogram. Biophys J 13:911–926

Hari R, Aittoniemi M, Järvinen ML, Katila T, Varpula T (1980) Auditory evoked transient and sustained magnetic fields of the human brain. Exp Brain Res 40:237–240

Harrison JM, Howe ME (1974) Anatomy of the afferent auditory nervous system of mammals. In: Keidel WD, Neff WD (eds) Auditory system. Springer, Berlin Heidelberg New York, pp 283–336 (Handbook of sensory physiologie, vol 5/1)

Hoke M (1985) Auditory evoked magnetic fields. Paper presented at the First International Conference on Dynamics of cognitive and sensory processing in the brain, 18–22 August 1985, Berlin

Hoke M (1988a) Auditory-evoked magnetic fields. In: Başar E (ed) Dynamics of sensory and cognitive processing by the brain. Springer, Berlin Heidelberg New York Tokyo, pp. 311–318

Hoke M (1988b) SQID-based measuring techniques – A challenge for the functional diagnostics in medicine. In: Kramer B (ed) The Art of Precise Measurement in Physics and Medicine. Verlag Chemie, Weinheim, pp. 287–335

Hoke M, Lehnertz K, Lütkenhöner B, Pantev C (1988) Spatial distribution of auditory evoked neural activity over the scalp. In: Başar E, Bullock Th (eds) Dynamics of cognitive and sensory processing in the brain. Springer, Berlin Heidelberg New York Tokyo (in press)

Jervis BW, Nichols MJ, Johnson TE, Allen E, Hudson NR (1983) A fundamental investigation of the composition of auditory evoked potentials. IEEE Trans Biomed Eng 30:43–49

Khanna SM, Leonard DBG (1982) Basilar membrane tuning in the cat cochlea. Science 215:305–306

Mardia KV (1972) Statistics of directional data. Academic, London

Merzenich MM, Brugge JF (1973) Representation of the cochlear partition on the superior temporal plane of the macaque monkey. Brain Res 50:275–296

Merzenich MM, Knight PL, Roth GL (1975) Representation of the cochlea within the primary auditory cortex in cat. J Neurophysiol 38:231–249

Merzenich MM, Kaas JH, Roth GL (1976) Auditory cortex in the grey squirrel: tonotopic organisation and architectonic fields. J Comp Neurol 166:387–401

Okada Y (1983) Auditory evoked field. In: Williamson SJ, Romani GL, Kaufman L, Modena I (eds) Biomagnetism: an interdisciplinary approach. NATO ASI Series. Plenum, New York, pp 433–442

Pantev C, Hoke M, Lehnertz K (1986a) Randomized data acquisition paradigm for the measurements of auditory evoked magnetic fields. Acta Otolaryngol [Suppl] (Stockh) 431:21–25

Pantev C, Hoke M, Lütkenhöner B, Lehnertz K, Spittka J (1986b) Causes of differences in the input-output characteristics of simultaneously recorded auditory evoked magnetic fields and potentials. Audiology 25:263–276

Pantev C, Lütkenhöner B, Hoke M, Lehnertz K (1986c) Comparison between simultaneously recorded auditory-evoked magnetic fields and potentials elicited by ipsilateral, contralateral and binaural toneburst stimulation. Audiology 25:54–61

Pantev C, Hoke M, Lehnertz K, Lütkenhöner B, Anogianakis G, Wittkowski W (1988a) Tonotopic organisation of the human auditory cortex revealed by transient auditory evoked magnetic fields. Electroencephalogr Clin Neurophysiol 69:160–170

Pantev C, Hoke M, Lehnertz K, Lütkenhöner C (1988b) Neuromagnetic evidence of an amplitopic organization of the human auditory cortex. Electroencephalogr Clin Neurophysiol (in press)

Pantev C, Hoke M, Lütkenhöner C, Lehnertz K (1988c) Influence of stimulus intensity on the location of the equivalent current dipole in the human auditory cortex. In: Atsumi K, Kotani M, Ueno S, Katila T, Williamson SJ (eds) Biomagnetism '87. Denki University Press, Tokyo, pp 210–213

Phillips DP, Orman SS, Musicant AD, Wilson GF (1985) Neurons in the cat's primary auditory cortex distinguished by their responses to tones and wide-spectrum noise. Hear Res 18:73–87

Reite M, Edrich S, Zimmerman JT, Zimmerman JE (1978) Human magnetic auditory evoked fields. Electroencephalogr Clin Neurophysiol 41:114–117

Reite M, Zimmerman JT, Zimmerman JE (1981) Magnetic auditory evoked fields: interhemispheric asymmetry. Electroencephalogr Clin Neurophysiol 41:388–392

Romani GL, Williamson SJ, Kaufman L, Brenner D (1982) Characterization of the human auditory cortex by the neuromagnetic method. Exp Brain Res 47:381–393

Særmark K (1987) Magnetic fields from the auditory cortex. In: Basar E (ed) Dynamics of cognitive and sensory processing in the brain. Springer, Berlin Heidelberg New York (in press)

Sayers BMcA, Beagley HA (1974a) Objective evaluation of auditory evoked EEG responses. Nature 251:608–609

Sayers BMcA, Beagley HA, Henshall WR (1974b) Objective evaluation of auditory evoked EEG responses. Nature 247:481–483

Sayers BMcA, Beagley HA, Riha J (1979) Pattern analysis of auditory-evoked EEG potentials. Audiology 18:1–16

Scherg M, von Cramon D (1986) Evoked dipole source potentials of the human auditory cortex. Electroencephalogr Clin Neurophysiol 65:344–360

Suga N (1977) Amplitude spectrum representation in the Doppler-shifted-CF processing area of the auditory cortex of the mustache bat. Science 196:64–67

Mapping of MEG Amplitude Spectra: Its Significance for the Diagnosis of Focal Epilepsy

C.E. ELGER[1], M. HOKE[2], K. LEHNERTZ[2], C. PANTEV[2], B. LÜTKENHÖNER[2], P.A. ANNINOS[3], and G. ANOGIANAKIS[4]

Introduction

An epileptic seizure is a paroxysmal disturbance of brain function resulting from highly synchronized pathological activities of groups of neurons. The epileptic event is characterized by typical clinical phenomena, normally accompanied by characteristic, steeply rising field potentials of high amplitude which can be picked up by surface electroencephalogram (EEG) recordings. However, several experimental and clinical studies have clearly demonstrated that epileptiform potentials in the surface EEG do not necessarily reflect epileptic events in deeper cortical layers or brain structures (Elger and Speckmann 1983; Wieser 1983). This holds true especially for epileptic foci in the limbic system, which most often give rise to a pharmacoresistant temporal lobe epilepsy (Wieser 1983).

The surgical therapy of pharmacoresistant focal epilepsies, especially of temporal lobe epilepsy, is meanwhile accepted and successful worldwide. An indispensable prerequisite for a surgical intervention, however, is precise knowledge about the location of the primary epileptic focus. This presurgical evaluation of epileptic patients referred to surgery is commonly performed using invasive techniques like electrocorticography, depth electrode recording or foramen ovale recording (cf. Wieser and Elger 1987). These interventions are not without risk for the patient and are very expensive and time-consuming. Metabolic imaging techniques like PET and SPECT, indicating the focal area in terms of a region of hypometabolism, have not fulfilled the hope that they would reliably localize the focus in the more difficult cases referred to surgery (cf. Engel 1987; Wieser and Elger 1987).

As shown by Hoke et al. (this volume), measurements of magnetic fields permit higher spatial resolution than can be achieved with electric potential measurements. This implies that for localizing epileptic foci in the depth of the cerebrum, the magnetic counterpart of the EEG, the magnetoencephalogram (MEG), should be superior to surface EEG recordings. The attempt to localize the primary epileptic focus in the interictal interval is therefore one of the greatest challenges for neuromagnetism.

Since the introduction of superconducting quantum interference device (SQUID) magnetic field sensors, a number of attempts have been made to

---
[1] Clinic of Neurology and Epilepsy, University of Bonn, Federal Republic of Germany
[2] Institute of Experimental Audiology, University of Münster, Federal Republic of Germany
[3] Department of Physiology, University of Thessaloniki, Greece
[4] Department of Neurology, University of Thraki, Greece

localize the epileptic focus. Barth et al. (1982, 1984) mapped the magnetic field distribution after averaging a sufficient number of interictal spikes triggered by the EEG in patients mainly suffering from focal (partial) seizures, with the focus mainly located in the temporal or frontotemporal region. Mapping at successive instants revealed, in some cases, the existence of two sequential equivalent magnetic sources. Sato et al. (1985) computed field maps from manually-selected individual spikes in one patient with partial complex seizures, and found a dipolar source located in the right temporal area. Another technique, developed by Chapman et al. (1983, 1984) and later confirmed by Ricci et al. (1985), consists in mapping a statistical quantity, the relative covariance between the magnetic signal and the simultaneously recorded electric signal. Using a single-dipole-in-a-sphere model, the authors found satisfactory results for central, parietal and occipital locations, but the results were questionable for frontal locations and incorrect for source locations in the temporal region.

The latter fact would be fatal if surgical interventions were planned on the basis of incorrect localizations. Sutherling et al. (1985) noted that pitfalls like these usually arise from the inverse problem, an explanation also given by Ricci et al. (1985). We believe that the inverse problem is not the major source of error. Rather, we believe that a single dipole model is not appropriate for epileptic activity, for the following reasons:

1. An epileptic focus generates different types of epileptic activity the occurrence of which is unpredictable. The pattern may be a spike, a sharp wave or a spike-wave complex. All patterns may occur singularly or in trains.
2. The brain area generating a single epileptic discharge is varying and different neuronal populations may contribute to a single epileptic pattern, most of them with a *similar* field potential.
3. The synchronized action potentials of "epileptic" neurons discharging with high frequency give rise to synchronized projected synaptic activity, resulting in a number of new current dipoles.
4. The interictal activity is known to be of localizing value only in a very limited number of epileptic patients. Whether this is due to problems inherent in field potential recordings or is based on the epileptic process itself is an unanswered question.

These difficulties led us to test an alternative approach, namely use of the MEG for the presurgical evaluation of epileptic patients. Instead of studying the surface distribution of the time domain MEG, we chose to investigate the surface distribution of frequency domain aspects of the interictal MEG. Our hypothesis was that the surface distribution of spectral energy in specified frequency bands would exhibit patterns specific for specified locations or primary epileptic foci, patterns which would not be present in normal subjects. If correlation of a specified pattern with the (invasively determined) location of an epileptic focus could be established, an "atlas" of typical cortical projections of interictal epileptic activity would be extremely helpful in planning the strategy of presurgical invasive evaluation of epileptic patients, reducing the investigation time and the risk for the patient.

Methods

The method used has been described in detail elsewhere (Hohe et al. 1988). In brief, 32 MEG epochs of 1024 ms duration were recorded from each of up to 70 sampling positions in temporal and frontal regions with a second-order gradiometer coupled to a single-channel DC SQUID (BTi). Measurements were carried out in a magnetically unshielded environment (noise level approximately 30–50 $fT/\sqrt{Hz}$). The data were stored on a computer hard disk after filtering and analog/digital conversion, and averaged amplitude spectra were calculated off line for each sampling position. Isocontour maps displaying areas of equal spectral amplitude (iso-SA maps) were then calculated for specified frequency bands chosen according to those used in the conventional EEG (compound delta/theta band: 2–7 Hz; alpha band: 8–13 Hz; beta band: 14–25 Hz). So far, 22 patients suffering from temporal or frontal lobe epilepsy and four normal subjects have been investigated. The majority of the patients suffered from drug-resistant temporal or frontal lobe epilepsy and underwent thorough epileptologic investigation (sphenoidal electrodes, but no invasive methods).

Results

Figure 1 shows typical results obtained in one normal subject and one epileptic patient. In normal subjects, the spontaneous MEG activity exhibits an amplitude spectrum similar to that of the conventional EEG. While in occipital recordings high amplitudes are found in the alpha band, only low activity is found in other cortical regions. The delta/theta and beta bands do not show accumulations of spectral energy. The iso-SA maps in epileptic patients, however, are significantly different: Alpha activity is generally less pronounced. The iso-SA maps computed for the compound delta/theta range (2–7 Hz), however, show distinct accumulations of spectral energy and steep gradients over temporal or frontal regions of the scanned surface of the scalp. The beta band is again uncharacteristic. Comparison of the localization of the presumed epileptic focus as determined by conventional methods with the location of the accumulation of spectral energy in the iso-SA maps of the MEG showed sufficiently good coincidence in quite a high proportion of cases.

In order to test whether the isocontour maps exhibit a constant pattern, repeated measurements were performed in several patients. A typical result is shown in Fig. 2, from which two phenomena are obvious. Firstly, the recorded patterns are obviously stable over time at the site of the presumed epileptic focus. Though data acquisition for one map was performed sequentially at different sampling positions (single-channel SQUID) and measurements were done on different days at different times of day, the calculated iso-SA maps are very similar: the patterns of the iso-SA maps do not change, accumulations of the spectral energy in the delta/theta band occur over the same brain area. Secondly the iso-SA map of the brain area contralateral to the epileptic focus

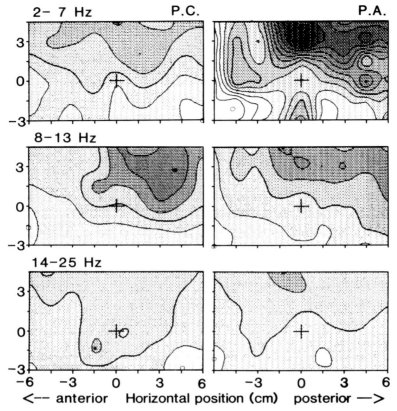

Fig. 1. Iso-SA maps (left temporal region) of a normal subject (P.C., *left*) and an epileptic patient (P.A., *right*) computed for different frequency bands. Spectral amplitudes are encoded using a gray scale. Areas between isocontour lines are shaded according to spectral amplitude. *Darker* areas designate higher amplitudes, *brighter* ones lower amplitudes. The *cross* indicates the origin of the sampling matrix (T3)

also shows some accumulation of spectral energy, but the follow-up recording yields a different pattern, indicating that no stable activity is generated in this brain area.

Conclusions

The technique for analysis of spectral features of the MEG presented here differs from previous approaches insofar as no dipole localization is attempted (cf. Barth et al. 1982, 1984; Ricci et al. 1985; Sato et al. 1985; Sutherling et al. 1985). It is not intended to solve the inverse problem, so no model assumptions have to be made. We rather postulate that there exist, in the iso-SA maps,

Mapping of MEG Amplitude Spectra

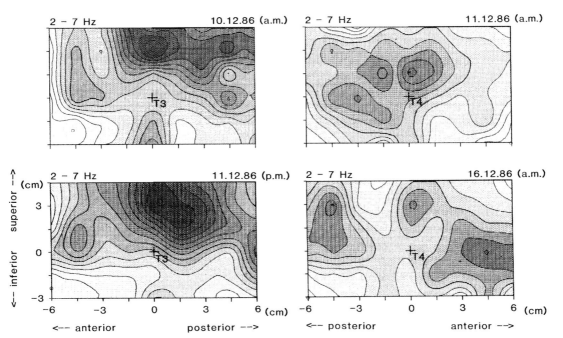

Fig. 2. Reproducibility of measurements: iso-SA maps measured on different days at different times of day (left and right temporal region, frequency band 2–7 Hz) of a patient (P.A.) suffering from pharmacoresistant focal epilepsy of left temporal origin

typical patterns of low-frequency spectral activity (2–7 Hz band) which are characteristic of specified locations of primary epileptic foci. These patterns are assumed to represent cortical projections of such foci located in deeper brain structures. Follow-up studies revealed that the patterns are stable over time, i.e., the long-term MEG activity in the interictal interval can be assumed to be quasi-stationary. We expect that an "atlas" of typical patterns of cortical projections of primary epileptic foci (localized precisely using invasive techniques) would be extremely helpful for precise planning of the strategy of presurgical invasive evaluation in patients suffering from pharmacoresistant epilepsy. The technique described also seems useful for control of long-term antiepileptic medication.

References

Barth DS, Sutherling W, Engel J Jr, Beatty J (1982) Neuromagnetic localization of epileptic spike activity in the human brain. Science 218:891–894

Barth DS, Sutherling W, Engel J Jr, Beatty J (1984) Neuromagnetic evidence of spatially distributed sources underlying epileptic spikes in the human brain. Science 223:293–296

Chapman RM, Romani GL, Barbanera S, Leoni R, Modena I, Ricci GB, Campitelli F (1983) SQUID instrumentation and the relative covariance method for magnetic 3D localization of pathological cerebral sources. Lett Nuovo Cimento 38:549–554

Chapman RM, Ilmoniemi RJ, Barbarena S, Romani GL (1984) Selective localization of alpha activity with neuromagnetic measurements. Electroencephalogr Clin Neurophysiol 58:569–572

Elger CE, Speckmann E-J (1983) Penicillin-induced epileptic foci in the motor cortex: vertical inhibition. Electroencephalogr Clin Neurophysiol 56:604–622

Engel J Jr (1987) Surgical treatment of the epilepsies. Raven, New York

Hoke M, Elger CE, Lehnertz K, Pantev C, Lütkenhöner B, Anogianakis G, Anninos P (1988) Epileptic activity analyzed by two-dimensional spectral analysis of MEG data. In: Atsumi K, Kotani M, Ueno S, Katila T, Williamson SJ (eds) Biomagnetism '87. Denki University Press, Tokyo, pp. 210–213

Ricci GB, Leoni R, Romani GL, Campitelli F, Buonomo S, Modena I (1985) 3-D neuromagnetic localization of sources of interictal activity in cases of focal epilepsy. In: Weinberg H, Stroink G, Katila T (eds) Biomagnetism: applications and theory. Pergamon, New York, pp 304–310

Sato S, Douglas R, Roger P (1985) Single magnetic spike mapping. In: Weinberg H, Stroink G, Katila T (eds) Biomagnetism: applications and theory. Pergamon, New York, pp 261–265

Sutherling W, Barth DS, Beatty J (1985) Magnetic fields of epileptic spike foci: equivalent localization and propagation. In: Weinberg H, Stroink G, Katila T (eds) Biomagnetism: applications and theory. Pergamon, New York, pp 249–260

Wieser HG (1983) Electroclinical features of the psychomotor seizure. Fischer, Stuttgart/Butterworth, London

Wieser HG, Elger CE (eds) (1987) Presurgical evaluation of epileptics. Springer, Berlin Heidelberg New York

Subject Index

abnormality
- detection 29ff.
- non-normal distribution 30

adaptive segmentation 72
Addison's disease 285
adrenocorticotropine 285
AEP 29, 458
- age dependent alterations 460
- brainstem 256
- click 20
- magnetic field 555, 537

aging 219
- pathological 220
- physiological 214

alcohol 26, 101
alcuronium 259
algorithm 6, 35, 197
aliasing 121, 130
alpha blocking 136
alpha rhythm 12
- attenuation response (AAR) 311
- blocking 136, 303
- power 137
- time locked 35

Alzheimer's disease 37, 233, 461–464
amblitopic organization 547, 562
amblyopia 201
amplifier 13, 147
amygdala 417, 422, 458, 472
analog-to-digital converter 129, 131
analysis of variance (ANOVA) 66, 99, 285, 442
anergic-anhedonic syndrome 518
anterior cerebral artery 97
anteriorization 233
antidepressive drugs 259, 485
- imipramine 485
antihypoxidotics 489
aphasia 16
apraxia 168
arachnoid cyste 469
area display technique 366
arecoline 518
artifact 4, 20, 28, 31, 131
- control 9
- electrode 4, 8
- eye blink 4, 8, 31

- eye movement 4, 8, 31, 34
- muscle 4, 6, 8, 31
- removal 8

attentional disturbances 424
autonomic orienting response 422

back ground activity 20
- alpha 16
- beta 16
- delta 16
- theta 16

background noise 36
band pass filtering 5
barbiturate 482
baseline 56, 60
Bavatron 14
behavioral studies 118
benzodiazepines 259
Bereitschaftspotential (BP) 314, 324
Binswanger's disease 236
bioavailability 482, 492
bioequipotency 492
blindness 176
"blink holidays" 9, 31
blood gas analyses 527
brachial plexus 81
brain 265
- infarction 265
- tumor 265, 273, 278
- - astrocytoma 279
- - ependymoma 279
- - glioblastoma 279

brain electrical activity mapping (BEAM) 22, 327
brain mapping 12, 15, 73
- imaging 15
brainstem auditory evoked potentials (BAEP) 194, 256, 407
brainstem generator 82
Brief Cognitive Rating Scale (BPRS) 242, 461
bulbocavernosus reflex 412
burst suppression 259, 262
buzzer 121

calcarine fissure 341
calibration 7, 147

carbamazepine 176
carotid artery 95
– stenosis 187
carrier waves 125
Carrol Scale 475
cartographie du sommeil lent d'après-midi 329
cartography 19, 329
– dream 329
– sleep 329
– wakefullness 329
cartoon 329
cartooned images 21
center of gravity 538
central nervous system (CNS) 11
cerebral blood flow 278
cerebrovascular diseases 94, 185
checkerboard 63, 64
check-size 404
chlorpromazine equivalent 459
cholinergic-adrenergic-balance hypothesis 518
cholinergic overactivity 518
choppy activity 507
chromophobia 28
"closed field" system 77
cocain
cognitive evaluation 90
– function 326
– impairment 219
– paradigms VI
– task 159
cognitive SEP components 86
– VEP components 337
coherence mapping 451
collodium 31
color graphics 5, 23
coma 26, 192
computed axial tomography (CT) 15, 124, 183, 278, 423
computer VI
contingent negative variation (CNV) 37, 311, 324
contour lines 55
– plots 363
corneal reflex 262
corpus callosum 424
cortex 383
– primary somatosensory 383
cortical activation 153
covariance 153, 298
– normalized 298
craniopharyngeome 400
cranioscopy 11
Creutzfeldt-Jacob's disease 239
cross correlation 152
– function 345

data reduction 65, 136
DC baseline 37
deglitching 32
delusion 425
dementia 168, 219
– degenerative 223
– senile Alzheimer type 233, 241, 458, 459
– vascular 223
demyelinating plaques 256
depression 32, 33, 35, 41, 101, 102
depth recording 265, 371, 381
desipramine type 293
desynchronization 305, 326
dexfen-fluramine chlorhydrate 288
diabetes 26
differential discriminant analysis 99
dipole 141
– best-fit 58
– computation 338
– current dipole 537
– equivalent dipole 141, 144, 338, 390, 407, 538
– localizing method (DLM) 407, 538
– orientation 365
– point dipole 141, 362
– radial dipole 141, 363, 407
– source 50, 171, 362, 407
direct memory access (DMA) 129
discriminant function 9, 28
dominance 90
– eye 90
– foot 90
– hand 90
dopamine 472
dorsal nerve of penis (DNP) 412
dose-efficacy ralations 492
Down's syndrome 296
dream report 330
drowsiness 9, 31, 32, 33
drug obuse 26
DSM-III 241, 296, 451
dynamic random-dot correlogram (DRDC) 398
dyslexia 37, 201, 296, 522
dysphasia 168

eating behaviour 288
EEG 77
– activity, spontaneous 53
– amplifier 13
– dynamic cartography 329, 333
– quantification 13
– topography 11
EKG 34
electroconvulsive therapy (ECT) 259, 474–481

Subject Index

electrode 21
- application 8
- cap 210, 304
- location 5
- number 21, 23
- pad electrodes 150
- placement 4, 5, 23
electrodermal orienting response 424
electrophysiology V
electroretinogram 266
encephalitis 26
encephalomalacia 265
encephalopathy 6, 23, 33, 38
encephaloscope 14
endogenous waves 458
epilepsy 19, 26, 173, 249, 565
- seizures 152, 279
- - complex partial (CPS) 249
- - generalized (GS) 249
- - simple partial (SPS) 249
epileptic focus 6
- fit 178
epileptic spikes VI
equipotential lines 343
erectile dysfunction (ED) 412
event-related desynchronization (ERD) 303–313
event-related potentials (ERPs) 273, 522
evoked potentials 3, 76, 458–473
- early, middle latency 192
- farfield 77
- nearfield 77
- postsynaptic 76
- stereoscopically 353
excitatory postsynaptic potentials 77
exogenous waves 458
exploratory data analysis (EDA)
eye movements 5
- - horizontal 5, 33
- - midline 5
- - vertical 5

factor analysis 297
factor analysis procedure 105
- general factors 107, 108
- specific factors 106, 107
false negatives 90
false positives 90, 92
fast Fourier transform (FFT) 22, 54, 58, 65, 137, 167, 438
Feldeigenströme (area specific currents) 14
fissure of Rolando 86
fluid-mosaic model of the membrane 247
fluorodeoxyglucose (FDG) 471
fluoxetine 293
fluvoxamine 293
foveal stimulation 202

frontal intermittent rhythmic delta activity (FIRDA) 231
frontal midline theta wave (Fmθ) 231
F-test 507
- wave 267

galvanic skin response 326
gamma range 124, 125
gaussian distribution 7, 91
gaussianity 30, 91
Glasgow Coma Scale 194
global dissimilarity 58
global dysfunction score 99
global field power 56, 57, 66, 68, 338, 342, 348
graphein 11
grapheme-phoneme conversion 522
gray scale 21
group grand average 104
growth hormone 287
guidelines 3–10

Hachinski's score 219, 241
hallucination 425
Hamburg-Wechsler Intelligence Scale for Children (HAWIK) 296
Hamilton's scale 219, 475
hand tracking 159
handedness 303
hard disk 8, 130
hardwave 19
head format 132
- model 539
- vertex view 10
head injuries 273
head model 390
- identification 390
- three-concentric-shell 390
hemiretina 63, 339
- EP field 63
- lower 69
- stimulation 63–65, 343
- upper 69
hemisphere imbalance syndrome 425
- scale 426
Hexamethyl-propyleneamineoxime (SPECT) 159
high pressure nervous syndrome (HPNS) 230
hippocampal formation 88, 244
hippocampus 192, 417, 422, 458, 472
holothane 263
hydrocortisone 285
hyperarousal state 516
hyperfrontal flow distribution 470
hyperfrontality 246, 472
hyperkinetic-inattention syndrome 296

hyperventilation 252
hypofrontality 423, 456, 471
hypoxia 527
– model 527
hypoxic hypoxidosis 533

ICD-9 241, 296, 451
immunological system 326
impotence 412
intelligence 17
intensive care medicine 192
interpolation 6, 21, 54, 132, 384
– bidimensional spline interpolation method 390
– four-point linear 6, 132, 168, 305
– inverse distance 6
– polynominal approximation 6
– surface spline 132
– three-point linear 6, 21, 22
– triangular 385
interstimulus interval (ISI) 194
inverse problem 338
ischemia 195
– ischemic cerebral vascular attacks (ICVA) 185
– transient ischemic attacks (TIA) 185, 209
isocontour maps 567
isoelectric EEG 259
isoflurane 259

jack-knife replication 97, 101

Kanisza figures 70
keyboard 4

Lagrangian multipliers 198
"landscapes" 53, 73
Laplace's equation 197
laterality 425
learning difficulties 176, 297
learning tasks 323
limbic system 565
lobectomy 265
long-latency evoked potentials 20
low-pass filter 130

magnetencephalography (MEG) VII, 62, 124, 391, 537, 565
magnetic field 537
– auditory evoked 537
magnetic resonance imaging 183, 396
Mahalanobis distance feature 92, 97
major depressive disorder 259, 285, 459, 466–468, 475
malformation, arteriovenous 265, 278, 279
Mann Whitney U-test 242
map hilliness 74

"map movie" 102
McNemar test 309
meningeoma 178, 274
meningitis 26
mental events 12
middle cerebral artery 209
mini mental state 219
minimal brain damage (MBD) 296
mismatch negativity 195
morphine 482
motor task 159
– performance 159
mouse 4
movie 329
multi infarct dementia (MID) 241
multiple sclerosis 256, 318, 342, 400
multivariate statistical analysis 92, 116, 185
multivariate statistics VII, 185
muscarinic agonist 519
musicality 17
μ rhythm 310

narcotherapy 263
– isoflurane 263
neuroleptics 483
– chlorprotixene 483, 500
neuronal activity 53
– circadian activity 53
– maturational stage 53
– metabolic condition 53
– motivational stage 53
neurophysiology 19
Niquist constraints 54, 60
nootropic therapy 233, 489–492
normalization 7
normative data bank 3, 7, 25, 90
nuclear magnetic resonance imaging (NMI) 124, 256
nystagmus 31
– vertical 31

obesity 288
olfactory system 120
"open field" system 76
optic nerve neuropathy 396
orienting response 195

P 300 88, 177, 192, 241, 356, 422, 458, 479
– coma 192
– depression 479
– P3a, P3b 192
– schizophrenia 432
– topography 356
– visually elicited 318
panic attacks 34
paradoxial lateralization phenomenon 271
Parkinson's disease 233

Subject Index

penicillamine 463
performance disorder 296, 297
perimetry 404
perineal electromyography 412
personal computer 129–135
pharmaco-EEG 16, 482–506
pharmacopsychiatry 483
phase coherence 555
phosphatidylserine 238, 459
photic stimulation 252
phrenology 11
physostigmine 518
piracetam 234
pixel 132, 391
positron emission tomography 124, 217, 246, 278, 515, 565
posterior cerebral artery 37
potential 318
– differentiating 318
– processing 318
– terminating 318
power spectrum 131
practical significance mapping (PSM) 511
present state examination 426
prestimulus epoch 36
principal component analysis (PCA) 361
probability level 29
prolactine 287
psychiatric disorders 94, 99–102
psychopharmacology 224, 458, 482–506
psychosis 16
psychostimulants 503
pyritinol 234, 241, 242, 483, 489, 527–543

quantified EEG V
quantitative-EEG (Q-EEG) 483

rabbit 220
– cortex 220
random-dot stereograms (RDS) 351
readyness potential, see Bereitschaftspotential
recording 77
– bipolar 77
– multichannel 357
reference 6, 21, 54, 60, 78, 537
– average reference 6, 21, 60, 311, 345, 398
– bipolar 311
– cephalic 366
– Laplacian transformation 6, 311
– linked earlobe 269
– location 6, 23
– noncephalic 77, 366
– reference-free 6, 24, 60
– source derivation 23, 62
– unipolar 311
regional cerebral blood flow (rCBF) 94, 159, 311, 439, 515

Reisberg's global deterioration scale 219
REM 63, 331, 518
reticular formation 192
rolandic fissure 391

sampling rate 4, 129
Sandoz Clinical Assessment-Geriatric Score (SCAG) 496
scalp current density (SCD) 390
scalp topography 338
schizoaffective psychosis 465, 471
schizophrenia 16, 26, 37, 101, 421–437, 438–450
– evoked potentials 458
– hebephrenic subtype 459, 508
– limbic hypothesis 422, 465
– negative symptoms 425, 439
– paranoid subtype 459, 508
– positive symptoms 425
– residual subtype 459, 508
– topographic EEG data 507–517
– type I, II 438
school problems 38
scopolamine 482
selective attention 474
selective attention task 86
SEP-generators 77
– subcortical 78
septicaemia 173
short latency auditory response 20
short-term memory 192
signal-to-noise-ratio 67, 71, 78, 105, 362
significance probability mapping (SPM) 16, 21, 25, 28, 30, 32, 167
simple topographic electrical activity mapping (STEAM) 147
single-dipole-in-a-sphere model 566
single equivalent current dipole, see dipole
sinusoidal luminance profile 397
sleep 330
– paradoxical 330
– stages I, II, III and IV 330
– study 330
slow negative cortical potential shift 314
– attention 318
– floating 318
– sustained 318
– transient 318
slow negative potentials shift (SP) 159
slow wave 356
slowing 29
– focal 29
– generalized 29
software 19, 129
somatosensory evoked potentials 76, 383–389, 458
– brain averaged response 76

somatosensory evoked potentials, early components 79, 383, 390
– long latency 412
– nearfield neural generator 81
– P 300 88
– prerolandic SEP 86
– spinal averaged response 76
source extension 141
– localization 24, 235
– model 539
space oriented segmentation 70
spatial frequency 348
SPECT 217, 284, 565
spectral analysis 4, 20
spectrally analyzed EEG 3
spike 19, 20, 29, 65, 154
– topography 44
square root spectra 7
standard deviation 20, 28
stimulus 351
– half field 357, 370
– non-target 459
– stereoscopic 351
– target 459
strabismus 201
stress 326
striate cortex 365, 381
– peristriate 381
stroke 26, 189
Student's t-test 30
subarachnoid hemorrhage (SAH) 97
subtraction maps 87
succinylcholine 259
super controls 27
superconducting quantum interference device (SQUID) 565–566
superconductivity VII
superior colliculus 84, 371
sylvian region 391, 538
sylvian seizure syndrome 48–49

task
– paired association 323
– reading 309
– recognition 309
– spatial 314
– verbal 314ff.
temporal lobe epilepsy 32, 41
temporolimbic system 422
thalamic lesions (SEP) 83
thalamus 192, 371, 417

thiopental 259
time efficacy relation 496
tonotopic organization 541
– chrono-topogramm 15
– topogramm 15
topographic mapping V, 3, 19, 21
– cognitive processing 354
– color display 5, 23
– data collection 5
– guidelines 3–10
– neurometric 90
– operating environment 4
– teaching 147
topographic pharmaco-AEP 300, 459, 468
topos 11
toposcope 14, 482
tracer 162
trajectories 119
tranquilizers 27, 503
– diazepam 503
transient ischemic attack 94, 209
trigeminus stimulation 384
t-statistic 4, 31, 167, 242

underwater experiment 226
U-test 57

Vector EEG 407
VEP 29, 337–359, 458
– cognitive components 337
– flash 29, 116, 168, 201, 265
– pattern reversal 168, 201, 318, 360, 366, 396
– red light emitting diode (LED) 373–382
vibration stimulus 211
visual cortex 120
visuo-oculomotor activity 310
voltage gradient 61
volume conduction 76

wakefulness 329
Wechsler intelligence scale for children (WISC) 296
weighting factor 21
Wilcoxon test 442
Wilson's disease 459, 463
Würzburg Conference V, VII

zimelidine 293
Z-transformation 4, 30, 31, 90, 91, 94, 111, 115, 167